Diagnostic Breast Imaging
2nd edition

Diagnostic Breast Imaging

Mammography, Sonography, Magnetic Resonance Imaging, and Interventional Procedures

Second edition, enlarged and revised

Sylvia H. Heywang-Köbrunner, M.D.
Associate Professor and Substitute Director
Department of Diagnostic Radiology
Martin Luther University Halle-Wittenberg
Halle, Germany

D. David Dershaw, M.D.
Director, Breast Imaging Section
Department of Radiology
Memorial Sloan-Kettering Cancer Center
New York, NY USA

Ingrid Schreer, M.D.
Assistant Professor
Breast Center
University Hospital
Kiel, Germany

In collaboration with Professor Roland Bässler, M.D.

843 illustrations

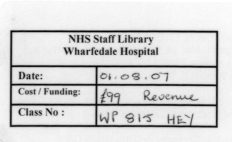
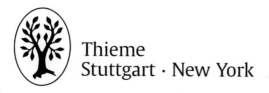

Thieme
Stuttgart · New York

Library of Congress Cataloging-in-Publication Data

Heywang-Köbrunner, Sylvia H., 1956-
  [Bildgebende mammadiagnostik. English]
  Diagnostic breast imaging : mammography, sonography, magnetic resonance imaging, and interventional procedures / Sylvia Heywang-Köbrunner, Ingrid Schreer, D. David Dershaw ; in collaboration with Roland Bässler ; translated by Peter F. Winter.— 2nd ed., enlarged and rev.
    p. ; cm.
  Includes bibliographical references and index.
  ISBN 3131028920—ISBN 1-58890-033-9
    1. Breast—Imaging. 2. Breast—Diseases—Diagnosis. I. Schreer, Ingrid. II. Dershaw, D. David. III. Title.
    [DNLM: 1. Breast—pathology. 2. Breast Diseases—diagnosis. 3. Biopsy—methods. 4. Magnetic Resonance Imaging. 5. Mammography. 6. Ultrasonography, Mammary. WP 815 H622b 2000a]
  RG493.5D52 H49 I3 2000
  618.1'90754—dc21   00-048876

Collaborator:

Roland Bässler, M.D.
Professor, Institute of Pathology
Municipal Clinics
Fulda, Germany

1st German edition 1996
1st English edition 1997

This book is an enlarged and revised new edition of the authorized translation of the German edition, published and copyrighted 1996 by Georg Thieme Verlag, Stuttgart, Germany.
Title of the German edition: Bildgebende Mammadiagnostik: Untersuchungstechnik, Befundmuster und Differentialdiagnostik in Mammographie, Sonographie und Kernspintomographie

First edition translated by Peter F. Winter, M. D.

Important Note: Medicine is an ever-changing science undergoing continual development. Research and clinical experience are continually expanding our knowledge, in particular our knowledge of proper treatment and drug therapy. Insofar as this book mentions any dosage or application, readers may rest assured that the authors, editors, and publishers have made every effort to ensure that such references are in accordance with *the state of knowledge at the time of production of the book.*

Nevertheless, this does not involve, imply, or express any guarantee or responsibility on the part of the publishers in respect to any dosage instructions and forms of application stated in the book. Every user is requested to examine carefully the manufacturer's leaflets accompanying each drug and to check, if necessary in consultation with a physician or specialist, whether the dosage schedules mentioned therein or the contraindications stated by the manufacturer differ from the statements made in the present book. Such examination is particularly important with drugs that are either rarely used or have been newly released on the market. **Every dosage schedule or every form of application used is entirely at the user's own risk and responsibility.** The authors and publishers request every user to report to the publishers any discrepancies or inaccuracies noticed.

© 2001 Georg Thieme Verlag
Rüdigerstrasse 14, 70469 Stuttgart, Germany
Thieme New York, 333 Seventh Avenue,
New York, N.Y. 10001 USA

Typesetting by primustype Robert Hurler GmbH
73274 Notzingen, Germany

Printed in Germany by Druckhaus Götz,
Ludwigsburg

ISBN 3-13-102892-0 (GTV)
ISBN 0-58890-033-9 (TNY)   2 3 4 5

Preface

The authors present a second edition of this book, encouraged by the success of the first edition. The second edition became necessary due to the technologic progress, increasing clinical data, as well as evolving, and new clinical and imaging strategies.

During the last years data has continued to accumulate on the value of screening mammography for reduction of breast cancer mortality in the 50–70-year age group. Furthermore, increasing proof now exists that similar results can also be achieved by screening women aged 40–49. Simultaneously, other imaging modalities as well as various methods for percutaneous biopsy have been further developed and improved. These increasingly supplement mammography in cases of diagnostic difficulties and in the assessment and management of women with breast disease. In addition to standard two-view mammography and clinical examination, special mammographic views and sonography are an important part of the imaging workup of these women. For selected indications MR imaging increasingly proves to provide valuable additional information. Percutaneous biopsy techniques under imaging guidance have become an indispensable tool for minimally invasive diagnosis of imaging detected abnormalities.

In this second edition, the authors have again attempted to present to the reader a cogent approach to imaging of the breast, updating the information available in the first edition. Again, the value of imaging is analyzed for both the symptomatic patient and the asymptomatic woman. The latest results of breast cancer screening (including younger age groups and latest discussions concerning the overall value) and the value of other imaging techniques in this clinical context are reviewed. New information concerning genetic and other risk factors are included to provide sufficient background for proper application and interpretation of imaging studies in these patients. The latest technologic progress in mammography, ultrasound, MRI, and percutaneous biopsy techniques has been included, and its present and future impact on diagnostic strategies are considered. A critical analysis of new modalities under investigation has been added.

Based on both technologic progress in mammography, ultrasound, MRI, and percutaneous biopsy and based on evidence from increasing study-proven data, standards and strategies of workup undergo continuous evolution and adaptation. The authors have presented algorithms for patient management based on this new material. These algorithms take into account the constantly increasing knowledge in this field, and they reflect state-of-the-art technology and clinical knowledge in mid-2000.

As in the first edition, the authors have reviewed the clinical, histopathologic, and imaging issues of breast disease together, in order to provide the necessary background for a sensible approach. The book is not designed to replace interdisciplinary work. Rather, it is hoped it will create an understanding of the value of close interdisciplinary cooperation, which is needed to achieve an optimum diagnosis and treatment for the patient with breast disease. For those involved in breast imaging this text presents findings associated with breast diseases and the differential diagnosis for each of these. The authors also have suggested algorithms for the workup of a variety of clinical and imaging dilemmas. These chapters are designed to assist in the workup of the symptomatic women and the interpretation of abnormal imaging studies.

This text is also designed to review for non-radiologist physicians the role of breast-imaging technologies in the workup of their patients and the concepts involved in the interpretation of these studies. Additonally, the authors also hope that this work will be useful to technologists who wish to add depth to their understanding of the images they create.

Finally it should be pointed out that this work has grown out of an international collaboration. Although the philosophy of which technologies are best used in which settings can vary from nation to nation, as well as from office to office, the fear of breast cancer and its impact on individual women affected by this disease and those who share their lives is without borders. We have attempted to present a rational approach to the early diagnosis of this disease for women of all nations.

Acknowledgements

The production of this book represents not only the time and effort of the authors whose names appear on the cover, but multiple other individuals. We would all like to thank the technologists with whom we work on a daily basis for their tireless efforts and constant compassion in producing the images that appear on these pages. We would also like to express our appreciation to Cliff Bergman at Thieme who helped us create the first edition of this text and guided us through the second edition. In addition, each of us would like to thank special individuals who have made this project possible.

Sylvia H. Heywang-Köbrunner would like to express her sincere thanks to those colleagues who have accompanied her for many years and who have made high-quality work and research possible by their constant support, enthusiasm, and their care for the patient: Dr. Rainer Beck, Dr. Thomas Hilbertz, Dr. Petra Viehweg, Dr. Anke Heinig and numerous other young colleagues and students, who joined us in our efforts and supported our work. She is very greatful for the unique cooperation with her clinical partners from gynecology, breast surgery, and pathology: Prof. Dr. W. Permanetter, Prof. Dr. H. Hepp, Prof. Dr. F.-W. Rath, PD Dr. J. Buchmann, Dr. D. Lampe, and Prof. Dr. H. Kölbl. Deep appreciation goes to Prof. Dr. R. Bässler, who reviewed crucial parts of this book. A special note of gratitude is addressed to the technologists at the University of Halle, particularly Ms. Klemme and Ms. Theuerkorn, for whom quality and patient care have always been the most important goal and who have constantly supported research and teaching at our institution. A special note of gratitude must be accorded to Ms. A. Fulbrecht, who typed major parts of the manuscript. Sincere thanks go to Prof. Dr. Dr. J. Lissner and Prof. Dr. R. P. Spielmann, who supported this work. Finally the author would like to express her deep gratitude to Deutsche Krebshilfe (German Cancer Foundation) for continuous support of both education and research associated with numerous projects.

D. David Dershaw would like to acknowledge the constant support, intellectual stimulation, and forbearance of his colleagues in breast imaging at Memorial Sloan-Kettering Cancer Center in New York: Drs. Andrea Abramson, Linda LaTrenta, Laura Liberman, and Elizabeth Morris. Their constant love, humor, devotion to quality, and good taste make each day at work special; without them, it never would have happened. And to the Radiology Department at Memorial that has supported the academic endeavors of the Breast Imaging Section for many years, thanks again. To our many fellows, who work so hard, ask so many difficult questions and keep us thinking, you are deeply appreciated, fondly remembered, and often missed. Thanks to Beckie, Bruce, Brewster, John, Alan, and Andrea, who have made it possible to get through it all. And for Ryan, a special thanks.

Ingrid Schreer would like to express her gratitude for the excellent collaboration within the multidisciplinary team of physicians, technologists, and other coworkers at the University of Kiel. Special thanks go to the breast imaging team, in particular to Ms. M. Dickhaut and Ms. A. Große, who continuously supported the daily clinical and scientific work with all their effort and with empathy with the patients. This work would not have been possible without them. Deep appreciations go to Prof. H.-J. Frischbier, whose work and support constituted an essential basis for this book.

Sylvia H. Heywang-Köbrunner, M.D.
D. David Dershaw, M.D.
Ingrid Schreer, M.D.

Contents

I Methods

1. Patient History and Communication with the Patient   2

Scheduling 2
Patient Information 2
Patient History 3
References 7

2. Clinical Findings   9

Visual Inspection 9
Palpation 10
References 13

3. Mammography   14

Purpose, Accuracy, Possibilities, and Limitations 14
  Indications 14
  Accuracy 14
  Screening 15
  Problem Solving 15
Mammographic Technique 16
Components of the Mammographic Imaging Technique 17
Specific Requirements and Solutions ... 26
  Image Sharpness 26
  Contrast 27
  Noise 36
  Radiation Dose 36
Positioning and Compression 39
  Compression 39
  Positioning for Standard Views 41
  Positioning for Additional Views 45
Film Labelling 50
  Spot Compression and Magnification Technique 52
Positioning of Breasts
  with Implants 56
  Specimen Radiography 59
Quality Factors 60
  Hardware Factors that Influence Image Quality 60
  Influence of the Screen–Film System and Film Processing on Image Quality 62
  Quality Assurance in Mammography 63
Reporting and Documentation Findings 65
  Clinical Findings 65
  Mammography Report 65
Digital Mammography 71
Galactography 74
  Appendix: Sonographic Imaging of Lactiferous Ducts 78
Pneumocystography 81
  References 83

4. Sonography   87

Purpose, Accuracy, Possibilities, and Limitations 87
Diagnosing Cysts 87
Differentiating Solid Lesions 87
Diagnosing Carcinoma 87
Younger Women 88
Screening with Sonography 88
Equipment Requirements 88
Transducer 88

Image Quality 89
Examination Technique 92
Time-gain Compensation 92
Focusing 93
Examination Technique 93
Interpreting Sonographic Findings 96
Normal Sonographic Findings 96
Focal Sonographic Lesions 97
References 102

5. Magnetic Resonance Imaging (MRI)   103

Purpose, Accuracy, Possibilities, and Limitations 103
Accuracy 103
Indications 104
Technical Requirements 106
Examination Procedure 108

Planning the Examination 108
Examination Procedure 109
Interpretation Criteria and
Documentation of Findings 109
Interpretation Criteria 110
References 125

6. Breast Imaging Techniques under Investigation   128

Scintimammography 128
Positron Emission Tomography 129

Other Methods 129
References 130

7. Percutaneous Biopsy   132

Purpose 132
Definitions 132
Accuracy 133
Possibilities and Limitations 134
Contraindications 135
Complications 135
Patient Information, Patient Preparation, and Postbiopsy Care 136
Techniques for Biopsy and Biopsy
Guidance 136

Fine Needle Aspiration 136
Core Needle Biopsy 137
Vacuum-Suction Biopsy 137
Ultrasound-Guided Biopsy 140
Stereotactic Biopsy 141
MR-Guided Percutaneous Biopsy 146
References 150

8. Preoperative Localization   152

Purpose, Definition, Indications, and Side Effects 152
Methods and Technique 153
Mammographically Guided Localization Techniques 153
Ultrasound-Guided Localization 155

MR-Guided Localization 157
Galactographically Guided Localization 158
Localization Materials 158
Problems and Their Solutions 159
References 160

II Appearance

9. The Normal Breast   162

Anatomy 162
The Adolescent Female Breast 163
    Histology 163
    Clinical Examination 163
    Mammography 163
The Mature Female Breast 163
    Histology 163
    Sonography 163
    Clinical Examination 163
    Mammography 165
    Sonography 166
    Magnetic Resonance Imaging 168
Involution 170
    Histology 170
    Clinical Examination 170
    Mammography 170
    Sonography 170
    Magnetic Resonance Imaging 170
Abnormalities 171
Asymmetry 171
    Clinical Examination 171
    Mammography 171
Accessory Breast Tissue (Polymastia) 173
    Clinical Examination 173

Macromastia 173
    Clinical Examination 173
    Mammography 173
    Sonography 173
    Mammography 173
    Sonography and Magnetic Resonance
    Imaging 173
Inverted Nipple 174
    Clinical Examination 174
    Mammography 174
    Sonography 174
    Magnetic Resonance Imaging 174
Pregnancy and Lactation 175
    Histology 175
    Clinical Examination 175
    Mammography 175
Breast Response with Hormone Replace-
ment Therapy 177
    Sonography 177
    Magnetic Resonance Imaging 177
    Mammography 177
    Sonography 180
    Magnetic Resonance Imaging 180
    Percutaneous Biopsy 180
    References 180

10. Benign Breast Disorders   181

Pathogenesis 181
Incidence 181
Histopathology 181
Clinical Findings 183
Diagnostic Strategy and Objectives .. 183

Mammography 184
Sonography 191
Magnetic Resonance Imaging 192
Percutaneous Biopsy 195
References 196

11. Cysts   197

Histology 197
Medical History and Clinical Find-
ings 197
Breast Examination 197
Objectives of Diagnostic Studies 198
Diagnostic Strategy 198
Sonography 198

Aspiration of the Cyst 201
Pneumocystography 202
Mammography 202
Magnetic Resonance Imaging 202
Appendix: Galactoceles and Oil Cysts 205
References 208

12. Benign Tumors

Hamartoma or Adenofibrolipoma 209
    Histology 209
    Clinical Findings 209
    Diagnostic Strategy 209
    Mammography 209
    Sonography 209
Fibroepithelial Mixed Tumors 210
    Fibroadenoma, Adenofibroma, Juvenile
    or Giant Fibroadenoma 210
        Percutaneous Biopsy 210
        Magnetic Resonance Imaging 210
        Histology 211
        History 211
        Clinical Findings 211
        Mammography 211
        Sonography 217
        Percutaneous Biopsy 222
        Magnetic Resonance Imaging 222
        Diagnostic Goals 223
        Overview of the Diagnostic Strategy . 223
    Papilloma 224
        Histopathology 224
        Clinical Findings 225
        Cytology of Nipple Discharge 225
        Diagnostic Strategy and Goals 225
        Mammography 226
        Galactography 227
        Sonography 227
        Magnetic Resonance Imaging 227
        Percutaneous Biopsy 229
    Lipoma 230
        Clinical Findings 230
        Diagnostic Strategy 230

        Mammography 230
        Sonography, Magnetic Resonance
        Imaging, or Needle Biopsy 230
    Lipoma 231
        Clinical Findings 231
        Diagnostic Strategy 231
        Mammography 231
        Sonography, Magnetic Resonance
        Imaging, or Needle Biopsy 231
Rare Benign Tumors 231
    Leiomyoma, Neurofibroma, Neurilem-
    moma, Benign Spindle Cell Tumor,
    Chondroma, Osteoma 231
    Angiomas 231
Benign Fibroses 232
    Diabetic Mastopathy or Fibrosis 232
        Histology 232
    Granular Cell Tumor (Myoblastoma) 232
        Clinical Findings 232
        Diagnostic Strategy 232
        Mammography 232
    Granular Cell Tumor (Myoblastoma) 233
        Sonography 233
        Magnetic Resonance Imaging 233
        Percutaneous Biopsy 233
    Focal Fibrous Disease or Fibrosis
    Mammae 233
    Intramammary Lymph Nodes 234
        Histology 234
        Clinical Findings 234
        Diagnostic Strategy and Goals 234
        Imaging 234
        Percutaneous Biopsy 234
        References 235

13. Inflammatory Conditions

Mastitis 236
    Etiology 236
    Clinical Findings 237
    Diagnostic Strategy and Goals 237
    Mammography 237
    Sonography 241
    Magnetic Resonance Imaging 241
    Biopsy Methods 241
Abscesses and Fistulae 242
    Histology 242
    Clinical Findings 242
    Diagnostic Strategy 242
    Sonography 243
    Mammography 243

    Magnetic Resonance Imaging 243
    Percutaneous Biopsy 245
    Percutaneous Drainage 245
Granulomatous Conditions 245
    Histologic and Microbiologic Confir-
    mation 245
    Clinical Findings 246
    Diagnostic Strategy 246
    Mammography 246
    Sonography 247
    Magnetic Resonance Imaging 249
    Percutaneous Biopsy 250
    References 250

14. Carcinoma in situ 252

Lobular Carcinoma in Situ (LCIS) 252
    Incidence 252
    Histology 252
    Clinical Presentation and History 253
    Mammography 253
    Sonography 253
    Magnetic Resonance Imaging 253
    Percutaneous Biopsy 253
    Therapeutic Decisions after Docu-
    mented LCIS, Goals and Value of Di-
    agnostic Methods 253

Ductal Carcinoma in Situ (DCIS)
(Intraductal Carcinoma) 254
    Incidence 254
    Histology 254
    Clinical Findings and History 255
    Diagnostic Methods: Value and
    Goals 256
    Mammography 256
    Sonography 262
    Magnetic Resonance Imaging 262
    References 264

15. Invasive Carcinoma 266

    Definition and Problems Posed 266
    Spectrum and Detectability 266
    Diagnostic Strategy and Goals 267
    Histology 270
    Clinical Presentation 273

    Mammography 274
    Sonography 295
    Magnetic Resonance Imaging 303
    Percutaneous Biopsy Methods 307
    References 310

16. Lymph Nodes 313

    The Role of Imaging 313
    Anatomy 313
    Normal Lymph Nodes 313
    Metastatic Adenopathy 315
    Other Causes of Adenopathy 319
    Nodal Calcifications 319

    Sentinel Node Imaging 320
    Percutaneous Biopsy 321
    New Techniques in Nodal Imaging:
    MRI and PET 321
    Internal Mammary Nodes 322
    References 323

17. Other Semi-malignant and Malignant Tumors 325

Phyllodes Tumor (Cystosarcoma Phyllodes) 325
    Histology 325
    Clinical Findings 325
    Diagnostic Strategy and Goals 325
    Mammography 326
    Sonography 326
    Magnetic Resonance Imaging 327
    Percutaneous Biopsy 327
Sarcomas 328
    Histology 328
    Clinical Findings 329
    Diagnostic Strategy and Goals 329
    Mammography 329
    Sonography 329
    Magnetic Resonance Imaging 330
    Percutaneous Biopsy 330

Malignancies of the Breast of Hematologic
Origin 332
    Clinical Findings 332
    Diagnostic Strategy and Goals 332
    Mammography 332
    Sonography 333
Metastases 334
    Magnetic Resonance Imaging 334
    Percutaneous Biopsy 334
    Magnetic Resonance Imaging 335
    Percutaneous Biopsy 335
    Histology 335
    Clinical Findings 335
    Diagnostic Strategy and Goals 335
    Mammography 335
    Sonography 336

Magnetic Resonance Imaging 336
Percutaneous Biopsy 337
Other Very Rare Tumors 337
Fibromatosis (= Extra-abdominal
Desmoid) 337

Hemangiopericytoma and Hemangioendothelioma 338
References 338

18. Post-traumatic, Post-surgical, and Post-therapeutic Changes 339

Post-traumatic and Post-surgical Changes .. 339
Histology 339
Clinical History and Findings 339
Diagnostic Strategy and Goals 339
Mammography 340
Sonography 342
Magnetic Resonance Imaging 347
Changes Following Breast-Conserving Ther-
apy without Irradiation 349
Definition 349
Percutaneous Biopsy 349
Clinical and Imaging Findings 349
Changes Following Breast-conserving Ther-
apy and Irradiation 350
Definition 350
Differential Diagnosis and Diagnostic
Strategy 350
Clinical Findings 350
Differential Diagnosis and Diagnostic
Strategy 351
Diagnostic Strategy and Goals 351

Mammography 351
Sonography 359
Magnetic Resonance Imaging 361
Percutaneous Biopsy 364
Changes Following Reconstruction,
Augmentation, and Reduction 364
Reconstruction 364
Diagnostic Strategy 365
Mammography 365
Sonography 368
Magnetic Resonance Imaging 368
Augmentation 368
Diagnostic Strategy 369
Mammography 370
Sonography 370
Magnetic Resonance Imaging 370
Percutaneous Biopsy 370
Reduction 371
Diagnostic Strategy 371
References 373

19. Skin Changes 375

Nodular Changes of the Skin and
Subcutaneous Tissue 375
Clinical Findings 375
Diagnostic Strategy 375
Mammography 375
Skin Thickening 375
Diagnostic Strategy 378

Clinical Findings 378
Mammography 379
Sonography 380
Contrast-enhanced MRI 380
Biopsy Methods 380
References 381

20. The Male Breast 382

Clinical Findings 382
Gynecomastia 382
Histology 382
Mammography 382
Clinical Findings 382
Diagnostic Strategy 382
Mammography 383
Other Methods 383

Breast Cancer in Men 384
Histology 384
Clinical Findings 385
Mammography 385
Sonography 385
References 386

III Application of Diagnostic Imaging of the Breast

21. Screening 388

Results of International Studies 388
    Randomized Studies 388
    Case Control Studies 389
Further Screening Studies 390
    Breast Cancer Demonstration
    Project 390
    United Kingdom Trial of Early
    Detection of Breast Cancer (TEDBC) . 391
    Controversies and Answers 391

Benefit–Risk/Benefit–Costs 392
    Benefit–Costs 393
Recommendations on the Basis
of the Trials 394
    References 394
    Suggested Reading 395

22. Additional Diagnostic Evaluation of Screening Findings and Solving of Problems in Symptomatic Patients 396

Pathognomonic Findings 396
Differential Diagnosis and Diagnostic
Workup 397
    Smoothly Outlined Density 397
    Lesions Not Smoothly Outlined 402
    Architectural Distortion 405
    Asymmetry 411
    The Radiographically Dense Breast 419
    Dense Breast in Asymptomatic
    Patients without Increased Risk 419
    Dense Breast in Asymptomatic
    Patients with High Risk 422
    Dense Breast with Palpable Finding . 428
    Dense Breast and Special
    Considerations 431
    Microcalcifications 434
    Possibilities and Limitations of
    Diagnostic Methods 434
    Analysis of Microcalcifications 436
    Microcalcifications Suggestive of
    Malignancy 436

    Definitely Benign Calcifications 440
    Indeterminate Microcalcifications ... 449
    Nipple Discharge 452
    Inflammatory Changes 454
The Young Patient 455
    Breast Changes in the Young Patient
    and Their Histology 455
    Risk of Breast Cancer 456
    Clinical Findings 456
    Mammography 457
    Sonography 459
    Percutaneous Biopsy 461
    Magnetic Resonance Imaging 464
    Diagnostic Strategy 464
    References 465
Appendix 1 469
    TNM Classification of Breast
    Carcinomas (1) 469
    References 469
Appendix II 470
    Definitions of Anatomic Locations (1) 470
    References 470

Index 469

I Methods

1. Patient History and Communication with the Patient

Providing the patient with some essential information concerning breast imaging may help gain her understanding and cooperation. Furthermore obtaining a limited history is very helpful both for separating screening patients from those who need a diagnostic breast study and to support image interpretation in diagnostic breast studies.

Both information about the patient and her history can be obtained orally or by use of an information sheet, a checklist, or a questionnaire.

■ Scheduling

The issue of whether mammography should be scheduled according to the menstrual cycle is controversial. Even though data exist which suggest an impact of the menstrual cycle on breast density and on the accuracy of mammography[1, 2], on the whole the patient's menstrual cycle is disregarded. At the University of Halle, it is routine to perform mammographic imaging during the first part of the menstrual cycle. During this time, the breast is more compressible, and compression is less painful, which is appreciated by the patients. Furthermore, due to less interstitial fluid during the follicular phase and to the better compression, the glandular tissue may even appear less dense on the mammogram, which facilitates diagnosis. Theoretically, it might even be possible to further decrease the radiation risk with such scheduling, since most cells tend to be in the G2 phase (in which they are more sensitive to radiation) during the luteal phase of the menstrual cycle, but not during the follicular (first) phase[3].

In contrast-enhanced (c.e.) magnetic resonance imaging (MRI), nonspecific enhancement in benign tissue may be encountered at the end of the menstrual cycle and during menses, while it is less frequent between days 6 to about 17 of the cycle. Therefore c.e. MRI should—if possible—be scheduled between days 6–17 of the cycle[4, 5].

■ Patient Information

If the patient asks specific questions, they should, of course, be discussed or answered by the technologist or physician. Furthermore, the following essentials concerning the imaging techniques involved may be helpful to gain the patient's understanding and cooperation.

■ Mammography

- The patient should understand the importance and necessity of compression. Adequate compression helps visualize small carcinomas since normal tissue usually can be spread out while carcinomas persist. Compression also helps to reduce the radiation dose (see Chapter 3, p. 29).
- Any fears that compression might cause cancer should be allayed.
- Possible fear of radiation exposure from mammography should be addressed by putting the risk into proper perspective. For example, the theoretical risk (so small that it can only be extrapolated) of dying from cancer caused by a mammogram is comparable to the risk of dying of lung cancer from smoking three cigarettes (see Chapter 3, p. 34).

As in any other radiologic examination, pregnancy should be excluded.

Patients who undergo screening mammography should understand that not all cancers can be detected by mammography. Therefore, they should be encouraged to continue to perform breast self-examinations. If a change is noted, even if it occurs shortly after screening mammography, the patient should contact her doctor.[6]

■ Sonography

Ultrasound examinations are generally very well accepted by patients. It should, however, be explained that, in general, ultrasonography cannot replace mammography for excluding the presence of cancer.

■ Magnetic Resonance Imaging with Contrast Medium

Contrast-enhanced MRI—like the other methods that do not use ionizing radiation—is well accepted by the patients except for those who suffer from claustrophobia. Contrast-enhanced MRI is used as an additional imaging modality for specific indications. Before performing c.e. MRI, ask for any contraindications and document their absence. These include cardiac pacemakers, intracerebral vascular clips, clips from surgery performed within the last 2 months, implantable drug infusion pumps, and certain types of cardiac valve prostheses.[7]

Finally, the patient should be informed of the necessity of injecting contrast medium. The few contraindications concern rare cases of allergy against paramagnetic contrast medium and severe hepatic or renal insufficiency. Extensive tolerance data are available for the paramagnetic contrast medium Gd-DTPA (studies in over 5 million patients).[8, 9] Tolerance of this contrast medium is excellent. Side effects occur significantly less frequently than with radiographic contrast media.

Paramagnetic MRI contrast media may even be used in the presence of an allergy against radiographic contrast medium since there is no allergic cross reaction.[8]

■ Interventions

When a puncture is planned (aspiration of a cyst, aspiration cytology or needle biopsy), the patient should be informed about possible hematoma formation and about the very low risk of infection. The patient should be questioned about any coagulatory disorders, aspirin intake, or anticoagulation treatment. Provided the direction of puncture is strictly parallel to the chest wall, injury to the chest wall can be excluded, and the very rare complication of iatrogenic pneumothorax need not be mentioned. If a silicone implant is present and might be damaged, the patient must also be informed. At some centers, it is routine to obtain informed consent before any of these procedures.

■ Patient History

To save time, many centers have the patient fill out a questionnaire (Fig. 1.1). The questions may concentrate on data that are significant for assessing risk and interpreting the images.

■ Risk Factors

A history of risk factors should be obtained in all patients. Even though improvement of the radiological mammographic reporting based on patient history has not been proven[10], knowledge of an increased risk may support the decision for additional imaging whenever mammography is difficult to assess. In the first place this would include supplementary ultrasound. In patients with hereditary breast cancer additional MRI may be an option, which for reasons of quality control and experience should be performed within one of the ongoing trials. Knowledge of risk factors may influence recommendations concerning the starting age for screening (see Chapter 22) and appropriate screening intervals. Finally, in cases with a strong personal or family history of breast cancer, genetic counselling may be recommended to the patient.

Even though risk factors are an indicator of increased risk for breast cancer, it is important to realize that an absence of risk factors does not exclude the occurence of breast cancer. In fact, 70 % of breast cancers occur in patients without any risk factors.[11]

The following risk factors for breast cancer have been described:

- Personal history: The personal history of an invasive or in situ breast carcinoma is significant, as is the history of breast disease with atypias (confirmed in earlier biopsies), particularly if a positive family history or other risk factors coexist. A personal history of an ovarian, endometrial, or colon cancer also increases the risk of breast cancer.[11–16]
  A very high risk of breast cancer exists in women with proven gene alterations, which are associated with hereditary breast cancer. These include mainly BRCA1 or 2 alterations, furthermore ataxia telangiectatica, Li-Fraumeni syndrome, HRAS-1 alterations, and other alterations.[13,16–23]
- Family history: A history of breast cancer in first or second-degree relatives, the number of members affected, their gender (male breast

Mammography Questionnaire for the Patient

Last name: _____ first name: _____ date of birth: _____

Address: _____

phone (home): _____ phone (work): _____ insurance provider: _____

referring physican: _____
(name, address): _____
last mammogram (date/facility): _____

Have you had cancer?   No ☐
☐ right breast when?_____ type?_____
☐ left breast when? _____ type?_____
☐ other cancer organ:_____ date: _____

Might you be pregnant?   yes ☐   no ☐

Are you currently nursing?   yes ☐   no ☐

first day of last menstruation? _____

menopause (since when?) _____ status after hysterectomy? Yes ☐   No ☐

Are you on hormones (oral contraceptives,
postmenopausal replacement)? _____ If yes, medication/dosage: _____ since when?_____

HISTORY
age of first menstruation: _____
Have you had severe breast infection? (age/which breast?) _____

Have you had breast surgery? _____
(Which breast/when/result) _____

Have you received radiation therapy?_____
a) to the breast (which breast, when)? _____
b) to the chest (when, why)? _____
c) multiple x-rays, CT's, fluoroscopy of the chest? _____
_____

Was your breast injured (accident?)

☐ right   ☐ left   when? _____

FAMILY HISTORY

family member (age)	breast cancer (age)	ovarian cancer (age)
_____	_____	_____
_____	_____	_____
_____	_____	_____
_____	_____	_____
_____	_____	_____
_____	_____	_____

other cancers in family (member/cancer):

Have you or your doctor noted an abnormality?   ☐ No

which abnormality?	right breast	left breast	since when?
pain	☐	☐	_____
lump breast	☐	☐	_____
thickening breast	☐	☐	_____
skin change?	☐	☐	_____
reddening ☐ retraction ☐	☐	☐	_____
change of nipple	☐	☐	_____
discharge: milky ☐ transparent ☐	☐	☐	
greenish ☐ red/brown ☐			

I have no further questions and consent to the proposed examination

Date: _____   Signature: _____

Fig. 1.**1**   Mammography Questionnaire for Patient History

Technical data

Patient name: _____ date/examination: _____

type of unit: _____ film/screen system _____

Standard views:

	cc:					mlo				
	KV	mAs	kp*	t/f**	AEC	KV	mAs	kpT/f	angle	AEC*
left:										
right:										

* compression   *target/filter   ** automatic exposed control: yes or no

Additional views:

breast/view	retake? (y/N)	KV	mAs	kp	t/f	AEC	spot?	magnification

reasons for inadequate views? _____

_____

problems? (pain, compliance?) _____

_____

Technologist: _____ Physician: _____

(physician's work sheet: see p. 9)

Table 1.1 Relative risk of breast cancer related to one or more risk factors (according to Maass[4] and Stoll,[5] used with permission)

Risk doubles
Menopause after age 50
Menarche before age 12
Nulliparity
Obesity in postmenopausal women
Epithelial hyperplasia

Risk increases by a factor of 2 to 4
First childbirth after age 30
Breast cancer in mother or sister
Combination of nulliparity and epithelial hyperplasia
Previous ovarian, endometrial, or colon cancer

Risk increases by factor of more than 4
Prior breast cancer
Breast cancer in mother and sister
Premenopausal bilateral breast cancer in the mother or sister
Atypical hyperplasia
Family history combined with late first pregnancy or nulliparity

Table 1.2 Criteria for Referral for Genetic Screening for Breast Cancer (modified from 18)

I   Women or men with a maternal or paternal relative who has previously been tested and found to have a clinically significant alteration in a breast cancer (BRCA) gene.

II. Women or men with a personal and family history as follows:
- Women with breast cancer < 50 plus
  - breast cancer in ≥ 1 first- or second-degree[1] relatives diagnosed at age < 50
- Women with breast cancer at any age plus
  - breast cancer in > 1 first- or second-degree relatives diagnosed at an age < 50, or
  - ovarian cancer in > 1 first- or second-degree relatives
- Women with ovarian cancer plus
  - breast cancer in ≥ 1 first- or second-degree relatives or
  - ovarian cancer in ≥ 1 first- or second-degree relatives
- Men with breast cancer plus breast and /or ovarian cancer in ≥ 1 first- or second degree relatives

III Women with a personal history (but no family history) of breast and/or ovarian cancer as follows:
- Breast cancer at age < 30, or
- Breast cancer at age < 40 and of Ashkenazic Jewish descent, or
- Ovarian cancer and of Ashkenazic Jewish descent, or
- Breast cancer and ovarian cancer, or
- Multiple primary breast cancers[1]

IV Women or men with a family history (but no personal history) of breast and/or ovarian cancer as follows:
- Breast cancer in
  - ≥ 1 first-degree and ≥ 1 second-degree relative, both diagnosed at age < 50
  - > 3 first- or second-degree relatives with at least 1 relative diagnosed at age < 50
- Ovarian cancer in ≥ first- or second-degree relatives
- Breast cancer ≥ 1 first- or second-degree relative

[1] First-degree relatives are parents, siblings, and children; second-degree relatives are aunts, uncles, grandparents, grandchildren, nieces, nephews, or half-siblings.
[2] Multiple primary breast cancer refers to tumors in both breasts or multiple tumors in one breast.

cancer!), age at detection (early age, premenopausal) are significant. Occurrence of ovarian cancer in first or second-degree relatives is also important information.
Presence of a proven clinically significant gene alteration in a family member.[11–13, 17, 18]
- Early menarche or late menopause, the frequency and duration of breast feeding, first childbirth after age 30, nulliparity, or the absence of breast feeding slightly influence the overall risk.[11, 12]

Estimates concerning the importance of these risk factors have been made for the general population. The importance of some of these factors, as derived from epidemiologic calculations, is summarized in Table 1.1.

Apart from the risk factors listed in Table 1.1, it is known that increased intake of n-6-polyunsaturated fatty acids and (less strongly) saturated fats increase the risk of breast cancer[24], whereas vegetable consumption and to a lesser degree fruit consumption decrease the risk of breast cancer.[25] Increased consumption of alcohol and tobacco elevate the individual risk.[17]

Taking oral contraceptives slightly increases the risk of breast cancer by about 25%; stopping taking oral contraceptives decreases the risk.[26, 27] Hormone replacement therapy appears to increase the risk of breast cancer. This increase de-

pends on the period of use and checking various additional biologic factors (such as android obesity, bone density, mammographic density, androgen and estrogen circulating levels, alcohol consumption, benign breast disease, risk factors) is recommended to carefully weigh the individual pros and cons.[28–30]

Whereas the risk of the vast majority of women can be sufficiently well assessed based on the above data concerning personal and family history, the risk in patients with hereditary breast cancer would be underestimated.[17] While the vast majority of breast cancers is sporadic, only 5–10% appear to be hereditary. Identification of such women may be useful, because genetic counselling should at least be offered to these patients. Genetic counselling may help the woman to correctly perceive her risk (most affected women indeed overestimate their true risk); to provide individual psychologic report; to choose an optimum schedule and combination of methods for early detection for the patient and, if desired, for her close relatives; and to inform the patient about the possibilities of preventive medication or prophylactic surgery.

Table 1.2 gives an overview of cases in which hereditary breast cancer should be suspected and genetic counselling offered at a specialized center.

■ Medical History Data Helpful for Image Interpretation

The following data may be helpful in image interpretation:

- Recent pregnancy or breast feeding. This can be the cause of extensive proliferation of glandular tissue, which may be misinterpreted if the physician is unaware of the patient's history.
- Administration of female hormones. In some postmenopausal patients, hormone replacement therapy may involve extensive proliferation of glandular tissue. Newly occurring or increasing densities can be mistaken for suggestive findings if the physician is unaware of the patient's history.
- Thyroid hormone. Published studies have described that administration of thyroid hormone can promote fibrocystic changes in the breast.
- Surgery or radiation therapy. Changes after surgery or radiation therapy can produce masses, distortions or microcalcifications that can simulate or obscure a carcinoma (see Chapter 16). Here, careful documentation of scars and their location in the breast is important. Architectural distortion outside the scar area may be a sign of malignancy. Knowledge of the period of time that has elapsed since

surgery or irradiation may also be valuable for correct image interpretation.

Furthermore the following symptoms may be a hint to malignancy:

- Any—even slight—changes of the nipple, such as a recent deviation or inversion of the nipple, are important. Even though deviation or inversion of the nipple can be congenital or can occur following inflammation, new development may be an important and early hint of malignancy.
- Spontaneous discharge. Significant factors here include color, occurrence over time (association with pregnancy), number of involved ducts (single versus multiple), and the results of cytologic smears where available.

Significant aspects of any clinical findings (skin dimpling, skin changes, palpable findings) include:

- Time when the condition was first noticed,
- Changes since the condition was first noticed (decrease, increase, time span)
- Results of previous examinations (such as surgical biopsy, core biopsy or cytology)

If *previous imaging studies* exist, ask for the name and, if known, the address of the physician who performed them. It may be useful to obtain these films for comparison. Whenever available, *compare findings with earlier imaging studies*, since this might improve diagnostic accuracy.

■ References

1 Baines CJ, Vidmar M, McKeown-Eyssen G, Tibshirani R. Impact of menstrual phase on false negative mammograms in the Canadian National Breast Screening Study. Cancer. 1997;80(4):720–4
2 White E, Velentgas P, Mandelson MT et al. Variation in breast density by time in menstrual cycle among women aged 40–49 years. J Natl Cancer Inst. 1998;90(12):906–10
3 Spratt JS. Re: Variation in mammographic breast density by time in menstrual cycle among women aged 40–49 years. J Natl. Cancer Inst 1999;91:90
4 Kuhl CK, Bieling HB, Gieseke J et al. Healthy premenopausal breast parenchyma in dynamic contrast-enhanced MR imaging of the breast: normal contrast medium enhancement and cyclical-phase dependency. Radiology. 1997;203:137–44
5 Müller-Schimpfle M, Ohmenhäuser K, Stoll P et al. Menstrual cycle and age: influence on parenchymal contrast medium enhancement in MR imaging of the breast. Radiology. 1997;203:145–9
6 Berlin L. Malpractice issues in radiology. AJR. 1999;173:1161–7
7 Stark DD, Bradley WG jr. Magnetic Resonsance Imaging. 3rded. St. Louis: Mosby; 1999

8 Niendorf HP, Alhassan A, Geens VR, Clauss W. Safety review of gadopentetate dimglumine: extended clinical experience after more than 5 million applications. Invest Radiol. 1995;29:179–82

9 Niendorf HP. Gadolinium-DTPA: a well-tolerated and safe contrast medium. Insert Eur Radiol. 1994;4:1–2

10 Elmore JG, Wells CK, Howard DH, Feinstein AR. The impact of clinical history on mammographic interpretations. JAMA 1997;277:49–52

11 Maass H. Mammakarzinom: Epidemiologie. Gynäkologe. 1994;27:3

12 Stoll BA. Defining breast cancer prevention. In: Stoll BA, ed. Approaches to breast cancer prevention. London: Kluwer; 1991

13 Easton D, Peto J. The contribution of inherited predisposition to cancer incidence. Cancer Surv. 1990;9:395

14 Friedrichs K. Genetische Aspekte des Mammakarzinoms. Gynäkologe. 1994;27:7

15 Prechtel K, Gehm O, Geiger G, Prechtel P. Die Histologie der Mastopathie und die kumulative ipsilaterale Mammakarzinomsequenz. Pathologe. 1994;15:158

16 Dupont WD, Page DL. Risk factors for breast cancer in women with proliferative disease. N Engl J Med. 1985;312:146

17 Weitzel JF. Genetic cancer risk assessment. Cancer suppl. Dec 1, 1999; 86(11):2483–92

18 Kutner SE. Breast Cancer Genetics and Managed Care. Cancer suppl. Dec 1, 1999;86:2570–4

19 Swift ML, Sholman L, Perry M, Chase C. Malignant neoplasms in the families of patients with ataxia – telangiectasia. Cancer Res. 1976;36:209

20 Malkin D, Li FP, Strong LC et al. Germline p 53 mutations in a familial syndrome of breast cancers, sarcomas and other neoplasms. Science. 1990;250:1233

21 Hall J, Ming KL, Newmann B et al. Linkage of early-onset familial breast cancer to chromosome 17q 21. Science. 1990;250:1990

22 Krontiris TG, Devlin B, Karp D et al. An association between the risk of cancer and mutations in the HRAS 1 minisatelite locus. N Engl J Med. 1993;329:517

23 Zuppan P, Hall JM, Lee MK et al. Possible linkage of the estrogen receptor gene to breast cancer in family with late onset disease. Am J Hum Genet. 1991;48:1065

24 Fay MP, Freedman LS. Meta-analyses of dietary fats and mammary neoplasms in rodent experiments. Breast Cancer Res Treat. 1997;46:215–23

25 Gandini S, Merzenich H, Robertson C, Boyle P. Meta-analysis on breast cancer risk and diet: the role of fruit and vegetable consumption and the intake of associated micronutrients. Eur J Cancer. 2000;36:636–46

26 Pathak DR, Osuch JR, He J. Breast carcinoma etiology: current knowledge and new insights into the effects of reproductive and hormonal risk factors in black and white populations. Cancer. 2000;1/88(suppl5):1230–8

27 Seifert M, Galid A. Oral contraceptives and breast cancer—a causal relationship? Gynäkol. Geburtshilfliche Rundsch. 1998;38(2):101–4

28 Beral V, Banks E, Reeves G, Appleby P. Use of HRT and the subsequent risk of cancer. J Epidemiol Biostat. 1999;4:191–210

29 Russo IH, Russo J. Role of hormones in mammary cancer initiation and progression. J Mammary Gland Biol Neoplasia. 1998;3(1):49–61

30 Chiechi LM, Secreto G. Factors of risk for breast cancer influencing post-menopausal long-term hormone replacement therapy. Tumori. 2000;86:12–16

2. Clinical Findings

A complete breast examination includes the physical examination as well as a mammogram. In a screening setting, about 10% of breast cancers will only be detectable by physical examination.

Additionally, it is important at the time of diagnostic mammography to correlate mammographic findings with physical findings and vice versa. Competence in physical examination of the breast is therefore a necessary skill for the mammographer.

■ Purpose

Initial examination of the breast involves visual inspection and palpation. When the physical examination is abnormal, subsequent diagnostic imaging studies should always be interpreted together with clinical findings. The physician must also ensure that the examination includes the marginal areas of the breast, namely the area close to the sternum, the inframammary fold, the lateral border of the glandular body, and the axilla, which may be poorly imaged at mammography.

Visual Inspection

■ Technique

Observe the breast with the patient's arm raised as well as with her hand placed on her hip. Alternatively, the patient may be seated with her arms extended, next to her body pressing on the edge of the table. Observe and document any findings with respect to:

- Breast size and symmetry
- Contour
- Skin changes
- Nipples

■ Findings

The *size* of the breast can vary considerably among individual patients. Small breasts are generally easy to examine clinically, while macromastia will limit the amount of information provided by palpation. It is important to determine whether asymmetry in breast size (anisomastia) is an indication of:

- Individual variation
- A postoperative condition

- Retraction in the presence of disseminated tumor (reduction in breast size combined with palpable thickening)

Normal *breast contour* is convex. Flattening or dimpling can result from surgery or from retraction due to a subjacent tumor.

Skin changes may be generalized or circumscribed. Examples of such changes include:

- Erythema (mastitis, inflammatory breast carcinoma, or acute radiation reaction)
- Skin thickening
- Peau d'orange (skin thickening with inversion of the pores indicative of lymphedema)
- Prominent veins (supraclavicular, infraclavicular, or mediastinal mass producing venous compression)
- Hyperpigmentation or telangiectasia (sequela of radiation therapy)

Circumscribed skin changes include:

- Verrucae
- Nevi
- Atheromas
- Fibroepitheliomas

- Sebaceous cysts
- Scars
- Long area of retraction associated with thrombophlebitis (Mondor disease)

Inversion of the nipple can be:

- Congenital
- Acquired as a result of surgery
- The result of breast inflammation or a malignant tumor
- Associated with retraction

Deviation of the nipple or lack of symmetry when compared to the opposite side can be an indication of beginning retraction. Asymmetric depigmentation of the nipple can occur as a result of radiation therapy.

Crusty deposits on the nipple can be a sign of pathologic discharge. Eczematous changes in the nipple can be a sign of Paget disease.

Any abnormalities in breast size or contour and any skin or nipple changes should be noted along with the probable causes suggested by the clinical examination or the patient's history. The radiologist should be aware of any benign skin lesions that might simulate a focal lesion at mammography. Cutaneous lesions may calcify, which should be considered in the mammographic differential diagnosis.

Precisely document any scars since they may explain mammographically detectable structural changes (Fig. 2.1).

Palpation

■ Technique

Palpation should be performed gently, allowing for the patient's individual sensitivity to pain.

- Using the fingertips of both hands, separate the glandular tissue from the underlying and surrounding tissue and palpate it
- Examine the breasts individually and systematically
- Assess the individual consistency of the gland, looking for circumscribed areas of altered (i. e., firmer) consistency
- Always palpate both breasts for comparison
- Assess the mobility of the nipple
- Also assess the mobility of the breast tissue with respect to the skin and chest wall

Move your fingers toward each other and grasp the glandular tissue to assess whether a plateau appears as a sign of a desmoplastic reaction in the subjacent tissue (the Jackson sign).

Palpation is initially performed with the patient standing, after which the examination is continued with the patient supine. The final procedure is the examination of the lymph drainage routes. These include the axillary tail of the breast, the axilla, the infraclavicular region, and the supraclavicular region. Palpate axillary lymph nodes by examining the patient with her arms hanging down. Move your fingertips as far superiorly into the axilla as possible. Applying moderate pressure against the lateral chest wall, move slowly down the lateral chest wall. Lymph nodes will typically slide away under the fingertips. Palpate the axillary tail, the infraclavicular region, and the supraclavicular region using the same technique as for glandular tissue.

■ Findings

Palpation provides information about:

- The structure of glandular tissue
- Possible asymmetry
- Lumps and their consistency and relation to the surrounding tissue, skin (the Jackson sign), pectoralis muscle, and painful sensation
- Nipple and the subareolar tissue
- Lymph drainage routes

The structure of the glandular tissue can be soft or, in the presence of breast disorders, firm or granular. Granular texture may be finely, medium, or coarsely nodular. Documenting these palpatory findings is very valuable for interpreting subsequent findings. Asymmetry can be an initial sign of a disseminated or focal carcinoma, but it can also be congenital.

For every circumscribed palpable finding, assess the following parameters:

- Consistency
- Contour
- Mobility and the relation to surrounding tissue (skin and pectoralis muscle). A malig-

Physician´s Work Sheet

Clinical findings:

Generally **soft** breast: _____   **Firm** glandular tissue: _____

Finely nodular glandular tissue: _____   **Coarseley nodular** glandular tissue: _____

Additional findings:
(please number if more than one)

– Mobile lumps: ○   – Immobile **lumps**:

– Inverted **nipple**:   △   – **Thickening**:

– **Retraction** (skin, nipple):   □   – **Scar**:

– Cutaneous **verruca**   ●
  or similar finding:

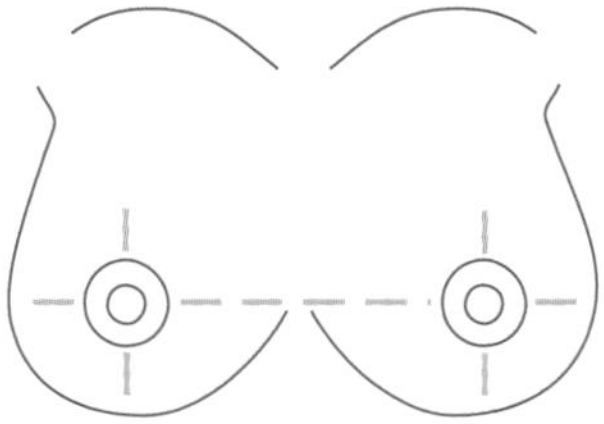

R   **L**

Finding number:	Approximate size:	First noticed when:	Change in size: ↑ ↓ —
1.	_____	_____	_____
2.	_____	_____	_____
3.	_____	_____	_____
4.	_____	_____	_____

Nipple discharge? N □

	number of ducts	color?	spontaneous?
right □	_____	____	_____
left □	_____	____	_____

pain?   N □

	symmetric?	localized*? (where)	type of pain
right □			
left □			

Status of lymph nodes: _____

_____

Physician: _____

Fig. 2.**1** Physician's Work Sheet

nant tumor can cause a desmoplastic reaction, and/or tumor infiltration may form a plateau accompanied by peau d'orange. This sign can be detected even before a tumor can be reliably palpated.

Circumscribed lumps can be soft (lipomas, fibroadenolipomas, partially filled cysts, or medullary and mucinous carcinomas) or of firmer consistency (cysts, fibroadenomas, or carcinomas).

Involuted fibroadenomas, oil cysts, and circumscribed scarring can have the same hard consistency as a carcinoma.

Fibrocystic masses, distended or chronically inflamed cysts, and hematomas are painful, whereas malignant tumors are less often so. Some women with good body perception will feel localized pain or sense a change at the site of a tumor that may not even be palpable. This may be due to the disturbed parenchymal structure and consistency caused by the tumor.

When the nipples are examined, mobility should be assessed. Mobility can be compromised by a tumor in the subjacent tissue or by subacute or chronic mastitis or scarring.

Small (i. e., ≤ 10 mm), smooth, mobile, generally firm lymph nodes can be normal findings in the axilla but are pathologic in the supraclavicular or infraclavicular regions. Enlarged lymph nodes and/or lymph nodes with poor mobility should be regarded as pathologic until proven otherwise.

Ectopic glandular tissue may be present in the axilla, above or below the breast. This will be apparent as relatively soft circumscribed palpable findings. The patient may report changes in size or painfulness related to the menstrual cycle.

■ Problems

Palpation can reveal small carcinomas in superficial sites or in small breasts. However, tumors exceeding 2 cm in diameter may go undetected in the deeper tissue of large or lumpy breasts. In fact, less than 50% of the tumors smaller than 1.5 cm

and even less than 50% of the tumors between 1 and 1.5 cm in size are palpable.[1, 2]

Palpating disseminated carcinomas such as disseminated invasive lobular carcinomas is particularly difficult. More than 90% of intraductal carcinomas are nonpalpable. Extensive nodular breast disorders can greatly limit the diagnostic accuracy of palpation.

Any atypical palpable findings and any findings suggestive of carcinoma should be further assessed by mammography or other diagnostic studies. A clinical examination conducted by a physician familiar with the mammographic findings will permit improved diagnostic interpretation of asymmetries or circumscribed areas of increased density.

■ Summary

Careful palpation is essential even with regular mammographic screening. The reasons for this are:

1. Mammography has limited sensitivity, especially in radiodense tissue. Approximately 10% of malignancies are only discovered because they are palpable. This means that palpable findings, even with negative mammography, may require further workup or biopsy.
2. Palpation can detect malignant processes along the periphery of the glandular body or in the axillary tail which may escape detection at mammography.

Mammography does not replace careful physical examination.[3–8] However, whenever a questionable or suggestive clinical findings exists, further workup (by mammography, possibly ultrasound and/or percutaneous biopsy) should follow to avoid missing nonpalpable additional lesions or causing unnecessary biopsy (of lipomas, definite fibroadenomas, hamartomas, oil cysts or simple cysts).

■ References

1 Ciatto S, Roselli-del-Turco M, Cantarzi et al. Causes of breast cancer misdiagnosis at physical examination. Neoplasma. 1991;38:523–31

2 Reintgen D, Berman C, Cox C et al. The anatomy of missed breast cancers. Surg Oncol. 1993;2:65–75

3 Barton MB, Harris R, Fletcher SW. Does this patient have breast cancer? The screening clinical breast examination: should it be done? How? JAMA. 1999;282:1270–80

4 Flegg KM, Rowling YJ. Clinical breast examination. A contentious issue in screening for breast cancer. Aust Fam Physician. 2000;29:343–6

5 Shapiro S. Periodic screening for breast cancer: the HIP randomized controlled trial. Journal of the National Cancer Institute. Monographs. 1997;22:27–30

6 Smart CR, Byrne C, Smith RA et al. Twenty-year follow-up of the breast cancers diagnosed during the Breast Cancer Detection Demonstration Project. CA Cancer J Clin. 1997;47:134–49

7 Miller AB, To T, Baines CB et al. The Canadian National Breast Screening Study: update on breast cancer mortality. Journal of the National Cancer Institute. Monographs. 1997;22:37–41

8 Alexander FE, Anderson TJ, Brown HK et al. 14 years follow-up from the Edinburgh randomised trial of breast-cancer screening. The Lancet. 1999;353:1903–8

3. Mammography

Purpose, Accuracy, Possibilities, and Limitations

■ Indications

Mammography is the single most important imaging method in diagnosing breast disease. Its areas of application include:

- Screening. Mammography is the only imaging method to date that is suitable for screening.
- Problem solving. Aside from a few exceptions (such as unequivocal sonographic diagnosis of a cyst, unequivocal clinical diagnosis of an abscess, and very young patients), mammography is always indicated as a diagnostic method in symptomatic patients. In applicable cases, it may be used with other methods.

A basic knowledge of the accuracy of mammography is an important prerequisite to properly judge its value in screening and clinical use.

■ Accuracy

■ General Aspects

The sensitivity and specificity of the method cannot be precisely quantified. While high image quality and experienced examiners are essential prerequisites, accuracy also depends on the following factors:

- Patient selection: Screening versus diagnostic problem solving, type of screening (number of views, use of clinical data, and screening interval), distribution of findings in the study group, and the extent to which other methods of preoperative diagnosis are used.
- The threshold of the individual examiner. Experience being equal, a low threshold will lead to a high sensitivity at the expense of specificity, whereas a high threshold increases specificity and the positive predictive value at the expense of sensitivity.[1]

The individual threshold represents a compromise arrived at by assessing the tradeoff between the false negative rate and the false positive rate. It is also influenced by other factors such as limited funds of a screening program, restrictions concerning the accepted rate of excisional diagnostic biopsies, or the accepted number of additional examinations.

■ Sensitivity

Realistically, mammography has a sensitivity of about 90%, i. e., about 10% of carcinomas, which are otherwise symptomatic at the time of the mammographic examination, are not detected initially by mammography. When mammographic screening is performed, about 25–35% of the carcinomas become apparent between screening examinations, usually by manifesting clinical symptoms. They are called interval carcinomas. Finally it is important to know that numerous carcinomas detected at screening are retrospectively visible on the previous examination, mostly as some uncharacteristic change.[2, 3, 4]

Thus mammography does not provide a 100% sensitivity. There exists a threshold for mammographic detection of malignancy, which depends on tumor size, tumor type, and surrounding tissue. These limitations must be kept in mind, particularly for diagnostic mammography.

For screening, however, mammography is the only method that allows reproducible and reliable detection of a prognostically relevant number of nonpalpable carcinomas at an acceptable rate of false positive calls and at acceptable expense.

Overall sensitivity of mammography in fatty tissue is excellent. It decreases as radiodensity increases. This means that mammography has a lower sensitivity in radiodense tissue and, therefore, a negative mammogram does not eliminate the need for further workup of otherwise indeterminate or suggestive palpable findings in dense tissue.[5, 6]

Mammography is highly sensitive in detecting carcinomas containing microcalcifications, and this sensitivity is largely uninfluenced by the radiodensity of the surrounding tissue. These carcinomas account for about 50% of all cancers, including approximately 30–40% of all invasive carcinomas and about 90% of carcinomas in situ currently detected. Since these are generally not palpable but have excellent cure rates, mammography plays a decisive role in early detection.

■ Specificity

Mammography is specific in only a few cases:

- Absence of malignancy can be diagnosed reliably in fatty breasts (provided the area in question is included on the mammogram).
- A definitive diagnosis of a benign lesion is possible for a typical oil cyst, a hamartoma, a lipoma, a typically calcified fibroadenoma or lymph nodes with typical mammographic features.
- A quite reliable diagnosis of a benign tumor or cyst (> 98% correct) is possible in the case of a typical well-circumscribed mass.

In the majority of clinically or mammographically detected changes, mammography, however, is nonspecific and only permits likelihood statements.[7, 8]

- The specificity of the diagnosis of a carcinoma is quite high for spiculated masses, as well as for pleomorphic and cast-like microcalcifications with ductal distribution. However, a spiculated mass can also be caused by an area of fat necrosis or a radial scar. (Rarely, even suspicious microcalcifications are associated with papillomatosis, papilloma, fibroadenoma, plasma cell mastitis or fat necrosis).

In addition to the factors already mentioned (threshold and selection of patients), the size of the findings decisively influences the expected specificity of the mammographic study. In fact, most nonpalpable carcinomas, in particular small carcinomas, appear as nonspecific changes.[1, 9, 10, 11, 12, 13] Unless the examiner is only looking for large, obvious findings, one has to be aware that only 1 of every 5 to 10 mammographically suspicious changes will correspond to malignancy.[1, 7, 10–12]

Further diagnostic studies, including additional views, sonography, and percutaneous biopsy, can improve this rate so that more than half of the excisional biopsies of nonpalpable abnormalities will be performed for a malignancy.[14]

■ Screening

Due to the high sensitivity of mammography in fatty tissue and its ability to reveal microcalcifications, mammography can detect small carcinomas at an early and prognostically favorable stage.

Mammographic screening has resulted in a 30–50% reduction in mortality (see Chapter 21). To date, neither physical examination nor chemotherapy or hormonal therapy has been able to achieve comparable results.

Mammography is the only imaging modality suitable for screening. In addition to good sensitivity and acceptable specificity, it offers the following important advantages:

- It is the most cost-effective noninvasive examination method.
- Mammographic studies are reproducible and easily documented.
- It requires relatively little physician time (in contrast to breast ultrasound).
- It is the only technique that reliably visualizes microcalcifications—which are associated with about 30% of the invasive breast cancers and almost all presently detected intraductal cancers.

Yet despite the many advantages, one should bear these points in mind:

- Negative screening results do not exclude a carcinoma. Supplementary studies are always indicated in the presence of new or existing problems.
- In screening as in diagnostic use, best results are achieved by evaluating the mammographic studies in conjunction with clinical data and the patient's medical history. Clinical examination and patient history should not be neglected. About 10% of breast cancers are detected only by physical examination.
- The results are highly dependent on image quality and the examiner's level of experience.

■ Problem Solving

Problem solving begins when clinical data, the patient's medical history, or imaging studies (usually mammography) reveal an abnormality. The most important objective is to verify or exclude the presence of a carcinoma with the highest possible degree of certainty. Considering the general risk of surgery and expense, the physiological and psychological stress on the patient, patient compliance and costs, biopsies of benign lesions should be avoided whenever possible. Furthermore, severe or multiple scars may impair later diagnosis. However, a high degree of certainty is necessary to exclude a suspected malignancy.

The following should be remembered for problem solving:

1. The sensitivity of mammography is excellent (approaching 100%) in fatty breasts or in all fatty areas of the breast. This means that in the absence of mammographic findings, malignancy can be excluded with a high degree of certainty even in the presence of palpable abnormality in this area.[15] This applies only if the palpable findings in question
   – have been included mammographically (note that the axillary tail and areas close to the chest wall can be a problem)
   – lie entirely within fatty tissue
   For this reason it is useful to place a radiopaque marker over palpable lesions to localize them on the mammogram.
2. It is particularly important to remember that the sensitivity of mammography is significantly reduced in areas containing a high proportion of glandular or connective tissue.[5, 6] Carcinomas without microcalcifications can be overlooked in such areas. Thus, in tissue that is not mammographically equivalent to fat, any suggestive palpable findings require further workup.
3. Only a few entities have such a distinct mammographic appearance that no further diagnostic studies are necessary. These include:
   - lipomas
   - typical hamartomas
   - characteristically calcified fibroadenomas
   - oil cysts and some galactoceles
   - intramammary lymph nodes
4. Whenever a mammographically, clinically or otherwise detected abnormality does not exhibit a pathognomonic appearance, further workup is necessary.

Another important task of mammography concerns detection of secondary lesions. For this reason, even with palpable lesions undergoing surgical biopsy, mammography is always indicated preoperatively to be certain that a second non-palpable lesion that requires biopsy is not present.

Mammographic Technique

Compared to radiographic studies of other parts of the body, mammography places particularly stringent demands on equipment and image quality. The stringent demands of technique and positioning make mammography one of the most difficult examinations in conventional radiology.

The specific requirements can be **summarized as follows:**

- Extremely fine microcalcifications and fibrotic strands (tiny structures with a size of about 100 μm with only slight differences in density to the surrounding tissue) must be imaged sharply, with high contrast and with a low level of image noise.
- Despite the highest possible contrast, mammography must permit adequate assessment of areas of greatly varying density. These include fatty areas behind the nipple or close to the skin in small breasts, areas of radiodense fibrocystic tissue in large breasts and the tissue overlying the pectoralis muscle. This requires an imaging system with a wide object range.
- In view of the sensitivity of mammary tissue to radiation (especially in younger women), the examination should involve the minimum dose of radiation sufficient to produce an image of acceptable quality.
- Imaging the complete body of the gland is imperative for an accurate assessment in both screening examinations and diagnostic problem solving. This is possible only with a consistent effort to achieve optimum standard positioning. Knowledge and application of additional views, whenever indicated, is necessary.

These stringent requirements apply to the choice of equipment and film as well as to the level of training and experience of physicians and technical staff. Radiologists and radiologic technologists must ensure a standard of image quality that permits detection of early malignancy.

It is therefore *essential that radiologists and radiologic technologists* be thoroughly familiar with mammographic technique and constantly monitor quality. Studies have shown that only optimal imaging technique ensures early detection of breast cancer.[16] Where this is not the case, early stage carcinomas with excellent cure rates will not be detected with sufficient certainty. This has serious negative repercussions because the mammographic examination will give the patient and her referring physician a false sense of security, and both may underestimate the significance of early clinical signs of malignancy.

Components of the Mammographic Imaging Technique

(Fig. **3.1**)

■ The X-ray Tube

Mammography requires *special tubes* that produce particularly *low-energy radiation* in comparison to other diagnostic X-ray tubes. This is achieved by use of special targets and filters. Mammography requires low-energy radiation to achieve the required high tissue contrast.

Since the radiation needed originates in a small focal spot and the exposure time should be as short as possible (to avoid motion blurring), the tubes used for mammography must be powerful.

■ Sharpness: Focal Spot Size and Geometry (Source to Image–Receptor Distance = SID)

To achieve the required sharpness (spatial resolution), mammography tubes must have an extremely small focal spot. A *nominal focal spot size smaller than 0.4* is required today.

Note: A nominal focal spot size of 0.4 means that the diameter in each direction will be between 0.4 mm–0.6 mm. The local projection of the width of the focal spot will vary according to:

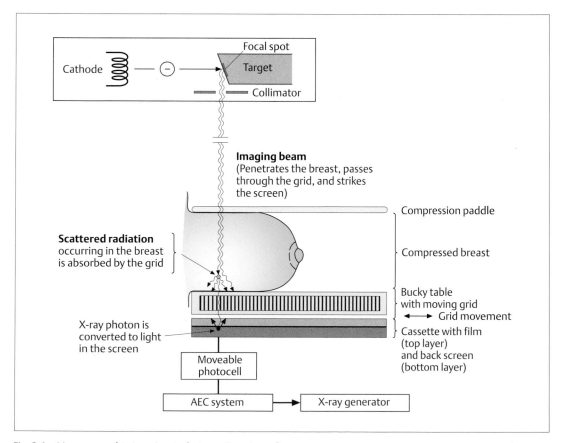

Fig. **3.1** Mammographic imaging technique. Overview of components

– its distance from the chest wall
– the angulation of the tube

In addition to minimal focal spot size, the proper geometric configuration of the focal spot, object, and image receptor is important in achieving the necessary sharpness. Use of a *small focal spot, the shortest possible distance between the object and the film and the longest possible distance between the focus and the film* will minimize the penumbra (geometric blurring) (Fig. 3.2).

■ Radiation Spectrum: Penetration and Contrast

The radiation produced in X-ray tubes is not monoenergetic but consists of a spectrum of radiation energies. This spectrum comprises X-ray bremsstrahlung and the characteristic radiation determined by the target material.

   Since the spectrum of imaging radiation greatly influences contrast and radiation dose, the following physical aspects should be considered:

– With *low-energy radiation,* slight differences in the radiodensity of soft tissue of the breast that would otherwise remain undetected can be visualized with *high contrast.*
– *Increasing energy* of the radiation *decreases soft-tissue contrast.*
– But, the radiation spectrum *must* have *sufficiently high energy for adequate penetration* of thick breasts and breasts with abundant fibrotic or glandular tissue.
– Radiation with insufficient energy will not penetrate the breast even with long exposure time. Such radiation is not suitable for imaging at all. It will unnecessarily increase the radiation dose and, since dense tissue cannot be penetrated, it will produce an inadequate image.

Thus, *higher-energy* radiation is required in *dense breasts* (in the presence of abundant fibrotic tissue, glandular tissue, or mastopathy) and in thick *breasts.*

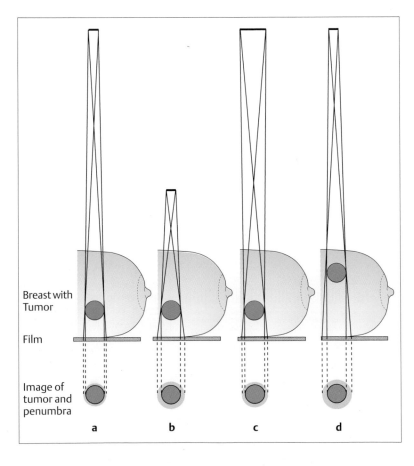

Breast with Tumor

Film

Image of tumor and penumbra

a   b   c   d

Fig. 3.2 A long SID (source-to-image receptor distance), small focal spot, and short distance between the object and the film minimize penumbra and optimize image definition (**a**). The penumbra increases with a short SID (**b**), large focal spot (**c**), and a long distance between object and film (**d**)

With the optimum radiation energy selected, the *absorption is higher in radiodense tissue (fibrotic tissue, glandular tissue, and malignant tissue) than in radiolucent tissue (fat or loose connective tissue).* These *differences in absorption* produce the image pattern.

Since too large a component of high energy reduces the contrast and too high a component of low energy results in excessive radiation exposure, it is advisable to adapt the radiation spectrum as closely as possible to the thickness and density of the breast.

The radiation spectrum is determined by the following factors:

1. The *target/filter combination* of the X-ray tube
2. The *peak kilovoltage (kVp)* setting on the X-ray unit

■ Target/Filter Combination

The radiation spectrum created at the target depends on the *kVp setting* and on the *target material.*

The radiation spectrum of molybdenum targets contains a higher proportion of low-energy radiation (including characteristic peaks at 17.5 and 19.6 keV) than do the spectra of tungsten or rhodium tubes.

Selective filtering is used to adapt the radiation spectrum of a given target as closely as possible to the specific requirements.

Selective filtering:

- Suppresses the low-energy components of the spectrum that would represent unnecessary radiation exposure because they are absorbed in the breast (like the standard aluminum filter)
- Reduces the energy components above the K absorption edge characteristic of the selected filter material, essentially permitting a narrow spectral range directly below the K absorption edge to pass. Any filter is particularly efficient at absorbing that part of the radiation whose energy exceeds a limit, referred to as the K absorption edge, specific to the filter material.

The effective spectral range can thus be defined by selecting the target and filter material and the thickness of the filter (Fig. 3.**3**).[17, 18]

Commercially available *target/filter combinations* include molybdenum/molybdenum, molybdenum/rhodium, rhodium/rhodium or tungsten/molybdenum, and tungsten/rhodium.

- The radiation quality from a molybdenum/molybdenum or tungsten/molybdenum target/filter combination is suitable for most breasts.
- The combinations tungsten/molybdenum, molybdenum/rhodium, tungsten/rhodium, and rhodium/rhodium provide, in this order, increasingly high-energy radiation spectra. They permit better penetration of large and mastopathic breasts with abundant glandular, fibrotic, and connective tissue, resulting in higher image quality and a reduction in unnecessary radiation exposure.

■ Peak Kilovoltage (kVp)

A higher kVp setting increases the relative proportion of high-energy radiation in the respective spectrum, whereas a lower kVp setting increases the relative proportion of low-energy radiation.

Selecting the proper kVp setting, target material, and filter material according to breast thickness and density: Since the optimum kVp for a target/filter combination is not applicable to others, automatic exposure control systems are provided to make it easier to match kVp to breast thickness and density. Depending on the manufacturer, the system can select or suggest the proper settings (see pp. 25 and 32).

■ Penetration: Heel Effect

The heel effect of the X-ray tube is also exploited to compensate for varying penetration in the chest wall and nipple.

The heel effect (Fig. 3.**4**) means that the intensity of rays emitted by the target is not uniform throughout the beam.[19]

More of the rays that leave the target at obtuse angle will be absorbed by the target than those leaving the target at acute angle, due to the longer path they have to travel in the target.

Since the thickness of the breast is greater close to the chest wall than near the nipple, it is best when the area of maximum radiation intensity lies near the chest wall. This is achieved by positioning the target opposite the cathode, which is closer to the chest wall. The intensity distribution of the radiation can be influenced by slightly angling (i. e., tipping) the X-ray tube. However, this alters the projection of the focal spot.

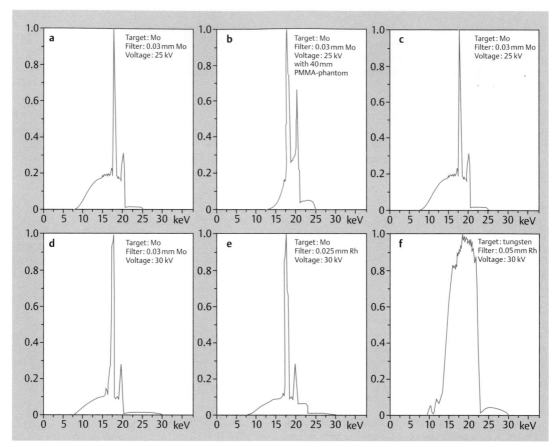

Fig. 3.**3 a–f** Radiation spectra of various target/filter combinations

a and **b** The illustration shows the photon spectrum of a molybdenum/0.030-mm molybdenum filter combination at 25 kV peak kilovoltage as it is emitted from the X-ray tube (**a**), and as it is measured at the image receptor after penetrating a 4-cm breast phantom (**b**). The respective spectra of radiation in the right and left pictures are normalized according to the maximum energy (= 100%) present in the respective spectrum.

Comparing the left and right illustration reveals that the low energies are absorbed in the breast. Thus, they cannot contribute to visualization but only increase the dose. The more breast thickness increases, the more low-energy components of the spectrum are absorbed in the glandular tissue.

Increasing the average energy of the spectrum in proportion to breast thickness and density is recommended to achieve sufficient penetration and avoid an excessive dose due to absorption of the low-energy radiation

c–f One way of increasing the high-energy components in the spectrum is to increase the kVp setting. Changing the filter material and/or filter thickness or choosing another target material make it possible to adapt the radiation spectrum even more closely to the thickness and density of the breast. (This increases the high-energy components in the spectrum and better filters out the low-energy components, which increase the dose, particularly in dense breasts.) This may be illustrated in the spectra of various target/filter combinations

■ **Scattered Radiation**

In every radiograph of the breast, *scattered radiation* is produced in the tissue. In denser and thicker glandular tissue, more scattered radiation occurs than in the thinner, fatty, transparent tissue. Increasing amounts of scattered radiation result in progressive loss of contrast.

■ **Scatter Reduction: Grids**

The grid is placed between the breast and the image receptor (screen–film system) to reduce undesired scattered radiation that impairs image quality.

Grids (Fig. 3.1) consist of strips of lead that absorb obliquely oriented radiation, whereas radiation parallel to the lead strips passes through. The lead strips are focused on the focal spot.

During the exposure, the grid rapidly moves perpendicular to the path of the beam and to the orientation of the strips to prevent the strips from appearing on the mammogram as thin lines that mar the image.

The efficiency of the grid depends on the height of the strips and the strip spacing. The ratio of strip height to strip spacing is known as the grid ratio. The larger the grid ratio, the greater the efficiency of the grid but also the greater the required radiation dose. For this reason, only grid ratios of 4:27 or 5:30 are recommended for mammography.[19, 20]

Since the grid absorbs both scattered radiation and a small proportion of useful radiation, it requires a longer exposure time and, therefore, an increased radiation dose. Exposures with a grid require a *grid exposure factor* of approximately 2.5. The use of more sensitive screen–film systems has compensated for this increased dose, compared with earlier gridless mammographic techniques.

The *significant increase in image quality* fully justifies the increased radiation dose required by the grid, and *grid mammography* has superseded gridless mammography.

Gridless mammography can only be performed without significant loss of quality in very small, compressed, and fatty breasts in the interest of reducing radiation exposure.

■ Scatter Reduction: Compression

The second important method of *reducing scattered radiation* consists of sufficient *compression of the breast.* By reducing breast thickness, compression reduces the proportion of scattered radiation, thus reducing the dose and improving the image contrast (see p. 31).[21, 20]

Other options for reducing scattered radiation include air-gap technique. The air gap, which is effective only in conjunction with good collimation, is used for scatter reduction in magnification mammography.[20] Slot mammography represents another effective method of scatter reduction (see p. 32).

■ Image Receptor System

After passing through the breast and the grid, the imaging radiation reaches the *image receptor system.* In modern screen–film mammography, this

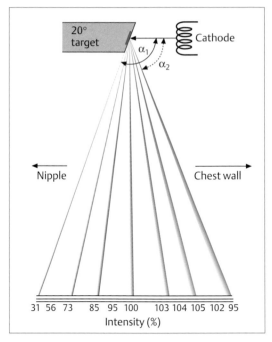

Fig. 3.**4** Heel effect
The beam created at the target focus is weaker on the target side than on the cathode aside. The illustration shows the radiation intensity referred to the central ray (100%). The intensity varies depending on the angle of egress of the radiation from the target. This effect is used in mammography by locating the cathode closer to the chest wall than the anode. Thus the radiation intensity will be greater close to the chest wall and less near the nipple, where the breast is thinner

system consists of *a single intensifying screen* with luminescent coating and *a special single-emulsion film* (Fig. 3.5 **a**).

The film emulsion and the coated side of the screen face each other. To obtain a sharp focus, the two must be in direct contact. Insufficient screen–film contact will cause significant local blurring.

Screen–film systems with dual-emulsion mammography films should not be used because the light photons, which are emitted from the film emulsion facing away from the screen, cause additional blurring (crossover effect). For reasons dictated by radiation geometry, the screen lies behind the film (back screen), maximizing image definition (Figs. 3.5 **b** and **c**).

Every quantum of radiation absorbed in the luminescent layer of the screen excites the phosphorus, causing it to emit several quanta of light. The resulting intensifying effect of the screen depends on the intensifying substance, the density

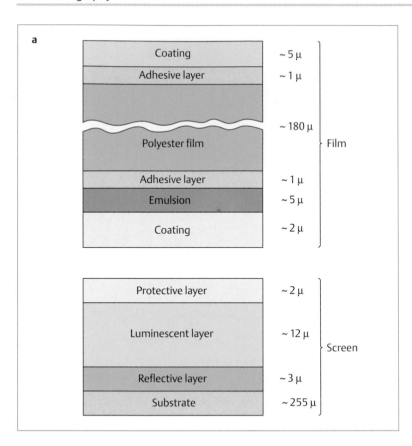

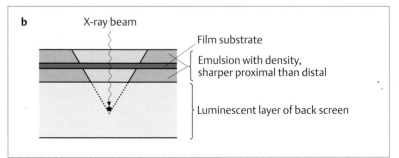

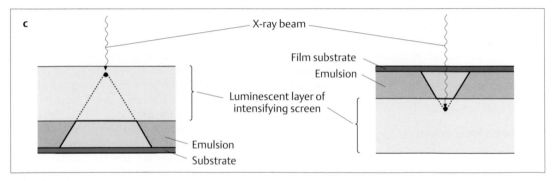

Fig. 3.**5b** and **c**

of the luminescent layer, the distribution of the coating, and the screen dye. All the currently available intensifying screens contain gadolinium oxysulfide as an intensifying substance.[19, 20]

While greater screen thickness and coarse crystal structures increase the intensifying effect of the screen, they also decrease the resolution. In addition to this, high intensification is accompanied by a significant increase in image noise (due to the lower number of X-ray photons that are needed). Thus to achieve the resolution required in mammography, only very high-definition intensifying screens (speed class 12) that achieve resolutions of 14–18 lines per millimeter should be used (see p. 27) for the importance of the screen–film system in optimizing resolution).[20, 22]

While the *sharpness* of a screen–film system is determined primarily *by the screen*, the *contrast* of the system is determined *by the film* and by the processing. Since the differences between the currently available high-resolution screens of the same class are slight, the sensitivity of a screen–film system and thus the required dose are then influenced by the choice of film.[22]

The contrast behavior of a mammographic film is shown in its respective *characteristic curve.* The characteristic curve shows the relationship between film density and the dose of radiation incident on the film. Optical density (blackening) is plotted against the logarithm of the radiation dose (Fig. 3.**6**).

The steeper the curve, the higher the contrast. The contrast is not only decisive in the medium density range. In dense breasts or dense areas of the breast, the contrast (and thus visualization) in the lower density range (0.5–1.5) is even more important.

For diagnostic purposes, uniformly high contrast in every density range would be desirable. Since the film curves flatten out significantly below an optical density of 0.6 and the human eye cannot distinguish differences at densities exceeding 2.2 (2.8–3.0 maximum in bright light), *the useful range of every film is limited to optical densities between 0.6 and 2.2–2.8.*

The exposure range (*x*-axis of Fig. 3.**6**) in which density differences can be visualized with good contrast, i. e., the useful optical density range (*y*-axis in Fig. 3.**6**), is known as the *imageable object range or latitude.*

If the film contrast is too high, the latitude will be too narrow. This means that the imageable object range will not include areas of very high or of very low density in the breast, and these areas can no longer be visualized in the useful density range. Density differences in these relatively *overexposed or underexposed areas* will no longer be adequately visualized (despite or because of the particularly high contrast in areas of medium density). Such overexposed or underexposed areas can appear particularly in large or dense breasts since their differences in absorption are especially high. To minimize these problems, the resulting contrast must be carefully optimized but should not be too high.[23]

The contrast is essentially determined by the choice of film, the quality of radiation (exposure voltage, target and filter), and the film processing.[20, 22]

■ Exposure

After selecting the proper film–screen system (FSS) and after adapting the radiation quality to the thickness and density of the breast, the film must be exposed in such a manner that all details relevant to the diagnosis are visualized in the optimum density range. This means that the mean optical density should lie approximately in the middle of the useful optical density range, i. e., between 1.4 and 1.8. (Recent studies have shown a mean density of 1.4–1.8 preferable to the mean density of 1.2–1.6 mentioned in medical guidelines.)[24]

Film density ranges below 0.6 and above 2.2 (or 2.8 in bright light) permit only limited visualization at best.

The *exposure* is the *product of tube current (mA) and exposure time (second)*, expressed as the

◁ Fig. 3.**5 b** The photons released from the luminescence centers of the intensifying screen are nondirectional in contrast to X-ray beams. For this reason, the diameter of the dense spot will increase with the distance between the film emulsion and the screen. This is illustrated by the diagram of a dual-emulsion film with a screen behind the film. Because of this phenomenon, only single-emulsion films are used in mammography

c Due to absorption of the X-ray beam within the intensifying screen, the majority of luminescence centers contributing to the image will be on that side of the screen, where the X-ray beam enters the screen. If a front screen were used, the majority of luminescence centers would be farther away from the film than if a back screen (behind the film) were used. Therefore, a front screen produces more blurring than a back screen. For this reason, only single-emulsion films with a back screen are used in mammography

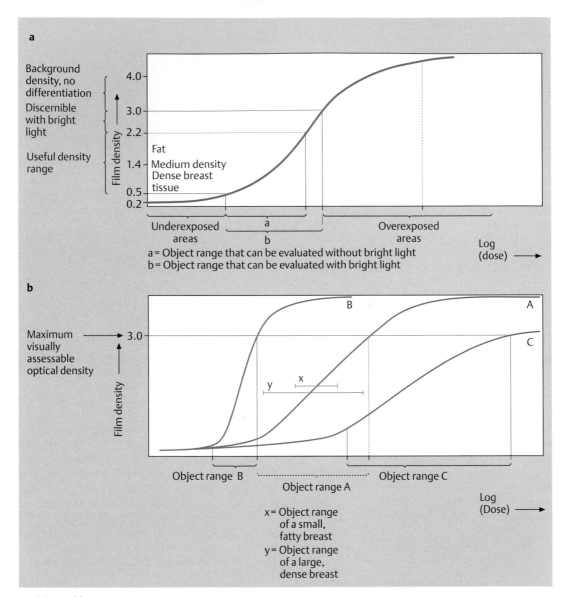

Fig. 3.**6 a** and **b**

milliampere–second product, or mAs product. One method of adjusting the exposure is by *selecting the settings manually*, i. e., all exposure parameters can be freely selected. However, this requires a fair amount of experience because the exposure varies with both breast thickness and breast density.

Even experienced radiologists and radiologic technologists will use *automatic exposure control systems* to minimize the chance of incorrect exposure. The purpose of an automatic exposure con-

trol system (a required feature on every mammography unit) is to ensure a reproducible mean optical density of 1.2–1.6 on the film regardless of breast thickness and density.

The automatic exposure control system (see Figs. 3.1 and 3.7) utilizes a *photocell* placed beneath the cassette containing the film and screen. The chamber measures the dose behind the image receptor in a representative area. When the *cutoff dose* for the selected mean optical film density is reached (this depends on the screen–

◁ Fig. 3.**6a** and **b**   The significance of characteristic curves
a Principle curve
b Exaggerated gradation curves of different films:
Film A shows a wide object range within which details are visualized with good contrast and can be easily discerned. *Film B* is more sensitive (left shifted) and images the details in the center section of the curve with greater contrast. However, its object range is narrower so that details beyond this range are visualized with poor contrast (underexposed or overexposed).
Film C requires a high dose yet images a narrower density range. In spite of this, it visualizes a wide object range with uniform albeit relatively low contrast.
Imaging a small breast requires a narrower object range than imaging a large, dense breast.
The mean exposure (center of the object range of the breast to be imaged) is adapted to the sensitivity of the screen–film system by selecting a higher or lower mAs product (right or left shift in the object range of the breast to be imaged). Changing the mAs product will not influence the width of the object range. This means that a small breast can be imaged with all three films. At optimum exposure settings, film B will produce the highest-contrast image. This image will be perceived as the sharpest, although there is no objective difference in the definition of films A, B, or C.
Film B cannot adequately image a dense breast. The object range of this film is narrower than that required for imaging dense breasts, and overexposed and underexposed areas will result. For this reason, film B should not be used although it produces better images of small breasts. Film A is the optimal film since it can image both large, dense breasts and small breasts with good contrast. Here, precise exposure settings are essential to avoid overexposed or underexposed areas since its object range is only slightly larger than a large, dense breast requires. Film C can image both small and large dense breasts in an acceptable range, albeit with slightly less contrast. This film should be considered if achieving precise exposure is a problem (as can occur with older automatic exposure control system with insufficient density compensation). Experience has shown that both microcalcifications and structures relevant to the diagnosis can be discerned, although they are less obvious.

film system used), the *system switches off the exposure.*
Since the sensitivity of the photocell varies with different radiation energies (that result from beam hardening behind breasts of different thickness or density and behind the image receptor), the automatic exposure control system must compensate for the variable breast thickness and density when determining the optimum cutoff dose.
The quality of the automatic exposure control system determines how well it can achieve a constant film density independent of breast thickness and density. (see pp. 32–34)[17, 25, 24, 20]
The position of the photocell has to be adjusted. To ensure that the automatic exposure control system will function optimally, position the *photocell* so that it lies *under a representative part of the glandular tissue (which is in the anterior third of the breast).* The correct position of the photocell will depend on the size of the breast. Improper positioning of the photocell will result in incorrect exposure. Problems may occur with very small breasts that cannot cover the photocell or with silicon implants (see p. 34).

■ Film Processing

Since deviations in chemical composition or developing time and temperature can cause problems with image contrast, noise, sensitivity, and fog, *it is essential to process the film strictly according to the manufacturer's recommendations and regularly monitor processing* (see pp. 35–36 and p. 39). Carefully controlled film processing becomes all the more important when it is understood that most acute changes in image quality are caused by deviations in film processing.[26, 27]

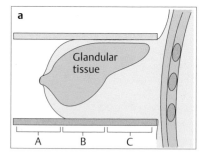
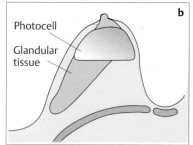

Fig. 3.**7a** and **b**   Positioning the photocell
a Lateral view of the compressed breast
Position A is poor (beam must pass through too much air). Position B is optimal.

Position C is poor (beam must pass through too much fat).
b View of breast from above showing optimal photocell position

Prolonging the developing time (for example from 90 to 180 seconds, i. e., extended processing) while keeping temperature constant can increase image quality with certain film types by increasing contrast and sensitivity. However, since many factors influence quality (including film type, the existing steepness of the gradation curve, film throughput, and so forth), no generalized recommendations can be made.[28]

■ **Viewing the Image**

Proper evaluation of the complete density range of a well exposed mammogram requires a viewbox that provides *homogeneous illumination at the required intensity.* Viewboxes must provide adjustable luminance in the range of 2000–3000 cd/m² at a color temperature of 4500–6500 K. An additional *bright spotlight* must be available for illuminating areas of high exposure. This light should provide luminance up to 20 000 cd/m². Focused illumination of images that cover a wide density range with bright light will make details in highly dense areas appear more readily visible. However, this is only possible up to an optical density of 2.8. Focused illumination provides important additional information, although this is always limited and is usually not able to compensate for incorrect exposure, an excessively high-contrast film, or excessively high contrast due to errors in processing the film.

All viewing areas for mammography, including the work area for technologists, should be furnished with identical illumination. All light bulbs should be changed routinely throughout these viewing areas and the viewboxes cleaned weekly. The films are to be read in a darkened room with masking of the viewbox to the size of the film, when possible. These latter techniques minimize ambient light and thereby increase contrast when viewing the films. A *magnifying lens* with magnification by at least a factor of 2 should be available for evaluating the mammogram.

Specific Requirements and Solutions

The ability to recognize structures on the mammogram is determined by:

- *Resolution*
- *Image noise*
- *Contrast*

These variables must be optimized using the lowest possible radiation dose.

The following sections will explain factors that influence these variables.

■ **Image Sharpness**

Image sharpness is determined by motion blur, geometric blurring, and the blurring of the image receptor system.[29, 20, 23] (Table 3.1)

Motion blurring is caused by patient motion and, less pronounced, by arterial pulsation. It can be minimized by:

Table 3.**1** Minimizing blurring

Goal	Recommendation	Limiting factors
Motion blurring	Short exposure time	Power
	Intense compression	Patient's pain tolerance
Geometric blurring	Long SID[1, 3]	Focus load rating, power
	Small focus	
	Intense compression (to reduce distance to objects farther from the film)	Patient's pain tolerance
Screen–film blurring	High-resolution screen,[2] sufficient dose (quantum noise), single-emulsion film	High radiation dose
	Good contact between film and screen	Exposure time

[1] SID, source-to-image receptor distance
[2] Rarely relevant
[3] Film granularity is not relevant because the screen blurring is always more important

- Adequate compression. This eliminates motion of the breast if the patient moves. Adequate compression will also suppress arterial pulsation (see p. 39–40).
- Short exposure time. This in turn depends on the X-ray tube rating, the size of the focal spot, the focus–film distance, the sensitivity of the screen–film system, and density and thickness of the object (breast compression!)

As a general rule, exposure times should not exceed 1 second (some guidelines still specify 2 seconds).

Geometric blurring can be reduced by:

- using a small focal spot
- maintaining the largest possible focus–film distance
- optimizing breast compression (Fig. 3.**2**).

Breast compression not only reduces motion blur (see above), it also reduces geometric blurring of structures that are farther away from the film by reducing the distance to the image receptor. The minimum focal spot size and maximum film-to-focus distance are limited by the capacity of the X-ray tube, the resulting extended exposure times, and the motion blurring that can occur.

When using a standard technique, according to the ACR standard,[30] the film-to-focus distance *should not be less than 55 cm* for a focal spot size of 0.4. For magnification imaging, the distance should be ≥60 cm. In magnification mammography, smaller focal spot sizes (0.1–0.15, depending on the power of magnification) are required to minimize the penumbra.

Today, low-dose screen–film systems are used almost exclusively as *image receptor systems* (see p. 19). The high-resolution industrial film used earlier is no longer acceptable due to the excessive radiation exposure associated with it. Few digital systems for diagnostic imaging have recently become commercially available, some are still in the development stage (see pp. 71–74).

The resolution of the screen–film system is primarily determined by the resolution of the intensifying screen, since film resolution is always higher than that of the screen. With very low-dose screen–film systems, the increased image noise that occurs can reduce the clarity of details (Fig. 3.**8**).

Differences between screens are almost always due to differing densities of the luminescent layer and the dye used for selective filtering of components of the green spectrum. Thinner,

more finely structured screens almost always produce *higher resolution* but are less sensitive, i. e., they require a *higher dose.*

Since the loss of definition resulting from the crossover effect is not acceptable for standard mammographic technique, only single-emulsion films with a back screen are used.

To minimize loss of definition due to *insufficient screen–film contact* between screen and film as the imaging radiation passes from the screen to the film, always wait at least 2 minutes after loading the cassette before performing mammography. Always ensure that a sufficient number of cassettes are available.

Most screen–film systems currently achieve a high-contrast resolution of 14–18 *line pairs per millimeter* (LP/mm), which can be verified using a lead line grid. This value matches the high-contrast resolution that mammography units achieve by adjusting focal spot size, film-to-focus distance, and object-to-film distance.[20]

However, the clarity of detail of microcalcifications is determined only in part by the spatial resolution. When present in areas of dense breast tissue, microcalcifications may show only very slight differences in density. Therefore, whether they can be detected is highly dependent on contrast and image noise. The clarity of details as a function of their size is expressed by the modulation transfer function, MTF (see Fig. 3.**9**).[19] This means that for a given image receptor system, large objects will appear with high contrast, whereas fine objects will be imaged with low contrast and will thus have poor resolution. Thus, despite its capability for a high-contrast resolution of 14–18 line pairs, an optimum technical system will be limited to detecting microcalcifications measuring *0.1–0.2 mm* or larger (corresponding to 10 or 5 LP/mm).

■ Contrast

Contrast can be defined as the relative difference in density between an object and its surroundings referred to the surrounding density:[19]

$$\text{Contrast} = \frac{\text{Density}_{obj.} - \text{Density}_{surroundings}}{\text{Density}_{surroundings}} \times 100$$

■ Fundamental Considerations

High contrast is always required to differentiate very fine structures with slight differences in density, such as microcalcifications. However, as was

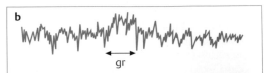

a

gr

b

gr

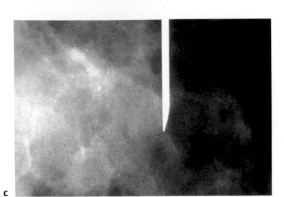

c

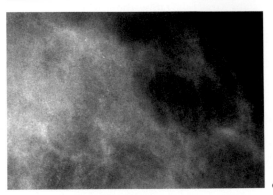

d

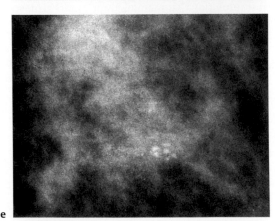

e

Fig. 3.**8a–f** Noise can interfere with the clarity of detail in particularly low-dose screen–film systems

a Theoretical principle of an image detail within a line

b The same detail as in (**a**) is much more difficult to discern in the presence of intense noise. If it were smaller, it might even go unnoticed

c and **d** Extremely fine microcalcifications, a sign of a ductal carcinoma, are readily apparent with a high-contrast and high-resolution screen–film system (**c**), but are hardly discernible with the low-dose screen–film system (**d**)

e View of a microcalcification cluster, using a particularly low-dose screen–film system. The high level of general noise and the extreme graininess interfere with identifying all of the microcalcifications. Only the larger calcifications are discernible

f Magnification mammography of a specimen of ductal carcinoma reveals surprisingly many microcalcifications, some of them relatively fine

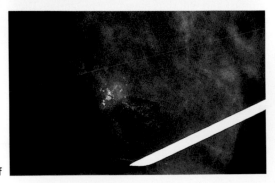

f

discussed on page 23, this contrast should *not be excessive* either. As described on pages 23–26, the flat part of the curve at the foot of the characteristic film curve (foot gradient) limits contrast in the low density range (dense breast tissue). In the high-density range, the eye can no longer per-

ceive differences over a density of 2.4. Even in bright light, recognition of differences is limited to densities below 2.8. Beyond the optimum exposure range (optimum density is 0.6 to approximately 2.4), image quality is significantly limited in that underexposed and overexposed areas begin to appear (Fig. 3.**6**). When high-contrast films are used, these limits are reached sooner, and details in the high and low density ranges can be lost due to underexposure or overexposure, respectively.[24]

Whereas low-contrast images appear to the eye to be "poor" or "flat," high-contrast images appear particularly "sharp." Here the physician must critically examine the images to verify that in the majority of breast studies, *no overexposed or underexposed areas appear*.

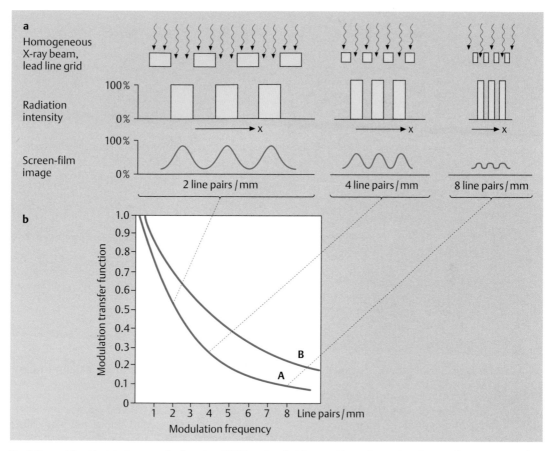

Fig. 3.**9a** and **b**   Modulation transfer function (MTF) and structural resolution

a A lead line grid imaged with a homogeneous beam. The radiation density in the image of the line grid is alternately 0 and 100%. Light scattering in the screen–film system in particular causes the sharp edges of the grid to appear fuzzy. The finer the grid, the more the differences in intensity will be equalized in the image

b The resulting relationship that renders structures less detectable as they become finer (local modulation frequency of intensity) is described by the modulation transfer function of a component (in this case, the screen–film system). As the fineness of the lines increases, the MTF decreases from an initial value of 1 (no loss of information), thus limiting the resolving power of the components.
Curve B shows a better modulation transfer function than curve A

■ **Factors that Determine Contrast**

Contrast is determined by various factors. These factors include (Table 3.**2**):

– Breast thickness and density of the breast tissue
– Radiation quality (target/filter combination, peak kilovoltage), breast compression, scatter-reducing techniques (such as grids), the choice of a suitable screen–film system, and film processing

Proper exposure is a prerequisite.

■ **Radiation Quality**

The *energy spectrum* of the X-ray radiation greatly influences radiation contrast. *Low-energy radiation increases the contrast.* However, if the radiation *energy is too low, penetration* of the breast will be significantly *poorer.* This means that in thick, dense breasts, even a long exposure time will fail to sufficiently expose the film, resulting in underexposure. Instead, this radiation is absorbed in the breast, and radiation exposure is increased unnecessarily.[17, 19, 20, 23]

Table 3.2 Optimizing contrast

Goal	Recommendation	Limiting factors
High-contrast image	1. Select a radiation spectrum with the lowest possible energy by using appropriate target material, filter material, and kVp setting	Unit design, breast penetration (dense breast), radiation exposure
	2. Compensate for breast thickness with compression (to reduce the density range that has to be imaged)	Compliance
	3. Reduce scattered radiation with compression, grid technique, low energy radiation	Patient compliance, penetration, radiation dose
	4. Air gap, (magnification mammography, see p. 52) Collimation (spot compression and magnification see p. 49)	Dose, small section
High film contrast	1. High-contrast film	Film latitude limited (overexposure, underexposure), limited exposure range, increased noise, fogging
	2. High-contrast development (time, temperature, activity of the chemicals)	
	3. Avoiding: – increased fog (film storage and processing) – Exposure to external light	

■ Target/Filter Combination

The energy spectrum of the radiation depends on the *target and filter material,* the thickness of the filter, and the *kVp applied.*

Whereas normal-sized and small breasts of moderate density usually can be optimally imaged with a *molybdenum target* and a *0.03 -mm molybdenum filter* at 25–30 kVp, the combinations molybdenum/rhodium, tungsten/molybdenum, rhodium/rhodium, or tungsten/rhodium may improve the image in large and dense breasts (Fig. 3.10).[17, 18] Recently developed units with bifocal tubes permit the selection of different target/filter combinations for thick and dense breasts or normal-sized and less dense ones. This means that the quality of the radiation is optimized not only by preselecting the maximum voltage, but also by selecting the most suitable target/filter combination.

■ Peak Kilovoltage (kVp)

Increasing the kVp setting increases the mean energy of the radiation and thus its penetrating power, whereas *decreasing the kVp setting* decreases the mean energy and penetrating power. However, *contrast is increased at a low kVp.*

■ Choosing the Optimum Target/Filter Combination and kVp Setting

A sophisticated automatic exposure control system is usually provided to aid the radiologic technologist in selecting a target/filter combination and the corresponding kVp setting appropriate to the respective breast density and compressed thickness.[31, 25, 18] One manufacturer, for example, provides a system that automatically selects the target and filter material, kVp, and mAs product (according to low-dose, standard, or high-contrast exposure settings) after a short test exposure. Other manufacturers provide push-button program selection (for fatty, normal, or dense tissue). Once the selection is made, the unit suggests the suitable target/filter combination and corresponding kVp, taking into account the compressed breast thickness. As usual, the beam is switched off as soon as the mAs product required for the correct mean film density has been reached.

In the semiautomatic mode, the radiologic technologist selects the target and filter material and the kVp, and the automatic exposure control system then selects the mAs product as usual. Finally, all mammography units must permit manual exposure control, whereby the radiologic technologist can freely select every parameter. This feature is useful in special cases, such as very

Fig. 3.**10 a** and **b**
The breast image obtained using a molybdenum target and rhodium filter at automatic exposure control settings of 29 kV, and 51 mAs shows a slight improvement in penetrating dense areas over the image obtained using a molybdenum target and molybdenum filter at automatic settings of 29 kV and 78 mAs. In this case, the rhodium filter system achieved a slightly higher-quality image with a dose reduction of approximately 40%. Published studies report dose reductions in dense breasts of up to 50% over molybdenum/molybdenum images at the same kVp setting, depending on the composition of the glandular tissue.[17, 18]
a Craniocaudal mammogram, molybdenum/molybdenum
b Craniocaudal mammogram, molybdenum/rhodium

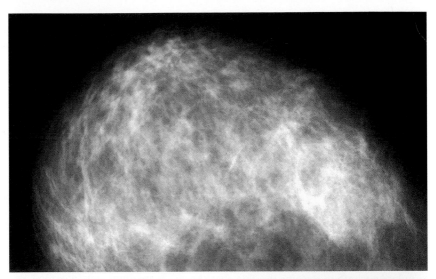

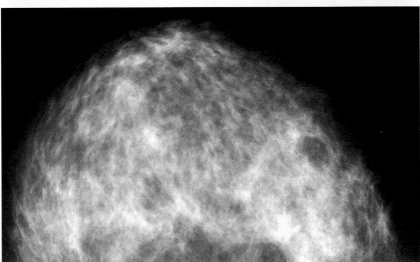

small breasts that do not cover the photocell or with augmentation implants, but considerable experience is required.

■ Reducing Scattered Radiation

Scattered radiation is an undesirable effect in breast imaging, since it causes opacification without diagnostic information and thus limits the information available on the film. Most of the scattered radiation is produced as the beam penetrates the breast tissue.

The most important means of effectively reducing scatter radiation are adequate breast compression and use of grid technique or collimation

(spot compression and air-gap magnification mammography, p. 32).

■ Breast Compression

The best possible breast compression contributes decisively to increasing contrast:

– It reduces the thickness through which the beam passes, significantly reducing scattered radiation, thus improving contrast. According to model calculations by Barnes, the ratio of scattered radiation to primary radiation in a breast compressed in thickness from 6 cm to 3 cm decreases from 1.0 to 0.4, resulting in an

improvement in contrast by a factor of 1.43.[32]
- In addition to this, healthy tissue usually spreads, whereas true masses will persist. This improves visualization of true masses and diminishes the likelihood of falsely identifying a lesion.
- It decreases motion of the breast during the X-ray exposure.
- Finally, breast compression also permits a significant reduction in radiation dosage (see p. 38).

■ **Grid Technique**

The grid technique significantly reduces scattered radiation (see Fig. 3.**11**). This makes this technique indispensable with glandular, normal-sized, and large breasts; it is indicated as the standard technique despite the fact that the required radiation dose is increased by a factor of about 2.5 (Fig. 3.**11**).[33, 23, 28, 34]

Gridless mammography may be considered only in small, low-density breasts in light of the lesser quantities of scattered radiation encountered in these patients.[20] However, in most centers the grid is only removed during magnification mammography.

Grids are not used in magnification mammography because a significant reduction in scattered radiation can be achieved with the air gap in conjunction with good collimation[33] (see p. 55).

In standard mammographic technique, however, the increased dose required by the grid is acceptable in light of the significant improvement in image quality, and it is more than offset by the reduced dose requirements of current screen–film systems.

■ **Other Techniques for Scatter Reduction**

When spot films using a contact technique (coned-down views without collimation) are done, the scattered radiation from the surrounding tissue is reduced by the collimation to a small area of interest.

In *magnification mammography,* good collimation in combination with the air gap effectively reduces scattered radiation, which is why this technique does not require a grid. The grid would only increase the dose unnecessarily and require significantly longer exposure times, leading to motion blurring (see p. 55).[33]

Slot mammography: This technique produces an image by exposing the breast line-by-line through a slit. Each exposed line is read behind the breast by an image receptor, which is collimated to the slit. By moving the slit over the breast, the complete breast is scanned. The technique effectively reduces scatter, thus improving image contrast. The additional dose, which is needed by a grid due to absorption within the grid, can be reduced. This technique is presently integrated in a fullfield digital mammography system, for which approval is filed (information from manufacturer).

■ **Correct Exposure as a Prerequisite for Good Contrast**

Once a suitable target/filter combination and kVp setting ensuring sufficient tissue penetration and contrast have been selected, *correct film exposure* is important to exploit the full contrast range of the film.

The exposure is regulated by adjusting the *intensity and duration of the radiation* (mAs product) and depends on the sensitivity of the screen–film system.

Since reproducibility of the correct mean density is greater with automatic than with manual exposure, the exposure is commonly set with the aid of an *automatic exposure control system.* For this reason, automatic exposure control systems are required on all mammography units, as are manual controls. Manual exposure may be required for patients with very small breasts or with implants.

■ **Automatic Exposure Control System**

The *automatic exposure control system* uses a *photocell placed underneath the cassette,* to determine the radiation dose. The photocell switches the beam off once the dosage required for a mean optical film density of 1.4–1.8 has been reached[24].

The automatic exposure control system is adjusted to match the sensitivity of the screen–film system.

With respect to automatic exposure control system, there are definite *differences in quality* that influence image quality.[31, 25] Not every automatic exposure control system is equally effective in achieving the desired optimum mean optical density on the film irrespective of the energy spectrum of the incident radiation behind the screen–film system. There are two reasons for this:

Fig. 3.**11 a** and **b**
The comparison shows that the significantly reduced scattered radiation in grid mammography permits significantly better visualization of the structures in the glandular tissue and of microcalcifications, which are located in the glandular tissue
a Mammogram without grid
b Mammogram taken 1 year later with grid

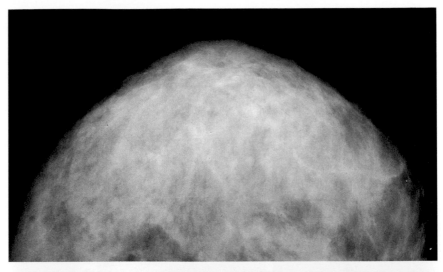

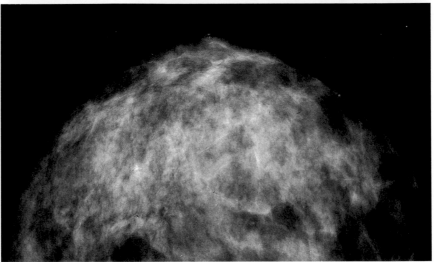

1. The required radiation energies vary with each patient due to differences in the thickness and density of the breasts imaged. In particular, the degree to which the lower-energy components of this spectrum are weakened depends on breast thickness and density. This means that the extent to which the radiation is hardened in the breast varies. To varying degrees, the radiation also undergoes further hardening in the grid table and cassette before it enters the photocell. Since the sensitivity of the photocell is dependent on the energy spectrum of the incident radiation, failure to compensate for thickness in dense and thick breasts will cause the unit to switch off too soon, producing an underexposed image.

2. With longer exposure times, the optical density of the film no longer increases in proportion to the exposure time (reciprocity law failure, see p. 38).[19] This means that insufficient optical density is achieved with long exposure times, i. e., the image is underexposed.

The design of modern automatic exposure control systems attempts to compensate for both effects as successfully as possible. Only such a compensation mechanism can ensure that the mean optical density of the images will remain largely constant regardless of the thickness and density of the breast and exposure time. Phantom images can be used to verify the quality of compensation achieved and thus the quality of the automatic ex-

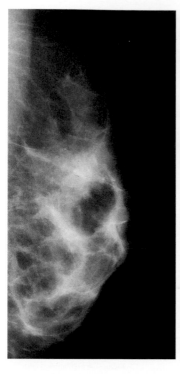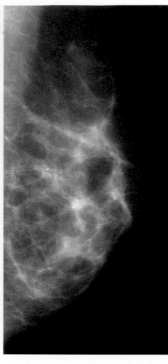

Fig. 3.**12 a** and **b**   Breast images using a high-contrast film (**a**) and a lower-contrast film (**b**)
a The high-contrast film shows parts of the glandular tissue in the relatively flat section of the characteristic curve. Contrast within the glandular tissue is therefore low, making these areas difficult to diagnose although the breast as a whole is correctly exposed. (The subcutaneous tissue is just barely discernible with the bright light.)
b The glandular tissue can be much better evaluated with the slightly lower-contrast film. (Note that positioning is significantly better than in **a**)

posure control system. The mean film density should only vary within narrow limits in images of plexiglass sheets of varying thickness produced with varying kVp.[20] Imaging thick and dense breasts using an older automatic exposure control system will require that the radiologic technologist make manual adjustments with the correction button according to his or her experience.

■ Positioning the Photocell

It is important to position the photocell under a *representative part of the glandular tissue.* Never position the photocell so that the breast does not completely cover it. Otherwise the photocell will receive full-strength radiation and will switch off too soon, producing an underexposed image. The central part of the anterior third of the breast has proven to be the optimum region for placing the photocell since it usually contains relatively uniform glandular tissue. In contrast, variations in the distribution of glandular and fatty tissue are greater in the areas close to the chest wall, increasing the risk that the photocell would lie under an area not representative of the rest of the breast (see also Fig. 3.**7**). Improper positioning of the photocell (unfortunately sometimes due to

the design of the unit) is the most frequent source of error that causes incorrect exposure.

■ Manual Exposure

Since very *small breasts* and breasts with *silicone implants* do not generally permit positioning the photocell under a representative area, manual exposure is required. When adjusting the exposure manually, the radiologic technologist sets the mAs product according to breast thickness and the estimated radiodensity. In the absence of previous mammograms, the radiologic technologist essentially estimates radiodensity according to tissue consistency. This requires experience. Recorded exposure values from previous examinations are helpful. This is one reason why it is worthwhile to record the thickness and degree of compression, the mAs product, kVp setting, and the target/filter combination at every mammographic examination. If breasts with implants are radiographed, the exposure setting that provides optimum exposure of the glandular tissue adjacent to the implant should be selected. The soft radiation cannot penetrate a silicone-filled implant. Adequate penetration of a silicone-filled implant would cause overpenetration of the glandular breast tissue. The same principle applies to saline-filled implants.

■ Film Selection

When selecting the film, *high contrast is important for visualizing details, but excessive contrast will limit the visibility of details in the areas of high and low density.* Especially in large and dense breasts, excessive contrast will manifest itself in the simultaneous presence of underexposed and overexposed areas (overexposed tissue in thin areas near the skin and underexposed in dense areas of the breast tissue (Fig. 3.**12**). Moreover, a very high-contrast screen–film system will be more sensitive to slight fluctuations in the development process, to an automatic exposure control system with less than optimum thickness and density equalization, and to suboptimal photocell positioning. This means that even slight deviations will lead to incorrect exposures that can affect the diagnosis (i. e., exposure tolerance is reduced).[23] For these reasons, *high-contrast films require an optimally adjusted automatic exposure control system, a precisely positioned photocell, and constantly optimized film processing.*

It is also important to understand that the increased image noise associated with particularly *low-dose screen–film systems* (screen noise and quantum noise) diminishes the clarity of detail (Fig. 3.**8**). Sometimes the very short exposures (necessary for small breast) are not possible on some equipment, leading to overexposure. Finally, with extremely short exposure times, the grid strips themselves will often be imaged when the grid does not move fast enough for the short exposure time (Fig. 3.**13**).[20] If problems of this sort occur, a slightly lower voltage or a less sensitive screen–film system must be used. If this does not solve the problem, then the mammography unit should be upgraded.

Screen–film systems with extremely low sensitivity can result in disproportionately *long exposure times* when used with high breast densities and low voltage (reciprocity failure law, see p. 38).[19] Since low-sensitivity films are no longer used today, these problems will only occur when a radiation energy is selected that is too low for breast thickness and density. In magnification mammography, long exposure times may occur due to the reduced power of the small tube focal spot. Particularly with low kVp setting when the automatic exposure control system does not compensate sufficiently, this can lead to incorrect ex-

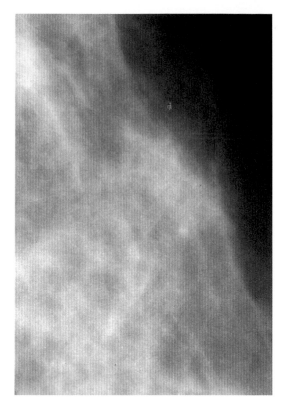

Fig. 3.**13** Particularly when imaging thin and fatty breast, using extremely sensitive films may result in the grid strips themselves being imaged as parallel lines due to the short exposure times required (partial view)

posure (as explained above) or it can result in motion blurring. Problems of this nature can be compensated for by selecting a higher voltage or by using a more sensitive screen–film system.

■ Film Processing

Film processing influences contrast, fog, sensitivity, and noise.[26, 27]

The rule is that increasing developing time or temperature will increase fog, noise, and film sensitivity, whereas contrast reaches its maximum at a certain development temperature and time. It follows from this that the *optimized processing parameters recommended by the manufacturer* must be strictly observed. *Quality control testing should verify consistent processing daily.* It should be noted that a sufficient degree of consistency can only be achieved with a minimum throughput of over 20 films per day.

With some films, *extending the developing time* can *further increase contrast and sensitivity.* Since the maximum contrast varies with the type of film, consultation with the manufacturers regarding such decisions may be advisable. Aside from this, a film's maximum contrast does not necessarily represent the optimum that a specific mammography system requires. No generalized recommendations can be made.

Improper or defective darkroom lighting may be an additional factor that influences contrast. For this reason, darkroom light should be checked once every year.[36]

■ Noise

(See Table 3.**3**)

Above a certain level, noise reduces the clarity of detail and can interfere with the perception of slight differences in density and extremely fine structures (microcalcifications).

Noise is composed of the structural noise of the intensifying screen, the granularity of the film, and quantum noise.[19, 37]

- The *structural noise* of the screen generally increases with more sensitive screen–film systems (see p. 35).
- The same applies to the granularity of the film.
- *Quantum noise* occurs as a result of fluctuations that exist and become visible when only a few statistically attributed X-ray quanta hit the screen. With extremely sensitive (i. e., low-dose) screen–film systems, quantum noise can cause disturbances. This is even

more pronounced in areas of dense breast tissue, where even fewer X-ray quanta reach the film–screen system.

Noise becomes particularly apparent and can interfere with the diagnostic study especially in high-definition images and with high film contrast. Although the trained eye can learn to distinguish relevant differences in density, this is only possible to a limited extent (see Fig. 3.**8**).

For this reason, it is important that noise does not exceed a certain level, which may vary individually. This means that when considering extremely low-dose screen–film systems, the radiologist should carefully weigh the disadvantages of increased noise against the advantages of the reduced radiation dose.

■ Radiation Dose

Studies of patients whose breasts were exposed to high doses of radiation either for therapeutic reasons or following the atomic bomb explosions in Hiroshima and Nagasaki[38–56] have demonstrated that the *glandular tissue of the breast is sensitive to radiation.* As in other radiographic studies, it is important to keep the dose used in mammography as low as possible without compromising the quality required for diagnosis.

Regrettably, initial reports *greatly overestimated* the *presumed cancer risk.* This in turn has unfortunately caused a great deal of uncertainty about mammography on the part of some patients and physicians. For this reason, we shall explicitly address the risk of cancer from mammography.

Table 3.**3** Minimizing noise

Goal	Recommendation	Limiting factors
Minimizing screen noise	Screen with minimal structural noise	Type of luminescent material, crystal structure and arrangement
Minimizing film noise	– Film should not be too high in contrast*	Contrast
	– Film with minimal granularity	Required dose
	– Contrast not too high	Contrast
	– Film processing	
Minimizing quantum noise	– Use a less sensitive screen–film system – Suitable film contrast – Suitable screen sharpness	Required dose, contrast, image definition

*Noise will become more noticeable where film contrast and screen sharpness are too high

■ Radiation Dose from Mammography

A certain dose of radiation is necessary to obtain a high-quality mammogram.

The absorbed glandular dose depends on various individual factors, such as the thickness and density of the breast, and can be measured via the entrance exposure. It can also be estimated on the basis of phantom images when the thickness of the breast is known.

Applicable statutes and regulations require that mammography units, screen–film systems, imaging technique, and development be selected and monitored so that the radiation dose at the image receptor does not exceed 300 μGy for a normal breast image. This dose is very small. It is less than the dose previously required for screen-less film mammography by at least a factor of 10. Today, the total dose for mammography of a normal breast in two planes is approximately 2 mGy, equivalent to 0.2 rad.[51, 56]

■ Assessing the Risk

At such low radiation doses, a possible cancer risk could only be demonstrated by comparing several million patients with and without mammography, all other factors being kept equal. Obviously, this is not feasible.

Not surprisingly, previous comparative assessments involving several hundred thousand patients who underwent mammography have not demonstrated any increase in the incidence of cancer.

For this reason, we can only extrapolate from the data on high-dose exposure to low doses. However, this ignores the body's repair mechanisms that are possible at low-dose exposures. Thus the results of such estimates that assume a linear dose–response curve represent the worst case. In this worst case, mammography in two planes (5 mGy)—performed at age 50—theoretically could produce cancer in 1 of 100 000 patients.[56] Even if higher radiation doses have been assumed per 2-view mammogram (up to 8 mGy) a benefit-to-risk ratio of 100:1 has resulted for women beyond age 40.[54, 57]

There are several reasons for the fact that the risk of cancer associated with mammography (worst case) is now thought to be less than in previous estimates:

1. Reduction in the radiation dose required for mammography.

2. Awareness of the fact that the carcinogenicity of radiation is highly dependent on the age at exposure. This was not taken into consideration in the original extrapolation of the data from high-dose exposure (Hiroshima, tuberculosis examinations, and irradiation for mastitis), in which many young patients were exposed. Radiation sensitivity of breasts is greatest in women younger than 30 years and is at most negligable in women 40 years old and older.[55, 57, 58]

For women undergoing screening, the risk of dying of breast cancer induced by mammography is so slight that it is considered to be essentially too small to calculate. It is approximately equivalent to the risk of dying of lung cancer from smoking three cigarettes.

Annual mammographic examinations over a period of 20 years would, at worst, increase the risk of breast cancer insignificantly from 10% to 10.06%.[23] At the same time, early diagnosis with mammographic screening can reduce breast cancer mortality by approximately 30–50% (see Chapter 21).

These comparisons illustrate that:

– *The risk of cancer from mammography is negligible* in comparison with other risk of daily life.
– Moreover, in weighing benefits and risks, the *radiation dose cannot be an argument against performing mammography* even in screening examinations of asymptomatic women (age 40 and older). This applies all the more to the diagnostic workup in symptomatic patients.

Even in a 40-year-old patient, the youngest women who usually undergo routine screening, the theoretical radiation risk increases only by a factor of 2.5, in comparison with a 50-year-old patient.[56]

In patients *below* the age of 40 years, routine mammographic screening examinations are not usually recommended for the following reasons:

– The overall incidence of cancer is significantly less
– At the same time, the tissue is more sensitive to radiation
– Mammography may be less effective in young, dense tissue. If mammography is indicated before age 40, as may be the case for patients with high genetic risk, it is recommended that this mammogram is performed in centers with strict quality control and a high level of expertise.[59]

Table 3.**4** Minimizing dose

Goal	Recommendation	Limiting Factors
Minimizing dose	Sufficient radiation energy (appropriate selection of kVP and target/filter combination) for: – Good penetration – Avoiding reciprocity law failure	Depends on mammography unit
	Breast compression – Reduce the thickness to be penetrated	Compliance
	Use sufficient power to avoid reciprocity law failure	Depends on mammography unit
	Correct exposure – Avoiding overexposure – Avoiding repeats	Depends on mammography unit (automatic exposure control system) and technologist's experience
	Low-dose screen–film system	Noise, resolution of the screen, characteristic film curve
	Special film processing	Fog*, noise*, contrast*

* Changes in film processing may be made only in consultation with the film manufacturer

Mammography should not be dispensed with where clinical or diagnostic findings require clarification and a malignant process cannot be excluded.

■ **Dose-related Optimization of the Exposure Technique**

Exposure technique and strategy (for example, the number of images) should be optimized with respect to the dose for the reasons mentioned in the previous sections. At the same time, *quality should not be sacrificed to reduce the dose, and restricting the maximum number of images should never compromise the required information.*

The following section discusses *factors influencing the radiation dose* which, when optimized, permit further dose reduction (Table 3.**4**).

■ **Radiation Quality**

Selecting *optimum radiation quality* permits optimizing both image quality and dose. In particular, *too high a proportion of low-energy radiation* must be avoided since it tends to be absorbed in dense glandular tissue and in thick breasts and contributes only slightly, if at all, to information on the mammogram.

The quality of radiation depends on the *target/filter material* and on the selected *maximum tube voltage*.[17, 18] Optimum adjustment of radiation quality is most easily achieved using *newer mammography units* that permit *adjusting* both voltage and *target/filter material* to the respective type of breast. Here, it is important that the *mammography unit* has *sufficient capacity*. If the *output is too low* (as with some inexpensive units), the only way to achieve the dose necessary for the desired optical density is by extending the exposure time. Since the *optical density* at *long exposure times is no longer proportional to the dose* but *increases* slightly, *this disproportionately increases the exposure time and the necessary dose.* This relationship is referred to as the "reciprocity law failure." To avoid this, the capacity of a mammography unit should never be below 1 kW at 30 kV. This is only a minimal requirement. Units of higher capacity are important for achieving adequate image quality in dense breasts and for reducing the radiation dose.

■ **Breast Thickness**

The *dose* required to penetrate the breast is highly dependent on the *thickness and density of the breast.* The density increases with a high proportion of glandular tissue containing large quantities of cells, fluid, and/or connective tissue. Good compression can markedly reduce the thickness, *significantly reducing the required radiation dose.* Thus, penetrating a breast compressed to 4 cm requires only 80% of the dose required to penetrate a breast compressed to 4.5 cm.[20]

■ Film Density

Mammography should always try to achieve the recommended optimum *mean film density* of 1.4–1.8.[24] An optical density that is too low significantly limits the *content of diagnostic information*. An excessively high optical density can also limit the diagnostic information but in any case is associated with an *unnecessary increase in the required dose*.

■ Grid

Since the proportion of scattered radiation in thick and dense breasts is significant (see p. 20),[32] a *grid* is required. Although the grid *increases in dose by a factor of approximately 2.5*, it is indispensable for achieving adequate image quality in these breasts. The radiologist may consider reducing the dose in patients with small and fatty breasts by not using the grid technique.[20] However, practical considerations have prevented frequent switching between gridless and grid techniques from becoming common practice.

■ Screen–Film System

The selection of a screen–film system also has a decisive influence on the dose. The advent of screen–film combinations has *reduced the dose by at least a factor of 10* compared with screenless films.

Among the new screen–film systems, we differentiate between systems with *low* and *extremely low dose* (speed class: 12 or 25, respectively) requirements. The latter are often marketed as "screen–film systems for mammographic screening." The respective required doses differ by about a factor of 2. The *extremely low-dose* screen–film systems are subject to significantly higher noise levels, generally at very high contrast. This can impair visualization particularly in the lower density range of dense breast tissue. Here, image noise can interfere with detection of microcalcifications. Optimum exposure and film processing are more critical here than with other screen–film systems. Depending on the mammography unit, extremely short exposure time settings may fall below the unit's minimum switching intervals (resulting in incorrect exposure) or cause the visualization of grid lines

(see p. 35). This may make adequate imaging with these films difficult.

■ Film Processing

Extending the processing time or increasing the processing temperature can increase the sensitivity of some films, permitting a further *reduction in dose* by as much as one-third. However, since this is frequently associated with a *further increase in contrast*, such modifications are not always desirable and should be considered in relation to other factors determining contrast. Moreover, an increase in processing temperature is frequently accompanied by a decline in quality.

■ Number of Images

In the interest of *reducing the radiation dose*, an effort should be made to *avoid* repeating images by ensuring optimal technical conditions, continuous quality assurance, and well-trained personnel. When adjusting exposure manually, the technologist should initially take only one mammogram, with the remaining images taken only after correct exposure has been verified.

Sites that intend to perform screening will invariably require a grid table for large breasts in addition to the standard grid table. If mammograms of large breasts are routinely obtained by combining small films, significantly increased doses can result (for mammography in two planes, up to four times as much). This should be considered unacceptable.

Positioning and Compression

Mammographic positioning involves obtaining the *best possible compression* and correct *positioning* to ensure that the entire glandular body is imaged.

■ Compression

As explained in the previous sections, adequate *breast compression* is one of the most important prerequisites for obtaining high-quality mammograms with the best possible visualization of pathologic changes.[60]

The contributions of compression to quality mammography are summarized here:
● Good compression improves the *resolution* by reducing the distance between the image re-

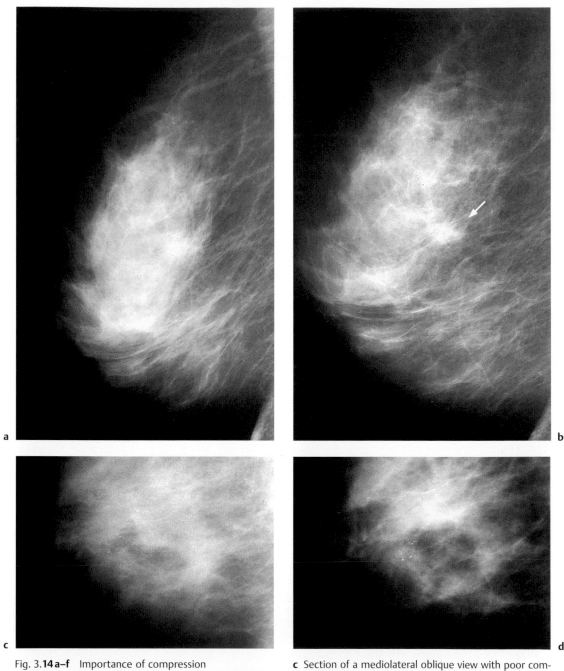

Fig. 3.**14 a–f**   Importance of compression

a Mediolateral mammogram with poor compression where the glandular tissue has not been sufficiently spread out. The carcinoma in the glandular tissue is difficult to discern

b With better compression and better spreading of the tissue, the carcinoma (arrow) and its spiculations are considerably easier to discern

c Section of a mediolateral oblique view with poor compression. The glandular tissue structures are dense and blurred because of insufficient compression. Several calcifications are faintly visible in the poorly compressed tissue

d A repeat mediolateral oblique view with good compression reveals significantly sharper visualization of the glandular tissue structures. Several more highly suggestive calcifications are now discernible.

ceptor and objects, which are farther from the image receptor. This reduces geometric blurring.

- It reduces motion blurring.
- It improves *contrast* since the reduced thickness of the breast significantly *reduces scattered radiation.*
- It improves *contrast* since low-energy radiation, which provides higher image contrast, can be utilized in penetrating tissue of reduced thickness.
- It permits higher *contrast* in the area of interest since by *equalizing the thickness of the tissue*, it reduces the necessary object range.
- It permits *visualization of small areas of pathology buried in the* glandular tissue since normal tissue can be spread, whereas malignant foci will persist due to their firmer consistency.
- It permits a significant *reduction in the dose* by reducing the thickness of tissue to be penetrated.

These mentioned advantages illustrate the importance of achieving the best possible *compression.* As an important prerequisite for high image quality, *early cancer detection* may depend on it (Figs. 3.**14 a–d**).

Naturally, the best possible breast compression can only be achieved with the patient's cooperation and must never be obtained against her will. Despite every effort to achieve optimum image quality, the technical staff must appreciate that the sensitivity of the glandular body to pressure varies. Patients differ in their willingness to endure pain or discomfort for good diagnostic results.

It is thus essential to *briefly discuss the need for compression* with the patient and to obtain her understanding, cooperation, and *motivation.* For this reason, the patient should be informed that some of the *smallest and earliest cancers can only be visualized with compression* and that compression significantly *reduces the dose of radiation.* She should be told that *there is no way in which compression can cause a carcinoma,* which is a common concern.

Since compression of tissue with low interstitial water content is less painful, and the density of the breast decreases and image quality improves as the water content decreases, *the mammographic examination may be more comfortable for women during the first half of the menstrual cycle.* When compressing the breast, it is important that all of the *glandular tissue is spread as* evenly as possible and that no skin folds are present.* Compression of unevenly distributed glandular tissue is more painful, and the folds may cause densities that interfere with the diagnosis.

■ Positioning for Standard Views

In mammography, we differentiate between *standard views* and *additional views.*

■ Number of Views in Standard Mammography

Except in unusual instances, all mammographic examinations should be obtained in two planes.

So-called single-view mammography, which essentially consists of only the mediolateral oblique view, has been used for screening, due to the lower costs involved. Because of its reduced sensitivity and specificity, most mammography experts do not regard single-view mammography as sufficient for diagnostic purposes or cost-effective. Many patients require repeated examinations.[59, 60] For this reason, mammography in only one plane should be reserved for exceptional cases (such as a limited examination in the presence of known findings, in young patients, or during pregnancy).

Whereas standard views permit reliable identification or exclusion of malignant processes in most patients, additional views should be used liberally whenever mammograms in the standard imaging planes are inconclusive or do not visualize the findings completely. Any additional view is preferable to an unnecessary biopsy or a carcinoma that goes undetected.

■ Standard Views

The *mediolateral oblique view* and the *craniocaudal view* used in combination have become the international standard views.[24, 60-65]

■ Mediolateral Oblique View

■ Purpose

The mediolateral oblique (MLO) view is regarded as the most important view since it best visualizes the tissue adjacent to the chest wall and the axillary tail. It is the view that is most likely to include all the breast tissue. It is designed to maximize visualization of the lower axilla and the upper outer quadrant. If tissue is not included on this view, it is most likely in the inferomedial breast. Most carcinomas can be visualized in the mediolateral oblique view.

■ Conducting the Examination

(Figs. 3.**15 a** and **b**)

Rotate the X-ray tube and the film holder to permit positioning the film cassette between the patient's pectoralis muscle and latissimus dorsi. This can be achieved with 30°–70° inclination, depending on the patient's habitus. For short, stocky women, positioning will be more horizontal, and for tall, lanky women more vertical. The beam will travel from medial and superior to lateral and inferior, hitting the film cassette perpendicularly. Positioning the cassette and compression paddle parallel to the pectoralis in this manner allows optimum mobilization of the glandular tissue away from the chest wall.

Place the cassette posterior to the anterior axillary line. Place it so that it mobilizes the lateral breast medially and up.[61] This makes it possible to pull the breast away from the chest wall to achieve optimum positioning. Placing the film cassette inferior to the breast or too far laterally increases the tension on the medial tissue, which is painful and prevents adequate pulling of the breast onto the film cassette.

Do not push the cassette too high into the axilla. This tenses the pectoralis, making it difficult to pull the breast forward. If part of the humerus appears on the image, it is a sign of inadequate compression. The arm should rest lightly on the cassette since this also permits better mobilization of the glandular tissue. Turn the patient so that she faces the mammography unit. Thus the medial parts of the breast tissue will be included, and the inframammary fold will become visible on the image. Now pull the breast forward firmly so that as much tissue as possible lies on the cassette. Unlike compression, pulling the breast forward is not painful but visualizes another centimeter of glandular tissue anterior to the chest wall. Pull the breast anteriorly and superiorly to separate the glandular tissue as much as possible.[20] Otherwise, small carcinomas will be easily concealed. Once the breast is spread out, it is easily compressible, and compression is less painful.

When lowering the compression paddle, the breast should be pulled until the compression paddle holds the breast in position. Make sure that the compression does not produce any folds

in the skin that might interfere with the diagnosis. Be certain that the inframammary fold is open and the abdomen is not superimposed.

■ Quality Criteria for Optimum Positioning in the Mediolateral Oblique View

(Fig. 3.**15 a–e**)

– The pectoralis muscle should be visible in the image at least to the level of the nipple.
– It should course superiorly along the lateral border of the image at an angle of about 20°.
– The inframammary fold should be included inferiorly. This is achieved by having the patient turn far enough toward the mammography unit.
– The glandular tissue should appear well spread out in the image.

■ Optimization

The view can be optimized by rotating the tube to an angle corresponding to the course of the pectoralis, lifting the breast, pulling it forward firmly, turning the patient toward the mammography unit, spreading out the glandular tissue, and achieving the best possible compression.

■ Craniocaudal View

■ Purpose

The mediolateral oblique view is routinely supplemented by the craniocaudal view in which the beam travels from superior to inferior (Figs. 3.**16 a–d**).

■ Conducting the Examination

To pull the breast as far away from the chest wall as possible, lift the breast from below to shift the inframammary fold as far superiorly as possible. It is possible to lift the inframammary fold by several centimeters. Then adjust the table to the height of the upward mobilized inframammary fold and lay the breast on the table. Pulling the breast forward and compressing it at the original height of the inframammary fold would increase tension on the skin and subcutaneous tissue superior to the nipple, limiting forward mobility. This also is painful. After achieving correct cassette and breast positioning, firmly pull the breast away from the chest wall until it is held in place by the compression paddle.

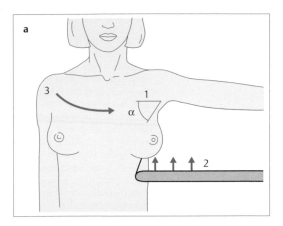

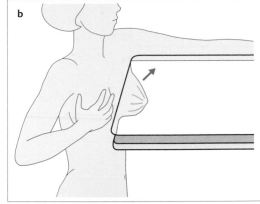

Fig. 3.**15 a–e**   Mediolateral oblique view
a Correct positioning is achieved by rotating the tube arm to an angle corresponding to the course of the pectoralis (1). Then the bucky is placed under the breast so as to mobilize the breast medially and superiorly as much as possible (2).
Finally (3), the patient is turned toward the unit and the technologist pulls the breast onto the film holder. That way as much medial breast tissue as possible is included, when the compression paddle (not shown) is lowered
b With the breast correctly positioned, the technologist pulls the breast tissue anteriorly and superiorly (arrow), moving it forward and spreading it as much as possible. The patient's ipsilateral arm (shown here) should rest on the film holder while she holds the contralateral breast back with her other hand

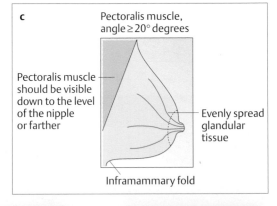

c A good mediolateral oblique view fulfills the following quality criteria: The pectoralis muscle should course diagonally along the superior and lateral border of the image (at an angle of at least 20°). The pectoralis should be visible in the image at least as far as the level of the nipple. The glandular tissue should appear well spread out, and the image should include the inframammary fold
Inclusion of the intramammary fold is an important sign that indicates sufficient visualization of the medial glandular tissue
d A small, not entirely smoothly contoured density close to the chest wall was only barely visualized in this poorly positioned mediolateral oblique view and thus was overlooked (the inframammary fold was not visualized)
e The medial lesion is readily discernible in the mediolateral oblique view with proper positioning (the patient was turned toward the mammography unit) (*Histology:* fibroadenoma)

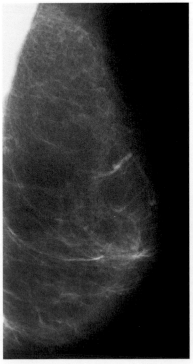

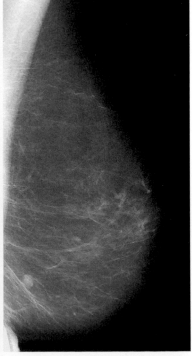

d

e

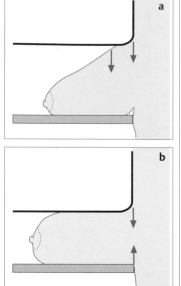

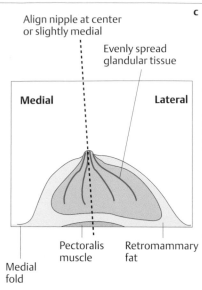

Align nipple at center
or slightly medial

Evenly spread
glandular tissue

Medial   **Lateral**

Pectoralis   Retromammary
muscle   fat

Medial
fold

Fig. 3.**16 a–d** Craniocaudal
(CC) view
a If the breast is not lifted,
compression will cause painful
tension (arrow) on the superior breast tissue, that also
hinders pulling the breast forward from the chest wall
b Correct positioning requires
mobilizing the breast as far superiorly as possible. Raise the
film holder accordingly. This
makes it possible to pull the
breast forward to achieve optimum positioning while
making compression far less
painful
c A good craniocaudal view
fulfills the following quality criteria: The image should include the entire body of the
gland with the retromammary
fat. This is best achieved with
the nipple centered or positioned slightly medially. In particularly high-quality images,
the pectoralis will just barely
be visible along the edge of
the mammogram and/or the
medial border of the image
will include the medial fold
d Craniocaudal view with
proper positioning

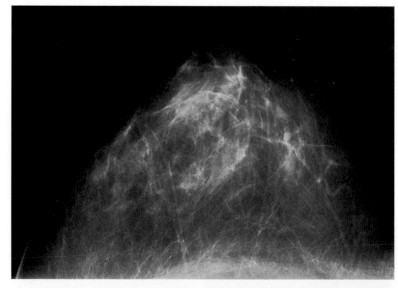

In the craniocaudal view, the nipple should be centered or pointing slightly medially. It is important to visualize the medial glandular tissue (which sometimes cannot be completely visualized in the mediolateral oblique view) as completely as possible. If this is problematic, it may be helpful to include the most medial aspect of the other breast to assure inclusion on the film of the breast being examined (see also cleavage view, p. 49). The craniocaudal view also serves as the second plane for imaging the axillary tail. This structure is rich in glandular tissue and should be carefully analyzed since it is a frequent site of cancer. To maximize visualization of the axillary tail, some authors recommend firmly pulling it forward before completely lowering the compression paddle. For this view, it is helpful to let the arm on the side being imaged hang down. This way, the outer quadrant of the relaxed pectoralis muscle will lie on the bucky, and it will be easier to pull it forward and visualize it. Here, too, make sure that the glandular tissue is well spread out before compression and that skin folds are avoided.

■ Quality Criteria

Ideally, the craniocaudal view should include the entire body of the gland with the medial and lateral retromammary fat. In particularly high-quality images, the pectoralis will just barely be visible along the edge of the mammogram. If the medial edge of the image includes the medial fold (which is not always possible), one can be sure that the body of the gland has been optimally visualized. Visualization of the medial breast is sometimes optimized by including the medial aspect of the opposite breast. If the pectoralis muscle is not included on the craniocaudal view, adequacy of inclusion of posterior tissues is determined by comparison with the MLO view. On the MLO view, measuring line is drawn at a 90° angle to the pectoralis muscle and through the nipple. The distance from the nipple to the posterior edge of the film on the craniocaudal view should be no less than 1 cm the length of the line drawn from the nipple to the pectoralis on the MLO view.

■ Positioning the Photocell

Once the correct settings have been selected, *choosing the proper position for the photocell is crucial to ensure proper functioning of the automatic exposure control system.* The photocell is optimally positioned under the *anterior third of the breast (behind the nipple)* since this area contains relatively uniform, representative glandular tissue. Make sure that the *photocell is completely covered by glandular tissue,* which should extend beyond the photocell by about 1 cm (Fig. 3.**7**).

■ Importance of Optimum Breast Positioning

Optimum positioning for standard views is important because:

- Compression is *less painful* whith good positioning.
- Good positioning will visualize considerably more tissue adjacent to the chest wall. In particular, since it is poorly accessible to palpation, this tissue is *especially important for early diagnosis* (Figs. 14.**1 a–c** and 14.**2 a** and **b**). The strip of fat usually present in this tissue makes it particularly suitable for detection of cancer by mammography.

Experienced staff can achieve very good positioning in as many as 90% of all cases. However, extensive scarring that does not permit sufficient mo-

bilization of the glandular tissue can cause problems. Similar problems can occur in the presence of chest deformities such as pectus excavatum or rotatory scoliosis. In patients with severe scoliosis this view may be more optimally positioned as a caudocranial view.

■ Further Procedure

No additional mammograms will be required if the standard views clearly reveal or exclude malignant findings and all breast tissue has been completely imaged. An additional view in the mediolateral (ML) projection is helpful even in the case of clear findings when a lesion is nonpalpable and preoperative needle marking is indicated.

However, if there is any uncertainty, obtaining additional views is the first step in arriving at a diagnosis.[63-65]

■ Positioning for Additional Views

The most important *additional views* include:

- Spot compression and magnification views (see p. 50)
- The 90° true lateral view
- The exaggerated lateral craniocaudal and the exaggerated medial craniocaudal view
- So-called rolled views
- The tangential view and oblique views with (customized) settings for visualizing findings in atypical locations

Rare applications include:

- The axillary view
- The so-called "cleavage" view

The special views required with implants are discussed on pp. 56–59.

■ 90° Lateral View

■ Significance

The 90° lateral view (Fig. 3.**17 a–c**) is used in the following situations:

- As a third imaging plane when a *questionable superimposed structure* cannot be clearly distinguished from a genuine lesion.
- For *initial assessment of indeterminate micro-calcifications.*The typical layering of milk of calcium in microcysts *(the so-called teacup phenomenon)* is only visible in a 90° lateral

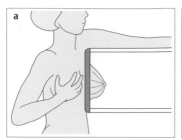 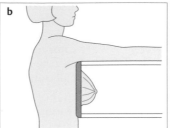 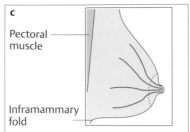

Fig. 3.**17 a–c** 90° lateral (true lateral) view
The 90° lateral mammogram is prepared using a medio-lateral or lateromedial beam with the mammography unit positioned at a 90° angle. Make sure to position the structures of interest as close to the film as possible
a Mediolateral view: The patient stands directly in front of the unit facing it. The upper outer corner of the bucky lies in the patient's axilla; her arm rests lightly on the film holder. Support the patient's back so that she will not withdraw when compression is applied. Lift the breast superiorly, pulling it away from the chest wall and spreading it to achieve good tissue separation until the breast is held in place by the compression paddle

b In the lateromedial view, the medial aspect of the patient's breast is positioned along the film holder. The arm of the side being imaged lies parallel to the upper edge of the compression cone. As in the mediolateral view, the technologist lifts the breast, pulls it forward, and holds it until it is held in place by the compression cone
c A good mediolateral view fulfills the following quality criteria: The image should include the entire body of the gland with the retromammary fat. The pectoralis should also be visible as a narrow band at least in the upper half of the image. The body of the gland should be well spread out, and the inframammary fold should be discernible

view. This pattern of layering is an important criterion for benign microcalcifications (see Chapter 10). For this reason, this projection (often with magnification) is frequently used in the assessment of microcalcifications.

– As an aid to localizing the true position of nonpalpable lesions in the breast prior to marking or percutaneous biopsy.

■ **Conducting the Examination**

When imaging the breast in the 90° projection, the *questionable structure* should be positioned as *close to the film* as possible to improve definition and minimize magnification. This means that a medial finding requires a *lateromedial (LM) view*, and a lateral finding requires a *mediolateral (ML) view*.

■ **Exaggerated Lateral Craniocaudal View**

(Figs. 3.**18 a** and **b**)

■ **Conducting the Examination**

The mammography unit is positioned as for the craniocaudal view parallel to the floor. However, the patient is turned so that the lateral breast is pulled onto the film cassette, compressed, and

imaged. The medial position of breast is, therefore sacrificed on the image.

■ **Purpose**

This view is used to visualize changes in the axillary tail of the breast in the craniocaudal plane. It is indicated in the presence of suspicious clinical findings in this area or to localize or further clarify uncertain or suspected findings which may be visible on the mediolateral oblique view but are not seen on the routine craniocaudal view.

Even in the absence of clinical findings, it can be used to supplement the standard views if these views do not adequately visualize the axillary tail.

■ **Exaggerated Medial Craniocaudal View**

■ **Purpose**

The exaggerated medial craniocaudal view can be used to image medial findings very close to the chest wall that are difficult to include on the correctly positioned craniocaudal view.

■ **Conducting the Examination**

The image is obtained with the mammography unit in the same position as for the craniocaudal

Fig. 3.18 a–c
a The laterally exaggerated craniocaudal view is performed like the CC view, but the patient is rotated and faces the film holder obliquely so that the lateral breast tissue is included in the field of view. In contrast to the routine craniocaudal view, the medial breast tissue is excluded
b The medially exaggerated view is performed with the patient rotated in the opposite direction to bring the medial breast tissue in the field of view
c This externally exaggerated CC view reveals a small breast carcinoma that was projected over the pectoral muscle in the mediolateral oblique view. Only the externally exaggerated view could exactly localize the small breast carcinoma by visualizing it in a second projection

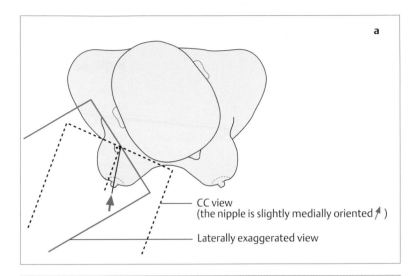

CC view
(the nipple is slightly medially oriented ↗)

Laterally exaggerated view

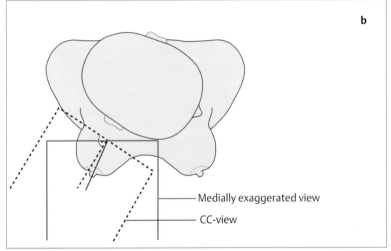

Medially exaggerated view

CC-view

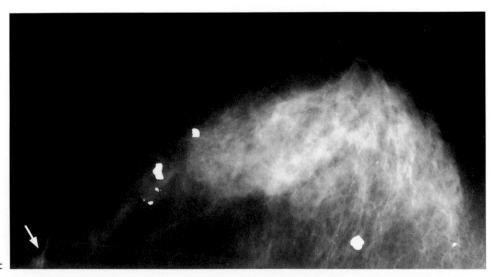

c

view. However, the patient is turned so that the medial breast is pulled onto the film holder, sacrificing the lateral aspect on the image.

■ Tangential View

■ Significance

Tangential views are valuable for detecting subcutaneous calcifications (Fig. 3.**19**). If the calcifications are in the skin or in the subcutaneous tissue, benign calcifications can be assumed. For this reason, definite intracutaneous or subcutaneous localization provides important information for the differential diagnosis of calcifications. The tangential view is also useful for displacing masses away from an overlying implant.

■ Conducting the Examination

When skin lesions are being assessed, phototiming may overexpose the skin. Therefore manually adjusting exposure settings may be appropriate in this situation.

There are various options available to localize calcifications in subcutaneous or cutaneous tissue clearly. One can attempt to find the true tangential view by taking several exposures. This method is not recommended because it is imprecise and exposes the patient to unnecessary radiation. Alternatively, a localizing plate with an alphanumeric grid can be used to compress the breast instead of the standard compression paddle. The selected breast projection (craniocaudal, caudocranial, mediolateral, or lateromedial) should have the area of calcifications nearest the fenestrated plate (Fig. 3.**19**). With the breast still compressed, this image is used as a guide and the area in which the calcifications are projected is marked. The gantry is then rotated and/or the breast rolled until this marker, with the localizing lights on, casts a shadow on the plate on which the breast is resting in this position. Then the beam is incident precisely tangential to the marked skin. If the calcifications in question are in the skin, they will be visualized in this location.

If only a small part of the body of the gland is fixed for a tangential view, *the breast may slip out of the compression device. A strip of double-sided adhesive tape, which is applied* to the compression paddle and/or grid holder, may be helpful to avoid this.

Cutaneous localization can also be achieved by stereotaxy. Using standard stereotactic images,

the z-axis of the target point is calculated as lying at the surface of the skin.

■ Oblique View with Customized Settings

Although positioning for the standard views should include all the glandular tissue in screening examinations, palpable changes occasionally occur in locations that render visualization next to impossible (especially in locations close to the chest wall). Here, the radiologist may use almost any *customized angle of the mammography unit and patient position* that can hold the breast in a fixed position and visualizes the findings in question for interpretation.

■ Axillary View

This view is used to evaluate findings in the lower portion of the axilla not visualized in the oblique view (this is rare). It is usually done as a 30° oblique, using a small, rectangular compression paddle. The chest wall is not included. The exposure can be phototimed.

■ Cleavage View

The cleavage view[20] (Fig. 3.**20**) is a rarely used one that visualizes the medial breast close to the chest wall particularly well. In this view, both breasts and the medial fold (cleavage) between them are compressed and imaged using a craniocaudal beam and a small compression cone. Since the photocell is not covered by the breast in this view, the exposure must be set manually.

■ Rolled Views

The rolled views[20] can be used to determine the depth of a lesion only detectable in one plane.

If, for example, we roll the upper breast medially from a craniocaudal position, lesions in the superior quadrants will move medially, that is in the direction of the roll, whereas lesions located in the inferior quadrants will move laterally in the opposite direction.

Today, the imaging modalities for determining the depth of a lesion detectable in only plane include mammographic stereotaxy, sonography, contrast-enhanced CT, and contrast-enhanced MRI. Rolled views can still be extremely helpful in determining whether dense areas detected primarily in one plane are real or represent superimposed structures (Figs. 3.**21 a–f**).

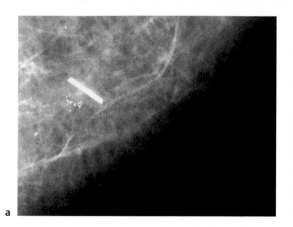

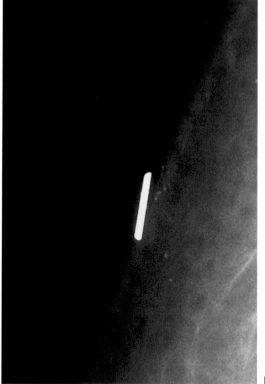

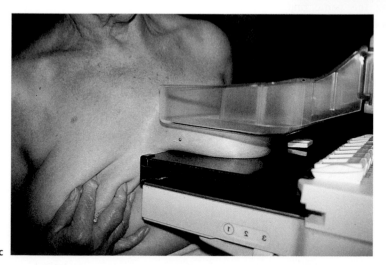

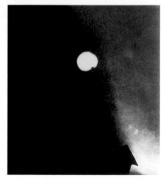

Fig. 3.**19 a–d** Mammogram demonstrating subcutaneous calcifications

a The mediolateral oblique view shows a small cluster of presumably benign microcalcifications very close to the chest wall (arrow), which in the craniocaudal view appeared to be in the medial glandular tissue

b To verify the subcutaneous location of the microcalcifications assumed on the basis of its morphology, the breast was compressed for a mediolateral oblique view. Using a fenestrated compression cone, a small marker was fixed against the skin above the cluster of microcalcifications

c Then another mammogram was performed with the patient positioned in a craniocaudal view with the tube at a 15° angle. The direction of the beam and compression was selected so that the skin marker was imaged tangentially to the beam next to the breast

d This craniocaudal view (magnifying a section of the skin) verifies that the microcalcifications are subcutaneous

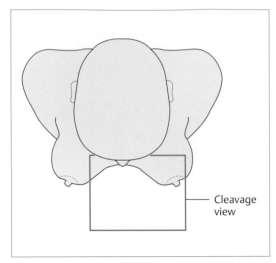

Fig. 3.**20** In the cleavage view, both breasts and the medial fold between them are compressed and imaged. This view visualizes medial lesions very close to the chest wall.

Film Labelling

The American College of Radiology (ACR) requires mammograms be labelled with a permanent identification label containing the name and address of the institution, the patient's name and a unique patient identification number (e. g., medical record number, social security number, date of birth), and the date of the examination. Each film should be labelled left or right and the view should be specified with radiopaque markers placed on the film near the axilla. The labelling abbreviations for positioning recommended by the ACR are:

Right	R
Left	L
Mediolateral oblique	MLO
Craniocaudal	CC
90° lateral:	
mediolateral	ML
lateromedial	LM
Magnification	M (used as a prefix before the projection)
Exaggerated craniocaudal	XCC
Cleavage	CV
Axillary tail	AT
Tangential	TAN
Roll:	
rolled lateral	RL
rolled medial	RM

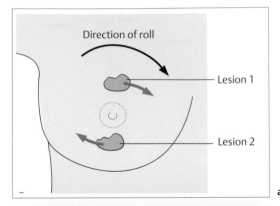

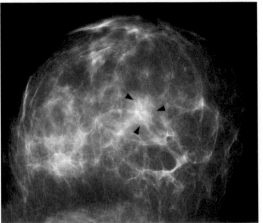

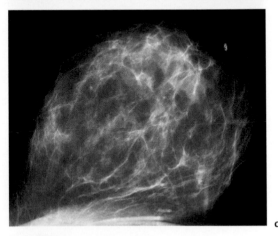

Fig. 3.**21 a–c**
a Principle of the rolled view shown with a craniocaudal view.
If the upper breast is rolled medially, superior lesions (lesion 1) will move in the direction of the roll, whereas inferior lesions (lesion 2) will move in the opposite direction
b Patient with an uncertain density that only appears in one plane
c The rolled view reveals that the density was caused by superimposition

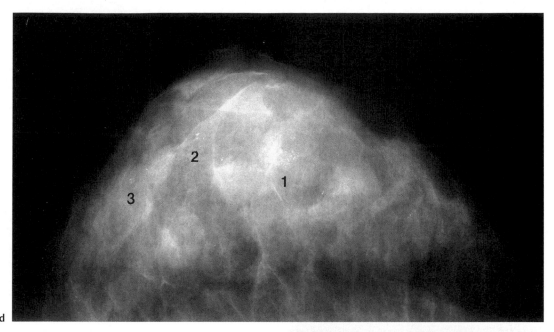

d

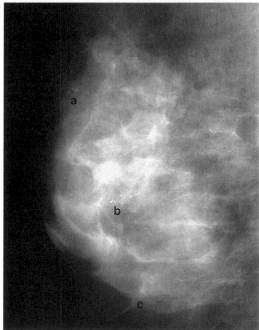

e

Fig. 3.**21 d–e**   This patient presented with three groups of indeterminate microcalcifications.
d Craniocaudal view shows three groups of microcalcifications: 1, 2, and 3.
e Oblique view also shows three groups of microcalcifications: a, b, and c. However based on the views and the morphology of the microcalcifications it was not clear which groups on the craniocaudal and oblique views corresponded. Thus, an exact localization was not possible. In order to choose the most appropriate approach for percutaneous biopsy, exact localization was, however, needed.

Caudocranial	FB (from below)
Lateromedial oblique	LMO
Superolateral to inferomedial oblique	SIO
Implant displaced (= Eklund view)	ID

For example, a right craniocaudal magnification view should be labelled RMCC.

The film should also be labelled with the unique initials of the technologist who performed the mammogram. Each screen should be labelled with a unique identifying number or letter, so that dusty or defective screens can be identified readily.

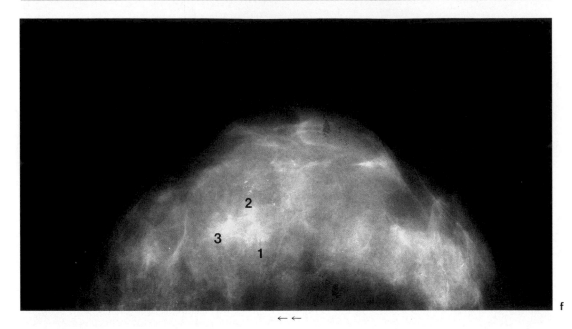

f

← ←

Fig. 3.**21 f** Therefore, another craniocaudal view was obtained, for which the upper breast was rolled medially (the double arrows indicate direction of rolling). Group 1 rolls medially and therefore corresponds to group a (in the upper breast); group 2 stays and therefore corresponds to group b (mid-breast); group 3 rolls laterally and therefore is located in the lower breast (corresponding to group c).

The ACR recommends, but does not require, that films also be labelled by flashing information on the film, rather than using a sticker. Technical factors (kVp, mAs, compression force, compressed breast thickness, and angle of obliquity on the MLO view) are also recommended to be included. If a facility has more than one unit, it is desirable to identify which unit was used. A paper sticker with the date of the examination is recommended so that different studies are easily identifiable.

■ Spot Compression and Magnification Technique

■ Spot Compression

■ Definition

In spot compression (Fig. 3.**22 a**), a small cone is used to compress only the area of the breast of interest, with the beam collimated on this small area of interest[66]. Spot compression can be performed in any imaging plane.

■ Advantages

– *Dense areas resulting from summation of superimposed images can be spread out;* malignant foci and architectural distortion will remain.
– Spreading of the surrounding parenchyma means that the outline of masses (possibly also of microcalcifications) is less obscured by superimposed tissue and may be better visualized. Note: Magnification may add information about the contours of masses.
– Better localized compression (reduction of the thickness to be penetrated) and, to a lesser extent, the collimation reduce scattered radiation and improve contrast.
– The increased compression makes its possible to decrease the distance between some structures and the image receptor and thus to decrease geometric blurring.
– Occasionally, findings close to the chest wall are more accessible with a small round cone.

■ Limits

Granularity and noise:

- Given the limited resolution of currently available screen–film systems, *magnification mammography* is better suited to *evaluating the contours of soft-tissue densities* and *analyzing microcalcifications.*

■ Indications

- Differentiating dense areas resulting from summation of superimposed structures from real masses (Figs. 3.**22 b, c** and Fig. 3.**23**).
- Imaging findings close to the chest wall.
- Evaluating the contours of focal lesions or microcalcifications only when magnification mammography is not available (Fig. 3.**24**).

■ Magnification Technique

■ Definition

Magnification mammography involves the following:

- The breast is placed on a platform located at a defined distance from the grid holder (Fig. 3.**24**).
- The area of interest is compressed and the image field is collimated as narrowly as possible to include only the area of interest as with spot compression.
- A small focal spot is selected and the grid removed.

■ Fundamental Considerations in Magnification Mammography

The total resolution (definition) in an unmagnified image is limited by geometric blurring, resolution of the screen–film system, and, in applicable cases, motion blurring.

Total resolution is also influenced by the contrast of the detail being imaged and by image noise.

Magnification mammography has the following effects:[22, 66]

1. Magnifying details by the factor *f* and projecting them on the screen–film system improves that proportion of the resolution (definition) determined by the screen–film system by precisely this factor *f*.

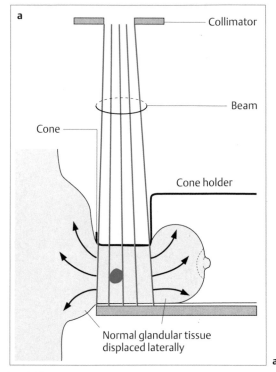

Fig. 3.**22 a–c**
a Spot compression (in the craniocaudal view)

2. Increasing the magnification while keeping the size of the focus constant would significantly increase the geometric blurring due to the larger penumbra (geometric blurring). The geometric threshold resolution has definitely been reached when the size of the penumbra equals or exceeds that of an imaged detail. For this reason, magnification mammography requires a *microfocus with a nominal maximum value of 0.1–0.15* (depending on the magnification factor). The size of the focus in turn limits the maximum feasible *magnification factor to 1.4–2.0* on standard units.
3. The minimal size of the focal spot is currently limited by the load rating of the microfocus.
4. Bearing in mind the limited power of the microfocus, we recommend the following measures to minimize exposure time (in the interest of reducing motion blurring and dose, and avoiding reciprocity law failure of the film):
   - Use a faster low-dose screen–film system (e. g., sensitivity class 25. At the given magnification factor, the screen–film system no longer influences maximum resolution).

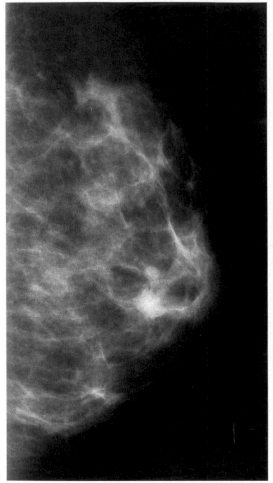

b

c

Fig. 3.**22 b** and **c** The mediolateral view shows an irregular retroareolar focal density measuring 6 mm in diameter (a). A spot compression view revealed this to be the result of superimposition (b)

- Increase kVp by approximately 2 kV compared with the corresponding nonmagnified exposure. This allows a decrease in the exposure time (mAs) while the density remains comparable to the nonmagnified view. Otherwise, the small focal spot would require a long exposure, and patient motion may be a problem.

5. To maintain an adequate signal-to-noise ratio, the dose required to produce the image increases as the square of magnification factor. If all other parameters are kept constant, magnifying the image by a factor of 1.4 will double the dose, and magnifying the image by a factor of 2 will quadruple the dose. Minimizing the dose is necessary in the interest of min-imizing the patient's exposure to radiation and to avoid exceeding the load rating of the microfocus. This is achieved by increasing the voltage by approximately 2 kV and eliminating the grid.

6. For magnification mammography, the grid is removed. This is necessary to limit the radiation dose to the breast and to reduce the exposure time, which otherwise might become very long (due to the increased dose required for magnification and due to the limited load rating of the small focus). To avoid motion blurring and the reciprocity law failure, the exposure time should not be too long. Removing the grid results in decreased radiation and shorter exposure time with less patient motion.

7. Scatter reduction, which improves contrast in magnification mammography, is achieved by the "air gap" combined with good collimation. The air gap itself allows reduction of scatter since part of the scattered radiation will pass beyond the film. Even though magnification without collimation is possible, good collimation significantly enhances the effect of the air gap. Only with good collimation (≤5 cm) can the lack of the grid be compensated by the air gap.

■ Advantages

– Improved resolution of fine details by overcoming blurring due to the screen–film system.
– Magnified details are easier to observe, i. e., there is more information on the film of the area imaged.
– When spot compression is used along with magnification, structures are less obscured by displacing the superimposed tissue.
– Dense areas representing summation of superimposed tissue can be differentiated from real findings (see also spot compression).

■ Disadvantages

– Magnification mammography increases the dose required, but this is largely compensated for by using a low-dose screen–film system, increasing the kVp, and eliminating the grid.

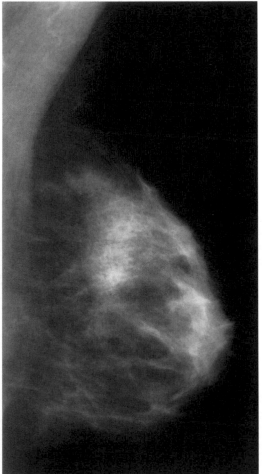

a

Fig. 3.**23 a–b**
a On the MLO view oblique view of this screening mammogram a discrete architectural distortion was noted about 4 cm behind the nipple
b On the craniocaudal view the architectural distortion cannot be clearly identified. Therefore, craniocaudal spot compression views were performed beginning laterally

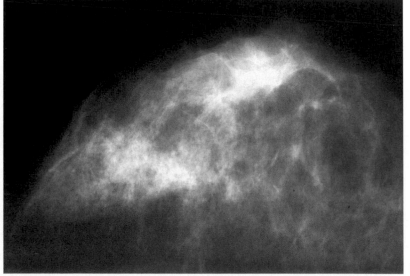

b

Fig. 3.**24** Magnification mammography

Collimation

Compression device
(paddle with holder)

a

b

Radiolucent table

Air gap
Good collimation
and a wide air gap
between breast and
cassette reduce
scattered radiation
in the image

Cassette holder
with cassette

Image

A small focal spot is necessary to
minimize the penumbra (see **Fig 3.2**)

Magnification factor f = $\dfrac{b}{a}$

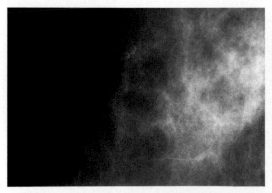

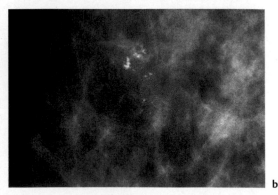

Fig. 3.**25 a** and **b** The craniocaudal view shows a group of pleomorphic microcalcifications at the margin of the parenchyma (**a**). An additional magnification view (**b**) clearly reveals them to be suggestive of malignancy

- Contrast could be decreased due to the lack of a grid and the higher kVp setting. This can largely be compensated for with good compression of the area of interest (pushing superimposed tissue aside) and good collimation (air gap reduces scattered radiation).

■ Indications

- Determining whether microcalcifications are present.
- Analyzing the geometry and distribution and of microcalcifications (Fig. 3.**25**).
- Detecting additional fine calcifications for improving the differential diagnosis of microcalcifications.
- Excluding or verifying the presence of multiple foci and assessing the extent of carcinomas with microcalcifications (Fig. 3.**26**).
- Analyzing the contours of masses, i. e., smooth, lobulated, spiculated (Fig. 3.**27**).
- Differentiating dense areas resulting from summation of superimposed structures from real masses (see also spot compression; Fig. 3.**22**).

■ New Developments

A new development that deserves attention is a special microfocus technique ("fine-focus"). With this technique an extremely small focus is obtained by means of electronic focusing. If such a focus is used, several-fold magnification is possible without significant geometric unsharpness. Such foci are presently used in certain systems for specimen radiography.[67]

■ Positioning of Breasts with Implants

Surgical technique and type and location of the implant determine the available mammographic imaging options. Following subcutaneous mastectomy and implant placement, usually only a small amount of tissue will remain around the implant. The distribution and architecture of the breast parenchyma can vary considerably. After augmentation mammoplasty, all of the breast tissue that was originally present will usually be superficial to the implant. Achieving good results in mammography depends upon the type of previous surgery and the type and position of implant material.

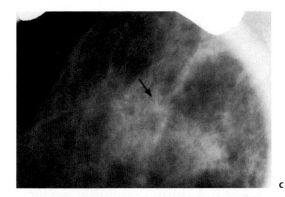

c

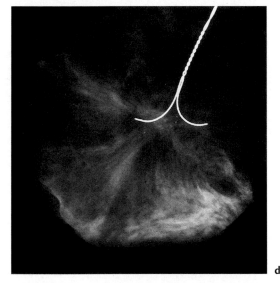

d

Fig. 3.**23 c–d**
c This craniocaudal compression view of the patient's left lateral breast allows identification of a star-like architectural distortion. The area was excised after preoperative wire localization
d The specimen radiograph demonstrates the architectural distortion even more clearly
Histology: radial scar with intermediate grade ductal carcinoma in situ

Standard mammography of these women usually requires manual exposure settings for those views that include the implants since the implant usually overlies the phototimer, attenuating the X-ray beam and causing the image to be overexposed.

The augmented breast should not be imaged as a screening study but always as a diagnostic mammogram. Full imaging of the augmented breast requires four views, not just the routine two views. MLO and craniocaudal views of the breasts, including the implant, are done to see

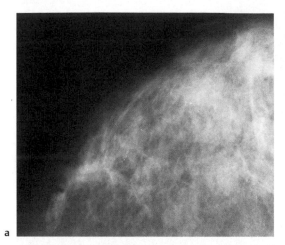

a

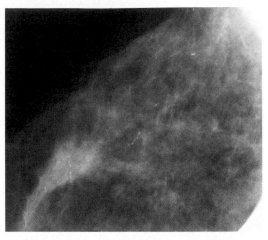

b

Fig. 3.**26 a** and **b** The craniocaudal view reveals a focal density with ill-defined contour with central and marginal microcalcification (**a**). The magnification mammogram (**b**) with spot compression clearly demonstrates highly suspicious spiculations. In addition to the above mentioned suspicious microcalcifications, more pleomorphic microcalcifications are shown on this magnification view extending toward the nipple

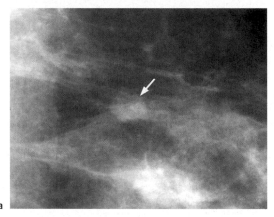

a

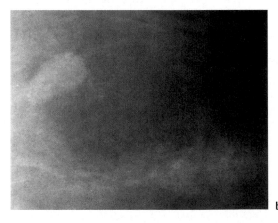

b

Fig. 3.**27 a** and **b** The mediolateral oblique view shows an indeterminate mass measuring 7 mm located at the superior margin of the parenchyma (**a**). Spot compression reveals this to be a smooth-contoured lesion, compatible with a lymph node

tissue back to the chest wall and to image the implant. Compression used should be adequate to stabilize the breast so there is no motion on the image. Compression beyond this should not be used for fear of rupturing the implant. An additional two views should be performed according to the procedure described by Eklund:[68] pull the glandular tissue anteriorly away from the implant, push the implant posteriorly, and gradually slide the compression paddle over the breast tissue anterior to the implant. This pushes the implant posteriorly, allowing better compression of the glandular tissue itself (Fig. 3.**28**). Imaging should be done in the craniocaudal and the MLO or 90° lateral projections. It should be possible to obtain these displacement views in about 80% of women with implants. In those women who have hard, noncompressable implants (capsular contracture) or for whom the displacement maneuver is painful, it will not be possible to obtain these additional two views. Since these views are done with the implant out of the way, phototiming can be used.

Mammography as described by Eklund is generally no longer possible after subcutaneous

Fig. 3.**28 a–d** Displacement method of imaging a breast with an implant following augmentation mammoplasty.
a The glandular tissue is pulled forward away from the implant, which
b is displaced posteriorly, as the technologist lowers the compression paddle over the breast tissue, and compresses it.
c This displaces the implant posteriorly so that it no longer covers the glandular tissue (as decribed by Eklund et al.[66])
d The nondisplaced view including the implant is shown.

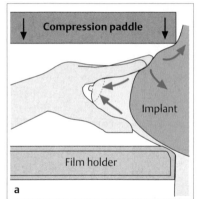

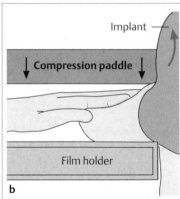

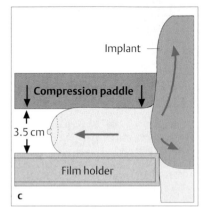

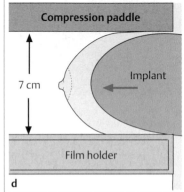

mastectomy and breast reconstruction. Mammography can still be performed to clarify clinical findings, but the radiologist should be aware that only the tissue layers tangential to the beam not obscured by the implant can be assessed. For this reason, mammography is usually performed in several planes, though it will not be possible to image all of the tissue surrounding the implant in these patients.

■ Specimen Radiography

Nonpalpable, mammographically confirmed lesions requiring excision must be localized preoperatively (see Chapter 8). After excision, specimen radiographs, i. e., radiographs of the surgical specimen, are obtained to verify whether it contains the mammographic findings leading to the excision and to identify the location of the lesion in the specimen for histologic analysis. If the biopsied lesion is malignant and it extends to the margin of the specimen, specimen radiography can also be used to suggest the need for further

surgical excision.[69-72] Specimen radiography can be performed using a mammography unit or a Faxitron, a tabletop X-ray unit designed for specimen radiography. If a mammography unit is used, manual settings instead of automatic exposure settings should be employed.

Compression of the specimen improves the image, especially when the biopsy has been performed for an uncalcified mass. Compression equalizes differences in thickness, reduces scattered radiation and spreads out the overlying tissue.

A radiograph in a second plane might help to localize small foci of disease or to determine if the lesion has been transsected during surgery. Due to the geometry of the specimen, a specimen radiograph in the second plane is, however, often not possible and is not standard. Areas in the specimen that require histologic analysis should be indicated for the pathologist so they will not be overlooked.

If microcalcifications are present, it is sometimes useful to include magnification in addition

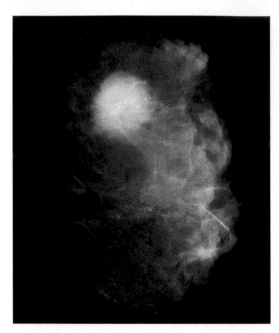

Fig. 3.**29** A magnification radiograph of a specimen clearly reveals not only the calcifications within the center of the tumor but two additional remote foci of microcalcifications

Histology: Highly fibrotic invasive ductal breast cancer measuring 17 mm; intraductal tumor is shown adjacent to the mass. Furthermore, another focal ductal carcinoma in situ was verified 15 mm distant from the invasive tumor

to the standard radiograph. This provides additional information about further extremely small microcalcifications and their relationship to the margins (Fig. 3.**29**). In breast-conserving treatment of carcinoma, this is important for determining the extent of tumor and its proximity to the margin of the excised specimen. However, assessment of a mass surrounded by dense breast tissue may be difficult. Furthermore, areas removed because of asymmetry may not be identified with certainly on the specimen radiograph.

It may also be very difficult to assess complete excision in case of larger areas of indeterminate microcalcifications. Finally, it must be remembered that in some cases the full extent of tumor may only be visible histologically. Therefore, correct and complete excision can only be assessed by combined evaluation of the preoperative mammogram, the specimen radiograph, and the histopathologic result.

Radiologic examination of the paraffin blocks is indicated whenever histopathologic examination of a biopsy performed for mammographically detected microcalcifications fails to reveal these calcifications since the standard procedure involves microscopic examination of only representative sections of the biopsy. Radiologic examination of the paraffin block will reveal whether microcalcifications are present in the part of the biopsy that was not examined under the microscope. If any doubts exist concerning correct or complete excision, a repeat mammogram is recommended.

Mammography may be performed in the early postoperative period without causing any undue pain. However, only compression sufficient to stabilize the breast should be used.

If, due to postoperative changes, removal of a mass or density in question is uncertain, MRI shortly after surgery (optimally within the first 10 days) may be helpful (see p. 104).

Quality Factors

■ Hardware Factors that Influence Image Quality

The ACR has recommended specifications for new mammography equipment.[30]

These requirements and other important hardware factors that influence image quality are summarized and discussed in the following section. More detailed information is available in the applicable literature.[20, 73, 74, 75]

■ Generator and Tube Power

Adequate generator or tube output is required to achieve sufficiently short exposure times, particularly for thick and dense breasts and for magnification mammography. Most quality mammography units achieve 4–5 kW.

The required power also depends on the target and filter material used. When tungsten and rhodium targets are used, the change in radiation quality is enough to penetrate even thick and dense breasts using less power than conventional molybdenum tubes and filters.

Insufficient power requires excessively long exposures times (>2 sec) that result in motion blurring. Moreover, insufficient power disproportionately increases the exposure time and radiation dose required for adequate optical density (reciprocity law failure). If the automatic exposure control system is unable to compensate for this effect, then an underexposed image will result.

Before installing a mammography unit, it is advisable to check the electrical system on the premises for voltage fluctuations. Mammography units cannot compensate for voltage drops; fluctuations in radiation quality will result, even when settings remain constant.

Because of the need to keep the voltage constant over time and, furthermore, because of the short exposure times required for low-dose film–screen systems, newer units are equipped with high-frequency generators.

■ Resolution

The ACR requires measurement of a bar pattern 45 mm above the breast support surface of the unit, within 1 cm of the chest wall and centered laterally. At this point resolution should be 11 line-pairs/mm when the pattern is oriented with the bars perpendicular to the cathode–anode axis of the X-ray tube, and 13 line-pairs/mm when parallel to this axis.

■ Magnification Technique

Magnification mammography has become increasingly important. Studies have demonstrated that magnification mammography permits better analysis of microcalcifications, better visualization of the extent of carcinomas, and more reliable exclusion of malignancy. Most importantly, magnification mammography can reduce the number of unnecessary diagnostic biopsies. For this reason, breast imaging facilities, which are used for problem solving, must be able to perform magnification mammography. This requires an additional focus with a rated size less than or equal to 0.1–0.15 depending on the magnification factor, an insert for positioning the breast at a distance from the cassette, and a collimator. Magnification should be between 1.5–2.0×. Greater magnification may result in blurring due to long exposure times and increased geometric blurring. The dose also may become excessive.

■ Radiation Quality

The requirement that voltage must be regulated emphasizes the importance of radiation quality adapted to match the thickness and density of the breast.

The voltage settings required to achieve a certain desired radiation quality will vary depending on the mammography unit, target, filter, and generator, and thus are not necessarily comparable.

The ACR recommends that the X-ray source assembly include a molybdenum target, a beryllium window of 1.5 mm thickness or less, and a molybdenum filter. Alternate combinations can be used if they can achieve comparable diagnostic quality with equal or reduced radiation dose.

The newest mammography units offer a choice of various target/filter combinations to achieve the ideal radiation energy for the breast thickness and density to be penetrated. An auto-select mode is provided to aid in selecting the optimum parameter combination.

■ Radiation Protection and Field Limitation

Use of a moving grid is specified in the regulations to achieve the reduction in scattered radiation necessary to ensure sufficient contrast.

Grid lines should not be evident and should not degrade images obtained of the ACR phantom. Grids should be available in both 18 × 24 cm and 24 × 30 cm sizes.

The required collimation of the useful beam is intended to protect the chest wall from excessive radiation exposure. This value is verified during the acceptance inspection and in routine quality control testing.

The film must be completely exposed on the side close to the chest. The X-ray field may not extend more than 3 mm beyond the edge of the image receptor on the chest wall side (to protect the chest wall from excessive radiation).

X-ray attenuation in the compression paddle, grid table, and film cassette vary between the manufacturers. Exact specifications should be obtained, since high attenuation in the grid table and film cassette unnecessarily increases the radiation exposure of the breast. The ACR recommends that all materials between the X-ray filter and the breast should not absorb the X-ray beam by more than 20%.

■ Exposure

The option of an automatic exposure control system is mandatory for mammography equipment, because it minimizes the number of incorrect exposures for routine mammography. The manual adjustment option is required as well. It is needed for achieving good exposure with small breasts that do not completely cover the photocell, and breasts with implants.

The quality of the automatic exposure control system greatly affects image quality. Only a good automatic exposure control system can achieve a reproducible, constant mean optical density regardless of the thickness and density of the breast. Failure to sufficiently equalize differences in thickness and density will mean that voluminous breasts and breasts with dense glandular tissue will be underexposed. Where the automatic exposure control system does not compensate sufficiently, an experienced radiologic technologist must make manual adjustment with the correction key. This makes it more difficult to achieve reproducible optimum exposure settings.

A medical physicist can verify the quality of an automatic exposure control system by using it to image plexiglass plates of varying thickness. Differences in the mean optical density may not exceed a certain limit (maximum fluctuations in optical density are $\pm$ 0.12 by ACR standards and should produce reproducible exposures with a variation coefficient of $\leq$4%).

Even an optimally functioning automatic exposure control system will only produce correctly exposed mammograms when the photocell lies under a representative area of the breast (generally in the anterior third of the breast). Unfortunately, sometimes the design of the unit itself restricts the options for positioning of the photocell. In routine use, these design restrictions can have a detrimental effect similar to that of an automatic exposure control system that cannot properly compensate for differences in breast thickness and density.

■ Influence of the Screen–Film System and Film Processing on Image Quality

In addition to hardware factors, the choice of screen–film system and proper film processing greatly influence image quality.

■ Screen–Film System

Visualization of fine details requires high contrast. Yet contrast must not be too high to avoid relative underexposure of those areas with low optical density. Low-contrast films must be used when less sophisticated automatic exposure control systems or problems in achieving consistent film processing cause the mean optical density to fluctuate. High-contrast film does not tolerate such fluctuations in mean optical density, and overexposed and underexposed areas will result.

Extremely sensitive screen–film systems, which usually are of very high-contrast, are marketed by manufacturers as so-called screening systems. They exhibit increased noise that is further intensified by the greater contrast. Excessive noise can make it difficult to discern details.

With their extremely short exposure time settings, highly sensitive screen–film systems can result in the grid itself being imaged, particularly when used in older mammography units. When their exposure time settings fall below the unit's minimum exposure times, small breasts can be overexposed.

There are differences in film quality. Sensitivity fluctuations between film batches should not exceed $\pm$ 10%, but the acceptable range for each manufacturer may vary. This range can be obtained from the film manufacturer. Inexpensive films may exhibit greater fluctuations in fog and sensitivity between film batches. They produce different optical densities at the same exposure settings that may interfere with the interpretation. Sensitometric testing is indicated whenever such fluctuations are suspected.

■ Film Processing

As has been mentioned, films should always be processed according to the manufacturer's recommendations. Since aberrations of the film processing are the most frequent cause of acute fluctuations in quality, consistent processing should be verified daily (p. 61). If the processor is used for both mammography films and other films, then consistency should always be established with mammography films as well as with the type of other films most often used.[76] Processor consistency should be checked before mammography begins each day.

Separate film processing for mammography has certain advantages because processing can be optimized for this specific film.

Processors for mammography films should be equipped with soft rubber rollers to minimize tears (pickoffs) in sensitive mammography films. Separate film processing for mammography is only recommended if at least 20 mammography films are developed per day because otherwise the chemicals cannot be maintained at a constant level of activity. To keep the darkroom free of dust it should be cleaned daily. Weekly cleaning of screens is also necessary, but they should be cleaned more often whenever dust appears on films.

■ **Additional Factors**

The minimum exposure times of the automatic exposure control system and the speed of the moving grid of a mammography unit are also important.

If particularly low-dose screen–film systems requiring extremely short exposure time are used, the system will image a slow-moving grid. This interferes with image interpretation and should always be avoided.

Exceeding the machine-specific minimum exposure time can lead to overexposure of small or fatty breasts.

If the mammography unit cannot fulfill these requirements for grid speed and grid switching time, a slightly less sensitive screen–film system should be used. If this does not solve the problem, the mammography unit should be upgraded.

■ # Quality Assurance in Mammography

In the United States quality assurance in mammography is controlled under the federal legislation entitled the Mammography Quality Assurance Act (MQSA), which is administered by the Food and Drug Administration (FDA). All mammography facilities in the United States must meet the criteria established under MQSA.

Quality assurance entails procedures that guarantee the quality of all facets of mammography practice. This includes equipment, radiation exposure, and film interpretation. A subset of this is quality control (QC), which involves the technical procedures that guarantee a quality mammogram. The steps involved in QC include acceptance testing, establishment of baseline performance of equipment, assessing the reasons for change in the performance of equipment before they impact on the quality of the image, and documentation that appropriate corrections have been made whenever necessary.

The quality assurance program of a facility has procedures that are the responsibility of the radiologist, the radiologic technologist, and the medical physicist. The QA requirements outlined here are those specified in the final preliminary requirements. Some alterations may occur when the final QA requirements are established by the

FDA for the MQSA. The ultimate responsibility for quality assurance lies with the radiologist. The radiologist's responsibilities include assuring that appropriate education and training have been met by all those involved in mammography, delegating appropriate responsibilities to technologists and medical physicists, being certain that QC measures have been carried out, assuring that established criteria are met by the facility, and keeping appropriate records.

The medical physicist's responsibilities include acceptance testing of equipment. Additionally, an annual examination of facility equipment includes assessment of the mammographic unit assembly, assessment of collimation, assessment of focal spot performance, testing of kVp accuracy and reproducibility, measuring the beam quality (half-value layer measurement), testing automatic exposure control, evaluating uniformity of screen speed, testing radiation dose, and an overall evaluation of image quality and of artifacts.

Radiologic technologists are responsible for a variety of tests. These include:

Daily: Evaluating darkroom cleanliness and processor quality control
Weekly: Cleaning screens and viewboxes and evaluating viewing conditions
Monthly: Testing phantom images and making a visual checklist
Quarterly: Critical analysis and analysis of fixture retention in film
Semiannually: Assessing darkroom fog, screen–film contact and compression

Documentation that quality control measures have been met is required by federal legislation. Facilities are subject to annual inspection to ensure that they meet the requirements established by law.

In addition to the quality control measures mandated in an ongoing fashion, the radiologist interpreting the films should monitor the quality of those images and institute corrective action as needed on the basis of image quality. The radiologist should also appreciate that the QC measures required by the radiologic technologist entail a significant amount of time and training. A technologist should be designated as the quality control technologist. This technologist should be given adequate time in his or her schedule to perform the required procedures.

Medical Physicist's Responsibilities

The medical physicist's responsibilities include the following:

1. Mammographic unit assembly evaluation. This is to determine that all locks, angulation indicators and the mechanical support of the system operates properly. This includes visual inspection of the entire assembly, verification that moving parts operate appropriately, testing of locks to be certain they prevent mechanical motion, determination that the image recepter holder assembly is secure and slides smoothly into appropriate position. Verification that the compressed breast thickness scale, if one is provided, is accurate to within ±0.5 cm at from 15 to 20 lb of compression, and to be certain that in normal operation neither patient nor operator is exposed to hazards from sharp or rough edges or dangerous electrical wiring.
2. Collimation assessment. This testing is done to ensure that the collimator or cone does not allow significant radiation beyond the edges of the imager receptor. Testing is done by placing four small coins just inside the light field with the coins touching the edge of the lightfield. The compression cone is positioned 6 cm from the breast support, and an attenuating sheet of acrylic or other material is placed above the cone to attenuate the X-ray beam. The film is exposed, and the position of coins on the image assessed.
3. Evaluation of focal spot performance. This is done by measuring the dimensions of the focal spot perpendicular and parallel to the anode–cathode axis. Slit camera measurement of the focal spot size is performed as well as high-contrast resolution pattern measurement.
4. kVp accuracy and reproducibility. This testing is done to assure that kVp is accurate within ± 5% of the indicated kVp and is reproducible with a coefficient of variability ≤ 0.02. Measurements are done using a test device capable of measuring kVp with an accurancy of ± 1.5 kVp and with a precision of 0.5 kVp within the kVp range of mammographic equipment.
5. Beam quality assessment (half-value layer measurement). This is done to determine that half-value layer of the X-ray beam is adequate so that radiation exposure of the patient is minimized without loss of necessary contrast. An ionization chamber and electrometer calibrated to the mammographic X-ray beam energies and sheets of 0.1 mm thick aluminum (or equivalent) are necessary for testing.
6. Automatic exposures control (AEC) system performance assessment. This is done to ensure that the AEC system performs appropriately. Testing is performed by evaluating imaging optical density on film exposed with various thicknesses of a phantom in a controlled fashion.
7. Uniformity of screen speed. This is done by testing optical density on film exposed in the standard fashion on various cassettes used for mammography.
8. Breast entrance exposure. Average glandular dose and automatic exposure control reproducibility. Testing is done with a radiation detector and phantom placed above the image receptor holder assembly. Variation in AEC reproducibility is 0.05. The average glandular dose to the breast should not exceed 0.3 rad.
9. Image quality evaluation. This is done to assess the quality of the mammographic image and to detect any changes over time in the quality of image. Phantom testing over time should show a consistency of optical density at established exposure parameters. Under established parameters, optical density should not change more than ± 0.20, and density difference should not change by more than 0.05. Exposure time and mAs on the generator read out should not change from exposure to exposure by more than ± 15%.
10. Artifact evaluation. Films should be assessed for the presence of artifacts and, if present, their source determined.

The Radiology Technologist's Responsibilities

The radiology technologist's responsibilities include:

1. Darkroom cleanliness. This minimizes film artifacts due to dirt and dust. Daily cleaning of the darkroom is required.
2. Processor quality control. This assures that the film processor chemical system is working optimally. Testing is done daily before the initiation of clinical imaging by inserting a sensitometric strip to check film density and base-plus-fog level. Additionally, processor quality control operating levels need to be es-

tablished when the quality control program is initiated or when there has been an important change made in film, chemicals, or processing conditions. To ascertain that the system is stable, testing of the processor should be conducted on five consecutive days after such changes are made.

3. Screen cleanliness. To minimize dust and dirt particles in the screen, it should be cleaned at least weekly.
4. Phantom images. Monthly testing with phantom images should be carried out once baseline levels of performance are established within a department. Requirements state that sensitometric control strips need to be run daily for the processor.
5. Darkroom fog. This testing is done to be certain that light inside and outside the darkroom does not fog mammographic films. A visual inspection of the darkroom should be done semiannually. Clinical films are also exposed to tests for film fogging.
6. Screen–film contact. This testing is to determine that optimal contact is maintained between the film, the screen and the cassette. A film is exposed with a copper mesh placed on top of the screen. No grid is used. Evaluation of the image quality is made.
7. Compression. Semiannual test of compression is made using a bathroom scale to measure pounds of compression. Compression force should range between 20 and 40 lb.
8. Repeat analysis. Determination of number and cause of repeated mammograms is made.
9. Viewbox viewing conditions. This is checked to be certain that viewbox and viewing conditions are optimal throughout the department. Viewboxes should be kept clean and illumination levels uniform.
10. Analysis of fixture retention in film. As an indicator of maintained quality, the quantity of residual fixture in process film is determined. Test solution is placed on film and compared with a standard to make this determination.
11. Visual checklist. This is done to determine that the mammography unit indicator light, displays, and locks are working appropriately. Visual inspection of the equipment is made.

Reporting and Documentation Findings

■ Clinical Findings

A complete breast examination involves a physical examination of the breast in addition to mammography. The physical examination begins with the *visual inspection*. The examiner physician inspects the breasts for asymmetry in size (anisomastia), changes in shape or contour, generalized skin changes (such as erythema, skin thickening, peau d'orange, dimpling, hyperpigmentation, or vascular anomalies), focal skin lesions (such as lipomas, atheromas, nevi, or warts), or scarring (localization and cause).

Palpation provides information on the structure of the glandular tissue (soft, thickened, nodular). It also provides information on possible differences between the breasts, namely location and consistency of lumps and the relationship of these lumps to the surrounding breast tissue, the skin (the Jackson sign), and to the pectoralis muscle. Palpation can also assess pain and mobility of the nipple and the region posterior to it, and it reveals palpable changes in the lymph drainage routes.

These findings should be recorded. Information from the findings on physical examination is useful in interpreting or tailoring the mammogram.

Documentation of any abnormalities will help to check (Figs. 3.**30a**, **b**):

– Whether an area of clinical abnormality (if present) was included on the mammogram
– Whether an imaging method is positive or negative in this area and whether this is reliable

The final report should include a discussion of specific questions addressed to the radiologist. It should include those clinical findings that are relevant to further assessment (e. g., "palpable mass, not visible on the mammogram, sonographically indeterminate, further workup, e. g., biopsy, necessary") or that may aid in interpreting diagnostic imaging studies (such as visible nevi or scars).

■ Mammography Report

The radiologist's role is to describe the radiologic morphology without using histologic terms. However, there are certain entities that

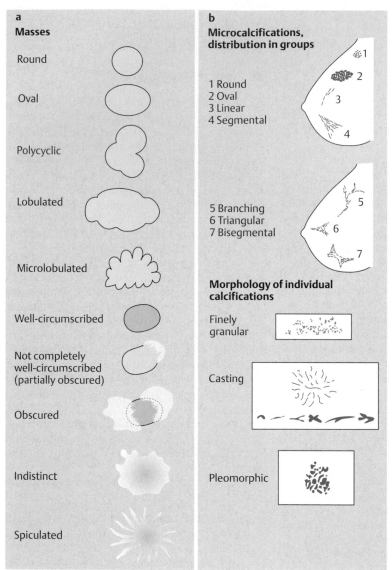

a
Masses

Round

Oval

Polycyclic

Lobulated

Microlobulated

Well-circumscribed

Not completely
well-circumscribed
(partially obscured)

Obscured

Indistinct

Spiculated

b
**Microcalcifications,
distribution in groups**

1 Round
2 Oval
3 Linear
4 Segmental

5 Branching
6 Triangular
7 Bisegmental

**Morphology of individual
calcifications**

Finely
granular

Casting

Pleomorphic

Fig. 3.**30 a** and **b**   Interpreting
and documenting findings
a Focal lesions
b Microcalcifications, in
clusters and solitary

have characteristic mammographic and sono-graphic findings allowing histologic diagnoses. These include lipoma, fibroadenolipoma, oil cysts, calcified fibroadenoma, and lymph nodes.

The radiologist must indicate the location of any significant mammographic finding based on the information from both mammographic views. This can be done by specifying the quadrant or, as is done with clinical findings, by the correspond-ing hour on the face of a clock.

The description of location should include the quadrant (see Appendix 2), whether the lesion is in the anterior, middle or posterior third of the breast, and the corresponding hour on the face of a clock.

Describing the location of the finding in the mammographic views, the radiologist records its position on an imaginary clock face. That means that a lesion located in the right upper outer breast would be between 9 and 12 o'clock, whereas one in the left upper outer breast would be between 12 and 3 o'clock. Findings located at 12 o'clock, 6 o'clock, 3 o'clock, 9 o'clock, or in the retroareolar region or the axillary tail are special cases. If only the craniocaudal and mediolateral oblique views are available, it is more difficult to

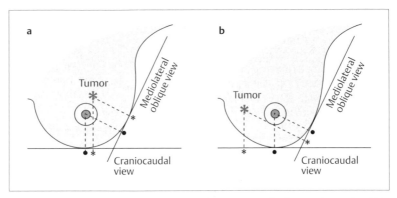

Fig. 3.**31 a** and **b** Localizing a tumor by means of the craniocaudal view and mediolateral oblique view. Aside from some uncertainty caused by the mobility of the breast parenchyma, the tumor can be localized by its different vertical projections in both views (**a**). It should be noted that a tumor located above and medial to the nipple can appear "below" the level of the nipple in the mediolateral oblique view (**b**).

define the correct position of the conspicuous finding. The quadrant can usually be determined by using a scheme as shown in Figure 3.**31**.

Importance of previous studies and follow-up: Whenever possible, the radiologist should compare the findings with previous mammograms (77). Comparison with mammograms that are 2 or more years old may be even more informative than the comparison with more recent mammograms. Discrete changes may go undetected with too short a follow-up period, whereas they become more obvious when older mammograms are compared, provided mammographic technique is comparable. Comparison with previous studies is useful for correct interpretation of asymmetries and for earliest possible detection of newly developing or increasing discrete densities or microcalcifications.

For example, a noncystic mass that has increased in size will require further workup even if it appears well circumscribed. Malignancy should be considered when a new mass develops, particularly in a postmenopausal patient. However, even an increasing or newly developing lesion cannot be considered as proof of a malignant process. New fibroadenomas can occur, particularly with hormone replacement therapy. Furthermore, hormone replacement can induce a changed parenchymal structure and an increased density.

Absence of a perceivable increase in size is not necessarily sufficient for excluding a malignant process, although it is true that absence of change with increasing time of follow-up makes a benign process more and more probable. It must,

however, be remembered that some cancers are slow growing and may show little or no change for several years. Also some malignant processes lead to retraction and even decrease in size.

Comparison with previous studies aids in detecting newly developing or increasing microcalcifications. However, the radiologist must be aware of other possible causes for a changed or stable mammographic appearance:

– Long-term stability of microcalcifications does not always exclude a malignant process
– Benign calcifications may increase or newly develop
– Ductal carcinoma in situ may remain unchanged for years or associated calcifications may only slowly increase over a period of years.

Given these considerations, careful analysis of morphology and arrangement of microcalcifications is even more important than follow-up.

The mammographic report should provide information about:

– Overall parenchymal pattern of the breasts
– Focal lesions, including their localization, size, density, and contour
– Calcifications, their localization, their distribution (presence of single or multiple) and their morphology
– Structural changes, including asymmetric densities and areas of architectural distortion

■ BI RADS Classification

Radiologists are encouraged to use in their reporting the terms recommended in the BI RADS (Breast Imaging Reporting and Data System) lexicon, published by the American College of Radiology.[78] The system has been developed to allow better standardization of mammography reporting and diagnosis.

■ Parenchymal Pattern

The overall composition of the breasts (for example, fatty, heterogeneously dense, extremely dense) should be described, as this will influence the sensitivity of mammography.

■ Masses

These are lesions seen on more than one view. A suspected mass seen only on a single view should be described as a density. A description of a mass should include:

– Size
– Contour
– Associated findings
– Presence or absence of associated calcifications
– Location
– An interval change

Descriptions for shape in the BI-RADS lexicon include:

– Oval or round
– Lobular
– Irregular
– Architectural distortion

Margins can be further described as:

– Circumscribed
– Microlobulated
– Obscured (partially hidden by adjacent structures)
– Indistinct or ill defined
– Spiculated

Density of a mass is described by comparing it with the density of normal breast tissue. It can be described as:

– High density
– Isodense or equal density
– Low density
– Fat-containing

Special cases which can be specifically described are:

– Solitary dilated duct
– Intramammary lymph node
– Asymmetric breast tissue
– Asymmetric focal density

The location of the lesion is indicated with respect to the quadrants or using a clock-face reference system (see preceding section). Any additional changes are also mentioned. These may include skin thickening or retraction, nipple retraction, or calcifications.

■ Calcifications

Localization, number, distribution pattern, and morphology of calcifications are described. Clusters of calcifications must be visualized in two planes to be regarded as genuine. If a "cluster" is visible in one plane only, it may not be a real cluster but caused by superimposition of single calcifications in different locations.

With respect to *localization,* a differentiation has to be made between calcifications outside the breast parenchyma (i. e., skin or subcutaneous tissue) and calcifications within the parenchyma.

If calcifications can be specifically characterized as benign, they should be described as such. These calcifications include:

– Skin calcifications
– Vascular calcifications
– Coarse, "popcorn" calcifications
– Large, rod-like calcifications
– Round calcifications—these can be described as punctate if they are smaller than 0.5 mm
– Centrally lucent calcifications
– Rim or (eggshell) calcifications—as seen in the walls of cysts
– Milk of calcium
– Suture calcifications
– Dystrophic calcifications

Calcifications classified as indeterminate include those that are amorphous or indistinct or fine granular. Calcifications suspicious for malignancy include pleomorphic or heterogeneous microcalcifications, as well as irregular linear, branching or casting calcifications.

The distribution of calcifications should be described as:

– Grouped or clustered: occupying less than 2 cm^3 of breast volume

Fig. 3.**32** Morphology of calcifications

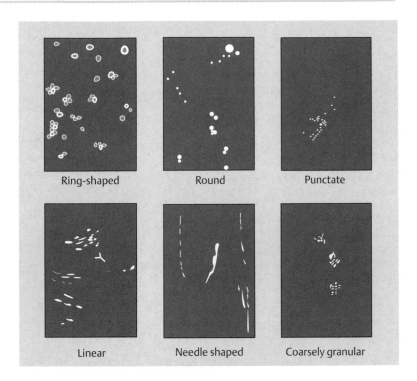

| Ring-shaped | Round | Punctate |
| Linear | Needle shaped | Coarsely granular |

- Segmental: occupying more than 2 cm³ but less than regional
- Regional: occupying a large volume of the breast, not in a ductal distribution, and not the entire breast
- Diffuse or scattered, distributed throughout the breast in a random fashion
- Linear, corresponding to a ductal pattern

Furthermore, a lobular distribution describes the presence of multiple punctate, generally round calcifications within a small area (2–3 mm). Such calcifications are usually located within the lobule and are arranged like a small morula or flower (rosette).

■ Associated Changes

These can be added to descriptions of masses or calcifications or can be used independently. They include:

- skin retraction
- skin thickening
- trabecular thickening
- nipple retraction
- axillary adenopathy
- architectural distortion
- increased vascularity

Additionally, the mammogram can show a diffuse increase in breast density. If previous studies are available, whether or not a finding represents an interval change, a new or increasing finding should be reported.

The final diagnosis should be categorized as:

Category 0: Additional imaging evaluation needed. This category should mainly be used in a screening situation and should rarely be used after full imaging workup. Recommendations of the ACR* for additional imaging include: use of spot compression, magnification or other special mammographic views, ultrasound, etc.

Category I: No findings, normal mammogram.

Category II: Focal benign findings, for which nothing further is required.

Category III: Probably benign finding, short interval follow-up suggested. A finding placed in this category should have a very high probability of being benign. It is not expected to change over the follow-up interval, but the radiologist would prefer to establish its stability.

Category IV: Indeterminate lesion, for which biopsy is recommended.

*ACR = American College of Radiology

Category V: Highly suggestive of malignancy and requiring biopsy.

If the mammogram is normal or benign, a recommendation regarding the interval for routine follow-up should be made. If a category III finding is diagnosed, the recommended interval for short-term follow-up (usually 6 months) should be explicitly stated. If a biopsy is recommended (usually category IV or V lesions), this should be clearly stated in the report. It should also be directly communicated to the referring physician and the patient. In the United States communication of results to the patient is required. It is advisable to document this communication in the written report. Finally, it may be helpful to give advice concerning the mode of histopathologic work-up (type of needle biopsy, open biopsy, preoperative wire localization).

■ **Interpreting and Documenting Screening Findings**

To reduce costs and save time, screening findings can be documented in a brief form to facilitate computer processing. The following categories (such as the BIRADS recommended in the United States for documenting findings) should be used: 1 = no pathologic findings, 2 = benign, 3 = probably benign, 4 = suggestive, and 5 = highly suggestive.

Categories 1 and 2 require only the standard follow-up examinations (in 1 or 2 years). Category 3 requires early follow-up examination (usually within 6 months). Category 4 means that a malignant process may be present and biopsy should be performed. Category 5 necessitates biopsy. The above implies that the number of false negative calls needs to be kept as low as possible for categories 1–3.[79] The BI RADS classification is certainly an important step forward toward improved standardization. However, continuous efforts and training are needed to further decrease interobserver variability.[80]Based on this knowledge screening programs may use double reading[81–83], which, however, only proves effective if at least one of the readers has special expertise.[84, 85]

Cost–benefit analysis is an important factor in evaluating screening mammography. A positive biopsy rate of 1 in 10 (malignant to benign), (i. e., positive predictive value of a biopsy recommendation of 10%) involves many unnecessary biopsies, i. e., biopsies of benign findings, which represent unacceptable costs. The other extreme, a rate of 1 : 1 (100% malignancies among the recommended biopsies), involves a significant risk of overlooking carcinomas, which would result in a high incidence of interval carcinomas because many indeterminate lesions, some of which are cancers, are not being sent for biopsy.

Screening involves more than documenting findings. It also requires documentation and evaluation of histologic results, of interval carcinomas and critical assessment of the positive predictive value, which should be in the 25–40% range, and of the accepted rate of so-called interval carcinomas. To assure that small cancers are appropriately diagnosed and not just large cancers for which diagnosis will not change the outcome, cancers diagnosed in a screening population should consist of more than 50% of diagnosed cancers as DCIS or invasive cancers ≤ 1,5 cm and less than 30% lymph node positive cancers.[86]

■ **Example Reports**

The asymptomatic patient: Compared to the previous examination of (date), the glandular tissue remains dense and nodular without evidence of focal lesions, calcifications, or structural changes.

Diagnosis: No mammographic evidence of malignancy. Follow-up examination in 1 year is recommended.

The patient with palpable findings: Corresponding to the palpable lesions is an ill-defined mass measuring 18 mm with pleomorphic microcalcifications in the left upper outer quadrant in the 2 o'clock axis in the mid-third of the breast. No associated findings.

Diagnosis: Highly suspicious mammographic findings corresponding to the palpable findings. Biopsy is required. No other focal lesion identified.

Another patient with a palpable mass: Dense and nodular parenchyma. Mammographic assessment is limited, no focal lesion identified. Additional ultrasound examination of the suspected mass is required for further evaluation.

Digital Mammography

Screen-film mammography is a high-resolution technique, enabling the radiologist to identify structures limited only by the size of the grains of silver in the film emulsion. However, screen-film imaging has limitations in contrast. The technique is optimized to display greater contrast among intermediate density tissues. This results in a limited dynamic range with limited contrast in high-density and low-density tissues, which can be most significant in the limited conspicuity of structures within dense breast tissue.

Inherent in recording images on film is the need to develop and store these images. Additionally, each examination generates only a single set of original images. Copied films invariably result in loss of information present on the original study and can compromise interpretation.

There are two possibilities of obtaining digital images:

1. Secondary digitization. This term describes production of a digital image from a screen-film mammogram.
2. Direct digital imaging. Here the image from the X-ray beam is directly captured on a digital image receiver.

Secondary digitization implies that the information recorded on a screen-film mammogram is transformed into a digital image. If performed with an appropriate scanner (sufficient light intensity, high resolution, high contrast, and sufficiently wide object range), good quality mammograms can be displayed with practically the same resolution and contrast as the original mammogram.[87, 88] However, no additional or new information can be gained (in over-exposed or under-exposed areas for example). Secondary image digitization might be useful for telemammographic consulting and has been used for the development and testing of programs for computer-assisted detection (CAD).[89, 90] Reproduction and storing of these images is possible with no loss of information. Since secondary digitization, however, is an additional step between mammogram and digital image, it does not offer all of the advantages and is more labor intensive than primary digital mammography.

Primary digital mammography captures the mammographic image electronically rather than on film using a screen. The information used to obtain the digital mammographic image is the same as that used in screen-film mammography and is the result of the passage of an X-ray beam through the breast. Thus, the physical characteristics of the breast that can be used for diagnosis are identical in these two types of images. Advantages and disadvantages of screen-film versus digital mammography concern visualization of these features (see pp. 72–73).

Primary digital image acquisition has already been successfully introduced for mammographic applications that require a small field of view:

– magnification mammography
– stereotactic imaging for interventions.

For this special purpose charge coupled devices (CCD) can be used, which allow a better resolution (up to about 10 line pairs) than digital luminescence or flat panel detectors. Furthermore, if magnification is used in addition, remaining limitations of the image detector may be completely overcome. Presently there is at least one system that allows a resolution up to 16 line pairs for spot views by combining a CCD receiver and magnification.

Fullfield digital mammography has proven to be technically more difficult. Several systems have so far been designed for fullfield digital mammography:[91, 92]

One type of digital mammography unit including the first approved unit are based on single-piece flat panel detector technology.[93] This technology offers very good image contrast and signal-to-noise, but is associated with a maximum detector resolution of presently only 5 lp/mm.

Another type of digital mammography equipment is based on an array of multiple CCDs.[94]

One manufacturer has combined such a receptor with a normal mammography unit. Another manufacturer has combined this receptor with a slot mammography unit.

This has the advantage of improved contrast without use of a grid, resulting in a decreased radiation dose. In this unit reduction of scattered radiation is achieved by a collimated moving slot. The CCDs provide high contrast and a much higher resolution than flat panel detectors, which does approach that of conventional mammography. However, the array is difficult to produce.

None of these systems has yet been approved. Phosphor storage screens can be used on conventional mammography units. The presently available phosphor storage screens allow a resolution of about 5 lp/mm and have not been generally accepted.[95,96] Another variant has been the combined use of phosphor storage screens and two-fold magnification. With this combination a resolution of about 10 lp/mm has been achieved.[97,98] However, interference of equipment geometry with patient positioning occurs with full-breast magnification. Furthermore, the radiation dose required for good-quality images is higher, largely due to the lower detection quantum efficiency (DQE[1]) of phosphor plates as compared to other receivers.[99] Lately the development of special high-resolution phosphor screens for breast imaging with up to 10 lp/mm resolution has been announced by one manufacturer and may become an interesting alternative to direct digital radiography.

Presently it is unclear which approach will lead to the best clinical results. In order to evaluate the significance of potential advantages and disadvantages of each system and of digital mammography compared to conventional screen film mammography, independent clinical studies are necessary.[100]

Digital mammography has several proven and potential advantages over film:[92]

- Digital imaging has a greater dynamic range than screen-film imaging. Due to the ability to window and level the image, subtle tissue-density differences that may be less evident on screen-film imaging can be appreciated with digital images. The wider dynamic range of digital imaging has a linear response that by far exceeds that of screen-film mammography.[91] This may make it possible to decrease the number of images required because of the necessity for retakes due to inappropriate penetration compromising tissue contrast. It may also cause some lesions that would otherwise not be visualized to be imaged mammographically. How this, as well as other advantages and limitations, may alter the success of screening studies to diagnose non-palpable breast cancer is as yet unknown.

- Postprocessing is necessary for adequate display of the full dynamic range of high contrast. Postprocessing refers mainly to optimized windowing and edge enhancement, enabled by various algorithms. However, more complicated techniques may also become feasible. They include dual-energy subtraction for improved visualization of microcalcifications,

digital subtraction, angiography for assessment of vascularization and tomosynthesis, which might help to overcome problems concerning superimposition.[101–102] The value of these additional possibilities is not yet known and requires fundamental investigation.

- The information from the examination is stored electronically and reproduced from the original image without loss of information. Information can be transferred electronically via telemammography so that monitoring and interpretation of the study can be done quickly at a site other than that where the image was obtained. Alternatively, these studies can be readily transferred elsewhere for an expert second opinion.

- Because the image is not stored on film, the need for processors, processor chemicals, and processor quality control may in the future be eliminated. Also, dark rooms, cassettes, and film will no longer be required. The savings from the elimination of film and film development are partially balanced by the higher cost of digital equipment, its maintenance, and the costs of digital storage. Nevertheless, in facilities in which other imaging procedures have been converted from film to picture archiving and communication systems (PACS), the use of full breast digital imaging could make it possible for a facility to completely eliminate the use of film.

- Finally, CAD can be readily applied to full breast digital imaging.[103–107] The digital image can automatically be fed through a computer system that can identify areas possibly representing carcinoma for special attention by the interpreting radiologist. This technology functionally operates as a second reading of the mammogram. Double reading of mammograms by radiologists has been shown to increase the detection rate for breast cancer of screening mammography by 9–10%.[108] It is possible, but not yet proven that CAD might have the same impact.[109] Application of this type of technology depends upon the ability of CAD systems to be reproducible. Additionally, the program may not identify more than an acceptable number of false–positive findings.

- Because CAD is only of value if it can detect carcinomas that would have been overlooked by the radiologist; it is not necessary for these systems to be able to identify every carcinoma that the radiologist sees. Expectations concerning the use of CAD have focused mainly on lesion detection. The usefulness of these systems for diagnosis appears currently to be more limited.[110, 111] This might be expected because of the ability of radiologists to characterize the level of suspicion of lesions they identify and because of the nonspecific nature of many mammographic findings.

Limitations of currently available full-breast digital technology include the following:

- A major limiting factor in the design of most digital systems[1], has been the problem of image resolution. Mammography requires both high contrast and extremely fine resolution to make detection of microcalcifications possible. Although not perfect[2,99] film meets these demands very well. For screen-film systems the limiting factor for resolution is the size of the silver grain in the film emulsion that makes it possible to obtain resolution of up to 16 line pairs per millimeter (lp/mm).[112] In digital imaging, resolution is determined by the size of the pixel in the digital detector. Resolution comparable to that of film would require a pixel size of 25 µm. Even when weighing specific advantages of digital imaging, such as greater dynamic range and postprocessing, optimum resolution for visualization of microcalcifications probably requires nevertheless a pixel size smaller than 50 µm. The sensors of some of today's fullfield mammography systems achieve a significantly lower resolution (see p. 71).
- Monitors must adequately display the high-resolution images. Those capable of 10 lp/mm resolution that can display the entire breast are currently too expensive for general medical use. Monitors with a resolution of 5 lp/mm (2000 x 2500 pixels) are also very expensive, but at least allow viewing of 10 lp/mm resolution on magnified parts of the breast.[91] Because of this problem digital images may need to be displayed on laser-printed film until high-resolution monitors are available at reasonable cost.
- While digital sensors are capable of displaying a dynamic contrast range of 12–14 bits, both the monitor and the laser printer truncate data displayed to 8–10 bits gray scale resolution. Sophisticated postprocessing is needed

to take advantage of the potentials of digital contrast capabilities. However, such postprocessing should not interfere with reading efficiency (both for reasons of cost-effectiveness and reader fatigue).
- Quality assurance programs for equipment, standardized examination technique, postprocessing, and documentation still need to be established or elaborated for digital imaging.[113]
- A general problem of high-resolution and high-contrast digital mammography is the large amount of data required. As compared to one CT or MR image (0.5–1.0 MByte), one single mammographic image (18 x 24 cm format)[3] requires up to 30 Mbyte (50 µm pixel size, 14 bit gray scale resolution). Assuming digital mammography would achieve this performance, we would then be faced with data storage and data transfer problems, and long transfer times and high costs would be associated with telemammographic transmission of whole breast studies.
- The costs for purchase and maintenance of digital systems presently exceed those of conventional systems by a factor of 3–5, which cannot be covered by reimbursement rates.

■ Summary

Digital imaging offers the potential of improved lesion detection based on the greater dynamic range of these systems compared with conventional screen-film imaging. This may make it possible to diagnose masses that are not apparent on film. However, there is a compromise in resolution with digital imaging. Very small structures, such as very fine microcalcifications, may be difficult—or in some cases even impossible—to appreciate with some digital mammography systems.

For imaging of a small field of view, resolution is not a problem, since high-resolution CCDs are available for this application. Maximum resolution and contrast can be achieved by magnification technique. The advantage of almost realtime imaging has become indispensable for stereotactically guided interventions.

Several designs exist for fullfield mammography, and it is difficult to predict which approach

---

[1] Description of the types of systems, see p. 71
[2] Imperfections of film mainly concern insufficient contrast within high or low density areas

[3] Formats for larger breasts (24×30 cm) are not yet available for digital mammography

will finally allow optimum use of potential advantages and offer a solution to the existing problems.

Despite the problems of existing technology, digital imaging is a promising technique. In the future it may allow elimination of film, processors, and processor chemicals. Storage space and file room support staff can be decreased. Telemammography will make it possible to send digital images of the breast to distant sites to monitor mammography off-site and to send images for second opinions. Because the reproduction of data from the original electronically-stored mammogram does not degrade the image, problems associated with loss of information on copied mammograms are also eliminated. Digital mammography also has the potential of being linked with CAD systems acting as second readers of mammograms, potentially increasing the detection rate of breast cancer at screening.

Problems that will require further investigation include resolution, image display (monitors and viewing), data reduction, handling, and quality assurance.

Galactography

■ Definition

Galactography refers to the examination of lactiferous ducts using a contrast medium.[114-116]

Injecting a water-soluble contrast medium permits mammographic imaging of the lactiferous duct system belonging to the excretory duct into which the needle is introduced. After the duct is filled with contrast medium, the breast is imaged in the craniocaudal and mediolateral planes. Oblique views or magnification mammograms may also be required. Galactography should only be performed in the presence of pathologic secretion, which itself makes it possible to detect the opening of the excretory duct. Absence of secretion precludes any ductal probing.

■ Indications

Galactography is indicated for the workup of pathologic discharge.

Pathologic discharge includes:

–   Spontaneous, nonmilky discharge (clear serous, cloudy, or brownish green) from a single or several ducts, usually unilateral. This does not include discharge that is expressed under firm pressure, since such a discharge can be provoked in many women.
–   Bloody discharge.
–   Discharge with suggestive cytologic findings (Groups IV or V).

Galactography is not indicated in the presence of:

–   Galactorrhea, i. e., milky discharge that is not due to pregnancy or breast feeding.
    Galactorrhea is always a sequelae of primary and/or secondary hyperprolactinemia and may occur bilaterally or unilaterally.
–   Bilateral, bloodless discharge from multiple ducts (serous or brownish green) without cytologic abnormality. This too can be the result of hormonal imbalance or duct ectasia with chronic inflammation.

■ Contraindications

Galactography is contraindicated in the presence of inflammation, which can be exacerbated by the procedure.

Hypersensitivity to contrast medium is a relative contraindication. The indication should be reviewed and the galactography only performed when clearly indicated and appropriate precautionary measures are taken (adrenaline, antihistamines, corticosteroids, or anesthesia standby). The physician may also consider intraoperative probing of the duct or, after injecting methylene blue, excision of the lactiferous duct without galactography.

■ Side Effects

Since a pathologic discharge is usually associated with duct ectasia, galactography can lead to *galactophoritis* or mastitis. This has only been observed in rare cases since the introduction of water-soluble contrast media.

Allergic reactions to contrast media are rare with galactography. Prophylactic antihistamine therapy may be considered in patients with known allergies to contrast media. Furthermore, the indication should be checked and appropriate precautionary measures taken (see previous section).

If a mild, acute reaction occurs, it can be treated with antihistamines. Severe reactions should be treated with intravenous cortisone and, in applicable cases, intravenous epinephrine, as with other contrast reactions.

If the injection pressure is too high or if too much contrast medium has been instilled, extravasation of contrast medium can occur, with contrast medium seen outside the duct system in breast parenchyma. In this setting lymphatic vessels may be imaged. The patient will usually perceive this as *pain*, although this has no serious effects other than insufficient or obscured visualization. The galactogram needs to be terminated, if this occurs. Contrast medium will be reabsorbed and the procedure can be repeated after a few days.

■ Procedure

Comfortable patient positioning and good lighting are important for this procedure. A magnifying lens or an eyepiece mounted on an eyeglass frame can be helpful in locating the excretory duct.

- Cytologic smears of the discharge may be taken before galactography.
- In the presence of profuse discharge, the breast should be expressed prior to galactography to remove coagulated blood or thickened secretion that might interfere with contrast medium injection or appear as filling defects that can lead to misdiagnosis.
- After disinfecting the nipple and the surrounding skin, the physician carefully inserts the probe into the nipple, first pressing out a small drop of secretion to better locate the opening of the secreting lactiferous sinus. Once the orifice is located, the physician will be able to insert the cannula without any difficulty. Use a thin (25–30 gauge), blunt, short cannula (such as the lymphography cannula or galactography catheter, or a 30-gauge sialography needle). Using a thin cannula minimizes the necessity for painful dilatation of the orifice. The tubing connecting the cannula to the syringe containing the contrast medium should be filled with contrast medium and free of air bubbles before positioning in the duct.
- Local anesthesia may be applied to the nipple in particularly anxious patients. After applying a topical anesthetic, the physician inserts a thin needle next to the areola and injects a local anesthetic behind the areola. After about 10 minutes, the nipple is completely insensitive, and the physician can begin the cannulation.
- Using a nonionic contrast medium is recommended because of its very low incidence of allergic reactions and particularly good patient tolerance. Nonionic contrast media have the added advantage of causing the least amount of unpleasant sensations during the examination.
- After the canula has been positioned in the duct, it can be secured in place with adhesive tape.
- Next, 0.1–0.5 ml of contrast medium without air bubbles is injected slowly into the duct.
- A helpful procedure is to compress the excretory duct with a swab during mammography until the moment of exposure. If the ductal system is only mildly dilated, it can be closed with vaseline or 4% collodion.
- Next, mammograms are obtained in two planes with additional magnification mammograms if necessary.
- It is important to use only moderate compression in galactography. Excessive compression can displace secretion from the ducts in the central breast (where compression is best) and simulate filling defects.
- If the ductal system is not sufficiently filled with contrast medium, the filming is repeated using a slightly greater quantity of contrast medium.
- Insufficient filling with contrast medium can be due to debris or coagulated blood within the ductal system. If this is the case, the ductal system should be expressed and again injected with contrast medium.
- Care should be taken not to introduce any air when injecting the contrast medium. If air has been inadvertently injected, the bubbles can be identified by their bead-like arrangement along the superior margin of the lactiferous duct in the lateral plane. For this reason, we prefer to use the 90° lateral view as the second imaging plane as opposed to the mediolateral oblique view. If any doubt remains, air bubbles can be identified by their mobility after a second injection.

■ Difficulties and Possible Solutions

Unsuccessful *cannulation* may be due to *an intraductal mass located near the nipple*. This will cause rapid reflux of the injected contrast medium.

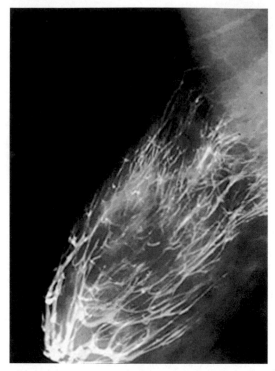

Fig. 3.**33** Normal galactogram. The segment of ducts belonging to the injected lactiferous duct will appear as a tree-shaped structure that extends from the excretory duct and divides into increasingly narrower branches towards the periphery

Sometimes the excretory ducts are extremely narrow or go into spasm when cannulation is attempted. In this case, we recommend applying a warm moist towel to relax the muscles.

Lifting the nipple helps extend a *kinked lactiferous duct* behind the nipple and facilitates cannulation.

Galactography is usually difficult in *retracted nipples.* Here, an attempt should be made to pull the nipple outward or spread out the areola with two fingers so that the orifice becomes visible.

■ **Findings**

Pathologic secretion can be caused by chronic inflammation, papilloma, papillomatosis, or, rarely, an intraductal or invasive carcinoma.

In Kindermann's material (1694 galactographies), no intraductal mass but only duct ectasia was present in 65% of the cases. Biopsies were done in 35% of all cases, and malignant tumors were found in only 4.3%. The majority of patho-

logic findings were caused by papillomas or papillomatosis. With bloody secretion, the incidence of malignancy increased to as high as 37%.[116]

The principal findings are:
- Normal ductal system (Fig. 3.**33**).
- Duct ectasia (Figs. 3.**34a** and **b**). This condition involves more or less pronounced distension of the ducts up to cystic distension. It occurs primarily in the presence of fibrocystic changes and subacute or chronic plasma cell mastitis (a preliminary stage of the familar calcifying plasma cell mastitis) or secretory disease.
- Filling defects or cutoff of the duct (Figs. 3.**35a** and **b**). Once filling defects due to debris are excluded, inflammatory changes or proliferative mastopathy should be considered, including papillomatosis, papilloma, and carcinoma.

Galactography is not suitable for diagnosing the nature of the filling defect. These changes require excision and histopathologic examination. However, galactography can be useful in localizing the site of the lesion causing the nipple discharge.

■ **Preoperative Marking of Galactographic Findings**

There are essentially two ways of marking nonpalpable galactographic findings:

1. The physician can perform repeat galactography of the suspicious duct immediately preoperatively. The duct is filled with a mixture of 50% contrast medium and 50% methylene blue. Since methylene blue diffuses rapidly, the blue-dyed ductal system must be excised shortly after injection.
2. After a repeat galactography with contrast and methylene blue has been performed, the galactographically suspicious area is marked under mammographic guidance (see mammographic localization procedure, Chapter 8). If a wire or carbon solution (the latter is only approved in several European countries) is used for marking, timing of surgery directly after the marking (with a well-positioned and fixed wire) is not as critical as it is if methylene blue is used.

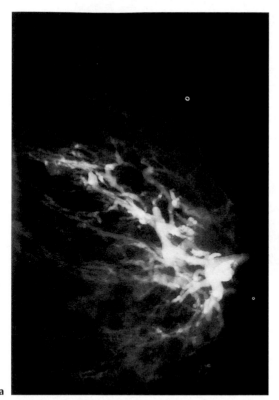

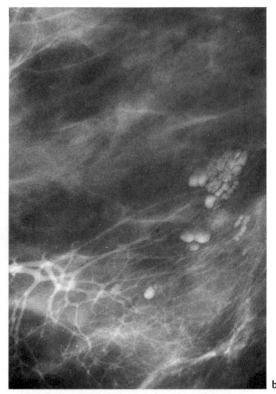

Fig. 3.**34a** and **b**
a Duct ectasia. No evidence of an intraductal mass

b Besides normal ducts a conglomerate of small cysts as well as several further small cysts are filled with contrast agent

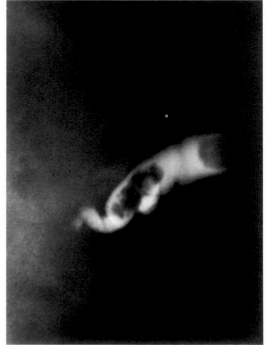

Fig. 3.**35a** and **b**
a Intraductal masses lead to isolated or multiple filling defects, i. e., the contrast medium flows around the intraductal mass in an arc-shaped pattern

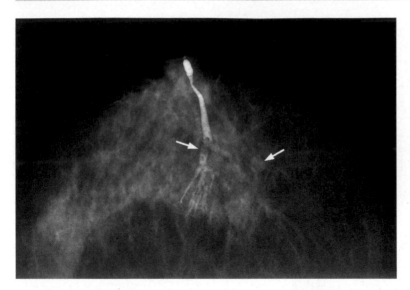

Fig. 3.**35 b** Multiple round filling defects in a distended lactiferous duct, histologically confirmed papillomatosis. The small, smooth-contoured, focal lesion in the parenchyma also corresponds to a papilloma

■ **Summary**

Galactography provides a simple and very reliable contrast-medium examination for the localization of intraductal masses. It may also help to better assess the extent of these lesions. Only when nipple discharge is due to duct ectasia can a definitive diagnosis be made. Biopsy is indicated for any intraductal mass detected by galactography because this imaging modality cannot reliably distinguish between benign and malignant filling defects.

■ **Appendix: Sonographic Imaging of Lactiferous Ducts**

Initial work has been done in using high-frequency ultrasound transducers in diagnosing intraductal masses. The higher resolution permits better sonographic imaging of ducts, particularly those located close to the nipple, than before. Sometimes it is possible to detect even small intraductal masses (Figs. 3.36–3.40 a and b). However, since sonography as a cross-sectional imaging modality cannot reliably visualize every segment of a winding duct and since it will not allow the necessary overview of the complete tree of a secreting ductal system, it cannot replace galactography.

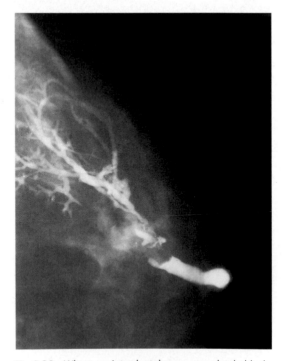

Fig. 3.**36** Where an intraductal mass completely blocks the respective lactiferous duct, the galactogram will show a filling defect with partial truncation of the duct

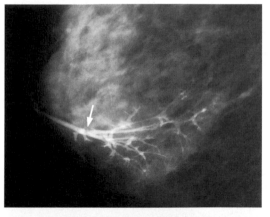

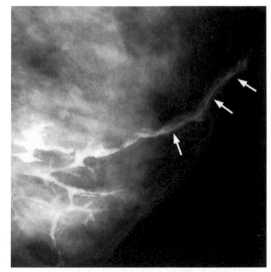

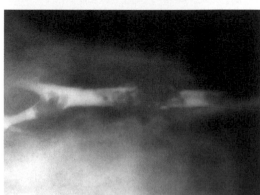

Fig. 3.**37 a–c** Various intraductal processes are shown
a Marginal filling defects that interrupt the contour of the wall: ductal carcinoma in situ
b Tiny round filling defects arranged like a string of beads in a main excretory duct
c Multiple irregular filling defects with loss of the contour of the wall: papillomatosis in transition to an invasive carcinoma

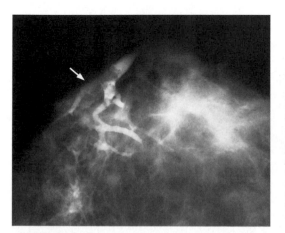

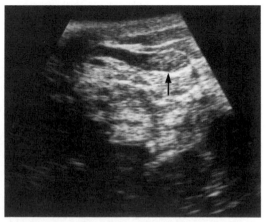

Fig. 3.**38 a** and **b**
a Lobulated filling defect in an ectatic lactiferous duct: papillomatosis

b Good sonographic image (13.5-MHz technique) of a distended duct containing a tiny hyperechoic mass

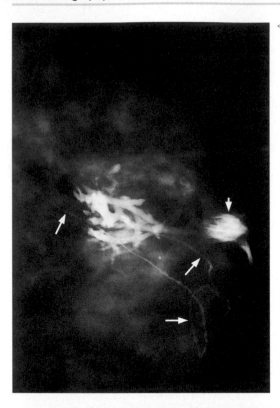

◁ Fig. 3.**39** Extravasation of constrast medium (short arrow) and several fine winding lymph vessels (long arrow)

Fig. 3.**40 a** and **b**
a Lobulated focal density is shown laterally on this mediolateral mammographic view
b Galactography revealed this to be a small convoluted cyst (arrow). Air bubbles in the lactiferous duct system can be identified by their uniform round shape and their varying localization on several views. On the mediolateral view, they can be identified by their localization along the superior wall of the ducts (double arrows). Leakage of contrast is seen in the inferior aspect of the breast
▽

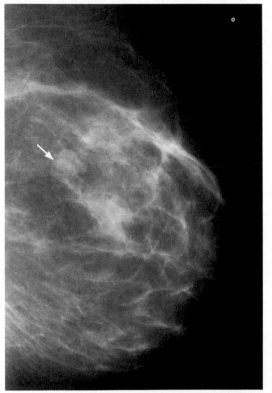

a

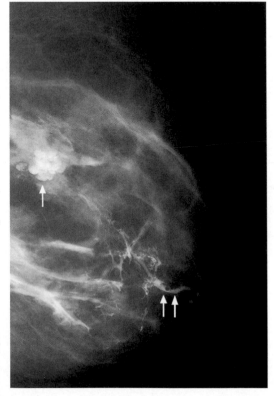

b

Pneumocystography

■ **Definition**

Pneumocystography refers to mammographic imaging of an aspirated cyst that has been filled with air. It has been used to diagnose and to treat cysts, i. e., bring about its involution.[117, 118]

■ **Indications**

With increasing capabilities of ultrasound, the application of pneumocystography for workup of *sonographic findings that are suspicious but inconclusive for cysts* decreases (uncertain differentiation between hyperechoic debris in the cyst, intracystic mass, and a hypoechoic solid mass). If a solid mass is suspected, core biopsy or excisional biopsy are usually indicated instead.

The use of pneumocystography for treatment of symptomatic cysts is controversial. Since large cysts can cause a sensation of pressure and pain, decompressing the cyst will relieve these symptoms. However, frequently after decompression of one cyst others will appear.

■ **Not Indications**

– Cysts with sonographically detected *irregularities in their walls* or intracystic masses. For these cases, pneumocystography has been replaced by biopsy.
  Aspirating a cyst containing a small intracystic mass can even be detrimental since surgery may become impossible if the mass is no longer palpable or visible in mammographic and sonographic images after aspiration and air absorption. However, this sort of complicated cyst will generally fill again if a papilloma or carcinoma is actually present, and the cyst will then again become visible for preoperative marking (possibly even palpable) in about 2 to 4 weeks.
– Unequivocal sonographic diagnosis of *asymptomatic* cysts. These cysts need no further assessment.

■ **Contraindications**

– Acute inflammation.
– Coagulopathies or anticoagulant therapy.

■ **Side Effects**

– Puncturing the skin is only slightly painful. Puncturing a hardened, chronically inflamed cyst wall may be painful. Filling the cyst with air sometimes causes painful tension in the breast.
– Inflammatory reaction after aspiration is extremely rare when the skin has been properly disinfected and sterile procedure has been observed.
– Hematomas due to injury of a vascular structure are rare but possible. The indication must be carefully checked in patients with coagulatory disorders or on anticoagulant therapy or aspirin.
– Pneumothorax has been observed in very rare cases in which the pleura was perforated while attempting to aspirate a deep cyst. For this reason, the needle should always be introduced parallel to the chest wall and never perpendicular to it. Perform the aspiration under sonographic guidance.

■ **Procedure**

● Palpable lumps can be aspirated without guidance.
● Aspiration under sonographic guidance is recommended for nonpalpable or confluent cysts. Aspiration under sonographic guidance is generally performed with the patient supine. In some cases with large palpable cysts, it is also possible to aspirate the cyst while the patient is seated. The fluid will collect at the bottom of the cyst and thus can be completely aspirated.
● Aspirate after disinfecting the skin. Select a needle that is not too thin (a 20-gauge needle will usually be sufficient) since the contents of the cyst may vary in viscosity.
● Empty the cyst completely. With the needle still in place, attach a new syringe and insufflate the cyst with a slightly smaller volume of air than the volume of fluid that was removed (note that the air will expand at body temperature). When doing so, the needle should not be dislocated to avoid perforating the opposite wall with the needle outside the cyst during subsequent insufflation.

- The contents of the cyst can be clear and serous, or it can be greenish, brownish, black, or cloudy, or tinged with blood following aspiration. If the cyst contains older blood (as opposed to fresh blood from an iatrogenic injury), excision should be considered to determine its cause.
- The rarely performed diagnostic pneumocystography (to differentiate between intracystic debris or masses, which is only used in sonographically inconclusive studies) should be performed in two imaging planes since smaller wall irregularities may not be visible when projected en face.

■ **Findings**

When the cyst is completely empty, it will appear as a well-circumscribed round or lobulated, thin-walled transparency (Figs. 3.**41 a–c**). Air inadvertently injected into the parenchyma will appear as transparent strips or bubbles of varying length on the mammogram (Fig. 3.**42**).

If the cyst is not completely empty, an air–fluid level may be visible (Fig. 3.**43**) or foam may appear showing up as multiple transparent bubbles. While this is not a pathologic sign, it may interfere with the diagnostic process.

Pneumocystography cannot reliably distinguish between benign and malignant intracystic masses. Overall, intracystic carcinomas are less frequent than papillomas. Like papillomas, they mammographically project into the lumen of the insufflated cyst (see Chapter 11).

Any suspicious intracystic mass is an indication for biopsy. Negative cytologic examination of the aspirated fluid should not prevent biopsy because false negative results are possible in the presence of necrotic material.

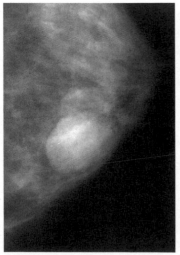

a

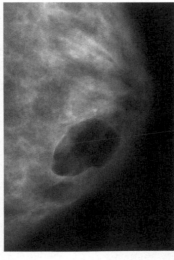

b

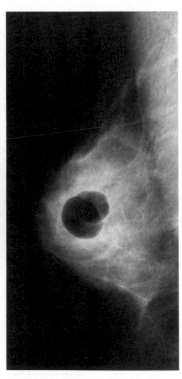

c

Fig. 3.**41 a–c**
a Mammography: Oval focal lesion with a halo, in the inferior half of the breast
b Pneumocystography: After aspiration and air insufflation, an oval, lobulated bright area with a faint halo is visible
c Pneumocystography of two communicating cysts

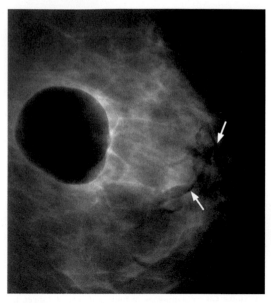

Fig. 3.**42** Curvilinear radiolucencies (arrow) in the parenchyma after pneumocystography, caused by interstitial air

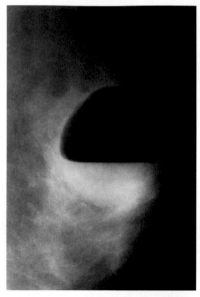

Fig. 3.**43** An air–fluid level is visible in the cyst that has not been completely emptied

■ Summary

If applied diagnostically, pneumocystography is used to verify the diagnosis of a cyst by aspirating it in the rare case of sonographically inconclusive findings. It may sometimes be used to decompress a painful cyst.

The introduction of air is believed by some to prevent refilling of the cyst by facilitating shrinkage of the cyst walls. If pneumocystography shows no pathologic findings, standard follow-up examinations will be sufficient.

When bloody fluid is aspirated from the cyst yet cytologic results are negative and pneumocystography shows no pathologic findings, a short interval (e. g., 3 months) follow-up sonographic examination may be desirable.

■ References

1 Kopans DB. Mammography screening for breast cancer. Cancer. 1993;72:1809
2 Bird RE, Wallace TW, Yankaskas BC. Analysis of cancers missed at screening mammography. Radiology. 1992;184:613
3 Van Dijck JAAM, Verbeek ALM, Hendricks JHCL, Holland R. The current detectability of breast cancer in a mammographic screening program. Cancer. 1993;72:1933
4 Sickles EA, Ominski SH, Sollitto RA et al. Medical audit of a rapid throughput mammography screening practice: methodology and results of 27 114 examinations. Radiology. 1990;175:323
5 Rosenberg RD, Hunt WC, Williamson MR et al. Effects of age, breast density, ethnicity, and estrogen replacement therapy on screening mammographic sensitivity and cancer stage at diagnosis: review of 183,134 screening mammograms in Albuquerque, New Mexico. Radiology. 1998;209:511–8
6 van Gils CH, Otten JD, Verbeck AL et al. Effect of mammographic breast density on breast cancer screening performance: a study in Nijmegen, The Netherlands. J Epidemiol Community Health. 1998;52:267–71
7 D'Orsi CJ. To follow or not to follow, that is the question. Radiology. 1992;184:306
8 Knutzen AM, Gisvold JJ. Likelihood of malignant disease for various categories of mammographically detected nonpalpable breast lesions. Radiology. 1993;189:927
9 Bjurstam N. Early carcinoma: the great mimick. Report of the Nicer Breast Imaging Course, Scandinavian Society of Mammography, August 24-28, 1994

10 Meyer J, Timothy J, Stomper P, Sonnenfield M. Biopsy of occult breast lesions: analysis of 1261 abnormalities. JAMA. 1990;263:2341
11. Elmore JG, Barton MB, Moceri VM et al. Ten-year risk of false positive screening mammograms and clinical breast examinations. N Engl J Med. 1995;338:1089–96
12. Hunt KA, Sickles EA. Effect of obesity on screening mammography: outcomes analysis of 88,346 consecutive examinations. AJR. 2000;174:1251–5
13. Liberman L, Abramson AF, Squires FB et al. The breast imaging reporting and data system: positive predictive value of mammographic features and final assessment categories. AJR. 1998;17:35–40
14 Rubin E. Critical pathways in the analysis of breast masses. Radiographics. 1995;15:925
15 Dershaw DD, Eddens G, Liberman L, Deutch BM, Abramson AF. Sonographic and clinical findings in women with palpable breast disease and negative mammography. Breast Dis. 1995;8:13–17
16 Boyd NF, Jong RA, Yaffe MJ et al. Critical appraisal of the Canadian National Breast Cancer Screening Study. Radiology. 1993;189:661
17 Aichinger H, Dierker J, Säbel M, Joite-Barfuß S. Bildqualität und Dosis in der Mammographie. Electromedica. 1994;62:7
18 Küchler A, Friedrich M. Fortschritte in der Mammographiethechnik – Bimetall-Anodenröhre und selektive Filtertechnik. Fortschr Rontgenstr. 1993;159:91
19 Christensen EE, Curry TS, Dowdey JE. An introduction to the physics of diagnostic radiology. Philadelphia: Lea Febinger 1978
20 Kimme-Smith C, Bassett LW, Gold RH. Workbook for quality mammography. Williams & Wilkins: Baltimore; 1992
21 Barnes GT, Brezovich IA. Contrast: effect of scattered radiation. In: Logan W W, Muntz EP eds. Reduced dose mammography. New York: Masson: 1979
22 Ranallo FN. Physics of screen–film mammography. In: Peters ME, Voegeli DR, Scanlan KA, eds. Handbook of breast imaging. New York: Churchill Livingstone; 1989:25
23 Friedrich M. Technik und Ergebnisse der Mammographie. Radiologe. 1993;33:243
24 Young KC, Wallis MG, Blansky RG, Moss SM. Influence of number of views and mammographic film density on the detection of invasive cancers: results from the NHS Breast Screening Programme. Br J Radiol. 1997;70:482–8
25 Frederick EE, Squillante MR, Cirignano LJ et al. Accurate automatic exposure controller for mammography: design and performance. Radiology. 1991;178:393
26 McKinney WE. Radiographic processing and quality control. Philadelphia: JB Lippincott; 1988
27 Yaffe MJ. Physics of mammography: image recording process. Radiographics. 1990;10:341
28 Kimme-Smith C, Rothschild PA, Bassett LW et al. Mammography film processor temperature, development time and chemistry; effect on dose, contrast and noise. AJR. 1989;152:35
29 Haus AG. Effects of geometric unsharpness in mammography and breast xeroradiography. In: Logan WW, Muntz WW, eds. Reduced dose mammography: New York: Massone; 1979
30 American College of Radiology. Recommended specifications for new mammography equipment. Screen-film x-ray systems, image receptors and film processors. Reston: American College of Radiology; 1995
31 Aichinger H, Joite-Barfuß S, Marhoff P. Die Belichtungsautomatik in der Mammographie. Electromedica. 1990; 58:61
32 Barnes GT. Mammography equipment: compression, scatter control and automatic exposure control. In: Haus AG, Yaffe MJ, eds. Syllabus: A categorical course in physics: Technical aspects of breast imaging, 3rd ed. Oak Brook: RSNA Publications; 1994:75
33 Friedrich M. Neue Entwicklungstendenzen der Mammographietechnik: Die Rastermammographie. Fortschr Rontgenstr. 1978;128:207
34 Dershaw DD, Masterson ME, Malik S, Cruz NM. Mammography using an ultrahigh strip density, stationary, focused grid. Radiology. 1985;156:541–544
35 Barnes GT, Moreland RF, Yester MV, Witten DM. The scanning grid: a novel and effective bucky movement. Radiology. 1980;135:765
36 Laubenberger T. Technik der medizinischen Radiologie. 6. Aufl. Köln: Dt Ärzteverlag; 1990
37 Yaffe MJ. Digital mammography. In: Haus AG, Yaffe MJ, eds. Syllabus: A categorical course in physics. Technical aspects of breast imaging. Oak Brook: RSNA Publications 1994:275
38 Baral E, Larrson LE, Mattson B. Breast cancer following irradiation of the breast. Cancer. 1977;40:2905–10
39 Boice JD, Land CE, Shore RE, Norman JE, Tokunaga M. Risk of breast cancer following low-dose radiation exposure. Radiology. 1979;131:589–97
40 Howe GR. Epidemiology of radiogenic breast cancer. In: Boice JD, Fraumeni JF, eds. Radiation carcinogenesis: epidemiology and biological dignificance. New York: Raven; 1984:119–30
41 Hrubec Z, Boice JD, Monson RR, Rosenstein R. Breast cancer after multiple chest fluoroscopies: second follow-up of Massachusetts women with tuberculosis. Cancer Res. 1989;49:229–34
42 Mettler FA, Hempelmann LH, Dutton AM, Pofer JW, Toyooka ET, Ames WR. Breast neoplasms in women treated with x-rays for acute postpartum mastitis: a pilot study. J Natl Cancer Inst. 1969;43:803–11
43 Miller AB, Howe GR, Sherman, GJ et al. Mortality from breast cancer after irradiation during fluoroscopic examinations in patients being treated for tuberculosis. N Engl J Med. 1989;321:1285–9
44 Shore RE, Hildreth N, Woodard ED, Dvoretsky P, Hempelmann L, Pasternack B. Breast cancer among women given x-ray therapy for acute postpartum mastitis. J Natl Cancer Inst. 1986;77:689–96
45 Kato H, Schull WJ. Studies of the mortality of A-bomb survivors. 7. Mortality, 1950–1978: I. Cancer mortality. Radiat Res. 1982;90:395–432
46 McGregor DH, Land CE, Choi K et al. Breast cancer incidence among atomic bomb survivors, Hiroshima and Nagasaki, 1950–1969. J Natl Cancer Inst. 1977;59:799–811
47 Preston DL, Kato H, Kopecky KJ, Fujita S. Studies of the mortality of A-bomb survivors. 8. Cancer mortality, 1950–1982. Radiat Res. 1987;111:151–78
48 Preston DL, Pierce DA. The effect of changes in dosimetry on cancer mortality risk estimates in atomic bomb survivors. Radiat Res. 1988;114:437–66
49 Shimizu Y, Kato H, Schull WJ, Preston DL, Fujita S, Pierce DA. Studies of the mortality of A-bomb survivors. 9. Mortality, 1950–1985: I. Comparison of risk coefficients for site-specific cancer mortality based on DS86 and T65 DR shielded kerma and organ doses. Radiat Res. 1989;118:502–24
50 Tokunaga M, Land CE, Yamamoto T et al. Incidence of female breast cancer among atomic bomb survivors, Hiroshima and Nagasaki, 1950–1980. Radiat Res. 1987;112:243–72

51 United Nations Scientific Committee on the Effects of Atomic Radiation. Sources and Effects of Ionizing Radiation. Annex C, Medical Radiation Exposures. 1993 report to the General Assembly. 1993 Vienna, Austria.

52 NRPB: Estimates of late radiation risks to the UK population. Documents of the NRPB. 1993: Vol. 4. No. 4: 66

53 National Academy of Sciences/National Research Council. Health effects of exposure to low levels of ionizing radiation. BEIR V. Washington, DC: National Academy Press, 1990.

54 Mettler FA, Upton AC, Kelsey CA et al. Benefits versus risks from mammography: a critical reassessment. Cancer. 1996;77:903–9

55 United Nations Scientific Committee on the Effects of Atomic Radiation (UNSCEAR). Epidemiological studies of radiation carcinogenesis. Report to the General Assembly. 1994 Vienna, Austria

56 Feig SA, Ehrlich SM. Estimation of radiation risk from screening mammography: recent trends and comparison with expected benefits. Radiology. 1990;174;638–47

57 Jung H. Mammography and radiation risk. Roe Fo. 1998,169:336–43

58 Feig SA, Hendrick RE. Radiation risk from screening mammography of women aged 40–49 years. J Natl Cancer Inst Monogr. 1997;22:119–24

59 Law J. Cancers detected and induced in mammographic screening: new screening schedules and younger women with family history. Br J Radiol. 1997;70:62–9

60 Tabar L, Dean PB. Optimum mammography technique: the annotate cookbook approach. Admin Radiol. 1989;54

61 Bassett LW, Bunnell D, Jahanshahi R et al. Breast cancer detection: one versus two views. Radiology. 1987;165:95

62 Muir BB, Kirkpatrick A, Roberts MM, Duffy SW. Oblique view mammography: adequacy for screening. Radiology. 1984;151:39

63 Eklund GW, Cardenosa G. The art of mammographic positioning. Radiol Clin North Am. 1992; 30:21

64 Logan WW, Janus J. Use of special mammographic views to maximize radiographic information. Radiol Clin North Am. 1987;25:953

65 Sickles EA. Practical solutions to common mammographic problems: tailoring the examination. AJR. 1988; 151:31

66 Berkowitz JE, Gatedwood OMB, Gayler BW. Equivocal mammographic findings: evaluation with spot compression. Radiology. 1989;171:369

67 Funke M, Breiter N, Hermann K et al. Magnification survey and spot view mammography with a new microfocus x-ray unit: detail resolution and radiation exposure. Eur Radiol. 1998;8:386–90

68 Eklund GW, Busby RC, Miller SH et al. Improved imaging of the augmented breast. AJR. 1988; 151:469

69 Fajardo LL, Jackson PJ, Hunter TB. Interventional procedures in diseases of the breast: needle biopsy, pneumocystography, and galactography. Am J Radiol. 1992; 1231-8

70 Rose A Osborne J, Wright G, Billson V. Is what you see what you get?
Breast specimen handling revisted: Australas Radiol. 1991; 35: 145

71 Samuels T, Kerenyi N, Taylor G. Practical aspect of mammographic pathological correlation: experience with needle localisation. Can Assoc Radiol J. 1990; 47: 127

72 Graham RA, Homer MJ, Sigler CJ. The efficacy of specimen radiography in evaluating surgical margins of impalpable breast carcinoma. AJR. 1994;162:33–6

73 Strauss KJ, Rossi RP. Specification, acceptance testing and quality control of mammography imaging equipment. In: Haus AG, Yaffe MJ, eds. Syllabus: A categorical course in physics. Technical aspects of breast imaging. Oak Brook: RSNA Publications; 1994:275

74 Yaffe M, Hendrick RE et al. Recommended specifications for mammography equipment. Reston: American College of Radiology; 1993

75 Linver MN, Osuch JR, Brenner RJ, Smith RA. The mammography audit: a primer for the Mammography Quality Standards Act (MQSA). AJR. 1995; 165: 19–25

76 Gray JE. Mammographic quality control for the technologist and the medical physicist as consultant to the technologist. In: Haus AG, Yaffe MJ, eds. Syllabus: A categorical course in physics. Technical aspects of breast imaging. Oak Brook: RSNA Publications; 1994:275

77 Harvey JA, Fajardo LL, Innis CA. Previous mammograms in patients with impalpable breast carcinoma: retrospective versus blinded interpretation: AJR. 1993; 161: 1167

78 Breast Imaging Reporting and Data System (BI-RADS™) 3rd ed. Reston, Va: © American College of Radiology; 1998

79 Lacquement MA, Mitchell D, Hollingsworth AB. Positive predictive value of the Breast Imaging Reporting and Data System. J Am Coll Surg. 1999;189:34–40

80 Berg WA, Campassi C, Langenberg P, Sexton MJ. Breast Imaging Reporting and Data System. Inter- and intraobserver variability in feature analysis and final assessment. AJR. 2000;174:1769–77

81 Blanks RG, Wallis MG, Given-Wilson RM. Observer variability in cancer detection during routine repeat (incident) mammographic screening in a study of two versus one view mammography. J Med Screen. 1999;6:152–8

82 Elmore JG, Wells CK, Lee CH et al. Variability in radiologists' interpretations of mammograms. N Engl J Med. 1994;331:1493–9

83 Johnston K, Brown J. Two view mammography at incident screens: cost effectiveness analysis of policy options. BMJ. 1999;319:1097–102

84 Anttinen J, Pamilo M, Soiva M, Roiha M. Double reading of mammography screening films—one radiologist or two? Clin Radiol. 1993;48:414–21

85 Taplin SH, Rutter CM, Elmore JG et al. Accuracy of screening mammography using single versus independant double interpretation. AJR. 2000;174:1257–62

86 Tabar L, Fagerberg G, Duffy SW, et al. Update of the Swedish two-county program of mammographic screening for breast cancer. Radiol Clin North Am 1992;30:187–210

87 Murphy JM, O'Hare NJ, Wheat D et al. Digitized mammograms: a preliminary clinical evaluation and the potential for telemammography. J Telemed Telecare. 1999;5:193–7

88 Chan HP, Niklason LT, Ikeda DM et al. Digitization requirements in mammography: effects on computer-aided detection of microcalcifications. Med Phys. 1994;21:1203–11

89 Leichter I, Lederman R, Bamberger P et al. The use of an interactive software program for quantitative characterization of microcalcifications on digitized film-screen mammograms. Invest Radiol 1999;34 394–400

90 Zheng B, Chang YH, Wang XH et al. Feature selection for computerized mass detection in digitized mammograms by using a genetic algorithm. Acad Radiol. 1999;6:327–32

91 Pisano ED, Yaffe MJ, Hemminger BM et al. Current status of full-field digital mammography. Acad Radiol. 2000;7:266–80

92 Feig SA, Yaffe MJ. Digital mammography. Radiographics. 1998;18:893–901

93 Muller S. Full-field digital mammography designed as a complete system. Eur J Radiol. 1999;31:25–34

94 Tesic MM, Piccaro MF, Munier B et al. Full field digital mammography scanner. Eur J Radiol. 1999;31:2–17

95 Gaspard-Bakhach S, Dilhuydy MH, Bonichon F et al. ROC analysis comparing screen film mammography and digital mammography. J Radiol. 2000;81:133–9

96 Kheddache S, Thilander-Klang A, Lanhede B et al. Storage phosphor and film-screen mammography: performance with different mammographic techniques. Eur Radiol. 1999;9:591–7

97 Fiedler E, Aichinger U, Bohner C et al. Image quality and radiation exposure in digital mammography with storage phosphor screens in a magnification technic. Rofo 1999;171:60–4

98 Funke M, Netsch T, Breiter N et al. Computer-assisted visualization of digital mammography images. Rofo Fortschr Geb Rontgenstr Neuen Bildgeb Verfahr. 1999;171:359–63

99 Säbel M, Aichinger U, Schulz-Wendtland R et al. Digitale Vollfeld-Mammographie: Physikalische Grundlagen und klinische Aspekte. Röntgenpraxis. 1999;52:171–7

100 Pisano ED. Current Status of Full-Field Digital Mammography. Radiology. 2000;21:26–8

101 Niklason LT, Christian BT, Niklason LE, et al. Digital tomosynthesis in breast imaging. Radiology. 1997;205:399–406

102 Webber RL, Underhill HA, Hemler PF et al. Nonlinear algorithm for task-specific tomosynthetic image reconstruction. In Boone JM, Dobbins JT, eds. Proc. SPIE Vol 3659;258–265. Med Imaging 1999 Physics of Medical Imaging

103 Zhong W, Yoshida H, Nishikawa RM et al. Optimally weighted wavelet transform based on supervised training for detection of microcalcifications in digital mammograms. Med Phys. 1998;25:949–956

104 Karssemeijer N, Veldkamp WJ, te Brake GM, Hendriks JH. Reading screening mammograms with the help of neural networks. Ned Tijdschr Geneeskd. 1999;143:2232–6

105 Lado MJ, Tahoces PG, Mendez AJ et al. A wavelet-based algorithm for detecting clustered microcalcifications in digital mammograms. Med Phys. 1999;26:1294–305

106 Qian W, Li L, Clarke L et al. Digital mammography: comparison of adaptive and nonadaptive CAD methods for mass detection. Acad Radiol. 1999;6:471–80

107 Nawano S, Murakami K, Moriyama N et al. Computer-aided diagnosis in full digital mammography. Invest Radiol. 1999;34:310–6

108 Thurfjell EL, Lernevall KA, Taube AAS. Benefit of independent double reading in a population-based mammography screening program. Radiology. 1994;191:241–4

109 Warren Burhenne LJ, Wood SA, D'Orsi CJ et al. Potential Contribution of Computer-aided Detection to the Sensitivity of Screening Mammography. Radiology. 2000; 215:554–562

110 Huo Z, Giger mediolateral, Vyborny CJ et al. Automated computerized classification of malignant and benign masses on digitized mammograms. Acad Radiol. 1998;5:155–68

111 Feig SA, Yaffe MJ. Current status of digital mammography. Semin Ultrasound CT MRI. 1996;17:424–443.

112 Williams MB, Fajardo LL. Digital mammography: performance considerations and current detector designs. Acad Radiol. 1996;3:429–437

113 Kimme-Smith C, Lewis C, Beifuss M et al. Establishing minimum performance standards, calibration intervals, and optimal exposure values for a whole breast digital mammography unit. Med Phys. 1998;25:2410–6 Pages 81–911.

114 Tabar L, Dean PB, Pentek Z. Galactography: the diagnostic procedure of choice for nipple discharge. Am J Radiol. 1983; 149: 31-8

115 Ciatto S, Bravetti P, Berni D, Catarzi S, Bianchi S. The role of galactography in the detection of breast cancer. Tumori. 1988; 74: 171–81

116 Kindermann G. Diagnostic value of galactography in the detection of breast cancer. In: Zander J, Baltzer J, eds. Early breast cancer. Berlin: Springer; 1985:136–9

117 Hoeffken W, Hintzen C. Die Diagnostik der Mammazysten durch Mammographie und Pneumozystographie. Fortsch Röntgenstr. 1970; 9–18

118 Tabar L, Pentek Z, Dean PB. The diagnostic and therapeutic value of breast cyst puncture and pneumocystography. Radiology. 1981; 141: 659-63

4. Sonography

After mammography, sonography is the most important breast imaging modality. Its most important roles include:

- Diagnosing cysts
- Characterizing masses that are incompletely assessed by mammography
- Characterizing palpable masses that are obscured by dense tissue on mammography
- Imaging guidance for percutaneous biopsy and localization

■ Diagnosing Cysts

Diagnosing cysts is one of the most important contributions of sonography to breast imaging. The diagnosis of a simple cyst makes it possible to assure that a mass is benign and requires no additional workup for definitive diagnosis. Sonography is essentially 100 % accurate in this diagnosis. Therefore, sonography is useful in the workup of any palpable or nonpalpable lesions that could be due to a simple cyst.[1, 2]

■ Differentiating Solid Lesions

Sonography is helpful as a modality in addition to mammography in assessing the internal texture and shape of the margins of masses that are partially or completely obscured by dense tissue on mammography. Palpable lesions that are located in dense tissue and cannot be clearly or completely visualized mammographically can often be further characterized by sonography.[3-5]

In interpreting sonographic results, the following considerations should be kept in mind:

- If a lesion is not a simple cyst and a mammogram has not been performed, this should be done to further characterize the mass, for example to demonstrate possible diagnostic patterns of calcifications.

- Benign sonographic findings in the presence of suspicious mammographic findings do not exclude malignancy.
- A mass that cannot be seen sonographically should be considered not to be a cyst and therefore solid. This implies that these lesions may also be caused by a carcinoma.
- If there are any doubts about the benignity of a lesion after complete imaging assessment, further diagnostic procedures (short-term follow-up or biopsy) are indicated.

■ Diagnosing Carcinoma

Although many carcinomas are seen sonographically as hypoechoic masses, the echogenicity of carcinoma is variable. Some carcinomas are isoechoic with breast tissue.

The sonographic visibility of carcinomas also depends on the surrounding tissue. Since fat is hypoechoic compared to glandular tissue (like most carcinomas, too), carcinomas may be missed sonographically within fatty tissue. Hypoechoic fat lobules may, furthermore, mimic malignancy.

Because of these factors, some cancers will not be seen with sonography, although they may be easily found mammographically.[6, 7]

This pitfall may occur in any type of breast tissue, but is more frequent within fatty breast tissue than in mixed breast tissue or dense hyperechoic glandular tissue.

Hypoechoic carcinomas are readily identified when they are located within more echogenic breast parenchyma. In these situations, where cancers may be obscured by surrounding breast tissue mammographically, sonography can be very useful, especially in assessing a palpable lesion.

Some anatomic structures in the breast can be confused with worrisome lesions. These include shadowing Cooper's ligaments and hypoechoic fatty lobules. Considerable time and effort is necessary in the sonographic examination of some breasts to reliably distinguish normal structures from malignancy. Diligent evaluation of sometimes numerous hypoechoic areas and shadowing is needed; this includes verification of the finding in two planes and compressibility checks.

■ Younger Women

In the imaging assessment of young women (usually those of 30 years or above), sonography is usually the first imaging study in the workup of a palpable mass. If diagnosis of a simple cyst is possible, no further workup is needed. If a simple cyst cannot be diagnosed, mammography should be performed to attempt to gain additional information before deciding upon the need for biopsy.

■ Screening with Sonography

The only imaging study that has been demonstrated to be effective for screening is mammography. Based on the limited sensitivity of ultrasound concerning the detection of small and in situ carcinomas—even if high-frequency transducers are used—ultrasound cannot replace mammography.[8-11] Only anecdotal evidence suggests that sonographic screening added to mammography[12-14] may allow detection of additional carcinomas. However, the existing results suggest that the false positive rate (recommendation for biopsy for lesions that are benign) may be unacceptably high with sonography.[12-14] The examination is also very operator dependent and time consuming.[15] Feasibility of a quality assurance (technique and reporting), which,however, would be indispensable for any type of ultrasound screening, is not established. Based on the existing evidence, there are no recommendations for the use of sonography for screening for breast cancer. In fact, the Standards of the American College of Radiology specifically state that sonography is not a screening study for the breast. Except in an experimental situation, sonography of the breast should only be used to further characterize focal lesions detected by physical examination or other imaging modality or as a guidance system for breast biopsy procedures.

■ Summary

Sonography is the most important breast imaging modality after mammography. It is excellent in diagnosing simple cysts, eliminating the need for biopsy of these masses.

Definitive sonographic diagnosis of solid masses is less certain, although certain characteristics can increase the likelihood that a mass is malignant or benign. In many cases biopsy will be required for a definitive diagnosis. When a mass is palpable and no focal sonographic findings are present, the lesion should be considered to be solid, increasing the possibility of it being malignant. When a cyst is seen to correspond to a palpable mass, care should be taken to make certain that the palpable lesion and the cyst are the same mass. When young women (30 years or below) present with a breast mass, the initial step in the evaluation of the mass is usually sonography. If the lesion is a cyst, no further imaging is needed. Because of its inability to reliably image microcalcifications and because of its very high false positive rate, sonography is not a proven tool for breast-cancer screening. Its use in this setting is not encouraged.

Equipment Requirements

■ Transducer

Breast sonography requires the use of hand-held, high-frequency, linear-array transducers. These should be able to be focused in the near field, and have a capacity for variable focus, so that the soundbeam can be focused at the level of interest in the breast. Transducer frequency should be at least 7.5 MHz. Transducers with a higher frequency may improve resolution. However, with increasing frequency the ability of the soundbeam to penetrate tissue decreases. Therefore, very high-frequency transducers may not be able to fully penetrate large breasts. They may also have a smaller configuration, decreasing the field of view.[16]

■ Image Quality

Factors determing the image quality of a breast sonography unit are: quality of resolution, image quality in the near field, and slice thickness.

■ Resolution

Resolution is determined by axial resolution, lateral resolution (Figs **4.1a–c**), and contrast resolution.

1. Axial resolution (resolution along the direction of sound travel) is determined by the length of the ultrasound pulse, which is generally about 2 wavelengths. The minimum axial resolution is half of this value. Generally, for a 7.5 MHz transducer, resolution is about 0.4 mm.

2. Lateral resolution (the width of the ultrasound pulse) is determined by the size of the transducer element or its aperture, the frequency, and the focus. Transducer designs have different abilities to focus the soundbeam. Fixed-focus transducers have a concave arrangement of transducer elements or use an acoustic lens. To change the focus of the soundbeam when using transducers of this configuration, the transducer must be changed. This design is largely archaic and is not part of modern ultrasound technology.

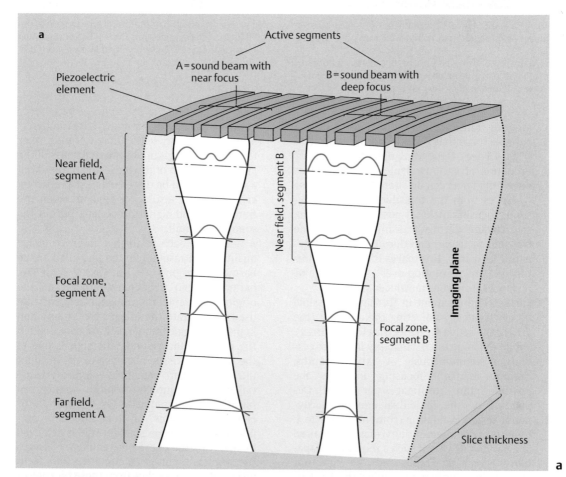

Fig. **4.1a** Schematic diagram showing the ultrasound beam emitted by a transducer. The depth of focus (shown here for segments A and B) is set by delaying the excitation of the respecitve central transducer element accordingly. The ultrasound signal (depicted in the diagram as individual echoes in the ultrasound beam) shows artifacts in the near field due to interference. A fixed focus can be achieved by a concave arrangement of the piezoelectric elements

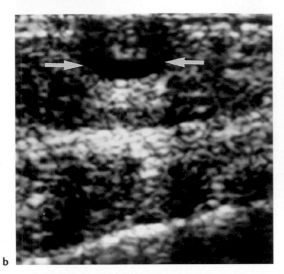

b

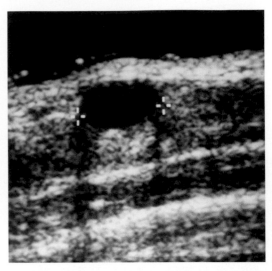

c

Fig. 4.1 b and c A small, subcutaneous cyst illustrates the impact of a stand-off pad in improved imaging in the near field

b A small cyst (arrows) is present, but there is suboptimal imaging of parts of the near wall. Additionally, axial resolution in the far wall of the cyst is poor

c Using a gel stand-off pad the cyst is now located in the area of focus of the soundbeam. There is better resolution of the wall of the cyst. A linear reverberation artifact is present in the leading edge of the cyst, just below the near wall

Modern transducers are designed to have a variable focus that is electronically controlled (Figs. 4.1 a–c). Depending upon the timing of excitation of various elements in the transducer, the focus can be altered to a variety of distances from the transducer surface. Electronic focusing makes it possible to focus the soundbeam during transmission (multiple transmit focusing) and during reception (dynamic focusing). This makes is possible to improve lateral resolution over a wide range of distances from the transducer surface.

Further improvement in focusing is possible by electronically adjusting the aperture (the area of the active piezoelectric element array). While dynamic focus capability improves resolution simultaneously at various depths, multiple transmit focusing decreases the possible frame rate (images per second). Depending on the individual equipment, dynamic lesion evaluation (compressibility test, monitoring of interventions) may be impaired at a varying degree. If such a multifocus capability is not desirable and therefore not chosen, the examiner must adjust the depth of the focus to the depth of the tissue area in question. Dynamic focusing is always active during reception and there is no control element necessary.

3. Contrast resolution is a major factor in determining the quality of the image. Among other factors, it is a measure of the sharpness of the lateral definition of the pulse and of how well a weak echo can be discerned next to a strong echo. Contrast resolution depends upon the transducer and signal processing within the sonographic unit.

A novel approach to further improve image quality of ultrasound is the so-called tissue harmonic imaging (THI) mode.[17,18] With THI, harmonic echo frequencies rather than the original (fundamental) transmit frequency are used to generate the image. The second and higher harmonic frequencies are contained in the reflected ultrasound echo signals due to the nonlinear tissue response to the incident ultrasound beam. The effect is improved spatial as well as contrast resolution in many applications. A prerequisite for THI is the efficient suppression of fundamental components in the echo signals. This is achieved by inverting the phase between two consecutive transmit pulses (phase inversion technique). When the echos from these two pulses are added, the fundamental echo components cancel each other and the harmonic echo signals are enhanced. This technique, of course, can only be achieved with high precision by

Fig. 4.**2** Reverberation echoes resulting from insufficient contract between stand-off pad and skin

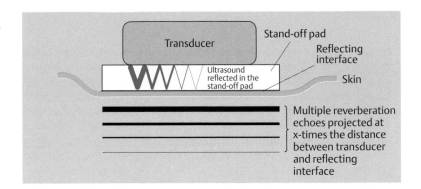

Transducer

Stand-off pad

Reflecting interface

Ultrasound reflected in the stand-off pad

Skin

Multiple reverberation echoes projected at x-times the distance between transducer and reflecting interface

all-digital beam-forming electronics, as provided by state-of-the-art high-end equipment. First interesting results have been reported in various indications and areas of the human body . The potential added value of this method for clinical breast ultrasound is being investigated.

■ Image Quality in the Near Field

Aside from optimal overall resolution, the image quality in the near field is important for breast sonography. Because the thickness of most breasts is only a few centimeters during sonography, many lesions will be located close to the transducer. High image quality in the near field is necessary to accurately assess these lesions. Unfortunately, transducer design and other factors can make it difficult to image these areas.

Because some transducers have difficulty focusing the soundbeam within a few millimeters of the transducer,with some it may be necessary to use a stand-off pad between the transducer and the breast to achieve good images of the subcutaneous tissues and the superficial breast tissue. These pads physically move the near field of the transducer away from the breast surface, placing the breast within a distance from the transducer at which the soundbeam can be reliably focused (Fig. 4.**1**).

When using a stand-off pad that is water-filled, it is important that the water be free of gas bubbles to ensure efficient sound transmission. This is not a problem with gel stand-off pads. For all pads, sufficient coupling agent (gel or oil) must be used to eliminate air between the transducer and the pad and between the pad the breast surface. Reverberation echoes can be caused by the repeated reflection of sound between the pad and

the transducer (Fig 4.**2**). These produce lines of echoes that run parallel to the transducer and repeat at one, two, three, or more times at a given distance from the transducer. They add artifact to the image, and compromise the ability to make an accurate diagnosis.

■ Slice Thickness

Slice thickness is a function of quality and design of the transducer and should be considered when purchasing equipment; furthermore, the appropriate transducer has to be chosen. If slice thickness is too thick, cysts that should appear echo free will not be reliably imaged due to the inclusion of adjacent solid tissue within the tissue slice. Accurate diagnosis may not be possible in these cases, particularly when cysts are small.

Compared with earlier sonographic units, newer units provide significantly finer gray-scale definition (4–8 bits, corresponding to 16–256 shades of gray). These units can produce high-contrast images of the varying echo intensities occurring in tissue and will elicit echoes within the cyst.

Special phantoms are available for assessing relevant image quality parameters for breast sonography.

■ Equipment Quality Control

Each facility should have in place a quality control program to maximize the quality of its breast sonography. Ongoing monitoring and evaluation of equipment should be a part of this program. A routine preventive maintenance program is desirable. Records should be kept to document this program. Efforts undertaken to improve quality of care should also be documented.

■ **Summary**

Linear transducers with a nominal frequency of at least 7.5 MHz should be used for breast sonography. Imaging detail is determined by axial, lateral, and contrast resolution. Lateral resolution is significantly influenced by focusing, which is most difficult in the near field. A stand-off pad is required during sonography if the transducer is not capable of adequately focusing the the near field.

Care must be taken to always image the area in question using the appropriate focus. This is possible by diligent manual adaptation of the focus depth, by use of multiple transmit focus or dynamic focusing. Slice thickness will also have an impact on the quality of the study, particularly when imaging small cysts. A quality control program is desirable to maximize patient care and safety.

Examination Technique

Sonography of the breast is usually best performed with the patient supine. When the outer quadrants are being scanned, the patient should extend the ispilateral arm over the head and elevate the ipsilateral shoulder (contralateral posterior oblique position). It is helpful to place a cushion or pillow under the ipsilateral shoulder to help the patient maintain this position. This positioning flattens the breast against the chest wall, decreasing the amount of tissue that must be penetrated by the soundbeam and reducing breast mobility. When the inner quadrants are being examined, a straight supine position accomplishes the same results for the inner quadrants.

When scanning a palpable mass, it can be helpful to bracket the lesion with two fingers of one hand and slip the transducer between these two fingers. This assures that the volume of the breast being imaged corresponds to the site of the palpable mass.

A sufficient amount of gel should be used between the transducer and the skin (and the stand-off pad, if one is being used) to eliminate air between these structures, thereby minimizing reverberation artifact. The use of slight compression on the transducer can also be helpful.

Slight compression and flat positioning of the breast also help to position tissue interfaces as parallel as possible to the transducer. Diagonal tissue interfaces such as Cooper's ligaments can cause part of the soundbeam to be reflected away from the transducer, resulting in acoustic shadowing. These shadows can be diagnostically confusing and can obscure lesions distal to the shadowing structures (Figs. 4.3 a and b).

■ Time-gain Compensation

Time-gain compensation adjusts the visual presentation of the reflected soundbeam to an image of equalized brightness and intensity, despite decreased energy of the beam as it travels farther from the transducer. For a 7.5 MHz beam, the soundbeam loses about 50% of its energy through every centimeter of tissue it traverses. Time-gain compensation allows the beam to appear to be at equal intensity at all distances from the transducer (Fig. 4.4). However, equalization of the intensity of echoes throughout the image requires matching image compensation to ultrasound absorption throughout the image. Although modern equipment is produced with programs to automatically compensate for decreasing intensity of the beam at greater distances from the transducer, variability in absorption patterns in different patients—due to the variable amounts of fatty, glandular, and fibrotic tissue in the individual breast—often require optimization of the image manually.

The echoes that make up the sonographic image are produced in two different ways. These are:

● *Specular echoes.* Specular echoes are strong echoes caused by reflection at interfaces with sufficient difference of impedance between two tissues. These interfaces must be sufficiently large (larger than the wavelength) and have a smooth surface. The angle of incidence equals the angle of reflection. Echoes striking diagonal interfaces can be reflected away from the transducer. Such echoes are not visualized on the ultrasound image.

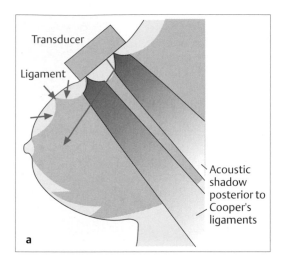

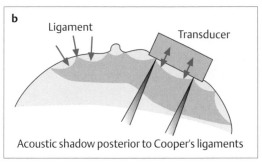

Fig. 4.**3a** and **b** Positioning the patient supine and applying slight compression helps to orient the interfaces parallel to the transducer (**b**). Less ultrasound energy is reflected away from the transducer than in a hanging breast (**a**)

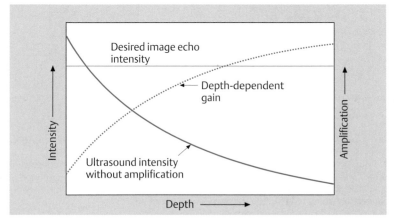

Fig. 4.**4** Time-gain compensation

● *Scatter echoes.* Scatter echoes occur at small interfaces with irregular surfaces. The size of these interfaces is of the same magnitude as the wavelength of the soundbeam. The sound wave is scattered in variable directions, and the intensity of the echo returned to the transducer is weak. Most echoes in glandular and fatty tissue are scatter echoes, produced by microscopic tissue interfaces.

■ Focusing

Optimal imaging of the lesion requires focusing the soundbeam at the depth from the transducer at which the lesion is located. This requires adjusting the focal zone to this site. As noted, this can be done by using a variable focus transducer and electronically adjusting the focal zone. In some cases, a stand-off pad will be required.

■ Examination Technique

Sonographic examination makes it possible to study the breast in an infinite number of planes. Standardization of the examination and appropriate labeling of images makes these studies interpretable by those who have not performed them, and also makes them reproducible.

Imaging in the radial and anti-radial planes (planes corresponding to spokes of a wheel extending from the nipple and right angle to these axes) corresponds to the normal pattern of ductal anatomy of the breast and to the labeling of lesions at o'clock axes. When needed, imaging in additional planes with appropriate annotation on the images can be performed. Imaging in at least two orthogonal planes usually makes it possible to differentiate real lesions from breast anatomy. For example, fat lobules typically appear as elon-

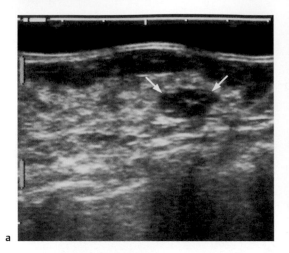
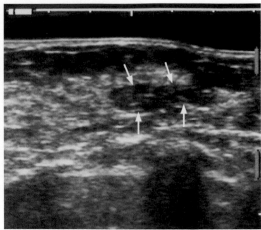

a

b

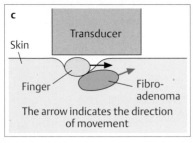

c

Transducer

Skin

Finger — — Fibro-
adenoma

The arrow indicates the direction
of movement

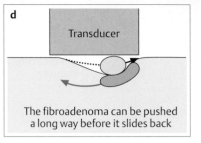

d

Transducer

The fibroadenoma can be pushed
a long way before it slides back

Fig. 4.**5 a–d**
a and **b** Imaging in two planes:
a Interspersed fat lobules can simulate a hypoechoic tumor
b As the transducer is turned, the same fat lobule appears as an elongated structure (arrow). The image in this plane also reveals that the fat lobule is connected to subcutaneous fat
c and **d** Assessing mobility (diagram). To assess mobility, insert a finger underneath the transducer. Fibroadenomas usually are far more mobile than carcinomas

gated structures in the second plane. Often, a connection to the subcutaneous or retromammary fat layers can be demonstrated (Figs. 4.5a and b).

Real-time imaging also makes it possible to determine mobility of a lesion. Fibroadenomas are typically excellently mobile. If this feature cannot be shown, malignancy should be suspected even in case of completely well-circumscribed lesions with homogeneous echogenicity[19] (Figs. 4.5c and d).

Compressibility of a lesion suggests that it is soft, often a cyst or other benign lesion. However, this characteristic should not be used to exclude the possibility of malignancy.

■ Doppler Imaging

Because breast carcinoma is hypervascular and many benign lesions are hypovascular, it was hoped that the determination of blood-flow patterns within a lesion would be helpful in differentiating malignant from benign processes. It has been suggested that breast cancers tend to show more vascularity. This pattern is usually that of vessels arising along the edge of the mass and extending into its center. These vessels are often branching and irregular. Smooth vessels paralleling the periphery of a mass are more characteristic of benign lesions, such as fibroadenomas. However, both patterns can be seen in benign and malignant processes. Additionally, benign lesions can be hypervascular and malignant lesions avascular (Figs. 4.6a and b, 4.7, 4.8). For this reason, the use of Doppler or power Doppler interrogation of breast masses has not been found to be useful by most experts in determining which lesions require biopsy and which are benign.[20–22]

The use of microbubble contrast agents has also been described in several studies in an at-

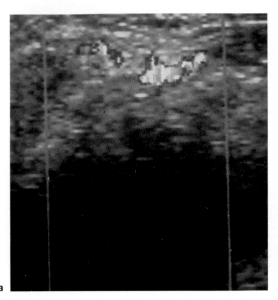

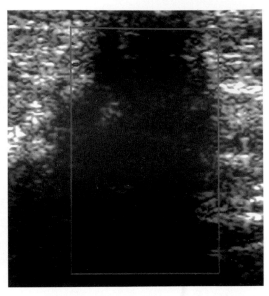

a

b

Fig. 4.**6 a** and **b** Doppler examination of breast carcinomas
a The hypoechoic and anechoic mass occupying the lower half of this image demonstrates prominent feeding vessels adjacent to it. This hypervascular pattern *should raise the suspicion of* a breast carcinoma

b This tall, hypoechoic, irregular, shadowing, infiltrating ductal carcinoma shows minimal vascularity. Some flow within the tumor mass is present and a few small, peripheral vessels are also seen

tempt to better define vascular patterns within lesions. Use of these agents remains experimental.[23]

■ **Image Labeling**

Due to the variabilities of examination technique that are possible during sonographic study, precise labeling of images is necessary so that sonographic examinations are reproducible and lesions can be found on repeat study. Labeling of sonographic studies of the breast should include:

- Patient identification: name and unique identifying number such as medical record number, birth date, or social security number
- Examination date
- Breast laterality (right or left)
- Breast quadrant
- Axis, indicated by o'clock designation
- Distance of the lesion from the nipple
- An indication if the lesion is palpable.

It is also desirable to include the initials or other identification of the technologist or physician performing the study.

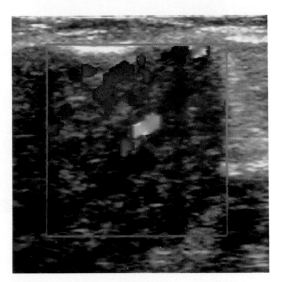

Fig. 4.**7** A solid, macrolobulated, well-defined mass shows large vessels in the *periphery* of the mass, penetrating deeply into it. Although this Doppler study demonstrates hypervascularity, the mass is benign; a fibroadenoma

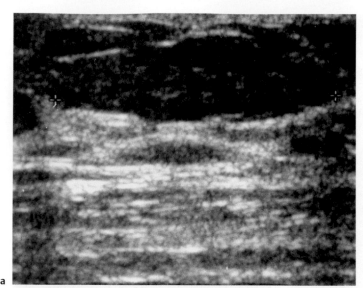

a

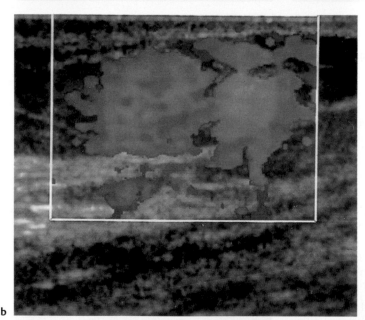

b

Fig. 4.**8a** and **b** This woman with a history of lung carcinoma presented with a new, palpable breast mass. She and her physician were concerned that this was malignant
a Sonography of the palpable mass shows an elongated, echogenic structure, marked by the electronic cursors
b Doppler interrogation demonstrates that this is a vascular structure, a varix

Interpreting Sonographic Findings

■ Normal Sonographic Findings

As in the mammographic pattern of the normal breast, there is a broad variation in the normal sonographic pattern of the breast. Subcutaneous fatty tissue appears hypoechoic with echogenic bands of Cooper's ligaments coursing through the fat. Glandular tissue has an echogenic pattern, interrupted by hypoechoic fatty lobules. Worrisome sonographic patterns can be caused by shadowing fibrous bands and by hypoechoic fat lobules mimicking a mass. Scanning in multiple projections will usually identify these findings as part the normal anatomy of the breast (Figs. 4.5a and **b**).

■ Focal Sonographic Lesions

■ Cysts

Simple cysts can be definitively diagnosed as benign lesions by sonography. Their characteristics include:

- Round or oval shape
- Smooth, thin wall
- Absence of internal echoes (except for artifactual echoes)
- Posterior enhancement of the soundbeam

When all of these findings are present throughout the lesion, a simple cyst can be definitively diagnosed (Fig. 4.9). In the breast, cysts commonly are clustered or have thin septations. Low-level echoes can be found throughout the cystic fluid, especially with high-resolution transducers. Under real-time study these will often be seen to be moving, representing debris within the cystic fluid. Sedimented debris in the dependent portion of the cyst will often move with a change in patient positioning.

Fig. 4.**9 a** This simple cyst can be definitively diagnosed sonographically due to its oval shape, thin wall, absence of internal echoes, and far wall enhancement of the soundbeam
b Complex cyst: This oval mass is smooth-walled and shows far wall enhancement of the soundbeam. However, internal multiple echos make this a complex cyst. This mass was a cyst with hemorrhage

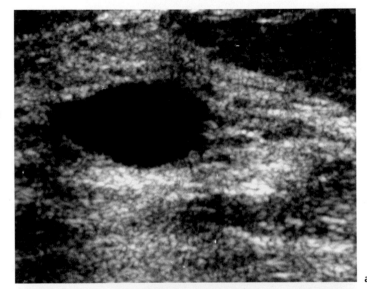

a

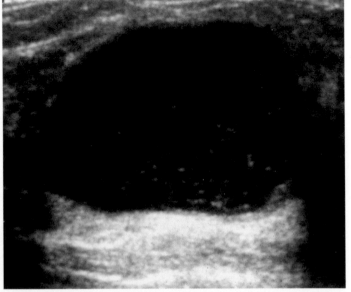

b

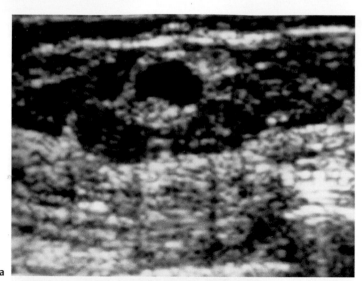

a

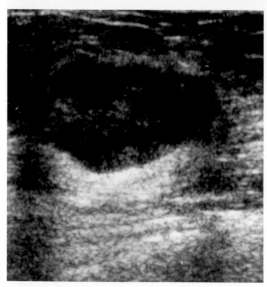

b

Fig. 4.**10 a** and **b** Masses that do not contain all the characteristics of simple cysts require additional workup to determine the diagnosis
a This round, hypoechoic mass is smooth-walled and shows far wall enhancement of the soundbeam. However, there is some irregularity to the far wall and internal echoes are present. This mass was due to lymphoma
b This complex mass has far wall enhancement of the soundbeam and a largely oval shape with most of its margins well-defined, and contains areas that are anechoic. However, the internal echo pattern is very heterogeneous and is inconsistent with a simple cyst. This mass was due to multiple myeloma involving the breast

peated. This should show that the mass has resolved.

Masses that do not contain all the characteristics of simple cysts require additional workup: cyst aspiration or (if the lesion proves to be solid) percutaneous biopsy (Fig. 4.**10**).

As noted above, when a palpable mass is scanned it can be bracketed with two fingers and the transducer slipped between the bracketing fingers to assure that the sonographically identified cyst corresponds to the palpable mass.

■ Solid Masses

Definitive diagnosis of the histology of a solid mass is usually not possible based on its sonographic pattern. However, certain characteristics are helpful in determining whether or not a solid mass might be malignant.[19,24,25] These include:

– shape
– height–width ratio
– margins
– internal echo pattern
– sound absorption (shadowing versus posterior enhancement)

A cystic mass that contains a focus of solid tissue or irregular mural thickening should be considered suspicious for carcinoma and undergo biopsy.

Cysts are common in the breast. It is important when a cyst is identified that the radiologist be certain that it corresponds to the worrisome lesion on mammography or physical examination. When the mass is seen on mammography, a marker can be placed over the mass seen on sonography, and the mammogram can be repeated. If there is still uncertainty, the cyst can be aspirated, and, if necessary, the mammogram may be re-

A systematic assessment of sonographic findings as an indicator of malignancy was done by Stavros and is based on a large number of verified lesions. These data provide evidence for the value of various sonographic features or their combinations.[25] However, no set of findings on sonography should be used to replace tissue sampling to diagnose carcinoma or any other entity.

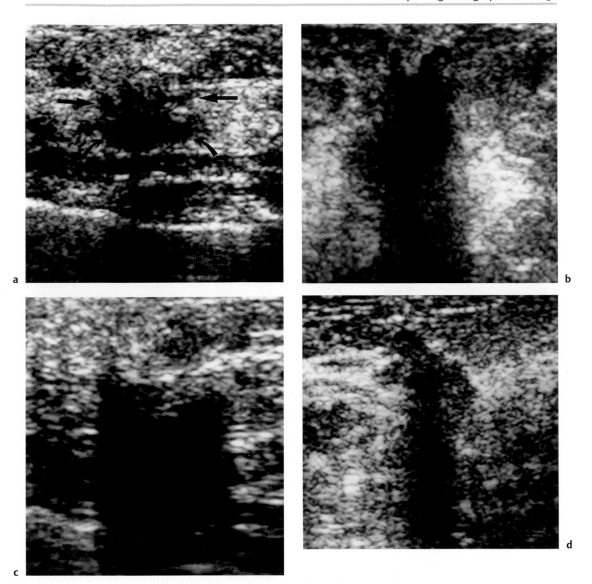

Fig. 4.**11 a–g** Sonographic patterns highly suspicious for malignant lesions

a This infiltrating ductal carcinoma shows relatively smooth walls posteriorly (curved arrows). However, the near margin (straight arrows) is spiculated, indicating an aggressive lesion

b Another infiltrating ductal carcinoma has spiculation of its near margin. It is also taller than it is wide, another characteristic of carcinomas. In addition, broad acoustic shadowing is seen

c This infiltrating ductal carcinoma shows many of the same characteritics as seen in Figure 4.**10b**. Additionally, the lateral margin of the lesion shows sharp angulation, suggestive of carcinoma. Significant acoustic shadowing is demonstrated

d The most striking feature of this small, infiltrating lobular carcinoma is that it is taller than it is wide. It also shows marked hypoechogenicity and acoustic shadowing, making it easily identifiable against the echogenic background pattern of the breast parenchyma, even though the lesion is only 1 cm in diameter

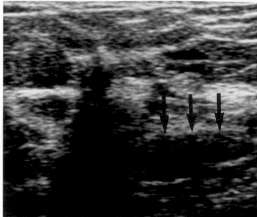

e

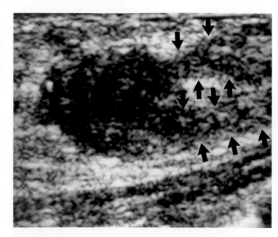

f

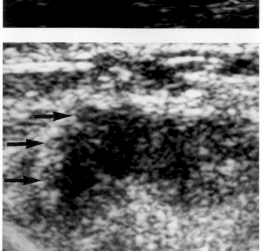

g

Fig. 4.**11 e** The lateral extension (arrows) of this carcinoma suggests ductal extension of the tumor

f This irregular tumor mass also shows ductal extension (arrows) arising from the upper and lower margins of the right side of the mass. The upper extension shows a branching pattern as it extends toward the right side of the image. Note the bright echo on the left side of the tumor mass, suggesting the presence of calcifications within this infiltrating ductal carcinoma. Note also that this carcinoma is wider than it is tall and shows no shadowing

g This very poorly defined tumor mass is grossly infiltrative along the right side of the lesion. The left side (arrows) shows a microlobulated contour, suggestive of the diagnosis of infiltrating ductal carcinoma

Sonographic findings that are most consistent with the diagnosis of malignancy are:[25]

– Spiculation of the margin or echogenic halo. (The echogenic halo in fact represents an increased number of interfaces caused by spiculations that extend into surrounding tissue.)
– Angulation of the margin (= margin that is acute, obtuse, or 90°)
– Lesion "taller than wide"
– Hypoechoic echo pattern
– Distal acoustic shadowing
– Sonographically evident punctate calcifications, visualized within a solid nodule
– Extension of the mass into a duct
– Branching
– Microlobulated contour

These findings are similar to mammographic patterns of irregular, multilobulated margins, spiculation, and ductal distribution of microcalcifications (Fig. 4.**11**).

Sonographic findings that are most consistent with a benign entity include (Fig. 4.**12**):[25]

– Absence of any characteristics of malignancy
– Intense homogeneous hyperechogenicity. (If the echotexture is not uniform or if it contains hypoechoic areas other than fat lobules that are larger than normal ducts or terminal ductal-lobular units (>4 mm), this criterion is not fulfilled.)
– Ellipsoid shape (smooth contours and lesion width >1.5 x height)
– Two or three gentle lobulations in contour
– Thin, echogenic pseudocapsule
– Excellent mobility of a mass[19]

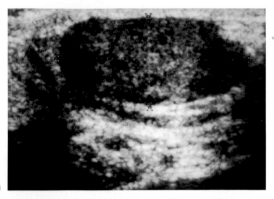

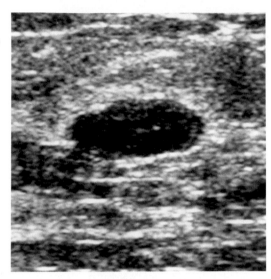

Fig. 4.**12 a** A well-defined mass is shown. With a single gentle lobulation, its homogeneous echotexture, its thin echogenic pseudocapsule, and excellent mobility (as checked during real-time imaging), it is a typical example of a benign fibroadenoma. Its oval shape and width greater than its height (ratio >1.5) further support this diagnosis

b This well-defined oval mass has a single, gentle macro-lobulation along its near wall. The internal echo pattern is heterogeneous, and the sonographic findings are nonspecific, although they suggest a benign lesion. This underwent biopsy and was found to be a benign phyllodes tumor

Fig. 4.**13** There can be a considerable overlap in the sonographic characteristics of benign and malignant lesions. In this patient the superficial mass (solid arrows) has an oval shape and is partially well-defined. However, there is a heterogeneous internal echo pattern, some irregularity of its margins, and microlobulation in the far wall. The deeper mass (curved, open arrows) has some lobulation of the near wall and a few internal echoes. These findings were due to a carcinoma adjacent to a silicone-filled augmentation prosthesis

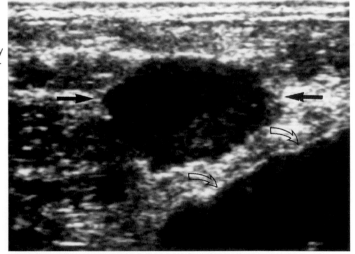

Other sonographic characteristics in solid lesions (homogeneous echo pattern, posterior enhancement, isoechogenicity) are of less value in differentiating benign from malignant solid masses. However, as with mammography, the radiologist should always remember that the definitive diagnosis of benign or malignant histology for indeterminate or highly suspicious lesions is based on tissue sampling, not on the imaging characteristics (Fig. 4.**13**).

■ References

1   Bassett LW, Kimme-Smith C. Breast sonography. AJR. 1991;156:449
2   Jackson VP. The role of US in breast imaging. Radiology. 1990;177:305
3   Harper P, Kelly-Fry E. Ultrasound visualizaton of the breast in symptomatic patients. Radiology. 1980;137:465
4   Dershaw DD, Eddens G, Liberman L, Deutch BM, Abramson AF. Sonographic and clinical findings in women with palpable breast disease and negative mammography. Breast Dis. 1995;8:13
5   Adler DD. Ultrasound of benign breast conditions. Semin Ultrasound CT MR. 1989;10:106
6   Feig SA. The role of ultrasound in a breast imaging center. Semin Ultrasound CT MR. 1989;10:90
7   Heywang SH, Dunner PS, Lipsit ER, Glassman LM. Advantages and pitfalls of ultrasound in the diagnosis of breast cancer. J Clin Ultrasound. 1985;13:525
8   Pamilo M, Soiva M, Anttinen J et al. Ultrasonography of breast lesions detected in mammography screening. Acta Radiol. 1991;32:220
9   Balu-Maestro C, Bruneton JN, Melia P et al. High frequency ultrasound detection of breast calcifications. Eur J Ultrasound. 1994;3:247
10 Ciatto S, Roselli-del-Turco M, Catarzis M et al. The diagnostic role of breast echography. Radiol Med (Torino). 1994;88:221
11 Potterton AJ, Peakman DH, Young IR. Ultrasound demonstration of small breast cancers detected by mammographic screening. Clin Radiol. 1994;49:808
12 Gordon PB, Goldenberg SL, Chan NHL. Malignant breast masses detected only by ultrasound: a retrospective review. Cancer. 1995;76:626–30
13 Kolb TM, Lichy J, Newhouse JH. Occult cancer in women with dense breasts: Detection with screening US–diagnostic yield and tumor characteristics. Radiology. 1998;207:191–9
14 Buchberger W, De Koekkoek-Doll P, Springer P et al. Incidental findings on sonography of the breast: clinical significance and diagnostic workup. AJR. 1999;173:921–7
15 Kopans DB. Breast-cancer screening with ultrasonography (letter). Lancet. 1999;354:2096
16 ACR standard for performance of the breast ultrasound examination. 1998 standards. American College of Radiology, Reston, VA; 1998;317.
17 Chapman CS, Lazenby JC. Ultrasound Imaging System employing phase inversion subtraction to enhance the image. U.S. patent number 5,632,277. 1997
18 Haerten R, Lowery C, Becker G, et al. Ensemble™ Tissue Harmonic Imaging. The technology and clinical utility. Electromedica. 1999;67:50–6
19 Tohno E, Cosgrove DO, Sloane UP. Ultrasound diagnosis of breast diseases. Edinburgh: Churchill Livingstone; 1994
20 McNicholas MMJ, Mercer PM, Miller JC, Mcdermott EWM, O'Higgins NJ, MacErlean DP. Color Doppler sonography in the evaluation of palpable breast masses. AJR. 1993;161:765
21 Cosgrove DO, Kedar RP, Bamber JC, Al-Murrani B, Davey JBN et al. Breast diseases: color Doppler US in differential diagnosis. Radiology. 1993;189:99
22 Raza S, Baum JK. Solid breast lesions: evaluation with power Doppler US. Radiology. 1997;203:164
23 Huber S, Helbich T, Kettenbach J, Dock W, Zuna I, Delorme S. Effects of microbubble contrast agent on breast tumors: computer-assisted quantitative assessment with color Doppler US–early experience. Radiology. 1998;208:485
24 Leucht D, Madjar H. Lehratlas der Mammasonographie. 2nded. Stuttgart: Thieme; 1995
25 Stavros AT, Thickman D, Rapp CL, Dennis MA, Parker SH, Sisney GA. Solid breast nodules: use of sonography to distinguish between benign and malignant lesions. Radiology. 1995;196:123

5. Magnetic Resonance Imaging (MRI)

Purpose, Accuracy, Possibilities, and Limitations

Contrast-enhanced (c.e.) MRI is the most sensitive additional imaging modality for supplementing mammography. Due to its moderate specificity, its applications should be restricted to selected indications.

Using contrast-enhanced MRI as the sole imaging modality or interpreting contrast-enhanced MRI without mammography does not represent sound diagnostic practice.

■ Accuracy

■ Contrast-enhanced MRI

Accuracy depends on the following factors:
- Technical factors:
  Field strength, use of an appropriate surface coil, appropriate pulse sequence, thin slices, dosage of contrast medium, and artifact suppression all influence accuracy. Standardization of technique and reporting and improved quality control remain important goals.[1, 2]
- Image interpretation criteria employed:
  C. e. breast MRI provides information concerning various tissue properties. This information is based on the presence of enhancement, morphology, and dynamics of enhancement. Various interpretation rules, which synthesize this information, have been suggested.[1-14] Using different combinations[3] of these parameters and different thresholds, rules optimizing sensitivity or specificity are possible. Very sensitive rules (sensitivity for invasive carcinomas >95%)[1,4,5] are usually associated with a lower specificity (30–50%, depending on the indications). Rules that provide better specificity (50–85%)[11-13] are, however, associated with lower sensitivities (90% for invasive malignancy).
  In order to obtain the most accurate diagnosis it is recommended

- to consider all available MR information
- to *always* make a final diagnosis based on MRI *and* conventional imaging
- to choose interpretation parameters that meet sensitivity and specificity requirements of the diagnostic question. For assessment of indeterminate lesions, sensitivity should be optimized to avoid false negative calls. For interpretation of lesions that are only detected by MRI, greater specificity is desirable to avoid too many false positive calls.

- Patient selection:
  MRI is a very sensitive method capable of detecting even small lesions not visualized by other methods. However, it is not specific. Therefore, its use should be limited to high-risk patients and to questions that cannot be adequately answered by the other imaging modalities or by percutaneous biopsy.[14]
  MRI is not recommended:
  - in a low-risk population (as in the usual patient with dense or nodular breast tissue): Here the prevalence of cancer is generally so low (3–5/1000 patients), that the additional workup of false positive MR findings that occur in 10–20% of the patients cannot be justified.
  - for differential diagnostic workup of lesions that are appropriately assessed by percutaneous biopsy. Due to its much higher rate of false positive results compared to percutaneous biopsy and due to the high rate of MR-detected incidental findings, which in the low-risk population mostly prove to be benign, MRI is not cost-effective.
  - for differentiation of benign entities from malignancy that are associated with unspecific enhancement: inflammatory changes, changes associated with mam-

mographically indeterminate or suspicious microcalcifications, patients with diffusely or patchy enhancing breast tissue that could not be positively influenced by hormonal changes (examination during correct phase of menstrual cycle or after discontinuation of hormone replacement therapy, see p. 108).

Excellent results have been achieved, when contrast-enhanced MRI was used as an additional method in cases or situations where a significant risk of breast cancer exists and where assessment by conventional imaging is impaired.

These situations include:
–   staging of the tumor extent within the breast and exclusion of multicentricity in the same or contralateral breast
–   assessment of scarring after breast-conserving therapy
–   evaluation of scarring after silicon implant
–   problem solving early after surgery
–   monitoring of neoadjuvant chemotherapy
–   search for primary tumor when the primary is unknown and breast cancer is suspected.

C.e. MRI may be helpful in some other selected cases, if using state-of-the-art workup the diagnostic question cannot be adequately answered (see pp. 105–6).

The role of MRI in screening women at high risk for breast cancer, e.g. BRCA-positive, is under investigation.

Experience with contrast-enhanced MRI has increased significantly since its first application in 1986.[15] Its role is now based on the published data of numerous authors, who mostly confirm good results. According to this experience[1-20], sensitivities of contrast-enhanced MRI to detect invasive carcinoma range from 90–98% and specificities from 30–85%. As noted above, rules that allow very high sensitivities (>95%) are usually associated with low specificities (30–50%), whereas very specific rules (70–85%) lead to decreased sensitivity (ranging around 90%).[11-13]

For DCIS sensitivities are generally lower than for invasive cancer and depend more on the diagnostic criteria used.[3, 20-25] Here sensitivities ranging from 50–90% have been reported, and low sensitivities for DCIS occur when the specificity is maximized.[3,24]

Since the majority of DCIS are detected today by the presence of microcalcifications found on mammography, the best diagnostic accuracy is achieved by combining information from mammography and MRI.

The advantages of strictly combined interpretation of all available information are apparent in a survey that included the results of 12,000 breast MR studies in six German universities.[14] Here MRI combined with mammography achieved sensitivities for invasive carcinoma between 98% and 99.5% and for in situ carcinomas between 80% and 99% and specificities of 50–85%, depending on the criteria applied and the patient selection.

In spite of the very good results achieved for the above-mentioned indications, for other indications experience remains limited.

Whether these results can be translated to a wider range of indications is not yet proven. As explained above, the major concern as to its use in a low-risk population is the expected number of false positive calls with respect to the number of cases where MRI can really add significant new information. Therefore, before recommending further indications, diligent testing will be needed.

Thus, the best results for breast MRI will be based on:

–   selection of appropriate interpretation criteria for the diagnostic situation,
–   interpretation of MRI together with other imaging modalities, and
–   strict selection of the appropriate indications.

■ Unenhanced MRI (for Visualisation of Implant Failure)

Today, noncontrast MRI is only used to assess breast implant for complications. In this setting it has the highest accuracy of all imaging modalities for determining implant rupture (sensitivity 90%, specificity ≥ 90%).[26-34]

Breast sonography can detect large leaks with high specificity. However, it is significantly inferior to MRI for demonstrating minor implant defects, especially in implants with many folds and in cases with severe scarring.

■ Indications

■ Contrast-enhanced MRI

Indications in which contrast-enhanced MRI has proven to provide valuable additional information include:

1. *Determination of multicentricity in the same or contralateral breast and preoperative assessment of the extent of the known tumor.* Therapeutically relevant new information (newly detected focus in the contralateral breast, evidence of multicentricity or larger than expected tumor volume) can be expected in 15–30% of patients.[1, 2, 5, 9, 35–37] Therefore, MRI should be considered in patients with non-fatty breast tissue, who—based on conventional diagnostics—are candidates for breast-conserving therapy. However, in case an enhancing lesion is detected, MR-guided needle localization or biopsy must be available for definitive diagnosis.

2. *Evaluation of scarring after breast-conserving therapy or breast reconstruction*
   a) *Breast-conserving therapy with irradiation*: C.e. MRI has proven particularly helpful later than 12 months after irradiation. By that time both hyperplastic enhancing breast tissue and post-therapeutic enhancing tissue have been replaced by non-enhancing fibrosis in >90% of the patients. Thus distinction between scarring and recurrence becomes excellent. This has been confirmed in over 500 cases.[38–46] Additionally, data on over 200 patients have shown that >45% of the recurrences were just MR-detected, and that recurrences detected by MRI were on average significantly smaller (9 mm) than those visible by other methods (17 mm).[46] Less than 12 months after irradiation, diffuse or focal unspecific enhancement can occur due to inflammatory reaction to irradiation. The degree to which diagnosis may be impaired by such enhancement is still debated.[46, 47] It is recommended that the indication for MRI during this timespan be considered on an individual basis.
   b) After *breast-conserving therapy without irradiation* enhancement due to granulation tissue usually subsides within 3–6 months of surgery. Evaluation of the scar after this period is usually excellent. Nonspecific enhancement due to hyperplastic or proliferative changes do, however, persist, even when no radiation was given.[48]
   c) In *patients with silicon implant* contrast-enhanced MRI adds new information that cannot be provided by other methods. It may therefore be recommended in patients with diagnostic problems due to

   severe scarring or increased risk (reconstructive surgery after T3 or T4 tumors, multifocal tumors, grade 3 tumors, status after previous recurrence). Even though published data are still limited, unequivocally a significant gain in sensitivity has been reported with the additional use of MRI.[49, 50]
   d) *Problem solving shortly after surgery.* As pointed out by several authors,[48, 51, 52] MRI may add important information if missed or residual tumor after surgery is suspected. For this indication it appears useful to use MRI as early after surgery as possible to forestall a false positive result due to the development of significant granulation tissue.[48]

3. *Monitoring of neoadjuvant chemotherapy.* First experiences in this field show that MRI is capable of recognizing nonresponders (no change of the enhancement curve, no decrease in size of the enhancing lesions) earlier than conventional breast imaging. Although it cannot exclude residual nests of tumor cells, it appears capable of demonstrating macroscopic areas of active tumor tissue.[53–56]

4. *Search for primary tumor* in cases with lymphnode or distant metastases of unknown origin. In a high percentage of cases contrast-enhanced MRI is capable of detecting a primary tumor. Therefore, it can be of value if mammography and sonography fail to discover the primary carcinoma.[57–59]

5. Evaluation of *high-risk patients* with mammographically dense tissue. Presently several studies are ongoing concerning the additional use of contrast-enhanced MRI in patients with a high genetic risk of breast cancer. First results[60–62] show that contrast-enhanced MRI may increase the detection rate of breast cancer in the mammographically dense breast tissue. However, a large experience is necessary to avoid causing a too high number of false positive calls, particularly in the younger patient groups and, if necessary, to take appropriate measures (for example by adapting the interpretation criteria).

Besides these major indications, contrast-enhanced MRI may be helpful in individual selected cases, if in experienced hands conventional imaging remains inconclusive or cannot answer a diagnostic question with sufficient certainty. Such indications may include progressive nipple retraction without known cause, nipple discharge if galactography is impossible, suspected lesion that cannot be localized in the third dimension. For reasons of cost-effectiveness contrast-enhanced MRI in these selected individual cases should be limited to those questions that cannot be solved by percutaneous biopsy.

■ Unenhanced MRI

Unenhanced MRI without contrast has become the method of choice for verifying and excluding defects in silicone prostheses.[26-34]

Technical Requirements

■ Contrast-enhanced MRI

Optimum technique is an important requirement to achieve high accuracy.

- Sufficient data on contrast-enhanced MRI of the breast are only available for field strengths of 0.5 tesla or higher. There is no information on whether the results obtained with these field strengths can be reproduced with lower field strengths.
- The use of dedicated breast coils is mandatory. Double breast imaging has the advantage of detecting additional unsuspected malignancy in the contralateral breast of women with breast cancer or other risk factors.
- The *slice thickness* should be ≤ 4 mm or, optimally, ≤ 2.5 mm. The reason is that small carcinomas tend to grow along ducts. If such a duct, filled with carcinoma, runs parallel to the slice, it may only partially fill the slice thickness. Then the signal increase after contrast agent will be reduced proportionally. The enhancement may be underestimated or undetected, and the carcinoma may go undiagnosed.
  For this reason, 3D sequences (i.e., pulse sequences with 3D data acquisition) should be used. These sequences permit imaging of thin slices with excellent signal-to-noise ratio and without gaps between the slices.
- In-plane resolution should be as good as possible . However, in general a compromise is necessary between in-plane resolution, field-of-view, and temporal resolution. Therefore, with double breast coils resolution mostly ranges around 1-1.5 mm, whereas with single breast imaging a resolution of 0.5-0.7 mm is possible.
- Temporal resolution is important for the following reasons: Early after contrast administration (1-3 min post injection) the best contrast exists between malignancy and surrounding tissue. Later, nonspecific enhance-

ment within benign tissue and decreasing enhancement of most malignancies may cause false negative and false positive calls. Early peripheral enhancement and early wash-out, both of which are important hints for malignancy, may only be detected by dynamic imaging. Optimum imaging time for dynamic imaging probably ranges around 60-120 sec for coverage of the complete breast tissue.[63,64] If increased emphasis is placed on evaluation of enhancement dynamics, specificity may be improved at the cost of sensitivity.

- Every effort should be made to avoid motion. For this reason:
  - Instruct the patient sufficiently (see p. 108)
  - Immobilize the breast as much as possible
- This is best done by using a breast coil with an integrated compression mechanism that allows breast immobilization by slight to moderate breast compression. If this is not available, cotton may be packed between the breast coil and the breast, but this is by far less effective. Commercially available add-on immobilization devices for existing breast coils may be expected in the near future.
- Care should be taken that cardiac artifacts are kept out of diagnostically important areas. This is done by switching the direction of frequency and phase encoding. Artifacts from cardiac motion can be efficiently avoided by imaging in the coronal plane. This can be done since in this plane cardiac artifacts run parallel to the spine and thus cross neither the breast nor the axilla.
- Fast 3D gradient-echo pulse sequences are the optimum method of visualizing small lesions (for example, FLASH 3D: TR = 14 ms, TE = 7 ms, FA = 25° at 1 Tesla or TR = 12 ms, TE = 5 ms, FA = 25° at 1.5 Tesla). The majority of published cases have been examined using these or similar gradient-echo pulse sequences.

- If other pulse sequences are used, their sensitivity for paramagnetic contrast media (e. g., Gd-DTPA) has to be tested. It is very important that the signal intensity in the dose range used increases close to linearly with the tissue uptake of Gd-DTPA. If this is not the case, saturation effects may occur and lesions with indeterminate and with strong uptake of Gd-DTPA may exhibit similar signal increase, leading to both false negative and false positive calls.

- Elimination of fat signal is desirable for improved detection of enhancement, since both enhancing lesions and fat display high signal intensity on postcontrast MR images. Detection of enhancement therefore depends on exact comparison of corresponding precontrast and postcontrast slices. Elimination of fat signal is possible either by use of spectrally selective fat saturation or water excitation, fat nulling (e.g. three-point Dixon)[65], or by image subtraction. Pulse sequences used for image subtraction have the advantage of being fast enough to allow good in-plane and temporal resolution.

Unless spectrally selective pulse sequences are used, breast MRI must be performed using an in-phase-condition. That is fat and water vectors need to point in the same direction.

If it is not fulfilled (in an opposed image), the fat and water vectors are opposite each other. If partial volume of fat and water occurs within the pixel (frequent with small carcinomas growing along ducts) due to changing cancellation effects in the precontrast and postcontrast images, Gd-DTPA uptake may become invisible. In fact, in small carcinomas and carcinomas in situ surrounded by fat, uptake of Gd-DTPA may lead to an increased signal, unchanged signal intensity, or even a decreased signal on the postcontrast image. This means that small carcinomas and carcinomas in situ may be undetectable on opposed images.

The in-phase condition is fulfilled when echo times of 4.8 ms ($\pm$ 25%) at 1.5 Tesla, of approximately 7.2 ms ($\pm$ 25%) at 1 Tesla, and of approximately 14 ms (or smaller than 3.5 ms) at 0.5 tesla are used.[1]

The dosage of Gd-DTPA ranges from 0.1 to 0.2 mmol/kg of body weight. Small lesions, in particular, may be better detected and differentiated at higher doses.[66]

- We strongly recommend *a standardized window setting* and *a standardized imaging order* for evaluating the large number of images.

- Quantitative evaluation of enhancement and enhancement dynamics can be valuable for lesions greater than 2 x the slice thickness. It may provide additional information.

The importance of high-quality imaging in contrast-enhanced MRI of the breast is comparable to its necessity in mammography. Optimum technique and the highest possible degree of standardization are prerequisites for good results.

■ Unenhanced MRI

Careful examination technique is essential for detection and diagnosis of small implant leaks. This includes:

- *Using thin slices.* The slice thickness should always be 5 mm or less. The protocol should contain at least one pulse sequence with slice thicknesses of 2 mm or less.

- *Images should be obtained in at least two imaging planes*, such as the coronal and the transverse planes or the sagittal plane if required.

- *A combination of pulse sequences is recommended*, such as:
  - T2-weighted sequence (thin slice) preferrably with fat saturation
  - T1-weighted sequence with or without fat saturation
  - A "silicone only" sequence with selective excitation of silicone may be helpful to differentiate fluid around the implants or in cysts from silicone deposits

Further possible combinations can be found in the relevant published studies.[26–34]

- Eliminating cardiac artifacts (see above).

Examination Procedure

■ Planning the Examination

■ Contrast-enhanced MRI

- *Strict criteria* should be applied to determine if contrast MRI is indicated (see p. 104–106). This is important not only to reduce costs, but also to minimize the incidence of false positive diagnoses that can result when clinical criteria are defined too loosely.
- *A short history and physical examination should be obtained.* High-quality mammographic studies (if indicated, additional mammograms or sonographic studies) are required to determine if MRI is indicated and to evaluate the results of MRI studies. This material must be available for the examination.
- Whenever possible, in premenopausal women the examination should be conducted between the 6th and 17th day of the menstrual cycle. Outside this time-frame, nonspecific, disseminated, and even focal enhancement may occur more frequently. This can lead to diagnostic errors.[67, 68] If indeterminate enhancement occurs outside the mentioned time-frame, we recommend repeating the examination between day 6 to 17 of the menstrual cycle.
    - Whereas oral contraceptives do not appear to have a negative influence on evaluation of contrast-enhanced MRI, post-menopausal hormone replacement therapy may be a cause of unspecific enhancement in up to 50% of patients. This effect can be eliminated, if hormone replacement therapy is stopped 6–8 weeks before contrast-enhanced MRI. Whether such a delay in diagnosis is acceptable must be decided on an individual basis.
    - Fresh scarring (< 6 months postoperatively or < 12 months after irradiation) can lead to diagnostically disturbing enhancement.[1, 48] Therefore, this information should be available for correct image interpretation. If possible, MRI should be scheduled >6 months after surgery or >12 months after irradiation.
    Previous FNA has not been reported to have a major effect on contrast-enhanced MRI, and core biopsy only rarely causes problems.[48] Nevertheless, we recommend

that the area within the breast and the time since biopsy is recorded.

- Before making an appointment, the physician should ask the patient if any absolute contraindications to MRI are present (these include cardiac pacemakers and certain cardiac valve implants, intracerebral ferromagnetic clips, vascular clips, and so forth; Chapter 1). We also recommend briefly asking the patient about claustrophobic reactions.
- The physician should discuss the procedure with the patient before beginning the examination itself.
    - The patient needs to be informed about the injection of the contrast agent and has to sign the consent form (see Chapter 1).
    - Absolute contraindications to MRI are excluded (see Chapter 1).
    - The purpose of the examination should be briefly explained to the patient.
    - The examination procedure should be described to the patient to familiarize her with it and address any fears she might have. The noise level during the study should be mentioned to her.
    - Finally, the patient should understand that she must remain completely still during the 10–15 min that the examination requires.

■ Unenhanced MRI

- Since unenhanced MRI is the method of choice for detecting implant defects, *no previous studies* (mammography or sonography) are required.
- Before the patient is scheduled, *absolute contraindications* to MRI should be excluded (see previous section). The absence of any absolute contraindications must be documented prior to the examination.
- Correct interpretation of the MR image requires the following information from the *patient's medical history*:
    - The *type of implant* if known (i.e., double-lumen or single-lumen).
    - Whether previous implants have *required replacement* (silicone leakage from earlier implants).
    - Whether any clinical symptoms are present (i.e., pain, inflammation, capsular fi-

brosis, or palpable findings). If a malignancy is suspected, a contrast-enhanced study should follow the unenhanced study.

- *The examination procedure should be briefly discussed* with the patient. She should be informed of the approximate *duration of the examination* (30–45 min) and her questions should be answered.

■ Examination Procedure

■ Contrast-enhanced MRI

- Establish *intravenous access.* Assure adequate length of the i. v. line, and position the patient prone on the patient table.
- *Both breasts (or one breast in case of single breast coil) should hang down into the plastic cup(s)*of the breast coil.
- To minimize breast motion during the examination, immobilize the breasts, preferrably by use of a dedicated immobilization mechanism.
- Next, slide the patient table *into the magnet.*
- Begin adjustment and measurements, which will take approximately 10 min.
- Prior to the injection of contrast medium, the breast is imaged using 2–4 mm slice thickness. Then the paramagnetic contrast medium followed by 30 ml saline is injected through the i. v. line.
- Immediately thereafter, the same slices are imaged another two or more times.
- *To increase the diagnostic reliability of images, the examination procedure should be standardized as much as possible.* This involves:
  - Using the same pulse sequence on the same unit
  - Using the same dosage of contrast medium per kg body weight for every patient
  - Using the same timing (i.e., injection speed, interval between beginning of measurement and injection of contrast)
  - Using standardized windowing
  - Using a standardized sequence of image documentation

After imaging is completed, the patient is taken out of the magnet.

■ Unenhanced MRI

- The patient must be positioned prone and the breasts should hang down into the plastic cups of the breast coil.

- The breasts should be immobilized with cotton or with a special compression device.
- The breast(s) should be examined in thin slices with different pulse sequences and in different imaging planes (see p. 107).

■ Interpretation Criteria and Documentation of Findings

■ Documentation of Findings

■ Contrast-enhanced MRI

Evaluation of the findings depends on the following factors:

- *MR unit* (field strength)
- *pulse sequence* used
- dosage of contrast medium
- *timing*

These values must be included in the report of the examination.

Field strength and pulse sequence are documented on the images. The dosage of contrast medium should be documented in the report. Timing should follow an established plan. Any deviations must be documented (these include deviations in duration of the administration of contrast medium or in the beginning and duration of contrast enhancement, as measured from the start of contrast injection).

The following patient history data should be obtained:

- Time of examination with respect to the patient's menstrual cycle, or postmenopausal examination
- Hormone therapy (especially postmenopausal)
- Recent surgery, needle core biopsy, or radiation therapy, specifying the approximate date of the procedure

Any additional data relevant to the finding should also be mentioned in the report.

- It is recommended to routinely document on hard copy the precontrast series as well as at least one early and one late series of postcontrast images. The same window setting should be used for precontrast and postcontrast images. The window chosen should be narrow enough to visualize slight enhancement, but wide enough to distinguish areas of intermediate and strong enhancement.

If subtraction images without motion artifacts exist, these should be imaged instead of the corresponding series of postcontrast images. A representative slice of each lesion should be documented on all pulse sequences, as well as an enhancement curve of each lesion. This allows optimum assessment of both lesion morphology and enhancement dynamics.

It is recommended to always document the images in the same systematic order.[1]

■ Unenhanced MRI

Thin slices, different *imaging planes*, and the suitable combination of *pulse sequences* are important for ensuring the accuracy of unenhanced MRI in detecting implant failure. For this reason, they should be documented accordingly.

■ Interpretation Criteria

■ Contrast-enhanced MRI

First compare all corresponding unenhanced and enhanced slices or—if good subtraction images are available—use subtraction images to *search for areas of enhancement.*

Detection of small foci and slight enhancement will depend on the technique used (i.e., pulse sequence, slice thickness, and dose of contrast medium; p. 106–7). Subtraction images are very helpful here. However, they are useable only in the absence of any patient motion.

The following factors should be considered when evaluating enhancement:

– *Presence* of contrast enhancement
– *Shape and morphology* of contrast enhancement curve
– *Rate of contrast enhancement (speed of uptake, washout)*

Even though different criteria have been used by various authors and standardized guidelines for image interpretation do not yet exist, the following general rules for image interpretation are widely accepted and should be known to those who perform c.e. MRI:

● *Presence of enhancement is the first and most frequent indicator of possible malignancy. However, this sign is not specific.* On the one hand >90% of invasive carcinomas enhance strongly. However, in approximately 10% of carcinomas only modest to moderate enhancement may occur. Also, numerous benign lesions (fibroadenomas, proliferative benign or inflammatory changes) enhance as well.

● The following *signs* unfrequently occur in benign disease and therefore should be considered *highly suspicious of malignancy*:
– Presence of enhancement within solid lesions, which is more pronounced peripherally (visible mostly on early postcontrast scans).
– Presence of early wash-out (decrease of signal intensity after a peak has been reached within about 3 min post injection.)

These two signs are highly suspicious, even if the lesion is well-circumscribed (exceptions include: cysts with distinct linear wall enhancement or lymph nodes with a fatty center)

● Furthermore, the following *signs* are often associated with malignancy and therefore need to be considered *suspicious until proven otherwise*:
– Presence of irregularly circumscribed, ill-defined or spiculated enhancement or presence of ductal or segmental enhancement. These signs may indicate malignancy even if enhancement is delayed.
– Rapid enhancement (peak within 3 min postinjection followed by a plateau) may also be indicative of malignancy. It is present in about 90% of the invasive carcinomas. In 40–50% it is associated with a wash-out and in the remaining cases with a plateau. For the latter signal curves, overlap exists with part of the enhancing fibroadenomas, proliferative changes, adenosis, or active inflammatory changes. Furthermore, up to 10% of carcinomas exhibit delayed enhancement.

● The following types of *enhancement* are *not typical for malignancy*:
– diffuse enhancement, usually indicating benign changes. However, diffuse enhancement may obscure a small enhancing malignancy or even indicate diffusely growing malignancy
– delayed enhancement (= continuous increase, peak later than 3 min postinjection), occurring most often within benign changes. However 5–10% of invasive malignancies and up to 50% of DCIS may exhibit delayed enhancement. Invasive malignancies with delayed enhancement

may include lobular carcinoma, tubular, medullary, papillary, or an occasionally not otherwise specified invasive ductal carcinoma
- well-circumscribed enhancement, most often occurring in fibroadenomas or papillomas. It is mostly delayed, but may be rapid as well. There do, however, exist some fairly well-circumscribed malignant lesions such as papillary, medullary, or invasive ductal carcinomas, DCIS, or rarely even lobular carcinoma. Many of them may exhibit delayed enhancement. If wash-out or ring enhancement is visible, the lesion must be considered suspicious
- The following findings are rare in malignancy and thus *support a benign process with high probability:*
  - Presence of low signal intensity septations within well-circumscribed or macrolobulated lesions are a quite reliable sign of benignity (rare exception: phylloides tumor)
  - Absence of enhancement. If this is the case, invasive malignancy can be excluded with a high degree of certainty. Exceptions to this rule occur in 1–2 % of invasive malignancies (scirrhous or diffusely growing type of lobular carcinoma, atypical mucinous carcinoma, atypical ductal carcinoma). However, 10–20 % of DCIS may also exhibit no enhancement.

As described above and as shown in Figures 5.1–5.4, some important clues exist concerning the presence or absence of malignancy. However, overlap also exists. *In order to obtain the most accurate diagnosis, combining information from conventional imaging and MRI is recommended.*

An algorithm for combining information of MRI and of convenional imaging in a systematic way is described in Table 5.1.

This algorithm is based on the following knowledge:

- *A definite enhancement with contrast is the most important sign of a malignant process.* However, even modest enhancement can occur in approximately 10 % of carcinomas. A number of benign lesions (fibroadenomas, proliferative benign disorders, and inflammation) can also show enhancement.
- *Focal enhancement with ill-defined or irregular borders or enhancement that follows ductal structures is suggestive of malignancy.* How-

ever, a similar appearance may occur in some cases with focal proliferative changes, adenosis, or, in rare cases, with focal inflammation or fat necrosis.
- *Well-defined focal enhancement* is indicative of a fibroadenoma (as in mammography), yet this does not exclude the possibility of a malignant process.
- *Diffuse milky or patchy enhancement* is most frequently associated with *proliferative benign breast disease.* However, this does not exclude the possibility of a diffusely growing malignancy or of a small malignancy surrounded by benign disease with similar enhancement.
- *Rapid enhancement is a strong indication of a malignant process* since most benign lesions enhance more slowly than carcinomas. However, *slow enhancement cannot exclude malignancy.* Delayed enhancement (maximum later than 3 min after administration of contrast medium) has been observed in approximately 10 % of malignancies.

On the basis of these results, the following application of MRI results is suggested:

- As previously mentioned, contrast-enhanced MRI should not be used for discrimination of palpable lesions or of those imaging detected lesions that can be worked-up by percutaneous biopsy.
- In the appropriate indications in the *absence of enhancement, an invasive carcinoma can be excluded with a high degree of certainty.* Exceptions to this rule occur in less than 1–2 % of invasive carcinomas. For this reason, we recommend a needle or open biopsy if carcinoma is strongly suspected. In the absence of this suspicion, we recommend standard mammographic and clinical follow-up. To minimize the chance of overlooking carcinomas in situ or a nonenhancing lobular carcinoma—which would generally be detected mammographically on the basis of microcalcifications or an architectural distortion not related to scarring—*MRI must always be combined with mammography.* Diagnostic decisions regarding microcalcifications, an architectural distortion not related to scarring, or any highly suspicious lesion should not be influenced by MRI.
- Ill-defined *focal enhancement,* focal enhancement that follows the ducts, any focal enhancement with early washout or early, more pronounced peripheral enhancement re-

Table 5.1 Guidelines for interpretation of contrast-enhanced MRI of the breast.

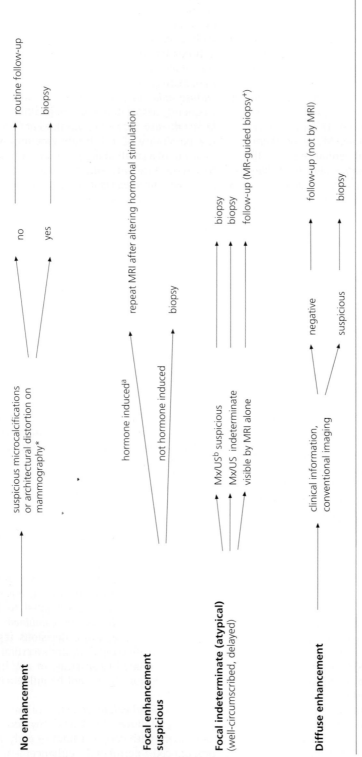

No enhancement
→ suspicious microcalcifications or architectural distortion on mammography*
→ no → routine follow-up
→ yes → biopsy

Focal enhancement suspicious
→ hormone induced[a] → repeat MRI after altering hormonal stimulation
→ not hormone induced → biopsy

Focal indeterminate (atypical)
(well-circumscribed, delayed)
→ Mx/US[b] suspicious → biopsy
→ Mx/US indeterminate → biopsy
→ visible by MRI alone → follow-up (MR-guided biopsy[+])

Diffuse enhancement
→ clinical information, conventional imaging
→ negative → follow-up (not by MRI)
→ suspicious → biopsy

* Potential signs of DCIS or lobular carcinoma, which may not enhance in about 20 % of the cases respectively
[a] Check hormonal influence: if MRI was performed during days 5–18 of menstrual cycle, repeat between days 6–17; if patient was receiving HRT, consider a repeat MRI 3 months after cessation of HRT
[b] MX = mammography; US = ultrasonography
[+] only in patients or conditions with a high risk of malignancy

Fig. 5.1   Findings are shown which on c-e MRI are *highly suspicious of malignancy.* They include *peripheral enhancement and wash-out*

a–d The leading lesion in this case is an ill-circumscribed mass with inhomogeneous enhancement. The enhancement is more pronounced in the periphery. Both morphology of the enhancement and the dynamic enhancement curve, which in this case also showed a wash-out, classify this lesion as highly suspicious of malignancy. Furthermore, a second very small lesion is seen at 9 o'clock. Due to its small size, both evaluation of lesion contours and of the dynamic curve (partial volume) is difficult. This lesion has to be considered indeterminate, possibly malignant

Histogy: The main lesion proved to be an invasive ductal carcinoma. The second focus was an otherwise occult focus of non-comedo DCIS

a Precontrast MRI

b Postcontrast MRI (second series after contrast agent; acquisition time of central k-space data: 130 sec p.i.)

c Subtraction image of image **b** minus image **a**. Whenever a curve is measured in such a lesion, the region of interest has to be placed into the area with the strongest and fastest enhancement. Care must be taken to avoid partial volume with surrounding tissue or with nonenhancing necrotic areas of the lesion

d The so-called enhancement curve shows the change of signal intensity (not the relative enhancement!) with time after injection, starting at 0 sec (= start of injection)

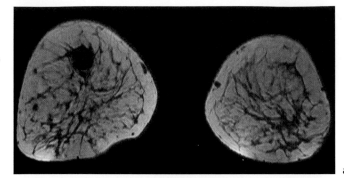

a

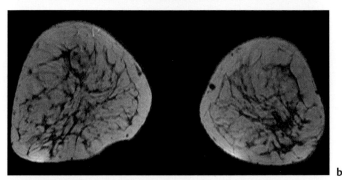

b

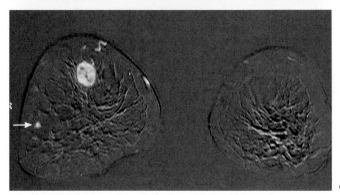

c

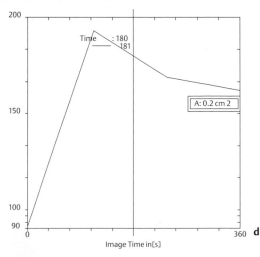

d

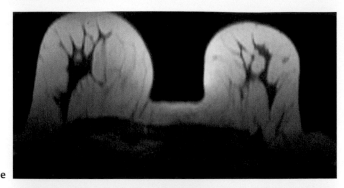

e

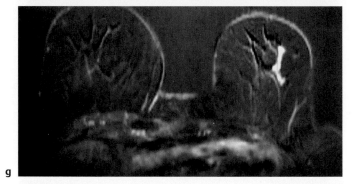

f

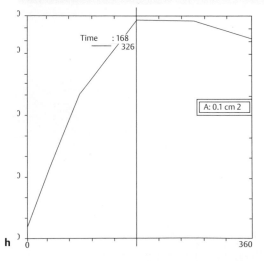

g

Fig. 5.**1e–h**   In this patient a strongly enhancing duct was detected by MRI alone (mammography and ultrasound did not show an abnormality). Furthermore the enhancement curve measured in this duct shows some wash-out. Based on the morphology (ductal enhancement) and the enhancement curve, this finding is highly suspicious. Histology: DCIS intermediate grade
Note some DCIS exhibit wash-out
e Precontrast MRI
f Postcontrast MRI (second series after contrast agent)
g Subtraction image of image **b** minus image **a**
h Enhancement curve shows wash-out

Time   : 168
        326

A: 0.1 cm 2

h   0   360

Fig. 5.**2** Findings that on dynamic contrast-enhanced MRI have to be *considered
suspicious for malignancy*, but may sometimes also occur in benign disease, include:
*ductal or segmental enhancement without
wash-out*. Based only on its typical morphology this type of enhancement often
indicates malignancy. Furthermore, *ill-circumscribed enhancement* may indicate
malignancy, but may sometimes also be
seen in benign changes.
a–d In this patient (status after breast-
conserving therapy on the right) segmental
enhancement was noted by chance in the
left breast laterally. Even though the enhancement curve shows a delayed plateau,
the lesion has to be considered suspicious
based on the segmental type of enhancement. Histology: intermediate grade DCIS
a Precontrast MRI
b Postcontrast MRI (second series after
contrast agent)
c Subtraction image of image **b** minus
image **a**
d Curve shows a delayed plateau-type enhancement

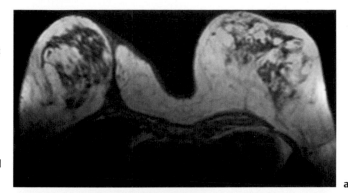

a

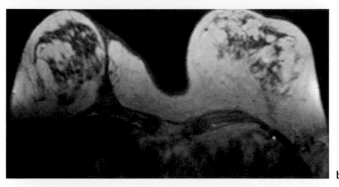

b

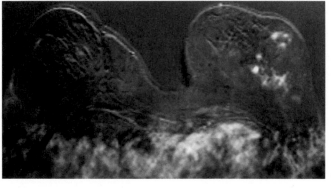

c

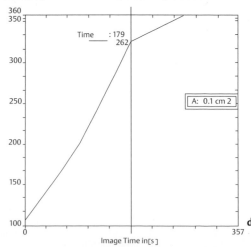

d

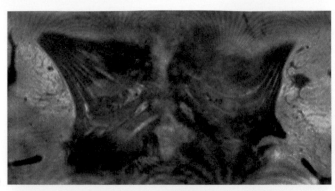

e

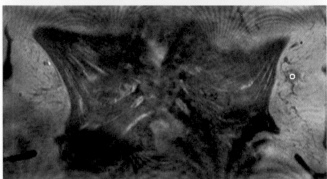

f

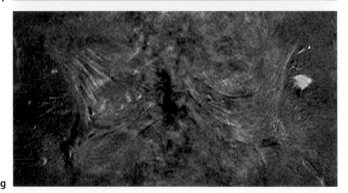

g

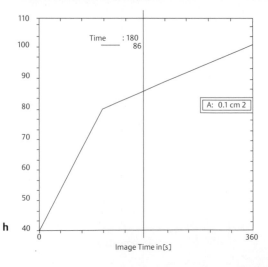

h

Fig. 5.**2e–h**   In this case an ill-circumscribed lesion was detected in the axillary
tail. Even though the enhancement curve is
delayed, the spiculated margin classifies
this lesion as suspicious
Histology: invasive ductal carcinoma T1, G2
e Precontrast MRI
f Postcontrast MRI (second series after
contrast agent)
g Subtraction image of image **b** minus
image **a**
h Curve shows delayed enhancement

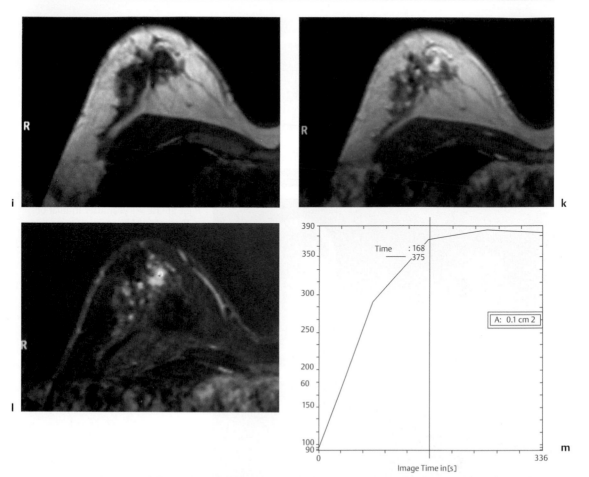

Fig. 5.**2 i–m** In this case a lobulated lesion with some-what irregular contours was detected by MRI. (The re-maining breast tissue shows monomorphous, evenly dis-tributed patchy enhancement, compatible with prolifera-tive changes). The enhancement curve shows a plateau and thus cannot rule out malignancy. Based on its con-tours and the indeterminate enhancement curve, the lobulated lesion was considered moderately suspicious and biopsy was recommended
Histology: sclerosing adenosis and papillomatosis
i Precontrast MRI
k Postcontrast MRI (second series after contrast agent)
l Subtraction image of image **b** minus image **a**
m Enhancement curve shows a plateau

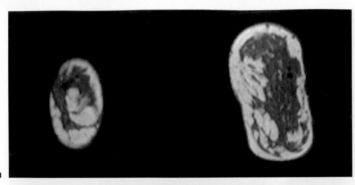

a

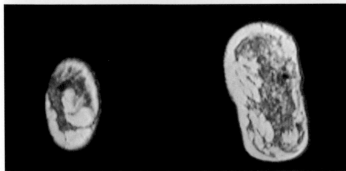

b

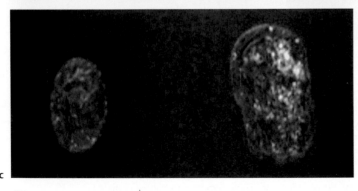

c

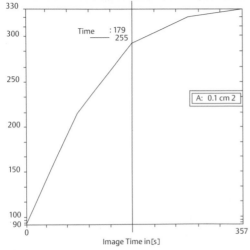

d

Fig. 5.3 Findings that are *atypical for malignancy, but may be seen in 5–10%* of malignancies, include: *delayed diffuse enhancement* and *delayed well-circumscribed enhancement.*

a–d In this patient, who was examined after breast-conserving therapy on the right, diffuse patchy enhancement was seen throughout the left breast (no segmental or ductal distribution). Follow-up confirmed this to be compatible with benign proliferative or hyperplastic changes, as they frequently also occur in normal breasts. Note: very little to no enhancement is seen in the right breast >1 year after irradiation.

a Precontrast MRI
b Postcontrast MRI (second series after contrast agent)
c Subtraction image of image **b** minus image **a**
d Enhancement curve shows delayed enhancement

Fig. 5.**3 e–h** This patient presented with a palpable thickening measuring about 4 cm in her right breast medially. The patient was on hormones and showed diffuse bilateral enhancement with a plateau-type curve. Generally, diffuse enhancement that does not show early enhancement or wash-out is very compatible with benign changes, particularly in a patient on hormone replacement therapy. However, malignancy can never be excluded in this type of tissue when a suspicious clinical or mammographic finding exists. Workup of the clinical finding must, therefore, be recommended

Histology (from bilateral mastectomy, as explicitly chosen by the patient): T2 infiltrating lobular carcinoma on the right medially, but not laterally, no sign of malignancy on the left

e Precontrast MRI

f Postcontrast MRI (second series after contrast agent)

g Subtraction image of image **b** minus image **a**

h Curve shows plateau-type enhancement

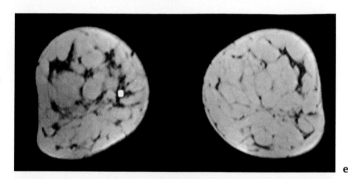

e

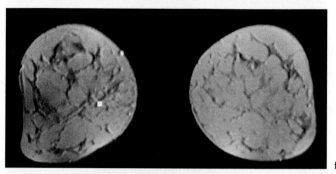

f

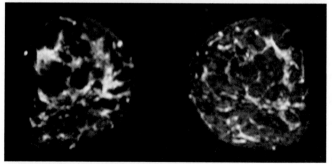

g

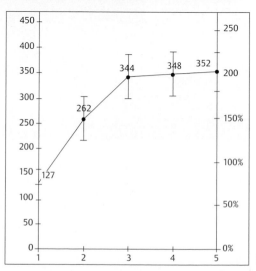

h

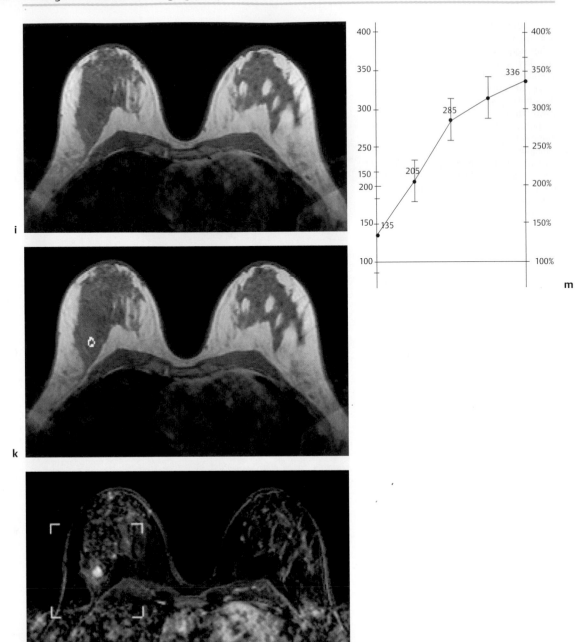

Fig. 5.3 i–m Well-circumscribed oval enhancing mass is shown. The smooth contours and delayed enhancement curve rule in a benign lesion, such as a fibroadenoma. Since the patient was at high risk and asked for a definitive diagnosis, MR-guided biopsy was performed on this MR-detected lesion

Histology: fibroadenoma
i Precontrast MRI
k Precontrast MRI showing the ROI measurement
l Subtraction image of image **b** minus image **a**
m Curve shows plateau-type enhancement

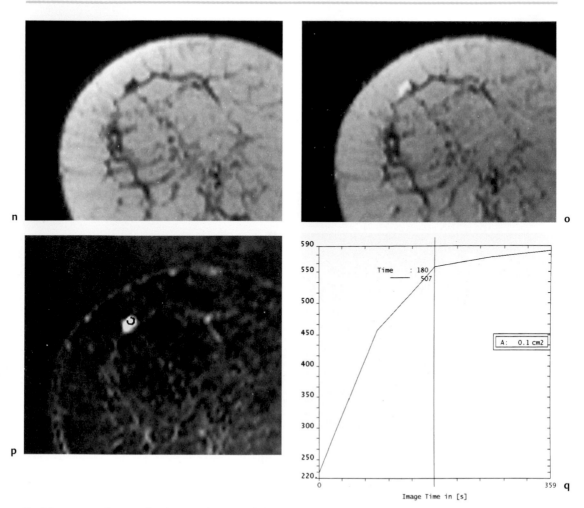

Fig. 5.**3 n–q** Another small enhancing lesion is shown. The curve is uncharacteristic and shows delayed enhancement. If such a lesion is detected by MRI alone, follow-up MRI would be recommended. In this case biopsy was performed because the patient was status after breast-conserving therapy on the left and because the lesion had newly appeared on a follow-up MRI
Histology: 5-mm ductal carcinoma G2

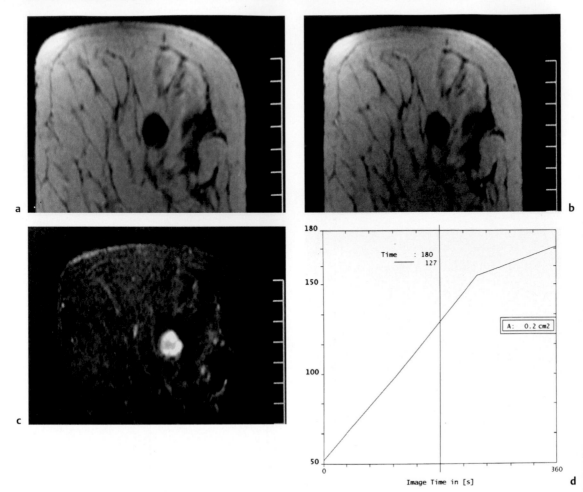

Fig. 5.4 Lesions or changes with a *high probability of being benign* include: *well-circumscribed* oval or lobulated lesions (< 3 gentle lobulations) *with fine internal septations* of low signal intensity (a–d). Furthermore, changes with *absent or minimal enhancement* are benign with a high probability, provided suspicious microcalcifications or an architectural distortion that is not explained by scarring are excluded (e–f).

a–d A completely well-circumscribed smooth and oval lesion is shown. The enhancement curve is delayed. On the postcontrast scan and on the subtraction image internal fine septations become faintly visible, ruling in a fibroadenoma. Benign lesion proven by follow-up
a Precontrast MRI
b Postcontrast MRI (second series after contrast agent)
c Subtraction image of image **b** minus image **a**
d Curve shows a delayed enhancement

Fig. 5.**4 e–f** This patient presented with a somewhat striking mammographic asymmetry, but no palpable abnormality. No enhancement is seen within either breast, ruling in benign asymmetry
Diagnosis proven by follow-up
e Precontrast MRI
f Postcontrast MRI (second series after contrast agent)
g Subtraction image of **b** minus **a**
h Curve shows no significant enhancement

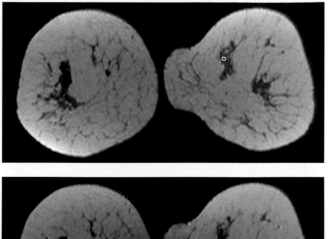

e

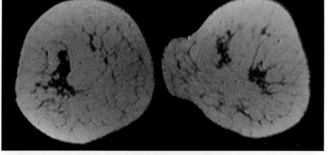

f

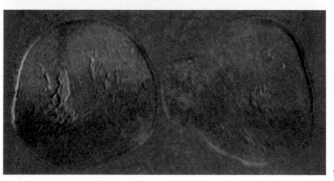

g

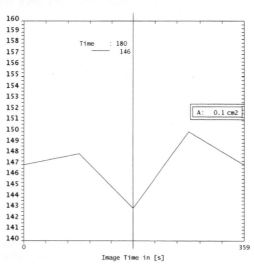

h

quires further workup, usually biopsy. This applies even if all other diagnostic examinations are negative.

- *Well-circumscribed enhancing lesions* visible with other imaging modalities and *not clearly benign* require further workup, usually percutaneous biopsy. If they are *detected* only by MRI, if no peripheral enhancement or early washout exists, and if no significantly increased risk of malignancy exists, we recommend a *follow-up MRI examination* after a period of 6 and 12–18 months. This procedure is necessary to avoid unnecessary biopsies of small, otherwise asymptomatic fibroadenomas, which are discovered with very high sensitivity by contrast-enhanced MRI.
- *MRI does not provide diagnostic information in the presence of diffuse enhancement.*

The high sensitivity of MRI is certainly its most important advantage. To make use of it, we recommend that a low threshold is selected for diagnosing any lesion that is visible by other methods as well (e. g., on one view) or that is clinically suspicious or indeterminate (e. g., nipple retraction). Sufficient specificity should be achieved by integrating information from mammography and clinical examination, follow-up examination, or needle core biopsy of indeterminate lesions.

For lesions that are only visible by MRI a higher threshold may be chosen, above which level or speed of enhancement will be regarded as suspicious. However, we must warn against generally improving specificity at the cost of sensitivity.[8, 12] Further research is required regarding the extent to which quantitative data from one unit may be transferred to another.

■ Unenhanced MRI

Knowledge of normal findings with a breast implant is an important prerequisite for correct diagnosis of implant failure.

■ Normal Findings in the Presence of a Breast Implant

The single-lumen implant consists of the very thin silicone plastic envelope containing either liquid silicone (silicone implant) or a saline solution (saline implant).

Double-lumen implants have a second smaller implant within the outer implant (which is generally filled with saline solution, rarely with silicone). The smaller inner implant is generally filled with silicone, rarely with saline solution. Some temporary implants have a valve through which the implant can be filled. Since this is magnetic, it will generally cause a large artifact.

The outer envelope of the implant is surrounded by a capsule of connective tissue that forms as the wound heals. Usually, the outer envelope will be in direct contact with the capsule of connective tissue so that a thin strip of low signal intensity (1–2 mm wide) will surround the implant.

In rare cases, fluid can accumulate between the outer envelope of the implant and the capsule of connective tissue (especially in folds). This fluid will appear as an area of high signal intensity in T2-weighted images and must be carefully distinguished from silicone leakage from the envelope of the implant (see below). Both the inner and outer implant envelopes can form folds.

■ Capsular Fibrosis (Contracture)

In capsular fibrosis, the capsule of connective tissue surrounding the implant contracts and may become hypertrophic. This produces a sensation of tension, sometimes pain, and causes the implant to assume a balloon-like shape. The diagnosis of capsular fibrosis is made clinically.

This balloon-like configuration is also seen by MRI. Thickening of the connective-tissue capsule only may be observed in some of these patients.

■ Implant Rupture

Rupture of a silicone-filled single-lumen implant or a silicone-filled outer implant envelope is recognizable by one of the following characteristic features:

- Silicone is present outside of the connective-tissue capsule (*extracapsular rupture*). Such extracapsular silicone depots are best visualized with a so-called "silicone-only" sequence or with a T2-weighted water saturation sequence, where they present as an area of high signal intensity outside the capsule (Fig. 5.**5a**).
- Silicone is present outside the implant folds, but still within the connective-tissue capsule (*intracapsular rupture*). With the aid of this sign (described in the literature as the *keyhole sign* or *reverse C sign*; Figs. 5.**5 a** and **b**), the examiner can detect even small implant defects.

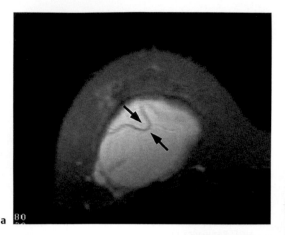 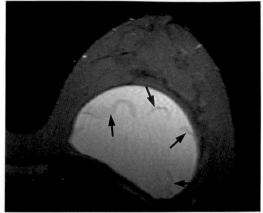

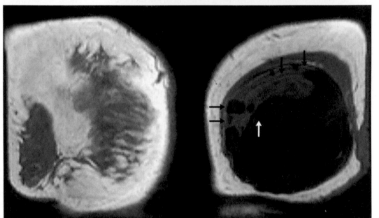

Fig. 5.**5a** and **b** Implant rupture
a Extracapsular rupture (open arrowheads) and intracapsular rupture (arrows). In the intracapsular rupture, silicone is present on both sides of the fold marked with the arrows. This is the "reverse C sign" referred to by Dr R Patt, Georgetown University
b "Linguini sign" in an intracapsular rupture. The torn outer envelope floats in the puddle of silicone fluid (similarly to linguini noodles) surrounded by the fibrous capsule
c "Salad oil sign". If the inner shell of a double lumen implant ruptures, both fluids (oily silicone and saline) mix and droplets (arrows) of one fluid are contained within the other fluid

- The outer envelope of the implant is completely ruptured and collapsed. It then appears as a thin, folded, linear structure floating in the puddle of silicone fluid, which is only surrounded by the connective-tissue capsule (so-called *linguini sign*).

If a saline-filled implant or the saline-filled outer envelope of an implant ruptures, it can usually be diagnosed clinically from the loss in volume.

If only the inner envelope of a double-lumen implant ruptures, the silicone and saline solutions will mix. This will produce droplets within the implant fluids as found when salad oil is mixed with vinegar (so-called *salad oil sign*).

■ References

1 Heywang-Köbrunner SH, Beck R. Contrast-enhanced MRI of the breast. New York: Springer; 1996
2 Fischer U. Lehratlas der MR-Mammographie. Stuttgart: Thieme 1999
3 Heywang-Köbrunner SH, Bick U, Bradley WG et al. International Investigation of breast MRI: results of a multicenter study (11 sites) concerning diagnostic parameters of contrast-enhanced MRI based on 519 histopathologically correlated lesions. Eur Radiology, in press.
4 Nunes LW, Schnall MD, Orel SG. Breast MR imaging interpretation model. Radiology. 1997;202:833–41
5 Harms SE, Flaming DP, Hesley KL et al. MR imaging of the breast with rotating delivery of excitation off resonance: Clinical experience with pathologic correlation. Radiology. 1993;187:493
6 Gilles R, Guinebretiere J, Lucidarme O et al. Non-palpable breast tumors: diagnosis with contrast-enhanced subtraction dynamic MR imaging. Radiology. 1994;191:625–31

7   Boetes C, Barentsz JO, Mus RD. MR characterisation of suspicious breast lesions with a Gd-enhanced Turbo-FLASH subtraction technique. Radiology. 1994;193:777–81

8   Kaiser WA. MRM promises earlier breast cancer diagnosis. Diagn Imaging Clin Med. 1992:88–93

9   Boetes C, Mus RD, Holland R et al. Breast tumors: Comparative accuracy of MR imaging relative to mammography and ultrasound for demonstrating extent. Radiology. 1995;197:743–7

10 Ikeda O, Yamashita Y, Morishita S et al. Characterization of breast masses by dynamic enhanced MR imaging. A logistic regression analysis. Acta Radiol. 1999;40:585–92

11 Kuhl CK, Mielcarek P, Klaschik S et al. Dynamic breast MR imaging: are signal intensity time course data useful for differential diagnosis of enhancing lesions. Radiology. 1999;211:101–10

12 Fischer U, Kopka L, Grabbe E. Breast carcinoma: effect of preoperative contrast-enhanced MR imaging on the therapeutic approach. Radiology. 1999;213:881–8

13 Heywang-Köbrunner SH, Viehweg P, Heinig A, Küchler Ch. Contrast-enhanced MRI of the breast: accuracy, value, controversies, solutions. Eur J Radiol. 1997;24:94–108

14 Heywang SH, Hahn D, Schmid H et al. MR imaging of the breast using Gadolinum-DTPA. J Comput Assist Tomogr. 1986;10:199–204

15 Boné B, Pentek Z, Perbeck L, Veress B. Diagnostic accuracy of mammography and contrast-enhanced MR-imaging in 238 histologically verified breast lesions. Acta Radiol. 1997;38:489–96

16 Brezina A, Schwaighofer BW. Magnetresonanztomographie (MRT) der Mamma bei Problempatientinnen. Wien Klin Wochenschau. 1994;106:584–9

17 Buchberger W, Koekkoek-Doll P de, Obrist P, Dunser M. Der Stellenwert der MR-Tomographie beim unklaren Mammographiebefund. Radiologe. 1997;37:702

18 Liu PF, Debatin JF, Caduff RF, Kacl G, Garzoli E, Krestin GP. Improved diagnostic accuracy in dynamic contrast enhanced MRI of the breast by combined quantitative and qualitative analysis. Br J Radiol. 1998;71:501–9

19 Sittek H, Kessler M, Heuck AF et al. Dynamische MR-Mammographie: Ist der Verlauf der Signalintensitätszunahme zur Differenzierung unterschiedlicher Formen der Mastopathie geeignet? RöFo. 1996;165:59–63

20 Heywang-Köbrunner SH, Viehweg P. Sensitivity of contrast-enhanced MR imaging of the breast. Magn Reson Imaging Clin N Am. 1994;2:527–38

21 Rubens D, Totterman S, Chacko AK et al. Gadopentetate dimeglumine-enhanced chemical-shift MR imaging of the breast. AJR. 1991;157:267–70

22 Gilles R, Zafrani B, Guinebretiere JM et al. Ductal carcinoma in situ. MR imaging-histopathologic correlation. Radiology. 1995;196:415–9

23 Soderstrom CE, Harms SE, Copit DS et al. Three-dimensional RODEO breast MR imaging of lesions containing ductal carcinoma in situ. Radiology. 1996;201:427–32

24 Westerhof JP, Fischer U, Moritz JD, Oestmann JW. MR Imaging of mammographically detected clustered microcalcifications; Is there any value? Radiology. 1998;207:675–81

25 Orel SG, Medonca MH, Reynolds C et al. MR imaging of ductal carcinoma in situ. Radiology. 1997;202:413–20

26 Brem RF, Tempany CMC, Zerhouni EA. MR detection of breast implant rupture. J Comput Assist Tomogr. 1992;16:157–9

27 Berg WA, Caskey CI, Hamper UM et al. Single- and Double-Lumen Silicone Breast Implant Integrity: Prospective Evaluation of MR and US Criteria. Radiology. 1995;197:45–52

28 De Angelis GA, Lange EE, Miller LR, Morgan RF. MR-imaging of Breast Implants. Radiographics. 1994;14:783–94

29 Everson LI, Parantainen H, Detlie T et al. Diagnosis of Breast Implant Rupture: Imaging Findings and relative Efficacies of Imaging Techniques. AJR. 163:57–60

30 Gorczyca DP, Sinha S, Ahn CY et al. Silicone Breast Implants in Vivo: MR Imaging. Radiology. 1992;185:407–10

31 Gorczyca DP, Brenner RJ. The Augmented Breast. Radiologic & Clinical Perspectives. New York, Stuttgart: Thieme; 1997

32 Piccoli CW, Greer JG, Mitchell DG. Breast MR Imaging for Cancer Detection and Implant Evaluation: Potential Pitfalls. Radiographics. 1996;16:63–75

33 Soo MS, Kornguth PJ, Walsh R et al. Complex Radial Folds Versus Subtle Sign of Intracapsular Rupture of Breast Implants: MR Findings with Surgical Correlation. AJR. 166:1421–7

34 Stroman PW, Rolland C, Dufour M et al. Appearance of Low Signal Intensity Lines in MRI of Silicone Breast Implants. Biomaterials.1996;17:983–8

35 Krämer S, Schulz-Wendtland R, Hagedorn K et al. Magnetic Resonance Imaging and its role in the diagnosis of multicentric breast cancer. Anticancer Research. 1998;18:2163–4

36 Oellinger H, Heins S, Sander B et al. Gd-DTPA-enhanced MR breast imaging: the most sensitive method for multicentric carcinomas of the female breast. Eur Radiol. 1993;3:223–8

37 Mumtaz H, Hall-Craigs MA, Davidson T et al. Staging of symptomatic primary breast cancer with MR imaging. AJR. 1997;169:417–24

38 Lewis-Jones HG, Whitehouse GH, Leistner SJ. The role of magnetic resonance imaging in the assessment of local recurrent breast carcinoma. Clin Radiol.1991;43:197–204

39 Dao TH, Rahmouni A, Campana F et al. Tumor recurrence versus fibrosis in the irradiated breast: differentiation with dynamic gadolinium-enhanced MR imaging. Radiology. 1993;187:751–5

40 Heywang-Köbrunner SH, Schlegel A, Beck R et al. Contrast-enhanced MRI of the breast after limited surgery and radiation therapy. J Comput Assist Tomogr. 1993;7:891–900

41 Gilles R, Guinebretiere JM, Shapeero LG et al. Assessment of breast cancer recurrence with contrast-enhanced subtraction MR imaging: preliminary results in 26 patients: Radiology. 1993;188:473–8

42 Mussurakis S, Buckley DL, Bowsley SJ et al. Dynamic contrast-enhanced magnetic resonance imaging of the breast combined with pharmacokinetic analysis of gadolinium-DTPA uptake in the diagnosis of local recurrence of early stage breast cancer. Investigative Radiology. 1995;30:650–62

43 Drew, PJ, Kerin MJ, Turnbull LW et al. Routine screening for local recurrence following breast-conserving therapy for cancer with dynamic contrast-enhanced magnetic resonance imaging of the breast. Ann Surg Oncol. 1998;5:265–70

44 Krämer S, Schulz-Wendtland R, Hagedorn K et al. Magnetic resonance imaging in the diagnosis of local recurrences in the breast cancer. Anticancer Res. 1998;18:2159–62

45 Rieber A, Merkle E, Zeitler H et al. Value of MR mammography in the detection and exclusion of recurrent breast carcinoma. J Comput Assist Tomogr. 1997;21:780–4

46 Viehweg P, Heinig A, Lampe D et al. Retrospective analysis for evaluation of the value of contrast-enhanced MRI in patients with breast conservative therapy. MAGMA (Magnetic Resonance Materials in Physics, Biology and Medicine). 1998;7:141–52

47 Müller RD, Barkhausen J, Sauerwein W, Langer R. Assessment of local recurrence after breast conserving therapy with MRI. JCAT. 1998;22:408–12

48 Fischer U, Kopka L, Grabbe E. Magnetic resonance guided localization and biopsy of suspicious breast lesions. Topics in Magnetic Resonance Imaging. 1998;9:44–59

49 Heinig A, Heywang-Köbrunner SH, Viehweg P et al. Wertigkeit der Kontrastmittel-Magnetresonanztomographie der Mamma bei Wiederaufbau mittels Implantat. Radiologe. 1997;37:710–7

50 Boné B, Aspelin P, Isberg B et al. Contrast-enhanced MR imaging of the breast in patients with silicon implants after cancer surgery. Acta Radiol. 1995;36:111–6.

51 Soderstrom CE, Harms SE, Farell RS et al. Detection with MR imaging of residual tumor in the breast soon after surgery. AJR. 1997;168:485–8

52 Orel SG, Reynolds C, Schnall MD et al. Breast carcinoma; MR imaging before reexcisional biopsy. Radiology. 1997;205:429–36

53 Abraham DC, Jones RC, Jones SE et al. Evaluation of locally advanced breast cancer by magnetic resonance imaging. Cancer. 1996;78:91–100

54 Mumtaz H, Davidson T, Spittle M et al. Breast surgery after neoadjuvant treatment. Is it necessary? Eur J Surg Oncol. 1996;22:335–41

55 Rieber A, Zeitler H, Rosenthal H et al. MRI of breast cancer: influence of chemotherapy on sensitivity. Br J Radiol. 1997;70:452–8

56 Kurtz JM, Spitalier JM, Almaric R et al. Results of wide excision for local recurrence after breast conserving therapy. Cancer. 1989;61:1969–72

57 Morris EA, Schwartz LH, Dershaw DD et al. MR imaging of the breast in patients with occult primary breast carcinoma. Radiology. 1997;205:437–40

58 Schorn C, Fischer U, Luftner-Nagel S et al. MRI of the breast in patients with metastatic disease of unknown primary. Eur Radiol. 1999;9:470–3

59 Orel SG, Weinstein SP, Schnall MD. Breast MR imaging in patients with axillary node metastases and unknown primary malignancy. Radiology. 1999;212:543–9

60 Kuhl CK, Schmutzler R, Leutner CC et al. Breast MR screening in women proved or suspected to be carriers of a breast cancer susceptibility gene: preliminary results. Radiology. 2000;215:267–76

61 Tilanus-Linthorst MM, Bartels CC, Obdejin AI, Oudkerk M. Earlier detection of breast cancer by surveillance of women at familial risk. Eur J Cancer. 2000;36:514–9

62 Stoutjesdijk MJ, Boetes C, Van Die LE et al. Magnetic resonance mammography for breast cancer screening of patients from high risk populations: results of a prospective pilot study. Radiology. 1999;213:454

63 Buckley DL, Mussarakis S, Horsman A. Effect of temporal resolution on the diagnostic efficacy of contrast-enhanced MRI in the conservatively treated breast. J Comput Assist Tomogr. 1998;22:47–51

64 Schorn C, Fischer U, Luftner-Nagel S, Grabbe E. Diagnostic potential of ultrafast contrast-enhanced MRI of the breast in hypervascularized lesions: are there advantages in comparison with standard dynamic MRI? J Comput Assist Tomogr. 1999;23:118–22

65 Daniel BL, Butts K, Glover GH et al. Breast cancer: Gadolinium-enhanced MR imaging with a 0.5 T open imager and three-point Dixon technique. Radiology. 1998;207:183–90

66 Heywang-Köbrunner SH, Haustein J, Pohl C et al. Contrast-enhanced MRI of the breast: comparison of two dosages. Radiology. 1994;191:639

67 Kuhl CK, Bieling HB, Gieseke J et al. Healthy premenopausal breast parenchyma in dynamic contrast-enhanced MR imaging of the breast: normal contrast medium enhancement and cyclical-phase dependency. Radiology. 1997;203:137–44.

68 Müller-Schimpfle M, Ohmenhäuser K, Stoll P et al. Menstrual cycle and age: influence on parenchymal contrast medium enhancement in MR imaging of the breast. Radiology. 1997;203:145–9.

6. Breast Imaging Techniques under Investigation

For those involved in breast imaging it is clear that significant progress has been made in this field during the last decades. Mammographic screening allows detection of malignancy at earlier stages and thus is able to reduce breast cancer mortality by at least 30%. By selective use of ultrasound, percutaneous biopsy and MRI workup of screening-detected indeterminate lesions, of problem cases and preoperative workup for treatment planning have been improved.

Nevertheless, mammography and these other methods still have limitations. Earlier detection might result in even higher mortality reduction. A decrease in the false negative and false positive rate of the diagnosis achieved by imaging and clinical examination would also be desirable.

With this perspective, research in various modalities continues. In this chapter the present state of imaging methods under investigation is summarized.

■ Scintimammography

Scintimammography provides functional information by evaluation of tracer uptake. Improved performance using technetium(Tc)-99 m Sestamibi has resulted in its replacing thallium 201 and Tc-99m-tetrofosmin as tracers.[1]

Sestamibi is a lipophilic complex, which is able to penetrate the cell membrane. Within the cell it is electrostatically bound to cytosole and membranes of mitochondria. Experimental studies indicate that Sestamibi accumulates preferentially in tumor cells.[2, 3] Although initial reports were enthusiastic, studies based on more patient data have demonstrated a usefulness on the whole limited to larger, often palpable cancers. These data have shown the following:[4-7]

1. For *palpable* lesions sensitivities of 83–97% have been reported
2. Specificities range from 70–90%

3. For lesions ≤1 cm, only a sensitivity of about 50% could be achieved in all studies
4. Detection of in situ carcinomas is unreliable

Among the breast imaging community it has been felt that *indications for scintimammography* cannot be deduced from the existing data.

Tumors ≤1 cm are prognostically most important since they have an excellent chance of being cured. A technology which misses a large number of these tumors cannot be considered useful for screening. Use of such a method for exclusion of malignancy can be harmful to the patient due to:(a) very unreliable diagnosis of early malignancy (which may be contained within a palpable abnormality)[8]; (b) the lower accuracy compared to surgery or percutaneous biopsy, even in the larger lesions.

Finally, there is no justification for using an additional method just for confirmation of a positive diagnosis.[8]

Also, radiation dose should be considered: with the usual dose of 740 MBc Tc-99 m for one Sestamibi study, about 2.5 mGy are applied to the breast. In addition, the radiation exposure of this intravenously injected tracer is transported to all organs of the body. The gonadal dosage is 6–9 mGy and the equivalent dosage to the whole body is about 6 mGy.[9,10]

Factors influencing the accuracy of scintimammography include:

1. tracer uptake (dependent on tumor histology)
2. lesion size
3. lesion depth (distance between lesion and camera and attenuation of radiation by tissue between lesion and camera)
4. resolution of the detector

The use of SPECT in addition to planar prone scintigraphy may minimally improve the technique.[11,12]It remains to be demonstrated whether reported improvement with special high-resolution cameras[13]will eventually result in the accuracy required for small lesions.

■ Positron Emission Tomography

Like scintigraphy or dynamic contrast-enhanced MRI, positron emission tomography (PET) is able to prositron functional information.

Compared to scintimammography it offers technological advantages: it can provide higher resolution than SPECT, and due to electronic collimation it allows a higher sensitivity for the tracer.[14] The two tracers mainly used for breast imaging have been 16-alpha [18F] fluoro-17-beta-estradiol (FES) and 2-[fluorine-18] fluoro-2-desoxy-p-glucose (FDG).

FES-PET is specific for the estrogen receptor, which is expressed by some breast cancers. It is thus capable of identifying receptor-positive tumor or metastases. Such information might be useful in predicting response to antiestrogens in metastasized patients (e. g., if different behavior of metastases and primary tumor might be expected).[15]

FDG is a glucose analogue and thus an indicator of increased metabolism. Uptake of FDG in tumors has been reported to be higher than that of Sestamibi.[1]

Based on first experiences, the accuracy of PET may be slightly higher than that of scintimammography. However, present data are still very limited.[14, 16, 17, 18] They predominantly concern large breast cancers ≥ 2 cm, while the detection rate for lesions ≤ 1 cm appears to be unsatisfactory for PET, as this is also the case for scintimammography.

Thus, as with scintimammography, PET cannot be recommended for detection or diagnosis of primary breast tumors. The radiation dosage (to the breast and whole body) resulting from a single injection of 740 MBc FDG even exceeds that of scintimammography: The dosage to the breast amounts to 6 mGy, the gonadal dose to 11 mGy, and the effective equivalent dosage to the body to 19 mGy.[10]

Thus, FDG-PET may be of value for assessing response of cancer treatment in selected cases. First studies reported a sensitivity of about 90 % and specificities of 74 and 91 % respectively for assessment of response to chemotherapy[19, 20], results that are comparable to those of MRI (see Chapter 5). A definite advantage of PET certainly is its capability to provide a fast overview of the whole body and to detect unsuspected metastases.[14]

■ Other Methods

Imaging of *tissue elasticity* is possible directly by ultrasound elastography, MR elastography, or indirectly by measuring ultrasound velocity using ultrasound CT or a method called CARI-sonography (clinical amplitude/velocity reconstructive imaging). With *ultrasound elastography*[21] shift of tissue structures with and without standardized slight compression is evaluated. *MR elastography*[22] promises to visualize tissue shifts exerted by a mechanical wave by use of motion-sensitive phase contrast imaging. Since ultrasound velocity correlates with tissue elasticity[23], imaging of ultrasound velocity by means of *ultrasound CT*[24, 25] or CARI sonography[26] also allows indirect imaging of tissue elasticity. *CARI sonography* is based on B-mode imaging of the compressed breast. The contralateral compression plate is imaged on the B-mode image as a reflexogen line underneath the breast tissue. Elevation of this line is an indicator of increased ultrasound velocity in the structures overlying the elevated part of the reflexogen line.

Preliminary data have shown that imaging of tissue elasticity may be of some value. However, false negative and false positive results occur. So far none of these methods is ready for clinical use.

Light transmission through breast tissue has been pursued for several decades. Clinical studies and extensive in vitro data have not yet shown a potenial clinical use.[27–29] Whether time-resolved transillumination, application, and development of new contrast media and optical tomography will allow a breakthrough remains to be seen.[27, 30–33]

MR spectroscopy is of interest because it is able to demonstrate changes of the concentration of certain metabolites within an anatomic area of interest. Using *phosphor spectroscopy* relative changes of the following compounds have been described for breast cancers: phosphomonoesters (PME), which include phosphocholine (PC) and phosphoethanolamine (PE), total phosphate (TP), phosphodiesters (PDE), and total nucleosidetriphosphates (TNTP).[34–36] Due to the technological difficulty of phosphor spectroscopy, it is limited to relatively large voxel sizes. Individual variations of changes in benign and malignant disease also occur.[37] At the present time the method has not proven sufficiently reliable for lesion differentiation. However, it may be useful in monitoring response to therapy in experimental settings. *Proton spectroscopy* has distinct advantages over phosphor spectroscopy, including the possibility of imaging smaller voxel sizes (down to about

1 cm³). Since phosphocholine can be detected by both 31 phosphorus- and H-spectroscopy, and since phosphocholine appears to be detectable in some malignancies, but unfrequently in benign processes, its use for lesion differentiation has been suggested. To date limited data exist.[38,39] They include false negative and some false positive findings. Studies on larger data sets will be needed to determine the potential clinical value of these findings.

Imaging of *dielectric properties and electrical impedance* of breast tissue is presently being investigated, since fundamental studies have shown that differences between benign and malignant breast tissues may exist.[40] Interesting preliminary results have been reported from measuring *static skin surface potentials*, which may be caused by a changed Na/K-relation around tumors.[41]

Another method (so-called *impedance imaging*) allows measurement of the impedance of breast tissue (conductivity and capacity), while a very small current is applied through an electrode distant to the breast. In contrast to initial reports[42, 43], overlap of benign and malignant changes does occur.[44] Improvements will be needed before there is any possibility for its clinical use.

So far all of the above-mentioned methods should be considered methods under investigation. Based on the established diagnostic methods, the prerequisites that need to be met for any new method are as follows:

–   If its exclusive or additional use for *screening* is considered, it must provide a sufficiently high sensitivity for nonpalpable lesions, especially those smaller than 1 cm. At the same time it must provide excellent specificity (>95%) in asymptomatic women. Otherwise, expensive workup would be caused making its use cost-ineffective. If it is to be used in addition to mammography, it must also add diagnostic information to mammography in a relevant number of prognostically significant (small) lesions.

–   If it is to be used to work up indeterminate lesions, it must provide excellent sensitivity for malignancy. If a new method with low sensitivity were used to exclude malignancy in such lesions, cancers (which had been detected by other methods!) will be misdiagnosed. Since this is unacceptable, methods with low sensitivity may not be used for this purpose. Over-

all, a new method for diagnostic workup would have to compete with the high sensitivity of percutaneous biopsy (>95%) and with its excellent specificity (almost 100%).

–   At this point it appears important to point out a frequent misunderstanding: a method with a high specificity does not necessarily classify cancers correctly. Specificity is defined as the rate of correctly classified *benign* changes only (true negatives divided by all benign lesions). Therefore, unless there is also a very good sensitivity (detection rate of cancers), a method which only has a high specificity is of little use for further differentiation, since cancers would be missed.

■ References

1   Williams MB, Pisano ED, Schnall MD, Fajardo LL. Future directions in imaging of breast diseases. Radiology. 1998; 206:297–300

2   Piwnica-Worms D, Holman BL. Noncardiac applications of hexakis (alkylisonitrile) technetium-99 m complexes. J Nucl Med. 1989;31:1166–7

3   Maublant JC, Zheng Z, Rapp M et al. In vitro uptake of Tc-99 m texoboroxime in carcinoma cell lines and normal cell lines: comparison with Tc-99 m Sestamibi and thallium-201. J Nucl Med. 1993;34:1949–52

4   Khalkhali I, Villanueva-Meyer J, Edell SL et al. Diagnostic accuracy of Tc-99m-Sestamibi breast imaging in breast cancer detection (abstr.) J Nucl Med. 1996;37:74P

5   Scopinaro F, Schillaci O, Ussof W et al. A three center study on the diagnostic accuracy of 99mTc-MIBI scintimammography. Anticancer Res. 1997;17:1631–4

6   Palmedo H, Biersack HJ, Lastoria S et al. Scintimammography with technetium-99 m methoxyisobutylisonitrile: results of a prospective European multicentre trial. Eur J Nucl Med. 1998;25:375–85

7   Prats E, Carril J, Herranz R et al. A Spanish multicenter scintigraphic study of the breast using Tc 99 m MIBI. Report of results. Rev Esp Med Nucl.1998;17:338–50

8   Klaus AJ, Klingensmith WC 3rd, Parker SH et al. Comparative value of 99mTc-Sestamibi scintimammography and sonography in the diagnostic workup of breast masses. AJR. 2000;174:1779–83

9   Tiling R. Mammakarzinom. Nuklearmedizinische und radiologische Diagnostik. Berlin, Heidelberg, New York: Springer; 1998

10 Radiation dose to patients from radiopharmaceuticals. Ann ICRP. 1998;28:1–126

11 Khalkhali I, Cutrone JA, Mena IG et al. Scintimammography: the complementary role of Tc-99 m Sestamibi prone breast imaging for the diagnosis of breast carcinoma. Radiology. 1995;196:421–6

12 Tiling R, Tatsch K, Sommer H et al. Technetium-99m-Sestamibi scintimammography for the detection of breast carcinoma: comparison between planar and SPECT imaging. J Nucl Med. 1998;39:849–56

13 Scopinaro F, Pani R, De Vincentis G, et al. High-resolution scintimammography improves the accuracy of technetium-99 m methoxyisobutylisonitrile scintimammography: use of a new dedicated gamma camera. Eur J Nucl Med. 1999;26:1279–88

14 Wahl RL. Overview of the current status of PET in breast cancer imaging. J Nucl Med. 1998;42:1–7

15 Dehdashti F, Flanagan FL, Mortimer JE et al. Positron emission tomographic assessment of „metabolic flare" to predict response of metastatic breast cancer to antiestrogen therapy. Eur Nucl Med. 1999;26:51–6

16 Avril N, Bense S, Ziegler SI et al. Breast imaging with fluorine-18-FDG PET: Quantitative image analysis. J Nucl Med. 1997;38:1186–91

17 Yutani K, Shiba E, Kusuoka H et al. Comparison of FDG-PET with MIBI-SPECT in the detection of breast cancer and axillary lymph node metastasis. J Comput Assist Tomogr. 2000;24:274–80

18 Scheidhauer K, Scharl A, Pietrzyk U et al. Qualitative [¹⁸F] FDG positron emission tomography in primary breast cancer: clinical relevance and practicability. Eur J Nucl Med. 1996;23:618–23

19 Schelling M, Avril N, Nahrig J et al. Positron emission tomography using [(18)F] Fluorodeoxyglucose for monitoring primary chemotherapy in breast cancer. J Clin Oncol. 2000;18:1689–95

20 Smith IC, Welch AE, Hutcheon AW et al. Positron emission tomography using [(18)F]-fluorodeoxy-D-glucose to predict the pathologic response of breast cancer to primary chemotherapy. J Clin Oncol. 2000;18:1676–88

21 Garra BS, Cespedes EI, Ophir J et al. Elastography of breast lesions: initial clinical results. Radiology. 1997;202:79–86

22 Wu T, Felmlee JP, Greenleaf JF et al. MR imaging of shear waves generated by focused ultrasound. Magn Reson Med. 2000;43:111–5

23 Weiwad W, Heinig A, Götz L et al. Direct in vitro measurement of sound velocity in carcinomas, fibrocystic changes, fibroadenomas and fatty tissue of the female breast. RoeFo. 1999;171:480–4

24 Greenleaf JF, Johnson SA, Lent AH. Measurement of spatial distribution of refractive index in tissues by ultrasonic computer assisted tomography. Ultrasound Med Biol. 1977;3:327–39

25 Scherzinger AL, Bergam RA, Carson PA et al. Assessment of ultrasonic computed tomography in symptomatic breast patients by discriminant analysis. Ultrasound Med Biol. 1989;15:21–8

26 Richter K, Heywang-Köbrunner SH. Sonographic differentiation of benign from malignant lesions: value of indirect measurement of ultrasound velocity. AJR. 1995;165:825–31

27 Alfano RR, Demos SG, Gayen SK. Advances in optical imaging of biomedical media. Ann N Y Acad Sci. 1997;820:248–70

28 Götz L, Heywang-Köbrunner SH, Schütz O, Siebold H et al. Optical mammography in preoperative patients. Aktuelle Radiol. 1998;8:31–3

29 Puls R, HeusmannH, Lampe D, Buchmann J, Heywang-Köbrunner SH. Spectral transillumination of the breast. RoeFo, submitted

30 Jarlman O, Berg R, Anderson-Engels S et al. Time-resolved white light transillumination for optical imaging. Acta Radiol. 1997;38:185–9

31 Michielsen K, De Raedt H, Garcia N. Computer simulation of time-gated transillumination and refection of biological tissues and tissue-like phantoms. Med Phys. 1997;24:1688–95

32 Riefke B, Licha K, Semmler W. Contrast media for optical mammography. Radiologe. 1997;37:749–55

33 NtziachristosV, Yodh AG, Schnall M, Chance B. Concurrent MRI and diffuse optical tomography of breast after indocyanine green enhancement. Proc Natl Acad Sci USA. 2000;97:2767–72

34 Redmond OM, Stack JP, O'Connor NG et al. 31P MRS as an early prognostic indicator of patient response to chemotherapy. Magn Reson Med. 1992;25:30–44

35 Leach MO, Verrill M, Glaholm J et al. Measurements of human breast cancer using magnetic resonance spectroscopy: a review of clinical measurements and a report of localized 31P measurements of response to treatment. NMR Biomed. 1998;11:314–40

36 Ting YR, Sherr D, Degani H. Variations in energy and phospholipid metabolism in normal and cancer mammary epithelial cells. Anticancer Res. 1996;16:1381–8

37 Twelves CJ, Lowry M, Porter DA et al. Phoshorus-31 metabolism of human breast: an in vivo magnetic resonance spectroscopic study at 1.5 Tesla. Br J Radiol. 1994;67:36–45

38 Roebuck JR, Cecil KM, Schnall MD et al. Human breast lesions: characterization with proton MR spectroscopy. Radiology. 1998;209:269–75

39 Kvistad KA, Bakken IJ, Gribbestad IS et al. Characterization of neoplastic and normal human breast tissues with in vivo (1)H MR spectroscopy. J Magn Reson Imaging. 1999;10:159–64

40 Surowiec AJ, Stuchly SS, Barr JR, Swarup A. Dielectric properties of breast carcinoma and the surrounding tissues. IEEE Transactions on Biomedical Engineering. 1988;35:257–63

41 Faupel M, Vanel D, Barth V et al. Electropotential evaluation as a new technique for diagnosing breast lesions. Eur J Radiol. 1997;24:33–8

42 Morimoto T, Kimura S, Konishi Y et al. A study of the electrical bio-impedance of tumors. J Invest Surg. 1993;6:25–32

43 Jossinet J. The impedivity of freshly excised human breast tissue. Physiol Meas. 1998;19:61–75

44 Melloul M, Paz A, Ohana G et al. Double-phase 99mTc-Sestamibi scintigraphy and trans-scan in diagnosing breast cancer. J Nucl Med. 1999;40:376–80

7. Percutaneous Biopsy

■ Purpose

The implementation of widespread mammographic screening has resulted in the discovery of a large number of nonpalpable lesions requiring tissue sampling. The ability to perform these biopsies percutaneously, rather than surgically, has multiple advantages. There is a considerable cost reduction and reduction of operation room (OR) time. Due to the smaller volume of tissue removed, morbidity is decreased; no cosmetically deforming scarring occurs, and no architectural distortion is seen on follow-up mammograms that can require additional biopsy to exclude carcinoma. Finally, in well-equipped breast centers biopsy can often be performed earlier, directly after imaging assessment has been completed.

■ Definitions

Percutaneous biopsy can be performed using a variety of biopsy techniques:

Fine needle aspiration allows sampling of cells, which are then cytologically analyzed. For fine needle aspiration a thin needle (e.g. 21 gauge) is used. The needle is introduced into the breast 3–5 times. During each needle introduction the volume of the lesion is sampled by 5–10 needle thrusts, fanned throughout the volume of the lesion.

Core needle biopsy yields larger tissue samples, which are analyzed histologically. Usually 3–10 tissue cores (each 20 mm long with a 2 mm diameter) are acquired using 14-gauge Trucut needles, which are shot into the lesion using a high-speed gun. Tissue acquisition is either performed by repeated needle insertion into the breast or by using a 13-gauge coaxial system, through which the needle is reinserted into the lesion 3–10 times.

Vacuum biopsy is a method that allows harvesting even larger amounts of tissue (usually >16 cores 20 mm in length and 3 mm in diameter using an 11-gauge vacuum needle). The vacuum needle is inserted into the lesion once. Then tissue is suctioned into the needle, cut off, and transported to the back end of the needle, where it is picked off. While the needle stays in place this is repeated 15–20 times and tissue is acquired from all directions around the clock by rotating the needle around its axis. That way, with a single needle insertion a contiguous volume of tissue (diameter about 15 mm) is acquired for histopathologic analysis, while bleeding is simultaneously suctioned out of the cavity.

Imaging guidance is indispensable for nonpalpable lesions.

Imaging guidance can also improve the accuracy of percutaneous biopsy of *palpable* lesions by directing the needle into the lesion or into proper areas within the lesion (for example avoiding nondiagnostic biopsies of necrotic areas).

Furthermore, correct needle position within the lesion can thus be verified and documented.

Imaging guidance of nonpalpable lesions should be performed stereotactically for mammographically visible lesions and sonographically for lesions visible by ultrasound. If a lesion is visible equally well by both methods, either can be utilized. The selection of guidance in an individual case will be a function of the imaging characteristics of the lesion, lesion location, breast configuration, the availability and cost of equipment, as well as the experience or preference of the physician and/or patient. If a lesion is detected and visible only by MRI, MR-guidance is needed for MR-guided localization or percutaneous biopsy. Whereas MR-guided localization should be available if breast MRI is performed, MR-guided percutaneous biopsy is presently still under development and sufficient experience can presently only be provided in few institutions (see p. 146–7).

The successful use of these procedures involves developing skills that enable the physician to perform these biopsy procedures safely and accurately. It also requires that the results of each biopsy be correlated with the imaging characteristics of the targeted lesion to be certain that the lesion has been sampled. Additionally, the physician must understand which benign lesions can be associated with carcinoma and require wider, surgical biopsy.

■ Accuracy

■ Fine Needle Biopsy

Fine needle aspiration biopsy has been the first method applied for percutaneous biopsy of breast abnormalities. Initially it was used for supplementary evaluation of palpable abnormalities together with mammography (so-called triple diagnosis). Fine needle aspiration biopsy has also come to be applied to the workup of nonpalpable mammographically or sonographically detected lesions.[1-13]

Swedish research groups have initiated these applications[1] and still have the largest experience in this area. They have reported a sensitivity of up to 100% and specificity of 96–100% under stereotactic guidance. A critical issue in interpreting literature data is whether nondiagnostic aspirations enter into the calculation. Another critical issue concerns the fact that the accuracy data of fine needle aspiration biopsy are corrected by correlation with imaging. Discrepancies between benign results of fine needle aspiration biopsy and imaging have mostly been considered an indication for further workup, mostly surgical biopsy, and have therefore been counted as a true positive call. If the above mode of evaluation is chosen, unrealistically high accuracy data may result.

It also has to be emphasized that the very high accuracy reported has only been achieved in highly specialized facilities with a highly specialized radiologist and cytopathologist and on-site availability of cytology evaluation.

By other authors and for widespread use these data could not be reproduced[2, 3] and the results published in the literature from other groups vary between 53–90% sensitivity (average of complete sensitivity* for stereotactic fine needle aspiration 83%, for US-guided fine needle aspiration 95%) and 91–100% specificity (average 98%).[2-13]

---

* Complete sensitivity is based on the true positive rate, if atypia, suspicious and malignant findings are considered true positive

■ Core Needle Biopsy

In contrast to aspiration cytology, core needle biopsy obtains cores of tissue and thus permits histologic diagnosis. It also permits receptor analysis. Core needle biopsy has become a well-established technique under mammographic stereotactic or sonographic guidance.

Based on comparative studies, both a large needle size (14 gauge) and a sufficient number of cores (3–10 cores) are a prerequisite for high accuracy.[14, 15]

Accuracy data of core needle biopsy are available from preoperative studies and from large series of patient examinations.[16-36] With few exceptions complete sensitivity of all studies ranges between 92–98% with a specificity of 100%. The exceptions concern few studies with lower sensitivity and one multicenter study with exceptionally good results. For the worse results obtained in the former studies influence of learning curve (early results) and insufficient standardization have been discussed. For the mentioned multicenter study relatively short follow-up exists.

Studies with sensitivity data for masses, architectural distortions, and microcalcifications have shown a higher sensitivity for masses (>97%) than for microcalcifications (85–95%, mean 88%) or for architectural distortion.[28, 31, 32, 14, 35, 36] In order to avoid a false negative diagnosis and delayed treatment, correlation of imaging and histopathology of core needle biopsy is indispensable. Part of the reported accuracy data refer to sensitivities obtained after correlation with imaging, so that a negative result of core needle biopsy is considered a true positive call if rebiopsy was initiated based on a discrepant correlation with imaging.

■ Vacuum-Suction Biopsy

Vacuum-suction biopsy is a method which—based on suction and its potential of removing larger areas of tissue—promises further improvement of accuracy.

Even though published data are presently limited to slightly less than 2000 cases, an improvement in accuracy (sensitivity 98–100%, specificity 100%) has been reported for vacuum-suction biopsy using 11-gauge needles.[37-45] Comparing results of different groups it may be suspected that accuracy decreases with a decreasing number of samples (< 16) and smaller probe size (14 gauge).[37-47]

Another interesting result of vacuum-suction biopsy as compared to core needle biopsy has been the significantly lower rate of ADH-underestimates (diagnosis of ADH instead of the correct final diagnosis of ductal carcinoma in situ or invasive carcinoma) and the lower rate of ductal carcinoma in situ underestimates (diagnosis of ductal carcinoma in situ instead of the correct diagnosis of invasive carcinoma).

The former has been reported to range between 0–26% for vacuum-suction biopsy versus 44–48% for core needle biopsy; the latter between 0–15% for vacuum-suction biopsy versus 16–35% for core needle biopsy. According to the present data the increased volume of tissue removed by vacuum-suction biopsy is not associated with any increase of complications, nor with any significant scarring.

■ Indications

Before any decision is made to perform tissue sampling, imaging workup must be complete. It is important to remember that biopsy should not be used to replace adequate imaging workup.

After this has been considered, various indications for percutaneous biopsy exist:

- The most frequent and cost-effective use of percutaneous needle biopsy procedures is in eliminating the performance of surgical biopsy. Therefore, in women in whom indeterminate lesions (BI-RADS category 4) are present, it may be possible to make a definite diagnosis of a benign entity. Thus it may be possible to spare the patient surgical biopsy.
- Percutaneous tissue sampling may be used for selected patients for whom short-term mammographic follow-up is recommended for probably benign lesions (BI-RADS category 3) but who cannot be relied on to return for follow-up or are too anxious to wait.
- When women have lesions that are highly suspicious for carcinoma (BI-RADS category 5) and for whom a two-stage surgical approach is planned (diagnostic surgical biopsy followed by a second therapeutic surgical procedure at a different date), needle biopsy can eliminate the initial surgery. A preoperative diagnosis of invasive malignancy will also be useful for treatment planning of the axilla and with the patient and her family for discussion of further treatment options.

- Finally, in the patient with a probable or proven carcinoma in whom more than one lesion is present, the ability to prove the presence of multiple sites of cancer makes it possible to plan for mastectomy.[56, 57] In the same setting, the ability to prove that only one worrisome area is malignant allows the surgeon and patient to plan for breast conservation.

■ Possibilities and Limitations

For choosing the appropriate biopsy technique in an individual lesion, based on published accuracies and the known possibilities and limitations of each technique, the following should be considered:

- The use of *fine needle aspiration biopsy* for workup of imaging-detected lesions must be viewed with caution. Very high expertise is an absolute prerequisite. Due to specificity data ranging between 91–100% even in experienced hands a cytologic diagnosis of malignancy is, in most countries, not accepted for decisions on important therapeutic measures (such as mastectomy, neoadjuvant chemotherapy, axillary dissection). Considering the very variable published sensitivity data of 53–100%, a negative cytologic finding may, in general, not be used to avoid surgical biopsy.
  However, some entities do exist where a cytologic diagnosis may be considered reliable. They include: diagnosis of malignant involvement of a lymph node and diagnosis of a fibroadenoma.
- *Core needle biopsy* is the standard method for the workup of masses, probably benign lesions, or for proving malignancy in suspicious lesions.
  Based on its excellent sensitivity and specificity, core needle biopsy is the method of choice for the workup of the majority of the masses. For workup of microcalcifications, core needle biopsy is not as reliable as it is for masses,[14, 28, 31, 32, 35, 58] even if—as recommended—up to 10 cores are taken. In order to reduce potential errors that may occur with core needle biopsy, systematic correlation of the histopathologic result of core needle biopsy with the imaging findings is required. Core needle biopsy is highly reliable if a socalled *specific* histologic diagnosis is possible: mainly carcinoma or fibroadenoma. Repeat

percutaneous biopsy or open surgical biopsy is needed in all cases with benign or border-line histopathology and discrepant imaging findings. Using accuracy data of core needle biopsy combined with imaging, an accuracy comparable to that of surgical biopsy has been reported.

The value of all percutaneous biopsy methods for the workup of architectural distortions is limited since only the positive diagnosis of malignancy is reliable. The benign diagnosis of a radial scar is unreliable, since in up to 25 % of radial scars a ductal carcinoma in situ or tubular carcinoma has been reported. Since malignancy associated with radial scars are mostly located in the periphery of the lesion, it may not be sampled by percutaneous biopsy.

– Present experience based on the data of almost 2000 cases acquired in studies[36–45] suggests that *vacuum-suction biopsy* is the most accurate biopsy technique for the workup of microcalcifications. Compared to the other biopsy techniques, it offers the following advantages:

- Since tissue is suctioned into the probe, errors caused by lesion shift during needle insertion, lesion shift due to bleeding, or needle deviation within dense tissue are minimized.
- Since, compared to the other methods, a much larger volume of tissue (up to 12–18 mm in diameter) can be acquired contiguously by vacuum-suction biopsy, sampling error can be strongly reduced.
- This advantage is most relevant for lesions in which malignant cells may be arranged dispersed (noncontiguous) within the area of interest. Such lesions include ductal carcinomas in situ and lobular carcinomas.
- Removal of a large part or even all of the lesion as well as the excellent visibility of the biopsy cavity allow direct proof of correct sampling in a high percentage of cases.

Based on these advantages and the available accuracy data, vacuum-suction biopsy appears to be ideally suited for the workup of microcalcifications. It also appears useful for the workup of indeterminate lesions, for which a correlation with imaging does not provide a reliable countercheck of histology.[40,41]

The value of vacuum-suction biopsy for workup of architectural distortion is not yet determined. Today the major limitation for a more widespread use of vacuum biopsy concerns the high cost of these biopsy probes.

If vacuum-suction biopsy completely removes the area of radiologic concern, the site of the lesion can be marked with a clip. In case the lesion proves to be malignant or rebiopsy is necessary, the clip will aid in finding the biopsy site again for correct re-excision.

■ Contraindications

Contraindications to these procedures are few. Inability of an individual patient to cooperate during the biopsy may make them impossible to perform. Many believe that coagulopathy, including compromise in coagulation due to drugs, contraindicates these procedures. However, the safe performance of these biopsies in these patients has been described.

In some patients stereotactic biopsy may be impossible if the breast is too thin to accomodate a biopsy needle (i. e., the tip of the needle and the acquisition chamber), or if a lesion is in a thin area of the breast. Also, lesions that are in the axilla or near the chest wall may not be able to be imaged, making it impossible to perform stereotactic procedures in these women.

■ Complications

Major complications are rare and consist of hemorrhage and infection. In one large series of stereotactic core biopsies, these occurred in 0.2 %.[33] In sonographically guided biopsies pneumothorax is a possible complication if the needle penetrates the chest wall. This rare complication may occur, since sonographically-guided biopsy is performed without a guidance mechanism that could prevent needle deviation toward the chest wall. Because the chest wall is out of the field of view in most stereotactic biopsies and because the needle is guided by a rigid mechanism, the needle cannot penetrate the chest wall during these procedures.

Minor complications are common after these biopsies. They include bruising and pain that may last a few days. For many women undergoing these procedures, anxiety about the possibility of a breast cancer diagnosis can be debilitating, compromising their ability to return to normal activities on the day of the procedure.

When a stereotactic biopsy is done with a patient sitting using an add-on unit, there is the possibility of vasovagal reaction. When the patient is prone on a stereotactic table or supine during a sonographically guided procedure, these reactions are very rare.

Possible side effects of local anesthetics (allergy, cardiac arrhythmia, rarely seizures) need to be considered, particularly in patients with cardiac disease, and the maximum dose must be strictly observed.

■ Patient Information, Patient Preparation, and Postbiopsy Care

Informed consent should be obtained before these procedures are performed. The patient should be aware of the possible complications, limitations, and risks of the procedure. She should understand how it will be performed and what she will experience during it.

For patients who are on medications that compromise coagulation, it is desirable to discontinue these drugs for a week before the procedure. The most common of these drugs include coumarin, heparin, as well as aspirin, ibuprofen, and vitamin E. It is rarely necessary to check the patient's coagulation profile unless abnormalities are expected (e. g., during/after coumarin therapy, chemotherapy, known coagulation defects). Because these are sterile procedures, prophylactic antibiotics for patients with cardiac valvular prostheses are unnecessary.

At the end of the procedure, hemostasis is established and the breast is bandaged. Following fine needle aspiration, patients can usually return to normal activity. After core needle or vacuum-suction biopsy, the patient should avoid certain analgesics and other drugs that can compromise coagulation for several days. Vigorous exercise, unnecessary manipulation of the breast, and hot bathing should also be avoided during the first 3 days after biopsy. The patient should be given postbiopsy instructions; it is helpful to review these orally and also give them to the patient in writing. These should include when to remove the bandage, how the results will be received, and what signs of possible complications to look for.

Techniques for Biopsy and Biopsy Guidance

■ Fine Needle Aspiration

Fine needle aspiration requires the least expensive materials. It removes cells from the area of suspicion that can be assessed cytologically. In some cases, it is possible to make a definitive diagnosis of certain benign processes, such as some fibroadenomas. Limitations in the use of fine needle aspiration include the inability to differentiate invasive from in situ carcinoma, a high rate of cellular atypia requiring surgical biopsy, and a high insufficient sampling rate.[2, 3, 59] The latter may be reduced by the presence of a cytopathologist or cytologist in the room at the time the fine needle aspiration is performed to evaluate the specimen for adequacy of cells retrieved.

Fine needle aspiration is performed by placing a small needle, 21–23 gauge, within the suspicious lesion, with the needle tip near the far edge of the lesion. (Fig. 7.1) Usually after applying negative pressure, the needle is moved within the lesion, fanning throughout the volume of the mass and applying a corkscrew movement to the needle. Usually 5–10 thrusts within the mass are performed during each fine needle aspiration. If cellular material or blood is seen within the needle hub, the needle is removed. It is customary to perform the aspiration at least 3–5 times.

The specimen can be placed on slides or directly injected into preservative. If slides are used, training is needed to correctly prepare these or the specimen may not be interpretable.

Cytologic analysis is also performed on specimens obtained at cyst aspiration. Aspiration of a cyst containing solid elements that could be malignant or cyst fluid that contains blood should be sent for cytologic analysis. For this sampling, the needle tip should be positioned within the center of the cyst and as much fluid as possible removed from the cyst. The specimen is prepared as for fine needle aspiration. If no solid material is obtained (only cyst fluid), no slides can be prepared, and the fluid is placed directly into preservative, as recommended by the individual cytopathologist.

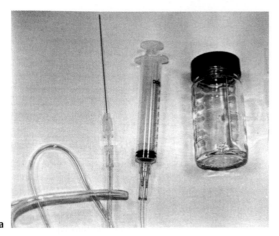

a

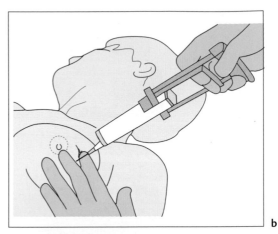

b

Fig. 7.**1 a** and **b**
a Equipment for fine needle aspiration. A small gauge needle can be attached to tubing and a 10-ml syringe. This makes it possible for a second set of hands to be used to apply negative pressure while the physician performing

the biopsy holds the ultrasound transducer and moves the needle. The specimen can placed on slides or in fixative
b Alternatively the Cameco handle can be used. The handle enables a negative pressure to be created without the need for another set of hands

■ Core Needle Biopsy

Core biopsies are commonly performed using needles of 14 gauge. They allow specimens to be obtained that can be analyzed histopathologically (Fig. 7.**2**).

A cutting needle is fired into the breast lesion, and a core of tissue is removed (Fig. 7. **2c**). The needle is removed after each biopsy and must be reinserted for another biopsy to be performed.

Gun-needle biopsy probes, usually paired with 14-gauge needles, are the most widely used type of biopsy probe for these procedures.

Studies have demonstrated that cutting needle size in gun-needle systems should be at least 14 gauge.[34] Smaller needles result in less diagnostic tissue specimens. The larger needle size does not result in a greater complication rate and does not significantly impact on the cost of performing these procedures. These systems are available in "long throw" and "short throw" configurations, describing the length the needle moves during the biopsy. Long throw systems move the needle at least 20 mm; short throw systems move the needle less than 15 mm. The long throw configuration is more effective in obtaining a diagnostic specimen.

Some use a coaxial system for easier reintroduction of the needle. These needles remove noncontiguous cores from the targeted site within the breast and function well for the biopsy of masses.

When microcalcifications undergo biopsy, especially if they are not tightly clustered or if they have similar shapes, targeting can be more difficult due to the need to direct the needle toward a single calcification.[14, 15, 28, 31, 32, 35, 58] Additionally, depending upon tissue resistance to the motion of the needle, the amount of deflection of the needle from its intended course can make it difficult to retrieve calcifications. With repetitive biopsy puncturing a small volume of the breast, the site becomes increasingly hemorrhagic, and tissue retrieval becomes more difficult.

Nevertheless, in most cases core biopsy will be successful in obtaining the accurate diagnosis. Considering the lower costs compared to vacuum biopsy or open biopsy, it may be considered first in appropriate situations.

■ Vacuum-Suction Biopsy

Vacuum-suction biopsy is the latest method of percutaneous biopsy. It appears to have the highest accuracy but is also associated with the highest costs. For the procedure first the needle is placed in the lesion in such a way that the lesion is centered at the acquisition chamber (Fig. 7.**3**). The chamber is opened. Tissue is then suctioned into the needle through the chamber (which is located on the side of the probe). Next, tissue is cut off by a rotating knife. Then, by means of a second vacuum, the tissue is transported within the

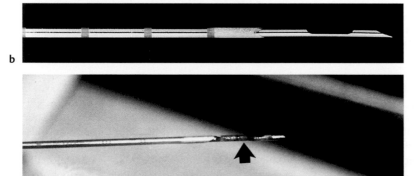

a

b

c

Fig. 7.**2a** and **b**
a Biopsy guns that use a spring mechanism to advance inner and outer parts of a needle at high speed
b Trucut needle for obtaining a tissue core: the inner needle has a notch, which traps the tissue as the inner needle is advanced. The outer needle closes over it, cutting and trapping the tissue core
c After the gun is fired and tissue is obtained, the needle is removed from the breast. Note that tissue fills the acquisition chamber of the biopsy needle (arrow)

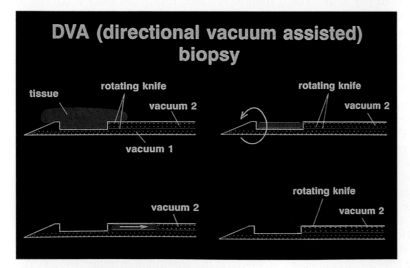

Fig. 7.**3** The principle of vacuum biopsy is shown: The first image illustrates placement of the probe into the lesion. The acquisition chamber at the side of the probe is opened and tissue is suctioned into the probe by means of vacuum 1.
The second image shows the closing of the acquisition chamber by moving the rotating knife forward. Thus a core is cut off. Before the core is transported back and while the acquisition chamber is still closed, the needle can be turned around its axis so that the next core can be acquired from a different direction.

The third image shows that by means of vacuum 2 the core can be pulled back to the far end of the probe, where it can be taken off by a forceps. (During this procedure only the parts within the probe move. The probe itself remains in the lesion throughout the procedure) The fourth image shows that, while the first core is transported to the far end of the needle, the acquisition chamber opens and the next core can be acquired. By repeating this procedure and turning the probe stepwise around the clock, lesions can be removed

needle to the far end of it, where it can be re-moved from the probe (Figs. 7.4 a,b). By repeating the procedure and by turning the needle around its axis, multiple tissue cores can be acquired from adjacent sites through a single probe inser-tion. That way focal areas of up to 15-mm diame-ter can be removed. Blood is also removed by con-tinuous suction. Based on this principle (suction, avoidance of hematoma, ample tissue acquisi-tion), errors caused by needle deviation, lesion shift due to hemorrhage, or local anesthetic can be compensated. Sampling error is reduced, and direct visualization of representative biopsy is possible by demonstrating removal of the entire imaging abnormality or a major part of it on a postbiopsy mammogram, which should be taken in two orthogonal planes.

Even though removal of an imaging abnor-mality is certainly the best proof of representative biopsy, it must be emphasized that so far no per-cutaneous biopsy method may be considered therapeutic in case of a malignant lesion or definitive in the diagnosis of atypical ductal hy-perplasia (ADH).[39–42] Reasons include: lacking capability of imaging to reliably assess the extent of malignancy or to detect residual microscopic disease.

Therefore, re-excision remains necessary in all cases where percutaneous biopsy yielded a di-agnosis of malignancy or ADH.

To avoid problems localizing the biopsy site, placement of a localizing clip or other marker at the biopsy site is recommended, unless an adja-cent landmark makes it possible to find the site[60, 61] (Fig. 7.5). This can be done by deploying a clip through the larger probes, e. g. 11 gauge. The clip will remain as a marker in the breast, while post-biopsy changes often last only a few days and, therefore, cannot be used for localization if re-ex-cision is necessary. Correct position must be checked by a mammogram, because in some cases the clip might be displaced because of the "accordian effect".*

The postbiopsy mammogram often allows direct visualization of the biopsy site (air, hema-toma, hole) in two planes and assessment of the extent of biopsy by removal of the entire or partial

---

* Because the breast is compressed in one direction when the clip is placed, the "accordian" effect on the breast when com-pression is released can result in the clip location being several centimeters from the biopsy site.

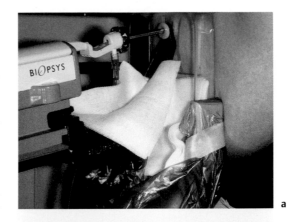

a

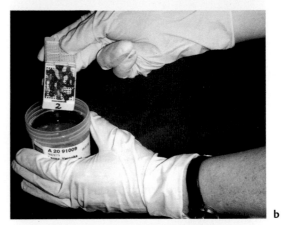

b

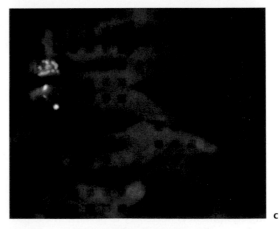

c

Fig. 7.**4 a-c** Specimen acquisition with vacuum-suction biopsy
a This image shows the needle in place during a pro-cedure. A specimen is visible in the acquisition chamber where it can be taken off
b The specimens of the first round are arranged in a sieve-like box and put into formalin
c The specimen radiograph showing the specimen in the box can be seen

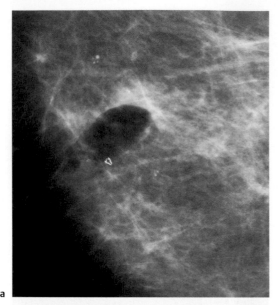

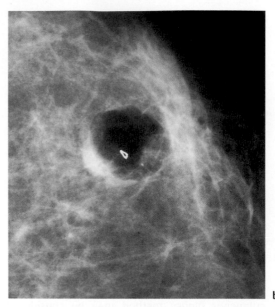

a

b

Fig. 7.**5 a** and **b** Localizing clip. A stereotactic biopsy was performed of a lesion that was removed completely with an 11-gauge vacuum-suction biopsy probe. In case repeat biopsy or surgical excision of the area is necessary, a clip is placed at the biopsy site to localize it. On a mammogram done immediately after the biopsy, the clip is shown to be in the wall of the cavity created by the biopsy on both the mediolateral and craniocaudal views

abnormality. Furthermore, it allows counter-checking and documenting the location of the clip to the biopsy site.

■ Ultrasound-Guided Biopsy

Biopsies performed with ultrasound guidance are appropriate for any lesions seen with ultrasound.[23, 59] Because calcifications are not reliably seen sonographically, this technique is usually not appropriate for the biopsy of calcifications. Ultrasound-guided biopsy is often faster to perform than stereotactic biopsies. However, biopsies of deeply situated and small lesions may be difficult and time-consuming.

The equipment needed for sonographic guidance should be available in all breast imaging facilites, so that no additional purchase of imaging equipment is necessary to perform these procedures. Ultrasound is also useful for biopsy guidance of the axilla, which is usually done using fine needle aspiration or 18–20 gauge Trucut biopsy needles. In women whose breasts under compression are too small to contain the core biopsy probe and in women with lesions in thin areas of the breast that will not accommodate the biopsy probe using stereotactic guidance, performance of biopsies under ultrasonographic guidance allows the biopsy to be performed, because the breast is flattened against the chest wall. Therefore, issues of breast thickness are eliminated. Finally, in experienced hands, biopsy of lesions near the chest wall and in areas that are difficult to position in the field of view of stereotactic systems may be possible. However, care must be taken not to violate the chest wall.

High-resolution linear-array transducers (7.5 MHz or higher) should be used for breast ultrasound and to perform these biopsies.

The patient should be positioned as for ultrasound, depending on lesion location (in the medial or lateral quadrants, see p. 92). Although an infinite number of approaches can be used, it is important to select an approach in which the lesion is well visualized.

If anesthetic is used, it should be purged of air, which will compromise sonographic imaging. The bolus of anesthetic can also obscure the lesion to be biopsied. The injection of anesthetic should be done under sonographic visualization to be certain that lesion conspicuity is not compromised.

When approaching the lesion, the needle should always be imaged in the long axis and the following should be observed:

- The needle needs to be exactly aligned with the plane of the transducer. Otherwise part of the needle will not be within the imaging plane. The image must, therefore, show the needle and the lesion in one plane.
- Imaging of the needle tip is of utmost importance. Only visualization of the needle tip allows avoidance of complications (inadvertant puncture of the chest wall).
- The biopsy should always be performed using a path that is as parallel to the chest wall as possible. There are two advantages to this:
  - Aiming the needle parallel to the chest wall minimizes the danger of injuries. This can be done by advancing the needle laterally beneath the lesion. The needle thus acts as a fulcrum to pick up the lesion (Figs. 7.**6**–7.**9**). Then the end of the needle is pressed down to lift the tip of the needle upward, i.e., away from the chest wall, before firing. Never fire a gun with the needle pointing toward the chest wall.
  - The needle is more readily visible since the ultrasound beam is reflected back to the transducer and not away from it. This makes it possible to image the entire length of the needle (Figs. 7.**6**–7.**9**).

For core and vacuum biopsy a small skin cut should be made to facilitate introduction of the needle. For fine needle aspiration the needle should be positioned within the mass near its far wall before negative pressure is applied. As described before, the needle will then be moved back and forth within the mass, fanning out within the mass (5–10 thrusts), during aspiration. This has to be repeated 4–5 times. For core biopsy the tip of the needle is placed at the deep lateral border of the lesion and the needle is fired, so that it will travel parallel to or away from the chest wall. Using 14 G needles, 3–5 good specimens should be obtained. Whenever multiple needlings are performed, pressure should be held over the biopsy site between samplings. If a vacuum-suction biopsy probe is used (which is not fired in the breast), the probe is positioned deep to the lesion (between it and the chest wall), performing a similar "fulcrum" motion as described for core needle positioning. Only if the probe is positioned deep to the lesion will the lesion not be obscured by shadowing of the probe.

Image recording during ultrasound-guided breast biopsy should include documentation of the lesion undergoing biopsy in orthogonal pro-

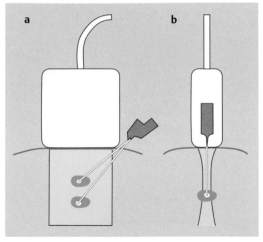

Fig. 7.**6a** and **b** Schematic diagram of ultrasound-guided biopsy (from [10])
a The needle is advanced toward the lesion under the transducer within the plane of the ultrasound-beam. Thus its entire length is visible. Anterior view
b Lateral view, i. e., in the direction of the biopsy

jections before biopsy is done, imaging with the needle in its prebiopsy and postbiopsy position for each tissue specimen obtained. These should be labelled core #1, core #2, etc. or fine needle aspiration #1, fine needle aspiration #2, etc. Film labelling should also include identification of the physician performing the biopsy, the date of the procedure, the location of the lesion within the breast, the name of the facility where the biopsy was done, the name of the patient, and a patient-identifying number (medical record number, birth date, social security number).

At the end of the procedure, adequate pressure should be maintained to obtain hemostasis. The site of needle introduction should be bandaged. The patient should be instructed how she will receive the results of her biopsy and how she should care for herself after the procedure (see p. 136).

■ Stereotactic Biopsy

Stereotaxis localizes the lesion through triangulation. Angled views make it possible to calculate the position of the lesion as defined in its location on a horizontal (x) axis, vertical (y) axis, and depth (z) axis (see Fig. 7.**10**).

Several configurations of stereotactic equipment are available. Add-on units that can be attached to mammographic machines can be used

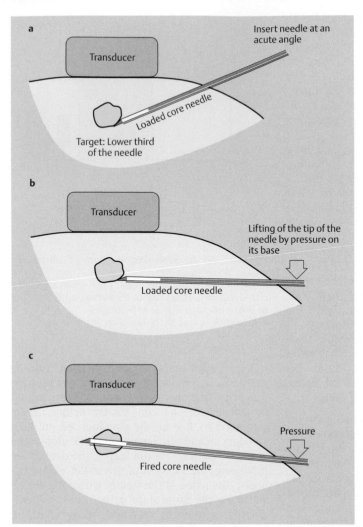

Fig. 7.**7 a–c**   Procedure for ultra-sound-guided needle biopsy:
a The needle is held at an acute angle to the surface of the breast. The needle points at the lower third of the lesion
b Pressing on the base of the needle lifts the tip of the needle upward
c This prevents injury to the chest wall when the device is fired

to convert these machines to stereotactic biopsy units. When these are used, the patient is usually biopsied in a sitting position and must remain motionless in position during the procedure. This can sometimes be difficult. Motion may compromise the examination. Maintaining this positioning may cause considerable discomfort in the patient's neck, back, and shoulders. There is minimal space available in this configuration of equipment to actually perform the biopsy. However, this is the least expensive configuration of stereotactic equipment. Also, with add-on units, in some cases it may be easier to position lesions near the chest wall or in the axilla in the field of view of the unit than with prone tables. In principle, it is also possible to biopsy patients in a lateral decubitus position, using mammography equipment and an add-on unit, if they are on a patient table adjusted to the height of the mammography equipment. However, this type of positioning is time-consuming and the position assumed is not very stable. To reduce imaging and waiting time (which is necessary for accurate biopsy without patient motion and for a minimum of patient comfort), digital receivers are becoming an increasingly important prerequisite for any type of stereotaxic percutaneous biopsy.

Dedicated prone tables position the patient face down with the breast hanging through a hole in the table in compression (Fig. 7.**11**). A mammographic unit is positioned under the table. The patient is less likely to move and is unlikely to faint with this equipment. There is a large amount of space for the physician to perform the biopsy.

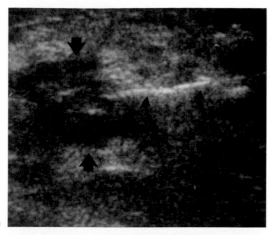 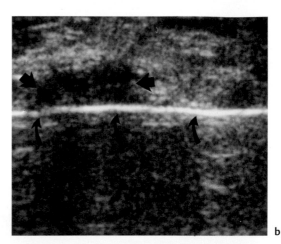

a · b

Fig. 7.**8a** and **b**   Core biopsy with sonographic guidance. An irregular mass was seen sonographically and is suspicious for carcinoma
a On the prefire image from the core biopsy, the cutting needle (curved arrows) is seen to be adjacent to the mass (arrows)

b On the postfire image, the needle (curved arrows) has passed through the mass (arrows), obtaining tissue from this infiltrating ductal carcinoma

Fig. 7.**9a** and **b**   Sonographically guided core biopsy
a After the skin has been cleaned and sterile gel or alcohol used as coupling agent for the transducer, anesthetic is injected under sonographic visualization
b The skin has been cut with a scalpel to ease entry of the cutting needle. The needle is then introduced along the long axis of the transducer. Alignment of the needle with the long axis of the transducer permits visualization of the length of the needle so it can be guided into the appropriate position

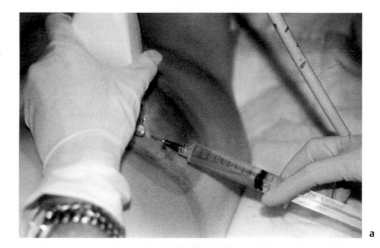

a

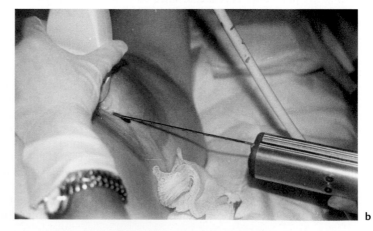

b

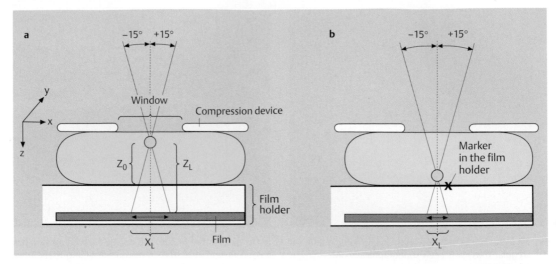

Fig. 7.**10 a** and **b**   Principle of depth localization
a First, the breast is compressed with a fenestrated compression plate. The opening needs to be precisely above the lesion to be sampled. Spot compression views are obtained by tilting the X-ray tube + 15° and – 15° out of the center
b Lesions closer to the film (**b**) will appear with less of a shift (X_L) on the film than lesions farther from the film (**a**). The mammography unit can calculate the depth of the lesion from the parallax shift of the lesion (X_L). The depth of the lesion (Z_L) is calculated using the following formula:

$$\frac{X_L}{2} = Z_L \cdot \tan 15°$$

or

$$Z_L = \frac{X_{L2}}{2 \cdot \tan 15°}$$

The formula can be adapted accordingly to determine the depth of the lesion with respect to the film holder. To do so, a reference point on the film holder is used and the formula is changed accordingly. This reference point is also used as a reference point for the lateral shift, since the film cassette is also moved manually between the + 15 and – 15 views to avoid exposing it twice

Some women may experience pain in their neck, back, or shoulders with this type of equipment. For many patients, however, psychologic stress during the procedure is reduced, since they cannot see the procedure and the biopsy equipment.

Stereotactic biopsies are appropriate for any lesions that can be seen mammographically and that can be approached using stereotactic equipment. Because calcifications are not reliably seen with sonography, when these are the target, the biopsy should be done under stereotactic guidance. As noted above, lesions that are too close to the chest wall, or lesions in breasts that are too thin under compression to contain the biopsy probe, cannot undergo stereotactic core biopsy. If ultrasound-guided biopsy is not possible either, open biopsy after wire localization (e. g., placing the wire so that the lesion is between the wire and chest wall) may have to be considered.

During stereotactic biopsy, a scout film without angulation is first done to document accurate positioning of the target in the field of view. Then the stereotactic pair is done moving the X-ray tube along the horizontal axis, and lesions will move to the right and left on these images (Fig. 7.**12a**). If the lesion is too close to the right or left side of the scout film, it will not appear on one of the stereotactic pairs. Therefore, an attempt should be made to position the target as close to the center of the x-axis as possible on the scout. After the stereotactic pair has been obtained, a cursor is placed over the identical site of interest to calculate the x, y, and z-axes. Great care is needed to identify exactly the same structure. If this is not possible (multiple similar calcifications, architectural distortion, which is imaged differently on different views), biopsy might be attempted in a different plane of compression

Fig. 7.**11** This image shows the patient position on a prone table during a procedure

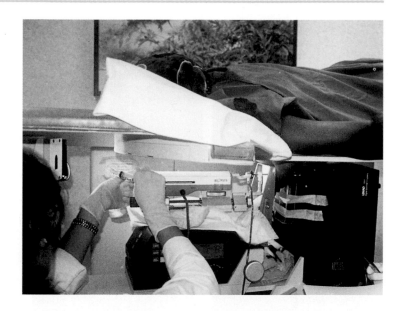

or percutaneous biopsy may not be possible using stereotaxis. In such rare cases ultrasound-guided percutaneous biopsy or open biopsy after wire localization should be considered. This precaution is necessary, since errors identifying the same structure on the stereotactic views will cause miscalculation of the lesion location on the z-axis. In order to recognize errors identifying the target, we recommend always counterchecking the calculated needle position with the position of the lesion in the two mammographic planes of the original mammogram. It is important to remember that (the center of) the lesion should be located at the center of the acquisition chamber of the biopsy probe (Fig. 7.**3**). Therefore, if core needle or vacuum-suction biopsy is performed, the needle or probe tip must be beyond the center of the lesion on the postfire images, since the lesion itself must be centered within the acquisition chamber of the needle or the probe. The depth of needle insertion always has to be adapted to the type of needle or probe and the center of the acquisition chamber with respect to the needle or probe tip (Figs. 7.**12 b,c**).

Before core biopsy needles or vacuum probes are introduced into the breast, a small cut (5 mm) is made in the skin after local anesthetic has been injected subcutaneously. Deep local anesthesia is also necessary for core biopsy, but it must be remembered that ample local anesthetic may obscure the lesion and cause lesion shift. If vacuum biopsy is performed, local anesthetic can be in-

jected in the deep tissues after the probe is fired into the lesion, because then the tissue is fixed by the probe itself. Minor shifts will be compensated by suction.

Before any tissue is obtained, a stereotactic pair should be obtained to ascertain if the needle is in good position. After the biopsy has been performed but before the needle is removed from the breast, another stereotactic pair is necessary to document that the needle has passed through the lesion or that tissue from the lesion has been obtained. These images should be obtained each time the probe is fired in the breast. (For vacuum-suction biopsy the needle will only be fired once per lesion in the great majority of cases.)

When calcifications are the object of biopsy, specimen radiography is necessary to confirm that calcifications have been obtained[59] (Fig. 7.**4 c**). The specimen radiograph should be taken during the biopsy procedure. The biopsy should be continued at least until calcifications are obtained or until tissue becomes so hemorrhagic that continued biopsy fails to obtain any useful tissue.[15, 38] The higher accuracy of vacuum biopsy with respect to diagnosis of microcalcifications may be explained by the better calcification retrieval rate (due to suction) and also by the fact that some cancers are located adjacent to, and not directly around, the calcifications.

Specimen radiography can be performed using magnification mammography, dedicated tabletop specimen radiography units, or digital imaging. If

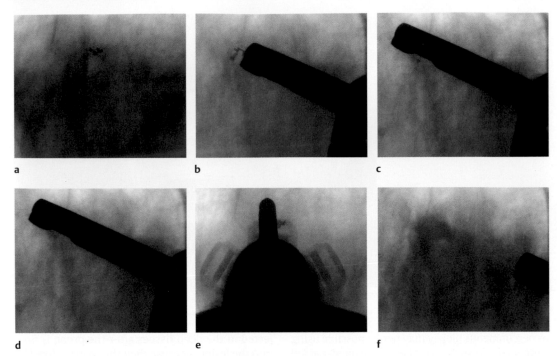

Fig. 7.12 a-f Images taken during a vacuum biopsy are shown
a The scout view shows an indeterminate group of micro-calcifications. From the three views (- 15°, 0°, and + 15°) the 0° and the − 15° views were selected for planning the procedure
b After planning, the needle, which is not yet fired, is introduced to the calculated „prefire" position. Its correct position is checked on this − 15° view

c Correct „prefire" position is also confirmed on the 0° view
d, e After the needle is fired into the lesion, needle position is once more checked on the - 15° and 0° view
f After withdrawing the needle, no more microcalcifications are visible at the biopsy site
Histology revealed ductal carcinoma in situ, which was confirmed after re-excision

magnification mammography is used, the lowest kVp and mAs settings on the unit should be used as the initial settings. Specimen radiographs should be kept as part of the medical record. A copy of the specimen radiograph may be appreciated by the pathologist.

As with ultrasound-guided biopsy, at the end of the procedure pressure should be held over the biopsy site to obtain hemostasis, the patient should be bandaged, and she should be given instruction on how to care for her breast after the biopsy and how she will receive the results.

■ MR-Guided Percutaneous Biopsy

Percutaneous biopsy of lesions, which are detected and only visible by MRI, is desirable for several reasons:

– Open surgery of benign MR-detected lesions could be avoided. (In most series 1 out of 2–4

lesions detected by MRI alone proves to be malignant.)
– Logistic problems due to difficult timing of MR localization procedure and surgery can be reduced.
– Since enhancing lesions cannot usually be visualized in a specimen MRI, specimen X-ray, or sonogram, uncertainties concerning correct excision of lesions visualized by MRI only may remain after surgery. Image-guided percutaneous removal could help to solve this problem.

Presently, experience with percutaneous core biopsy has been reported by a few authors.[62–66] Being a complicated procedure that is hampered by the inability to monitor the biopsy without major image artifacts, it has not been recommended for lesions < 1 cm and should still be considered to be "under development." MR-

Fig. 7.**13** a–g

a Equipment for MR-guided localization, core needle or vacuum biopsy. The housing of the biopsy coil is placed on the MR table. The patient has to lie prone on this housing, and the pending breast will be moderately compressed between the two compression plates (arrows). A ring coil is inserted between the bars of the compression plates. With her breast fixed, the patient has to lie still on this biopsy device throughout the procedure. For imaging she is moved into the bore, for biopsy she is moved out of the magnet. Based on the MR images, the transverse slice that contains the lesion can be identified. This is aligned with the aiming device that supports the biopsy gun. The height and depth of needle insertion is also determined from the transverse MR images and transferred to the aiming device. That way, by setting the aiming device to the calculated coordinates the lesion will be pierced by the biopsy probe and centered exactly at the acquisition window of the probe.

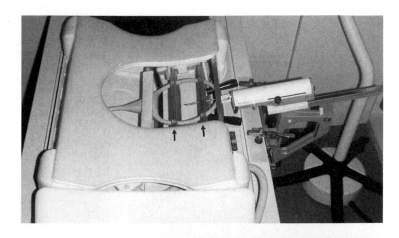

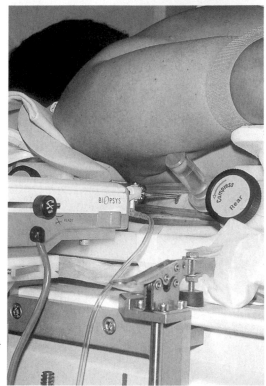

b Close-up images of an MR-guided vacuum biopsy. The ▷ patient lies prone on the biopsy coil. The vacuum biopsy probe is inserted into the patient's breast after the bars of the compression plate have been spread by a spacer

Fig. 7.**13** c–g   ▷

guided vacuum biopsy has proven much more promising, as confirmed by first experiences with over 200 examinations acquired in a European multicenter study[67, 68] (Fig. 7.**13**).

■ **Handling the Biopsy Specimen**

If the needle is removed from the breast and re-inserted, care should be taken not to place the needle in preservative and reintroduce it into the

breast (Fig. 7.**12**). For fine needle aspirations, a new needle should be used for each aspiration. If cores are undergoing specimen radiography, they should be kept moist with saline until they are placed in preservative so that drying artifact does not compromise the ability of the pathologist to make a diagnosis.

The pathologist should be supplied with adequate information to interpret the specimen. The lesion should be described, and the suspected di-

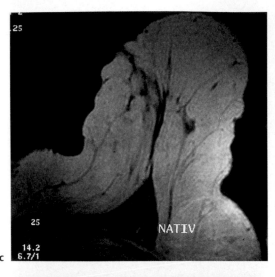

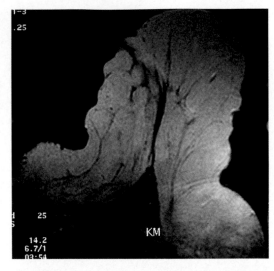

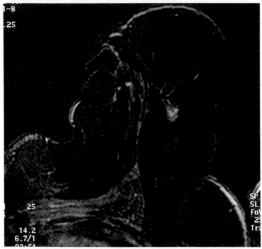

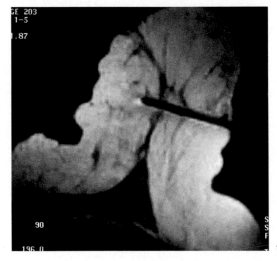

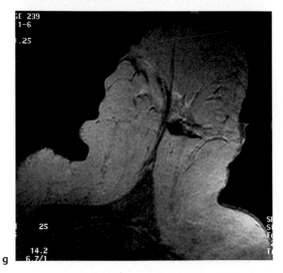

Fig. 7.**13 c–g** Representative images of an MR-guided vacuum biopsy. In this patient MRI was performed due to impaired assessment after breast-conserving therapy, because of overlying tissue (other slices) and scarring. A small enhancing focus was detected by MRI, which in retrospect could only be reproduced on one mammographic view

c Precontrast MR image of the lesion

d Postcontrast MR image. The lesion enhances and becomes almost isointense to fat

e Subtraction image of the lesion

f Based on the imaging coordinates of the lesion, first a thin MR-compatible substitute needle is inserted to the calculated position and checked by MRI. Then its correct position, which is shown here, is confirmed (in order to have the lesion at the acquisition chamber of the probe, the probe has to reach beyond the lesion). Then the patient is moved out of the MRI. The substitute needle is exchanged against the vacuum probe, and vacuum biopsy is performed at the calculated position

g Finally, correct removal is checked. This image shows that the cavity is in the exact place where the lesion had initially been

Histology: ductal carcinoma G2

agnosis should be included in the lesion description. If the lesion was calcifications the pathologist should be provided with the specimen radiograph or a copy. Any pertinent clinical history should also be provided.

■ Interpreting the Histologic Results

A pivotal step in the successful application of these biopsy procedures to patient care is the correlation of the biopsy results with the imaging pattern of the targeted lesion. This is the final determination of whether the suspicious lesion has been biopsied. For lesions that are BI-RADS category 3 and have benign histopathologies that are concordant with the imaging pattern, the biopsy can be assumed to have been successful.[27, 32] Concordance should, however, be checked very diligently in category 4 lesions. Furthermore, the type of biopsy (its reliability depending on the type of lesion), the individual accuracy of the radiologist (audit), and the success of the biopsy procedure (adequacy of the specimens, volume of tissue acquired, certainty or proof of correct needle placement or tissue acquisition, presence of hemorrhage) need to be taken into account. For lesions that are BI-RADS category 5 and have benign histopathologies, the need for rebiopsy should be strongly considered. Although some entities, such as focal fibrosis and scar, can have a spiculated pattern, rebiopsy may be appropriate to be certain that carcinoma is not present.[69]

Certain histopathologies are consistent with the imaging pattern but can be part of a focus of disease within the breast that can contain more aggressive diseases than those diagnosed at the time of biopsy. The most important of these is ductal atypia (atypical ductal hyperplasia, ADH), which is almost always evident as calcifications on mammography.[48–51] In the transformation of ductal epithelium from normal to malignant, the transitional phase is ADH. It may progress to ductal carcinoma in situ or to invasive cancer. The presence of ADH in biopsied ducts raises the possibility that part of the ductal epithelium near this lesion may have progressed to ductal carcinoma in situ or even invasive carcinoma. Furthermore, one focus of ADH may be indicative of multicentric disease which may be occult to imaging. The likelihood that ductal carcinoma in situ may be present increases as smaller amounts of tissue are removed due to the increased possibility of sampling error with small amounts of tissue (see accuracy of core biopsy and vacuum-suction biopsy, p. 134). Therefore, in all cases of core biopsy yielding a diagnosis of ductal atypia, surgical excision should be performed to evaluate for possible coexistent carcinoma.

Similar problems may occur, if ductal carcinoma in situ is diagnosed by percutaneous biopsy, since coexistent areas of invasive carcinoma can be present.[52–55] As with ductal atypia, this is a function of a histologically heterogenous lesion. Here, sampling at core biopsy may miss the most aggressive part of the lesion. As with ductal atypia, these so-called "underestimates" decrease with increasing tissue volume sampled. Since patients with ductal carcinoma in situ, like those with invasive carcinoma, always undergo surgical re-excision anyway, this has the following clinical significance:

– The need for possible surgical treatment or sampling of the axilla is not correctly assessed before re-excision of the lesion in those women with the incorrect diagnosis of ductal carcinoma in situ (instead of invasive carcinoma). Therefore, these women may need a second trip to the operating room for their axillary surgery after the final diagnosis of invasive carcinoma is established by surgical excision.
– In some of these women, preoperative consultation may incorrectly advise them that adjuvant chemotherapy is unnecessary.

Radial scar has been reported to have coexistent carcinoma present in up to 25 % of cases. This is usually located in the periphery of the lesion, and the cell type is usually tubular. Therefore, diagnosis of radial scar obtained from percutaneous biopsy raises the possibility of coexistent carcinoma and should result in surgical excision of the site.[69]

Controversy has surrounded the management of women with a core biopsy diagnosis of lobular carcinoma in situ.[70, 71] Because this lesion rarely has mammographic findings, it does not explain the cause of a mammographic abnormality that resulted in a biopsy recommendation. Therefore, another entity should be sought to explain the formation of the suspicious lesion. Without another reason for re-excision, lobular carcinoma in situ does not require wider, surgical excision. However, it is a marker for increased risk to develop breast cancer, and referral of the patient for high-risk management should be considered.

Some lesions will be difficult for the pathologist to diagnose based on tissue removed at core biopsy. Such difficulties may occur in differentiating phyllodes tumor from fibroadenoma. Furthermore, depending on the experience of individual pathologists, papillary lesions and lesions containing mucus may also be difficult for some pathologists to definitively diagnose as benign based on core specimens.[72] Finally other rare lesions can also be difficult for the pathologist to diagnose by core biopsy. The pathologist should note this difficulty in the pathology report and recommend surgical excision. When this occurs, patient management should be based on the pathologist's recommendation, and surgical excision of the lesion should be performed.

■ References

1   Azavedo E, Svane G, Auer G. Stereotactic fine-needle biopsy in 2594 mammographically detected non palpable lesions. Lancet I. 1998;1033–6

2   Pisano ED, Fajardo LL, Tsimikas J et al. Rate of insufficient samples for fine-needle aspiration for nonpalpable breast lesions in a multicenter clinical trial: The Radiologic Diagnostic Oncology Group 5 study. Cancer. 1998;82:678–88

3   NHS Breast Screening Programme. Guidelines for Cytology Procedures and Reporting in Breast Cancer Screening: Report by Cytology Sub-Group of the National Coordinating Committee for Breast Screening Pathology; NHSBSP Publication N. 22; Sept. 1993

4   Marcaccio MJ, O'Brien SE, Chen VS. Fine-needle aspiration cytology in breast lumps. Can J Surg. 1986;29:405–7

5   Dent DM, Kirkpatrick AE, McGoogan E, Chetty U, Anderson TJ. Stereotaxic localization and aspiration cytology of impalpable breast lesions. Clin Radiol. 1989;40:380–2

6   Dowlatshahi K, Yaremko ML, Kluskens LF, Jokich PM. Nonpalpable breast lesions: Findings of stereotaxic needle-core biopsy and finde-needle aspiration cytology. Radiology. 1991;185:639–40

7   Dempsey P, Rubin E. The roles of needle biopsy and periodic follow-up in the evaluation and diagnosis of breast lesions. Semin Roentgenol. 1993;28:252–8

8   Maestro C, Giudicelli T, Ettore F et al. Ultrasound-guided cytopuncture of impalpable solid breast lesions. J Radiol. 1994;75:497–503

9   Saalrela AO, Kiviniemi HO, Rissanen TJ, Paloneva TK. Nonpalpable breast lesions: pathologic correlation of ultrasonographically guided fine-needle aspiration biopsy. J Ultrasound Med. 1996;15:549–53

10 Lofgren M, Andersson I, Lindholm K. Stereotactic fine-needle aspiration for cytologic diagnosis of nonpalpable breast lesions. AJR. 1990;154:1191–5

11 Sarfati MR, Fox KA, Warneke JA et al. Stereotactic fine-needle aspiration cytology of nonpalpable breast lesions: an analysis of 258 consecutive aspirates. Am J Surg. 1994;168:529–31

12 Britton PD. Fine needle aspiration or core biopsy. Breast. 1999;8:1–4

13 Britton PD, McCann J. Needle biopsy in the NHS Breast Screening Programme 1996/97: How much and how accurate? Breast. 1999;8:5–11

14 Brenner RJ, Fajardo L, Fisher PR et al. Percutaneous core biopsy of the breast: effect of operator experience and number of samples on diagnostic accuracy. AJR. 1996;166:341–6

15 Liberman L, Evans WP, Dershaw DD et al. Specimen radiography of microcalcifications in stereotaxic mammary core biopsy specimens. Radiology. 1994;190:223–5

16 Parker SH, Lovin JD, Jobe WE et al. Nonpalpable breast lesions: stereotactic automated large-core biopsies. Radiology. 1991;180:403–7

17 Elvecrog EL, Lechner MC, Nelson MT. Nonpalpable breast lesions: correlation of stereotactic large-core needle biopsy and surgical biopsy results. Radiology. 1993; 188:453–5

18 Gisvold JJ, Goellner JR, Grant CS et al. Breast biopsy: a comparative study of stereotaxically guided core and excisional techniques. AJR. 1994;162:815–20

19 Dershaw DD, Morris EA, Liberman L, Abramson AF. Nondiagnostic core breast biopsy: results of rebiopsy. Radiology. 1996;198:323–5

20 Britton PD, Flower CD, Freeman AH et al. Changing to core biopsy in an NHS breast screening unit. Clin Radiol. 1997;52:764–7

21 Fornage BD, Coan JD, David CL. Ultrasound-guided needle biopsy of the breast and other interventional procedures. Radiol Clin North Am. 1992;30:167

22 Schulz-Wendtland R, Kramer S, Lang N, Bautz W. Ultrasonic guided microbiopsy in mammary diagnosis: indications, technique and results. Anticancer Res. 1998; 18:2145–6

23 Parker SH, Jobe WE, Dennis MA et al. US-guided automated large-core breast biopsy. Radiology. 1993;187:507–11

24 Fajardo LL, Jackson VP, Hunter TB. Interventional procedures in diseases of the breast: Needle biopsy, pneumocystography and galactography. AJR 1992; 158:1231–8

25 Nguyen M, Mc Combs MM, Ghandehari S et al. An update on core needle biopsy for radiologically detected breast lesions. Cancer. 1996;78:2340–5

26 Frayne J, Sterrett GF, Harvey J et al. Stereotactic 14 gauge core-biopsy of the breast: results from 101 patients. Aust N Z J Surg: 1996;66:585–91.

27 Lee Ch, Egglin TK, Philpotts LE et al. Cost-effectiveness of stereotactic core needle biopsy: analysis by means of mammographic findings. Radiology. 1997;202:849–54

28 Liberman L, Dershaw DD, Glassman JR et al. Analysis of cancers not diagnosed at stereotactic core breast biopsy. Radiology. 1997;203:151–7

29 Acheson MB, Patton RG, Howisey RL et al. Histologic correlation of image-guided core biopsy with excisional biopsy of nonpalpable breast lesions. Arch Surg. 1997;132:815–8 and 819–21

30 Fuhrman GM, Cederbom GJ, Bolton JS et al. Image-guided core needle breast biopsy is an accurate technique to evaluate patients with nonpalpable imaging abnormalities. Ann Surg. 1998;227:932–9

31 Meyer JE, Smith DN, Lester SC et al. Large core needle biopsy: nonmalignant breast abnormalities evaluated with surgical excision or repeat core biopsy. Radiology. 1998;206:717–9

32 Jackman RJ, Nowels KW, Rodriguez-Soto J et al. Stereotactic, automated, large-core needle biopsy of nonpalpable breast lesions: false-negative and histologic underestimation rates after long-term follow-up. Radiology. 1999;210:799–805

33 Parker SH, Burbank F, Jackman RJ et al. Percutaneous large-core breast biopsy: a multiinstitutional study. Radiology. 1994;193:359–64

34 Nath ME, Robinson TM, Tobon H et al. Automated large-core needle biopsy of surgically removed breast lesions: comparison of samples obtained with 14, 16, and 18 gauge needles. Radiology. 1995;197:739–42

35 Mainiero MB, Philpotts LE, Lee CH et al. Stereotaxic core needle biopsy of breast microcalcifications: correlation of target accuracy and diagnosis with lesion size. Radiology. 1996;198:665–9

36 Lee CH, Philpotts LE, Horvath LJ et al. Follow-up of breast lesions diagnosed as benign with stereotactic core-needle biopsy: frequency of mammographic change and false-negative rate. Radiology. 1999;212:189–94

37 Meyer JE, Smith DN, Dipiro PJ et al. Stereotactic breast biopsy of clustered microcalcifications with a directional, vacuum-assisted device. Radiology. 1997;204:575–6

38 Liberman L, Smolkin JH, Dershaw DD et al. Calcification retrieval at stereotactic 11-gauge vacuum-assisted breast biopsy. Radiology. 1998;208:251–60

39 Liberman L, Dershaw DD, Rosen PP et al. Percutaneous removal of malignant lesions at stereotactic vacuum-assisted biopsy. Radiology. 1998;206:711–5

40 Heywang-Köbrunner SH, Schaumlöffel U, Viehweg P et al. Minimally invasive stereotactic vacuum core breast biopsy. Eur Radiol. 1998;8;377–85

41 Götz L, Amaya B, Häntschel G et al. Mammographically guided vacuum biopsy: experiences with 700 cases. Eur Radiol. 2000;10(suppl):329

42 Jackman RJ, Marzoni FA, Nowels KW. Percutaneous removal of benign mammographic lesions: comparison of automated large-core and directional vacuum-assisted biopsy techniques. AJR. 1998;171:1325–30

43 Zannis VJ, Aliano KM. The evolving practice pattern of the breast surgeon with disappearance of open biopsy for nonpalpable lesions. Am J Surg. 1998;176:525–8

44 Philpotts LE, Shaheen NA, Carter D et al. Comparison of re-biopsy rates after stereotactic core needle biopsy of the breast with 11-gauge vacuum suction probe versus 14-gauge needle and automatic gun. AJR. 1999;172:683–7

45 Reynolds HE, Poon CM, Goulet RJ, Lazaridis CL. Biopsy of breast microcalcifications using an 11-gauge directional vacuum-assisted device. AJR. 1998;171:611–3

46 Liberman L, Hann LE, Dershaw DD et al. Mammographic findings after sterotaxic 14-gauge vacuum biopsy. Radiology. 1997;203:243–7

47 Berg WA, Krebs TL, Campassi C et al. Evaluation of 14- and 11-gauge directional, vacuum-assisted biopsy probes and 14-gauge biopsy guns in a breast parenchymal model. Radiology. 1997;205:203–8

48 Burbank F. Stereotactic breast biopsy of atypical ductal hyperplasia and ductal carcinoma in situ: improved accuracy with a directional, vacuum-assisted biopsy instrument. Radiology. 1997;202:843–8

49 Jackman RJ, Burbank F, Parker SH et al. Atypical ductal hyperplasia diagnosed at stereotactic breast biopsy: improved reliability with 14-gauge, directional, vacuum-assisted biopsy. Radiology. 1997;204:485–8

50 Liberman L, Cohen MA, Dershaw DD et al. Atypical ductal hyperplasia diagnosed at stereotaxic core biopsy of breast lesions: an indication for surgical biopsy. AJR. 1995;164:1111–3

51 Brem RF, Behrndt VS, Sanow L, Gatewood OMB. Atypical ductal hyperplasia: histologic underestimation of carcinoma in tissue harvested from impalpable breast lesions using 11-gauge stereotactically guided directional vacuum-assisted biopsy. AJR. 1999;172:1405–7

52 Won B, Reynolds H, Lazaridis CL, Jackson VP. Stereotactic biopsy of ductal carcinoma in situ using an 11 gauge vacuum-assisted device: persistent underestimation of disease. AJR. 1999;173:227–9

53 Götz L, Amaya B, Häntschel G et al. Comparison between histologic outcome in vacuum biopsy and re-excision. Eur Radiol. 2000;10(suppl1):2–10

54 Jackman RJ, Burbank FH, Parker SH et al. Accuracy of sampling ductal carcinoma in situ by three stereotactic breast biopsy methods (abstr). Radiology. 1998;209(P):197–8

55 Liberman L, Dershaw DD, Rosen PP et al. Stereotactic core biopsy of breast carcinoma: accuracy at predicting invasion. Radiology. 1995;194:379–81

56 Liberman L, Dershaw DD, Rosen PP et al. Core-needle biopsy of synchronous ipsilateral breast lesions: impact on treatment. AJR. 1996;166:1429–32

57 Rosenblatt R, Fineberg SA, Sparano JA, Kaleya RN. Stereotactic core needle biopsy of multiple sites in the breast: efficacy and effect on patient care. Radiology. 1996;201:67–70

58 Krämer S, Schulz-Wendtland R. Experiences with 400 core needle biopsies. Publication in preparation. Personal communication (April 2000)

59 Dershaw DD. Percutaneous biopsy of nonpalpable breast lesions: core or fine needle aspiration. In: Interventional Breast Procedures. Dershaw DD, ed. New York: Churchill Livingstone; 1996:103–6

60 Burbank F, Forcier N. Tissue marking clip for stereotactic breast biopsy: initial placement accuracy, long-term stability, and usefulness as a guide for wire localization. Radiology. 1997;205:407–15

61 Liberman L, Dershaw DD, Morris EA et al. Clip placement after stereotactic vacuum-assisted breast biopsy. Radiology. 1997;205:417–22

62 Heywang-Köbrunner SH, Hyynh AT, Viehweg P, Hanke W, Requardt H, Paprosch I. Prototype breast coil for MR-guided needle localization. J Comput Assist Tomogr. 1994;18:876–81

63 Orel SG, Schnall MD, Newman RW, Powell CM, Torosian MH, Rosato EF. MR imaging-guided localization and biopsy of breast lesions: initial experience. Radiology. 1994;193:97–102

64 Fischer U, Kopka L, Grabbe E. Magnetic resonance guided localization and biopsy of suspicious breast lesions. Top Magn Reson Imaging. 1998;9:44–59

65 Kuhl, C, Elevelt A, Leutner C, Gieseke J, Pakos E, Schild H. Interventional breast MR imaging: clinical use of a stereotactic localization and biopsy device. Radiology. 1997;204:667–75

66 Heywang-Köbrunner SH, Heinig A, Pickuth D, Alberich T, Spielmann RP. Interventional MRI of the breast: lesion localization and biopsy. Eur Radiol. 2000;10:36–45

67 Heywang-Köbrunner SH, Heinig A, Schaumlöffel U et al. MR-guided percutaneous excisional and incisional biopsy of breast lesions. Eur Radiol. 1999;9:1656–65

68 Perlet C, Sittek H, Prat X et al. Multicenter Study for evaluation of a new device for localisation and biopsy of MR-detected lesions. RoFo submitted (Study supported by EC Biomed 2 project).

69 Liberman L, Dershaw DD, Rosen PP et al. Stereotaxic core biopsy of impalpable spiculated breast masses. AJR. 1995;165:551–4

70 Liberman L, Sama M, Susnik B et al. Lobular carcinoma in situ at percutaneous breast biopsy: surgical biopsy findings. AJR.1999;173:291–9

71 Gabriel H. The dilemma of lobular carcinoma in situ at percutaneous biopsy: to excise or to monitor. AJR. 1999;173:300–2

72 Liberman L, Bracero N, Vuolo MA et al. Percutaneous large-core biopsy of papillary breast lesions. AJR. 1999;172:331–7

8. Preoperative Localization

Purpose, Definition, Indications, and Side Effects

■ Purpose

The increasing use of mammography has resulted in an increased rate of detection of clinically occult disease. Lesions requiring surgical excision that are only detected in diagnostic imaging studies, i. e., nonpalpable lesions, must be localized for the surgeon. Nonpalpable lesions can be localized under mammographic or ultrasound guidance or, less frequently, under CT or MRI guidance.

For image-guided localization only those imaging modalities should be chosen that clearly show the lesion. When several modalities fulfill this requirement, the modality that allows the fastest and easiest approach should be chosen.

There are several mammographically guided preoperative localization methods. They differ with respect to their technical requirements, the time required, their precision, and thus their accuracy.[1, 2]

Lesions that can be unequivocally identified by sonography can also be localized under sonographic guidance. On the whole, precision requires as much experience for ultrasound-guided localization as does mammographically guided localization. Ultrasound-guided localization of sufficiently large lesions can usually be performed more quickly than mammographic localization by experienced personnel.

Lesions that are only detected by contrast-enhanced MRI must be marked using contrast-enhanced MRI or CT. MR- or CT-guided localization can be performed with acceptable accuracy (± 5 to 10 mm) with the patient supine similar to the standard CT-guided biopsy of other organs. Special biopsy coils for percutaneous biopsy to mark lesions that were detected in MRI studies are meanwhile available and allow much better accuracy.

■ Definition

Preoperative localization refers to marking a nonpalpable lesion detected in a diagnostic imaging study for subsequent excision.

■ Indication

Any nonpalpable lesion requiring excision detected by mammography, sonography, or magnetic resonance imaging must be preoperatively localized and marked for the surgeon. Reliable excision and histologic examination of nonpalpable lesions can only be performed after such lesions have been correctly marked. Preoperative localization also enables the surgeon to excise a lesion with the removal of a minimal volume of breast tissue, minimizing postsurgical deformity.

■ Side Effects

The following side effects are possible:

- Pain
- Bleeding
- Vasovagal reaction[3]

The major pain perceived by the patient is felt during insertion of the needle through the skin itself. Advancing the needle or wire through the breast or injecting contrast solution (dye or carbon) is generally much less painful. The compression required in mammographically guided localization is also generally well tolerated, even with the needle in place. This assumes, of course, that the examiner proceeds gently.

Bleeding is only a problem when an artery is inadvertently injured during localization. If this occurs, firm compression has to be applied for a sufficient period of time (approximately 10 min).

The physician must always be prepared for vasovagal reactions since individual tolerance to the introduction of a needle into the breast varies greatly.

Methods and Technique

■ Mammographically Guided Localization Techniques

Before any preoperative localization, the radiologist should review the imaging studies to be certain a lesion exists and requires excision. Although lesions seen only on one view can be localized with stereotactic technique, an effort should be made to assess a lesion fully on two orthogonal views before scheduling needle localization. For this purpose it is recommended that a mediolateral or lateromedial view be obtained to supplement the craniocaudal and mediolateral oblique views. The true lateral gives a better sense of the depth of the lesion in the breast and thus helps to improve orientation.

Because the patient needs to cooperate during the localization procedure, she should not be premedicated. Local anesthetic is not given because its instillation is usually more painful than the insertion of a localizing wire into the breast.

■ Localizing Lesions Using a Perforated or Marked Compression Plate

Depending on the position of the lesion and the chosen way of access, a craniocaudal, caudocranial, mediolateral, or lateromedial view is obtained using a perforated plexiglass compression plate (Fig. 8.1) or a fenestrated compression plate with alphanumeric markings along its edge. The needle is to be inserted through the perforated or fenestrated compression plate and perpendicular to it. An initial image is taken with the patient's breast in compression between the localization plate. On this film the lesion must be imaged within the fenestration. The patient is held in compression while the film is developed. The point of needle insertion on the skin is chosen according to the coordinates of the lesion with reference to the markings. The skin over the lesion is cleansed and the needle is inserted into the breast, parallel to the chest wall. It is inserted beyond a depth calculated on the second orthogonal view, or as deep as possible if this depth cannot be exactly determined on the initial view. The needle should pass far enough through the lesion so that its tip will still penetrate the lesion after compression is removed and the breast relaxes. Next, a mammogram in the second orthogonal imaging plane is obtained. After this image compression on the breast is maintained. Based on this image, the depth of needle insertion is adjusted, if necessary. Once the needle is in the correct position, the wire is deployed or a marker solution injected. Correct needle insertion or correct placement and distribution of the marker solution is then also documented in two planes before the patient is sent to the operating room.

The *advantage* of this method is that it can easily be performed even by minimally experienced personnel and without expensive equipment. Because the approach is parallel to the chest wall, patients should never develop a pneumothorax.

The most relevant *disadvantage* is that it requires purchase of perforated or fenestrated plates. If so desired, an approach that approximates the probable surgical one can usually be achieved by careful selection of the initial plane of compression that is decisive for the direction of needle insertion. Even though the surgeon can approach a localized lesion independent of the position of the wire, some prefer to follow the path of the wire for the excision.

■ Stereotactic Localization

The accuracy that can be achieved with this procedure is comparable to that using a perforated compression plate, provided sufficient experience of possible pitfalls exists and the procedure is performed diligently. This is due to various hazards (see below) and the failure to readjust the needle depth on a second, orthogonal view before final deployment. The procedure is the same as in a stereotaxic biopsy (see p. 144–7). Once the correct position of the needle is verified, a marker wire is placed or a contrast solution injected. The needle usually just acts as a guide for

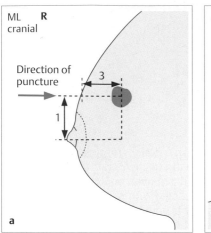

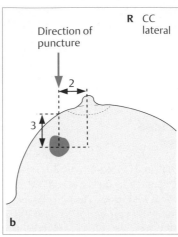

Fig. 8.**1 a–c** Schematic diagram of manual localization: The coordinates of the lesion in the horizontal (CC view) and vertical (ML view) direction (**a** and **b**) with reference to the nipple are marked on the skin of the breast and the depth of the lesion from the skin surface is measured

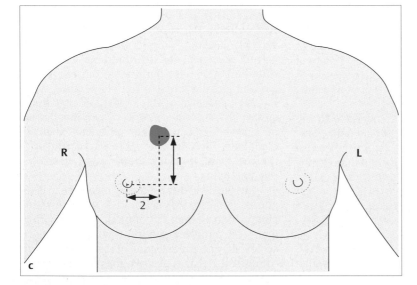

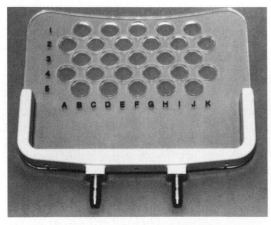

Fig. 8.**2** Perforated compression plate for localizing breast lesions

the wire and needs to be removed before releasing the compression on the breast. If the needle is to stay in place, an appropriate opening in the needle holder is necessary to allow detaching of the needle from it.

First the needle is placed in the same manner as for stereotaxic percutaneous biopsy. After the wire is placed, the proper position is first documented in the usual stereotaxic views (+ 15° and – 15°). After compression is released we strongly recommend that the correct wire placement be further documented in another plane perpendicular to the primary imaging plane (for example, in the mediolateral plane, if the first plane was the CC plane; Figs. 8.2 a–e). This is important because, particularly in dense breasts, tissue elasticity can cause the tip of the needle to lie above the lesion, not readily apparent in the stereotaxic views. A positioning error of a few millimeters in a compressed breast can correspond to a large positioning error (> 1 cm) in the relaxed breast.

To minimize the upward displacement of the needle that often occurs as a result of tissue elasticity, the needle may be placed 3–6 mm deeper than the calculated target point. This compensates for tissue elasticity, and once compression is relieved, the needle will usually lie at the desired location.

For localization, the stereotaxic method is comparable to localization procedures using a perforated compression plate. The major importance of stereotaxy is its use for percutaneous biopsy.

The following special problems can occur in stereotaxic needle localization:

- Due to the geometry of stereotaxy, slight deviations in the position of the needle in the targeting or documentation views can correspond to a significant deviation in depth localization. Localization errors can occur if the patient moves (in nondigital systems significant time may elapse for development of the localization views and for depth determination), or if the targets chosen on the + 15° and – 15° stereotaxic views prove not to be identical. This may occur with ill-defined lesions, for which it is difficult to identify the same structure on the + 15° and – 15° views or with multiple microcalcifications showing minimal pleomorphism.
- Even with the tip of the needle in the correct position, inserting the marker wire will usually push the denser breast tissue forward a few millimeters. The resulting positioning error in the compressed breast can result in a final positioning error in the relaxed breast of over 1 cm.

To minimize these problems, the following steps are recommended:

- Exercising extreme care in selecting the target point and in verifying it in the + 15° and – 15° views.
- Switching to another localization method if identical target points cannot be clearly located on the compression views.
- Always advancing the needle a few millimeters deeper than the target point to compensate for tissue elasticity.
- Always verifying the final result in two perpendicular planes.

- Always (with this method) using localization needles that can be repositioned in case of an unsatisfactory position.

■ Manual Localization

Manual localization was the first and simplest method for advancing a needle to a lesion under mammographic guidance. In most institutions, it has been replaced by the grid technique since an approach parallel to the chest wall is preferred. In the hands of an experienced radiologist it may, however, allow a fast approach to superficial lesions and to lesions which may be difficult to localize by the standard methods (retroareolar lesions).

The *advantages* are the simplicity and the fact that the point of entry lies directly anterior to the lesion, which often corresponds to the approach preferred by the surgeon.

Disadvantages are that it is generally not as precise as localizing with add-on devices with the necessity for corrections in a certain percentage of lesions, and it requires more practice and skill in three-dimensional visualization than other methods of localization. Finally, the axis of the needle is perpendicular to the chest wall, increasing the risk of injury to the chest wall when a lesion is located posteriorly.

Procedure: Figure 8.3 shows how the point of entry on the skin is selected based on the mammograms and how the depth of the lesion is measured. When transferring the coordinates of the lesion with respect to the nipple, the assistant must be careful to hold the breast in the same position as it was in the original mediolateral view. When inserting the needle, the physician places his or her other hand around the tissue into which the needle is to be inserted. This minimizes the risk of injury to the chest wall and brings the breast into a shape similar to that on the mediolateral view. The position of the needle is then verified in mammograms in two planes (craniocaudal and 90° mediolateral) and corrected if necessary. After verification of the correct needle position, a contrast solution is injected or a wire is placed through the needle.

■ Ultrasound-Guided Localization

Ultrasound-guided localization requires that the lesion be visualized via sonography. This means that it cannot be used with microcalcifications, yet it is very effective in localizing focal lesions. The procedure is similar to the ultrasound-guided per-

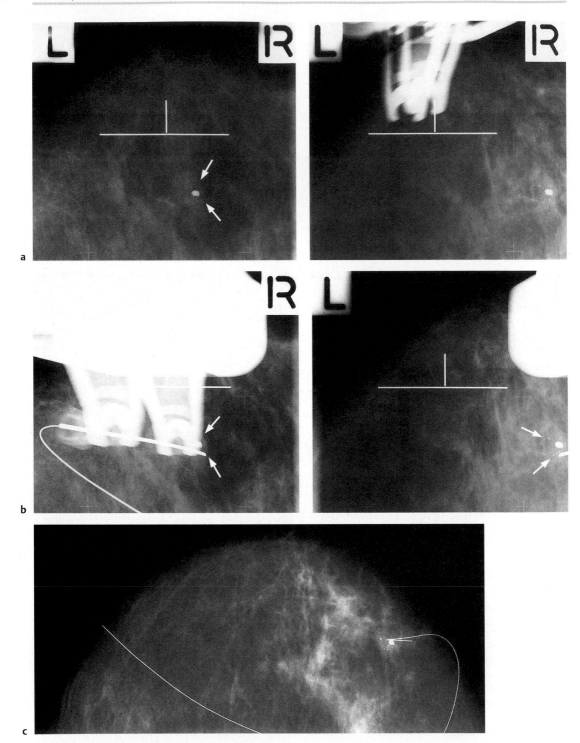

Fig. 8.**3 a–e**
a Two partial views with the tube tilted – 15° and + 15°
reveal a small focal lesion requiring localization or biopsy
b Demonstrating the tip of the needle in the center of the
focal lesion

c and **d** Documentation view demonstrating correct positioning of the localization wire
e Specimen radiography

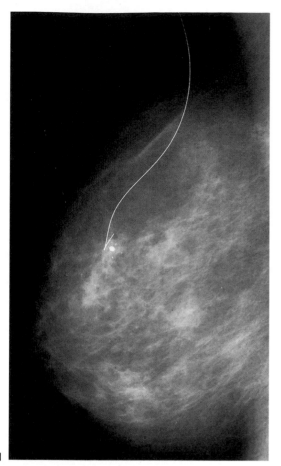

d

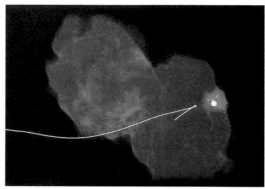

e

cutaneous biopsy (see p. 140-1). Instead of aspirating or performing a core biopsy, the radiologist deploys a marker wire through the needle. Contrast solutions are not generally used in ultrasound-guided localization. Sonographic verification of the correct needle position is mandatory (Fig. 8.4).

The *advantage* of ultrasound-guided localization over other methods of localization is that it takes the least amount of time. A *disadvantage* is that visualization of small or preinvasive lesions may be uncertain or impossible. Furthermore, it may sometimes be difficult to identify the lesion in a subsequent specimen sonogram.

■ MR-Guided Localization

Lesions detected by MRI alone must be preoperatively marked using contrast-enhanced MRI or contrast-enhanced CT. Ultrasound-guided localization by a physician experienced in both sonog-

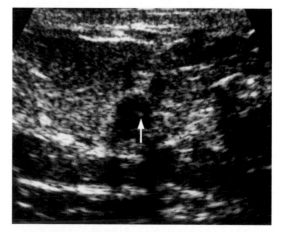

Fig. 8.**4** Documenting correct positioning of the needle after ultrasound-guided localization. The tip of the needle is visible as a hyperechoic point in the center of the lesion. Definite localization of the needle-tip position requires visualization of the needle in its long axis

raphy and MRI is recommended only where subsequent sonograms unequivocally demonstrate a lesion correlating with lesion the detected by MRI. Due to respiratory motion, a lesion detected by MRI can be localized with an accuracy of ± 1 cm using a CT or MRI unit without a special biopsy coil. Highly precise preoperative marking (and localization for core biopsy) is possible through the use of special "biopsy" or "localization" coils. Various devices for MR-guided localization are meanwhile available. The exact procedure varies with the device.[4–10]

■ Galactographically Guided Localization

If a lesion is only detected at galactography, repeat galactography will be required for preoperative localization of the lesion.

■ Technique

Several options for galactographically guided localization are available:

1. After galactography (see Chapter 3, p. 74–80) in the craniocaudal and mediolateral planes, the galactographic findings are localized using the standard mammographic localization techniques (i. e., manually, using a perforated plate, or by means of stereotaxy).
2. If only a single duct is involved, the duct may be galactographically visualized and delineated immediately preoperatively using a combination of contrast medium and patent blue. The blue-dyed ductal system must be excised immediately after instillation of contrast medium.
3. In the presence of significant duct ectasia, the lactiferous duct itself will sometimes be visible at mammography or sonography. In this case, mammographic or ultrasound localization is possible without the use of contrast media.

Localization Materials

The selection of localization materials depends on the interval between localization and surgery. Usually, localization is performed shortly before surgery.

In this case, some physicians elected to use low-cost *dye marking* with patent blue immediately preoperatively. Having verified correct needle position, the radiologist injects 0.2–0.3 ml of blue dye, such as methylene blue or patent blue, after which the surgeon removes the blue-stained parenchymal tissue. For mammographically guided localization, the radiologist adds 0.2–0.3 ml of a nonionic radiographic contrast medium. This is necessary for subsequent documentation of proper dispersion of the contrast solution on the two-view mammogram done after the localization has been completed. It is important to perform the surgery as quickly as possible after injecting the blue solution because within a few hours the solution can diffuse throughout large areas of the breast or even the entire breast, rendering precise localization impossible. If the interval between administration of the contrast solution and surgery cannot be limited to a few hours, the radiologist should choose a different localization procedure. Further disadvantages are that diffusion renders it impossible for the pathologist to identify the exact injection site, and in addition to contrast allergies, severe allergies to patent blue, although rare, have been known to occur.

Another simple procedure is to use a *carbon solution for marking the lesion.* The advantage of carbon is that it does not diffuse. Therefore it can be performed several days preoperatively since the carbon remains at the injection site until the surgeon removes it along with the lesion. However, even though inert and harmless, carbon solution is not approved in some countries (USA) for use in the breast.

This method has mainly been used for CT- and MR-guided localization since in these cases it is often difficult to coordinate the scheduling of the examination and surgery.

The sterile carbon solution, which can be prepared by most pharmacies (4 g of activated charcoal in 100 ml of 0.9% saline solution), in injected into the center of the lesion to be excised or directly proximal to it. Approximately 1–1.5 ml of solution have to be injected to achieve sufficient dispersion and visualization. For mammographically guided localization, 0.2–0.3 ml of nonionic radiographic contrast medium should be added to the solution for subsequent image documentation of correct dispersion. Then a fine line of carbon extending all the way to the skin is injected as the needle is withdrawn, to permit the surgeon to locate the lesion after the needle or wire has been removed. A particular advantage of this method is that the carbon also enables the pathologist to locate the injection site in the specimen.

Some surgeons prefer to have the needle left in place (suitable only if the mammography suite is close to the operating room) or have a marker wire placed through the localization needle to ·facilitate locating the lesion, which may be stained with dye or unstained.

Today *localization wires* are mostly used. They have the advantage of being more flexible and better anchored in the tissue. This minimizes the risk of wire migration.

There are various types of localization wires (Fig. 8.5). The tenacity of staying in place varies with their shape and the type of breast tissue. Dislocation can occur particularly in soft fatty tissue, whereby dislocation primarily occurs in the soft, fatty tissues. In rare cases, wires have been observed to migrate distally. This usually occurs only in wires whose form predisposes them to migrate in a certain direction, such as a simple 1-shaped hookwire. The so-called twist marker (which can also be retracted through tissue like a corkscrew), the Homer wire, and the Fixmarker (from BIP) are nondirectional. The particular advantage of these wires is that they can be withdrawn or retracted through the needle, making it possible to correct the position of the needle at any time.

Regardless of the wire chosen, the physician should ensure that the needle through which the wire is advanced is sufficiently stiff (it should not be too thin and flexible) because otherwise it can deviate considerably in dense tissue and seriously compromise the accuracy of localization. An adequate length of wire should extend beyond the skin and be securely taped to it to avoid retraction of the wire and its subsequent loss. During surgery, if the surgeon is dissecting along the length of the wire, he or she should be careful not to transsect it. It may then retract into the breast and be very difficult to locate.

Problems and Their Solutions

All methods require documentation of the final position of the localization wire or the contrast solution. This means that after mammographically guided localization, the position of the needle should be documented in two mammographic planes (craniocaudal and mediolateral). If the wire is improperly positioned but the distance between the tumor and the tip of the wire is still acceptable (i. e., does not exceed 10 mm), the radiologist may describe to the surgeon the exact

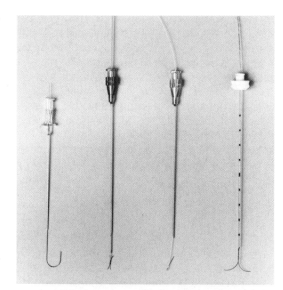

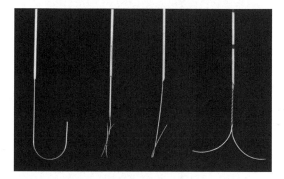

Fig. 8.**5** Various localization wires

position of the lesion in the image with respect to the tip of the wire. Large areas undergoing excision should have their margins marked with two wires. Multiple lesions can be needle localized for excision in one surgical procedure. Wires rather than dye should be used in this setting to avoid staining large areas of the breast.

The exact position of the wire or contrast solution should also be documented in MR-guided and ultrasound-guided localization. If improper positioning occurs, the necessary corrections should be discussed with the surgeon, assuming of course that the deviation is within acceptable limits. Sufficient experience and thorough discussion of the results are essential because precise localization is unfortunately not always possible. Furthermore, it is not always easy for the surgeon to find the contrast solution or marker wire, particularly in large breasts. Perioperative or intraoperative dislocation of the wire may occur. Close cooperation between radiologist and surgeon is essential for effective management, i. e., removal of the suspicious lesion with the smallest possible volume of breast tissue. Correct excision of microcalcifications and nonpalpable lesions detected at mammography should also be documented by specimen radiography.[11] Lesions detected only at sonography should be documented by specimen sonography whenever possible.

■ Summary

The increasing use of mammography has resulted in an increased rate of detection of clinically occult lesions. These lesions must be marked for the surgeon to ensure that they can be effectively removed. Several methods are available. Accepted methods involve use of a perforated or marked compression plate, stereotaxy or in selected cases manual localisation.

Focal lesions with correlating sonographic findings or focal lesions detected only at ultrasonography can be quickly and reliably marked using ultrasound-guided localization. Localization techniques guided by magnetic resonance imaging permit accurate marking of lesions that are detected only at MRI and require excision.

CT-guided localization after administration of contrast remains an alternative for marking nonpalpable MRI-detected lesions that are also visible by contrast-enhanced CT but not by conventional imaging. It is faster and easier than MR localization without a dedicated biopsy coil.

Due to the significant radiation dose and the lower accuracy, CT-guided localization should, however, in the future be replaced by MR-guided localization using dedicated coils.

The choice between needle marking, wire marking with various marker wires, or marking with carbon or methylene blue depends on the time interval between localization and surgery, the conditions under which the patient must be transported to the operating room and the surgeon's preferences.

■ References

1 Bauer M, Schulz-Wendtlandt R. Stereotaktische Lokalisation kleinster Mammaläsionen für Diagnostik und präoperative Markierung – Methodik, experimentelle Untersuchungen und klinische Ergebnisse bei 217 Patientinnen. Fortschr Rontgenstr. 1992;156:286–90

2 Homer MJ, Smith TJ, Safaii H. Prebiopsy needle localization. Methods, problems and expected results. In: Radiol Clin North Am. Breast imaging: current status and future directions. 1992;30(1):139–53

3 Helvie MA, Ikeda DM, Adler DD. Localization and needle aspiration of breast lesions: complications in 370 cases. AJR. 1991;157:711–14

4 Heywang-Köbrunner SH, Requardt H, Huynh AT et al. MRI of the breast: first experiences with a new localisation device. Eur Congr. Radiol. 1993;93:204

5 Heywang-Köbrunner SH. Work in progress: Prototype breast coil for MR-guided needle localization – first experiences. J Comput Assist Tomogr. 1994;18:876–81

6 Heywang-Köbrunner SH, Beck R. Contrast-enhanced MRI of the Breast. 2nd ed. Berlin: Springer; 1996

7 Orel SG, Schnall MD, Newman RW et al. MR imaging-guided localization and biopsy of breast lesions: Initial experience. Radiology. 1994;193:97–102

8 Fischer U, Kopka L, Grabbe E. Magnetic resonance guided localization and biopsy of suspicious breast lesions. Top Magn Reson Imaging. 1998;9:44–59

9 Kuhl C, Elevelt A, Leutner C, Gieseke J, Pakos E, Schild H. Interventional breast MR imaging: clinical use of a stereotactic localization and biopsy device. Radiology. 1997;204:667–75

10 Heywang-Köbrunner SH, Heinig A, Pickuth D, Alberich T, Spielmann RP. Interventional MRI of the breast: lesion localization and biopsy. Eur Radiol. 2000;10:36–45

11 Graham RA, Homer MJ, Sigler CJ, Safaii H, Schmid CH, Marchant DJ, Smith TJ. The efficacy of specimen radiography in evaluating the surgical margins of impalpable breast carcinoma. AJR. 1994;162:33–6

II Appearance

9. The Normal Breast

■ Anatomy

The mammary gland consists of 15 to 20 lobes with varying numbers of ducts and lobules. These structures are surrounded by collagenous connective tissue or stromal tissue. A lobule comprises approximately 30 terminal branches (acini or ductules) that form the parenchymal part of the lobule. Acini and terminal ducts are surrounded by loose mesenchyma. The lobule with

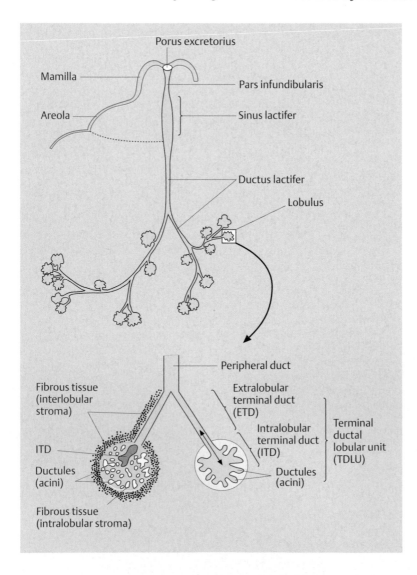

Fig. 9.**1** Schematic diagram and terminology of the lactiferous duct system[1]

Porus excretorius

Mamilla

Pars infundibularis

Areola

Sinus lactifer

Ductus lactifer

Lobulus

Peripheral duct

Fibrous tissue (interlobular stroma)

Extralobular terminal duct (ETD)

Intralobular terminal duct (ITD)

Terminal ductal lobular unit (TDLU)

ITD

Ductules (acini)

Ductules (acini)

Fibrous tissue (intralobular stroma)

its terminal branches, its short intralobular and longer extralobular duct form the terminal ductulobular unit (TDLU; Fig. 9.**1**). All terminal ducts open into a lactiferous duct that runs toward the nipple. The 15 to 20 main lactiferous ducts open in the nipple (Fig. 9.**1**).

The body of the gland is imbedded in fatty tissue. It is supplied by a network of blood and lymph vessels and is supported in the subcutaneous fatty tissue by connective-tissue structures known as Cooper ligaments. These ligaments arise from the stromal tissue of the body of the gland and insert into the prepectoral fascia and the skin. The body of the gland, which can vary greatly in form, size, and composition, converges toward the nipple, is generally symmetrical, and is particularly pronounced in the upper outer quadrants.

The Adolescent Female Breast

■ Histology

Histologically, the prepubescent breast consists of lactiferous ducts with adventitial alveoli comprised primarily of connective tissue and small amounts of fatty tissue. During puberty, the ducts increase in length, and the terminal alveoli increase in number. These later develop into lobules. Ductal growth triggers mesenchymal metaplasia and formation of connective tissue.

■ Clinical Examination

On palpation the breast is uniformly firm with readily palpable glandular tissue with a total absence of any nodular or finely granular consistency.

■ Mammography

The underdeveloped glandular body initially appears as a small nodule, later as a small tree-like glandular structure. The lactiferous ducts and connective tissue appear as a homogeneously dense, milky structure surrounded by a narrow layer of subcutaneous fatty tissue. Substructures are not usually discernible with the exception of some vessels and Cooper ligaments within the subcutaneous tissue (Fig. 9.**2**).

■ Sonography

The immature glandular tissue is initially relatively hypoechoic. The nodule of glandular tissue may appear as a hypoechoic nodule and should not be confused with a tumor. Even the developed glandular body is still relatively hypoechoic in adolescence and cannot always be distinguished from the surrounding hypoechoic fat. The echogenicity of the glandular tissue increases with maturity. However, local differences in the maturity of breast tissue can occur, producing alternating areas of predominantly hypoechoic and predominantly hyperechoic glandular tissue (Fig. 9.**3 a** and **b**).

The Mature Female Breast

■ Histology

Under the influence of estrogen, progesterone, prolactin, STH, ACTH, and corticoids, the ductal system becomes increasingly branched. A tree-like glandular structure with glandular lobules develops. This process of growth and differentiation continues until about age 30. The highest proportion of lobules are located far from the nipple along the periphery, particularly in the upper outer quadrant.

■ Clinical Examination

Physical examination of the normal female breast can vary considerably. Large, fatty breasts generally have a soft consistency. In rare cases, however, even fatty breasts will be firm and nodular on palpation. Glandular tissue with a high proportion of parenchymal or connective tissue usually feels firm. Generally, there will be less glandular tissue in the inner half of the breast than in the outer half. Therefore the breast is generally firmer in the upper outer quadrant due to the increased proportion of parenchymal tissue

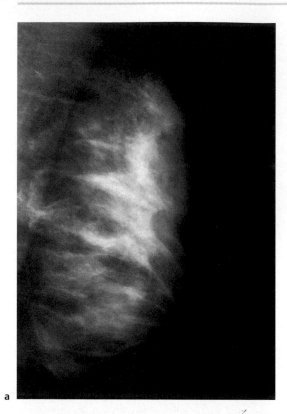

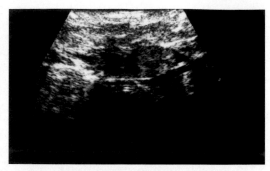

Fig. 9.2a and b
Mammography is usually not indicated in asymptomatic adolescent patients. An oblique single-view mammogram was obtained in this 15-year-old patient because of brownish discharge from the left nipple and because of a sonographic indeterminate hypoechoic finding behind the nipple
a Mammography reveals no abnormalities and shows the typical homogeneously dense breast tissue of a 15-year-old female
b Sonography: a hypoechoic area measuring 21 mm was noted about 1 cm behind the nipple. Considering the brownish discharge, the symptoms might well be compatible with juvenile papillomatosis, which typically cannot be discerned from the surrounding tissue mammographically. Further workup (puncture, cytology of the discharge) was refused by the patient

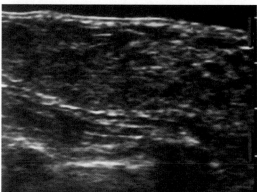

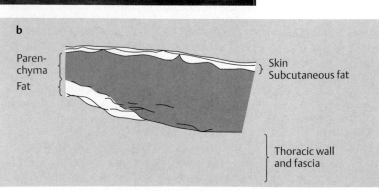

Paren-
chyma
Fat

Skin
Subcutaneous fat

Thoracic wall
and fascia

Fig. 9.3a and b Sonography of the adolescent breast
a The subcutaneous layer of fat seen here is narrow as in many adolescent breasts. The glandular tissue is still relatively hypoechoic and thus more difficult to differentiate from the subcutaneous fat than in an adult breast
b Diagram for Figure 9.3a

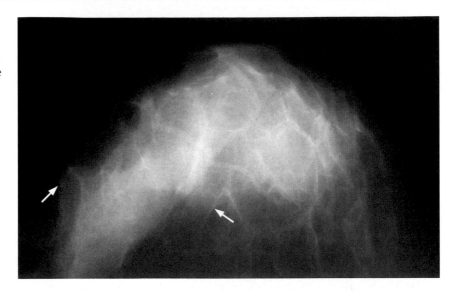

in this region. If fibrocystic changes develop, the uniformly soft to firm consistency of the breasts may change from a finely granular to coarsely nodular pattern on palpation.

The glandular tissue undergoes cyclical fluctuations, which may become apparent to the woman in the second half of the menstrual cycle as increased tissue tension or pain and enlargement of the breasts. This is due to the cyclical swelling of the lobular tissue. Temporary enlargement of the acini also occurs. For this reason, the glandular tissue of the breast in the second half of the cycle and especially immediately prior to menstruation will usually be firmer, more sensitive to pressure, and more painful.

■ Mammography

Normal glandular tissue (Fig. 9.**4**) will appear as a summation image of all microscopic parenchymal and connective-tissue structures, i. e., it will produce a homogeneous mammographic appearance. This homogeneous pattern will be interspersed with islands of fatty tissue appearing as round or curved radiolucencies in a wide variety of individual configurations. Often increased opacity corresponding to the physiologic distribution of parenchymal tissue will be seen in the upper outer quadrants.

Cooper ligaments appear in the mammogram as curved to linear densities. They extend from the cone of breast tissue through the fatty tissue to the skin. Depending on the specific composi-

tion of the breast, the glandular, connective, and fatty tissues, and the ligaments can be distinguished more or less clearly. Generally, Cooper ligaments are most prominent in the subcutaneous fatty tissue along the superior margin of the parenchyma on the oblique or mediolateral mammogram and in the prepectoral space.

The *lactiferous duct system* will not be visualized except for the large lactiferous ducts converging in the retroareolar region, where they are visible as band-like structures.

The density of the *parenchyma* may vary with the menstrual cycle. It may be denser in the premenstrual phase than in the postmenstrual phase. This means that the mammographic appearance of the parenchyma may vary both in terms of its structure and with respect to the phase of the menstrual cycle.

Parenchymal structures are always more easily discerned and their regular arrangement converging at the nipple more easily demonstrated when fatty tissue is present. Where less fatty tissue is interspersed, the parenchymal structures tend to blend into a homogeneous pattern of density that can hide small pathologic lesions.

In those women with increased premenstrual pain with resulting diminished compressibility of the glandular tissue and the increased premenstrual density with resulting poor visualization, mammography may be best performed in the postmenstrual phase of the cycle.

■ Sonography
(Figs. 9.5 a–i)

Glandular tissue generally appears hyperechoic, although its sonographic appearance may vary from moderately to highly echogenic. Surrounding or interspersed *fat* is hypoechoic. Rotating the transducer will usually identify these interspersed fat lobules as oblong hypoechoic areas to be distinguished from hypoechoic tumors. Sometimes a connection between the fat lobules and the subcutaneous fatty tissue allows their identification. Depending on the imaging plane, hypoechoic tubular or punctate structures traversing the glandular parenchyma will occasionally be visible. These structures are arranged regularly in the tissue and probably correspond to small ductal structures with periductal fibrosis or small foci of adenosis. Such findings represent a normal variant and do not require further workup. The examiner should verify that the layer of fatty tissue surrounding the body of the gland is completely intact and unchanged.

Cooper ligaments are hyperechoic and permeate the layer of fatty tissue, appearing as fine linear structures. Due to their orientation (almost parallel to the direction of sound propagation), Cooper ligaments can produce acoustic shadows that occur when the sound is reflected away from the transducer. These acoustic shadows can be recognized by the fact that they originate from Cooper ligaments. They can generally be eliminated by compression and do not represent a pathologic finding.

The skin itself appears as a hyperechoic line or, depending on the resolution of the transducer, as a double contour whose thickness generally does not exceed 3 mm except at the areola.

Since the retroareolar ducts run nearly parallel to the direction of sound propagation and periductal fibrosis is frequently present, the sound waves will often be reflected away from the transducer or absorbed behind the nipple. The acoustic shadow ("nipple shadow") thus produced does not represent a pathologic finding but a normal structure that can vary. This nipple shadow may impair visualization of the retroareolar region.

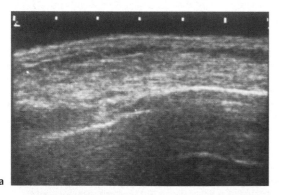

a

Fig. 9.**5 a–i** Sonography of the adult breast. Significant individual variations can occur both in the relative proportion of hyperechoic glandular tissue and more hypoechoic fatty tissue and in the echogenicity of the glandular tissue itself
a Breast with dense hyperechoic glandular tissue surrounded by a narrow layer of fat. The subcutaneous fascia is only partially visible. The prepectoral fascia is readily discernible
b Diagram for Figure 9.**5 a**

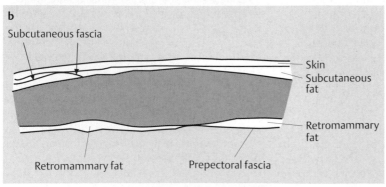

b
Subcutaneous fascia
Skin
Subcutaneous fat
Retromammary fat
Retromammary fat   Prepectoral fascia

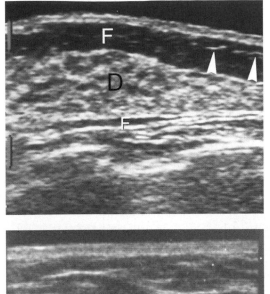

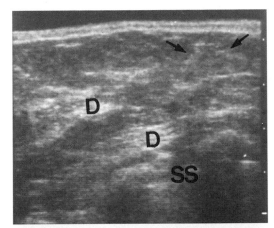

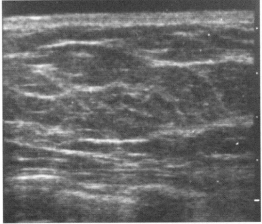

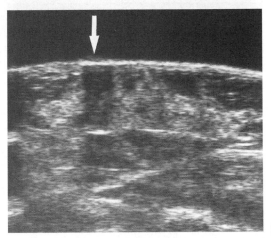

c In this breast, the hyperechoic glandular tissue (D) is permeated with extremely regular tubular hypoechoic structures. This image also represents a normal finding. The hypoechoic structures probably correspond to small ductal structures with periductal fibrosis or small foci of adenosis. Subcutaneous and retromammary fat (F) are visible as wide and very narrow hypoechoic strips. The subcutaneous fascia (arrowhead) is partly visible as a fine line of more distinct echoes

d This partially involuted breast contains abundant hypoechoic fatty tissue in addition to a smaller amount of remaining hyperechoic glandular tissue (D). Permeating this fatty tissue are thin hyperechoic ligamentous structures, which can produce discrete acoustic shadows (SS) depending on the direction of sound propagation. On the right, a fine Cooper ligament inserting into the skin (arrows) is visible

e Extremely fatty breasts appear hypoechoic on sonography. The hypoechoic fat is transversed only by thin hyperechoic linear ligamentous structures

f–i Sometimes it may be difficult to distinguish normal structures from pathologic changes. This may be the case for the nipple shadow (**f**), for acoustic shadows posterior to Cooper ligaments (**g** and **h**), or for interspersed fat lobules (**i**)

f The dense ductal structures posterior to the nipple often absorb sound or, if they lie parallel to the direction of sound propagation, reflect sound energy away from the transducer. This can produce a nipple shadow (arrow). In contrast to the shadow posterior to a mass, the nipple shadow begins posterior to the nipple and can vary in intensity. This shadow represents a normal structure.

Lesions in this poorly visualized area should always be carefully excluded by careful palpation and, if necessary, by tilting the transducer

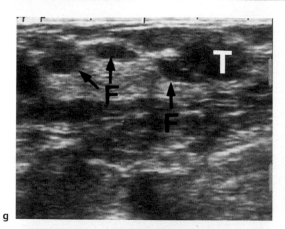

g

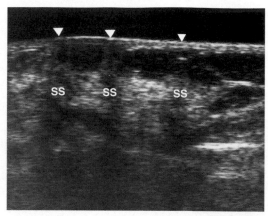

h

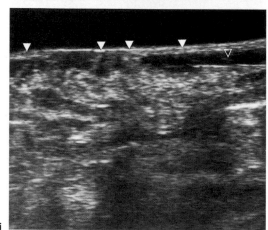

i

Fig. 9.**5 g** If hypoechoic fat lobules (F) are interspersed in the glandular tissue, they may simulate a tumor (T). The shown tumor proved to be a fibroadenoma. It is surrounded by multiple interspersed fat lobules (F). The main criteria for differentiation include:

1. Fat lobules are easily compressible
2. In the vertical plane, the fat lobules will generally appear as long structures that often are connected to the subcutaneous fat (see also Fig. 4.**5**)

h Acoustic shadows (SS) can occur at Cooper ligaments (arrowheads) if they are parallel to the direction of sound propagation. These shadows can be distinguished from pathologic shadows by their point of origin. These shadows also generally disappear when compression is increased or the transducer is tilted, i. e., they are not constant

i The same breast as in Figure 9.**5 h** with increased compression applied. The open arrowhead shows a Cooper ligament that does not cause an acoustic shadow regardless of whether compression is applied. The other Cooper ligaments produce obvious acoustic shadows without compression, which disappear when compression is applied

■ **Magnetic Resonance Imaging**
(Figs. 9.**6 a–d**)

MRI is not necessary for imaging the normal breast. However, normal breast tissue will often be incidentally visualized on MR images, or normal tissue will be diagnosed after a suspected pathologic change has been ruled out.

In T1-weighted spoiled-gradient echo sequences (FLASH, T1 FFE, and SP GRASS), fat has moderate signal intensity, whereas all glandular and ductal structures and fibrous connective tissue (with Cooper ligaments) are visualized with low signal intensity. After intravenous injection of the contrast medium gadolinium-DTPA, glandular, fatty, and connective tissue do not nor-

mally enhance, i. e., these structures appear identical in precontrast and postcontrast images. Only vascular structures can be traced through the images as small enhancing worm-like structures or punctate cross sections of high signal intensity. Contrast enhancement of the nipple itself occurs in approximately 50% of all patients and should not be regarded as pathologic in the absence of suggestive clinical findings. Occasionally, a milky or patchy diffuse enhancement, sometimes even focal enhancement, can appear in normal glandular tissue. This enhancement is probably due to hormonal changes and usually occurs in young patients with active glandular tissue or in postmenopausal patients receiving hormone therapy (particularly where preparations with a high pro-

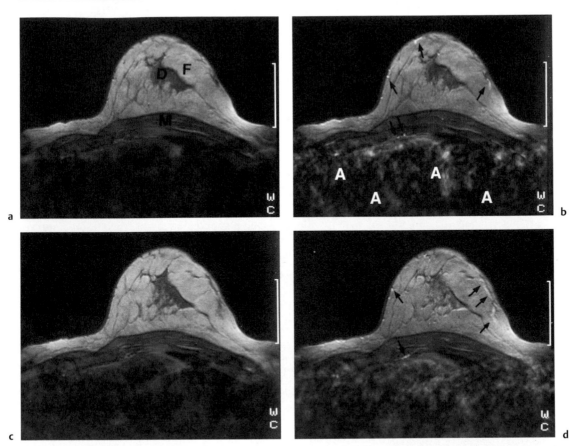

Fig. 9.**6 a–d** Contrast-enhanced MRI of a normal breast.
a On the T1-weighted transverse slice of the breast
(FLASH 3D), glandular and connective tissue (D) are visualized with low signal intensity, as is muscle (M). Fat (F)
shows moderate signal intensity.
b After application of contrast, normal glandular tissue
and fatty tissue only enhance slightly at the beginning of
the menstrual cycle (between the 6th and 16th days) and
in the postmenstrual phase. This means that the signal intensity hardly changes at all in comparison to the plain
image (**a**). Only the band of artifacts caused by blood
flowing through the heart (A) significantly increases in sig-

nal intensity, as do the vessels (arrow) that can be traced
through the images after contrast application as winding
or punctiform structures of high signal intensity
c and **d** In the second half of the menstrual cycle, slight to
intense diffuse or nodular enhancement patterns are
often seen in normal glandular tissue
c Comparable image of the same breast as in Figure 9.**6 a**
in the second half of the cycle before application of contrast
d After application of contrast in the second half of the
cycle, moderate diffuse enhancement may be seen (arrows indicate vascular structures)

gesterone content are used). It is usually transient
and more pronounced before and during menstruation. Since this enhancement can interfere
with the exclusion of malignancy and can lead to
false positive findings, we recommend to perform
contrast-enhanced MRI between day 6 to day 17

of the menstrual cycle, whenever possible. Also, it
should be performed in young patients (those
below the age of 30–35 years in whom the incidence of malignancy is typically very low and the
glandular tissue tends to be metabolically more
active) only if definitely indicated.[2, 3]

Involution

■ Histology

As ovarian function decreases, involution of the glandular body sets in. Lactiferous ducts, lobules and parenchyma become atrophic, and fatty and fibrous tissue dominate. Often ectasia of the large excretory ducts occurs.

■ Clinical Examination

The findings of the clinical examination vary considerably, depending on the extent of the parenchymal involution, the presence of structural changes due to benign breast disorders, and the extent of fibrosis.

■ Mammography

The formerly dense epithelial and mesenchymal parts of the glandular tissue that absorb radiation

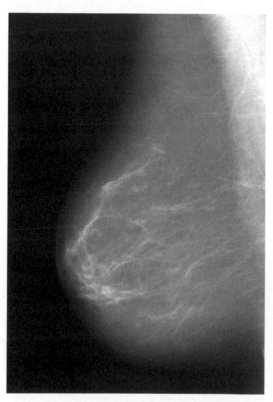

Fig. 9.**7**   Involution. Radiolucent glandular body only delineating Cooper ligaments, few glandular and ductal as well as vascular structures (MLO view)

are replaced with fat as involution progresses. The body of the gland itself becomes considerably more radiolucent and fibrous tissue, vascular structures, and remaining glandular lobules become more readily discernible, as do the large retroareolar ectatic lactiferous ducts (Fig. 9.7).

Involution begins in the inner half of the breast and involves the upper outer quadrant and the retroareolar region later. Thus mammography in the older woman will reveal residual glandular tissue primarily in the retroareolar region and in the upper outer quadrant. Involution improves the visualization of the breast. *In a completely involuted fatty breast, the sensitivity of mammography approaches 100%.*

■ Sonography

The fatty involuted breast appears hypoechoic on sonographic examination (Fig. 9.5 e). Only remaining islands of hyperechoic connective tissue and Cooper ligaments traverse the hypoechoic fatty tissue. Residual parenchyma generally appears as moderately echogenic islands in hypoechoic fat.

Over 90% of breast carcinomas are hypoechoic (similar to fatty tissue). Only some breast carcinomas have a distinctive posterior acoustic shadow or a hyperechoic peripheral rim. This comprises the *sensitivity of ultrasonography in the fatty breast.* Islands of fatty tissue with or without posterior shadowing due to fibrous septa can also be mistaken for tumors. To avoid both false positive and false negative calls the sonogram should generally be read in conjunction with mammography.

With the excellent sensitivity of mammography applied to the involuted breast, sonography is not necessary for detecting or excluding malignancy. *However, it is indicated for differentiating cysts from solid masses* since simple cysts can reliably be diagnosed even in the fatty breast.

■ Magnetic Resonance Imaging

In MR images, fatty tissue has high signal intensity before and after intravenous administration of contrast medium, whereas residual parenchyma and connective-tissue structures have low signal intensity. Due to the high sensitivity of mammography, contrast-enhanced MRI is not generally needed in the fatty breast.

■ Summary

The breast of an asymptomatic patient over the age of 40 is generally examined clinically and mammographically. In the presence of uncertain palpable and mammographic findings, ultrasound can provide additional information. Ultrasound as the first diagnostic imaging procedure is only indicated in younger women.

The physician should verify the clinical absence of:

– Palpable pathologic findings
– Asymmetry
– Skin or nipple retraction
– Pathologic discharge

In diagnostic imaging studies, special attention should be given to:

– Uniform skin thickness
– Visualization of fine Cooper ligaments
– Visualization of an undisturbed subcutaneous and retromammary layer of fat

– Symmetrical distribution of the body of the gland
– Regular configuration of ductal structures converging at the nipple

Furthermore, imaging studies serve to verify the absence of:

– Masses and densities
– Architectural distortion
– Suspicious microcalcification

Comparison with the contralateral breast is important both in light of the immense variety in size, arrangement, and density of the parenchyma among patients, and because clinical, mammographic, and sonographic detection of abnormality will depend on the recognition of sometimes subtle structural abnormalities. Comparison with previous diagnostic imaging studies (where available) is even more important.

Abnormalities

■ Definition

Breasts may vary considerably with respect to size, shape, and consistency. The following conditions are regarded as abnormalities:

– Asymmetry
– Macromastia
– Polymastia (for example in the axillary tail or axilla)
– Inverted nipple

Asymmetry

■ Clinical Examination

The most frequent abnormality is asymmetry in breast size (anisomastia).[4, 5] Depending on the severity of this condition, which can vary greatly, the difference in size will be more or less apparent upon visual inspection. The difference in palpable findings between the two breasts can vary accordingly. Patients will typically have long been aware of the asymmetry and, apart from cyclical fluctuations, no significant changes will be observed over time. This distinguishes anisomastia from pathologic asymmetry in size, such as can occur in the presence of benign masses (cysts, fibroadenomas, or phyllodes tumor) or when the consistency of one

breast gradually changes as a result of a disseminated malignant process. When this is accompanied by retraction and loss of volume—which in fact is typical for scirrhous breast cancers—malignancy must be considered highly probable until proven otherwise.

Asymmetry must always be assessed carefully because it may be the presenting sign of malignancy.

■ Mammography

Mammography will reveal asymmetric parenchymal distribution correlating with the clinical and anatomic asymmetry (Figs. 9.8 a–d).

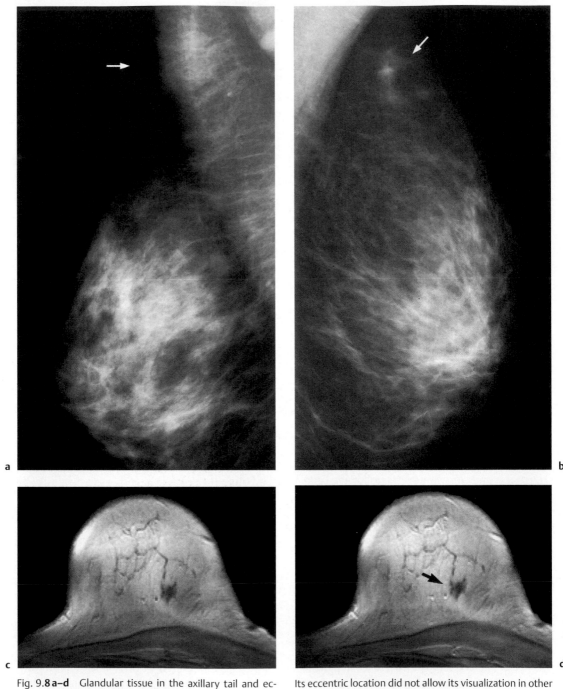

Fig. 9.**8 a–d** Glandular tissue in the axillary tail and ectopic glandular tissue (Fig. 9.**8 b–d** from [6])

a Glandular tissue in the axillary tail will generally have the same structure as glandular tissue within the breast. In the presence of regular architecture, mammography at usual follow-up intervals will generally be sufficient (negative sonography supports this diagnosis)

b–d In the presence of irregular structure, further workup with MRI or needle core biopsy is appropriate

b Irregularly shaped tissue is visualized in the axillary tail.

Its eccentric location did not allow its visualization in other imaging planes. It could not be identified sonographically

c Transverse MR section through the lesion prior to administration of contrast medium

d The same slice after intravenous injection of Gd-DTPA. In the absence of enhancement, malignancy could be excluded with a high degree of certainty. Follow-up examinations over 4 years even showed a slight decrease in density The finding is compatible with residual asymmetric glandular or benign breast tissue

Macromastia

■ Clinical Examination

Macromastia is a condition in which breast volume exceeds the physiologic value by 50%, i. e., when the weight of the breast exceeds 600 g. Macromastia occurs most frequently during puberty and is rare during pregnancy. A significant increase in breast size can accompany general obesity as increased fatty deposits are found in the breast. The same differences in tissue consistency are encountered as in normal patients. However, increased breast size can render clinical examination of deeper-lying tissue difficult or even impossible.

■ Mammography

Depending on the tissue composition, the mammographic appearance will vary between radiolucent in fatty breasts to radiopaque in breasts with a high proportion of glandular and connective tissue. Whereas mammography can achieve close to 100% sensitivity in detecting pathologic changes in the fatty breast, the sensitivity of mammography in dense and voluminous tissue is significantly reduced.

■ Sonography

The diagnostic value of sonography is often limited, particularly in very large breasts. It is difficult and often even impossible to image the entire glandular tissue. Furthermore, acoustic shadows and limited sound penetration may not permit sufficient visualization of the deeper-lying tissue. For this reason, sonography in large breasts should be used exclusively to assess focal findings.

Accessory Breast Tissue (Polymastia)

Circumscribed development of glandular parenchyma in the axilla is the most common site of accessory breast tissue. This tissue is either completely separate from the rest of the parenchyma (Figs. 9.8 a–d) or connected with the parenchymal tissue in the axillary tail. Glandular tissue extending far into the axillary tail can occur on one or both sides. Since breast cancer can also occur in ectopic glandular tissue, this tissue should always be carefully examined.

Supernumerary mammary glands are found along the milk line (mamma accessoria) and may or may not have an associated nipple (mamma aberrata). Polythelia refers to the presence of supernumerary nipples without mammary tissue.

■ Clinical Examination

Palpation will reveal what appears to be a soft tumor in the axilla, which may be isolated or adjacent to the glandular tissue in the axillary tail or at other locations. Sometimes the patient will report tenderness and fluctuations in size related to her menstrual cycle. Swelling may also occur during pregnancy and lactation.

■ Mammography

Corresponding parenchymal densities can be visualized mammographically with an oblique view in the axillary tail or in the axilla on an axillary view (Figs. 9.8 a and b). The criteria for assessment are the same as those for glandular tissue within the breast.

■ Sonography and Magnetic Resonance Imaging

Sonography (Figs. 9.8 c and d) also visualizes the asymmetrical configuration of normal or mastopathic glandular tissue. The same applies to MRI, where normal tissue and benign proliferative breast disorders normally will not enhance.

Due to its high sensitivity in detecting malignancy, MRI may be used for differential diagnostic problems caused by asymmetric tissue.

Inverted Nipple

(Figs. 9.9 a–d)

■ Clinical Examination

Unilateral or bilateral inverted nipples may represent normal variants. It is, however, important that the inversion exists since birth or is long-standing (unchanged for years). Recently occurring retraction and/or inversion can be the result of chronic inflammatory or malignant processes. Therefore, careful history is required to determine the need for workup of this finding.

■ Mammography

Depending on the projection, the inverted nipple can appear as a round, smooth-contoured mass mammographically. However, in most cases, the skin will be clearly seen to dip into this mass. The risk of confusing this condition with a lesion is minimal if the examiner is familiar with the clinical findings. Failure to image the nipple in profile may result in a false mammographic picture of nipple inversion.

■ Sonography

The inverted nipple itself can appear as a hypoechoic nodule with or without an acoustic shadow. Here, too, the risk of confusion is minimal if one knows the clinical findings and is familiar with the typical sonographic findings.

■ Magnetic Resonance Imaging

In MR imaging studies, the examiner should bear in mind that the normal inverted nipple can enhance.

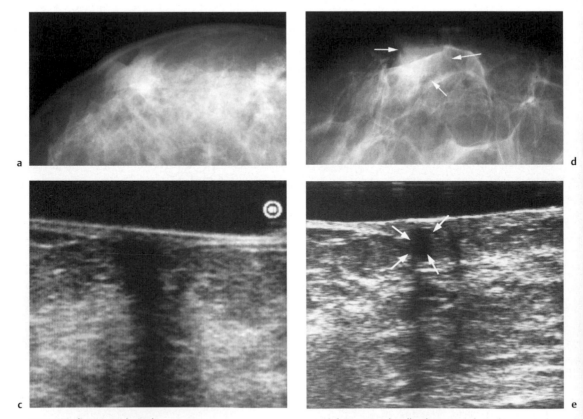

Fig. 9.9 a–d Inverted nipple
a and b Mammographically, the inverted nipple typically appears as a funnel-shaped density (a) or a mass (b)

c and d Sonographically, the inverted nipple can produce a pronounced nipple shadow (e) or it may appear as a hypoechoic nodule (d)

Summary

Asymmetry and polymastia are congenital conditions that will generally be identified with a careful history. The examiner must exclude significant changes that are not due to hormonal influences (i. e., pregnancy or menstrual cycle). If the breast examination is normal (revealing just increased glandular tissue, but no change in consistency, and no retraction) and mammographic appearance is normal (composition corresponds to normal glandular tissue), then it is highly probable that the condition represents a normal variant.

In the presence of uncertain densities, further diagnostic studies (mammography, ultrasound, MRI, and/or percutaneous biopsy) are indicated (see also Chapter 22).
Congenital inverted nipple is another normal variant which cannot be confused with a mass if the examiner is aware of the history and physical examination. This condition should be distinguished from recently occurring nipple inversion. Here, particular care should be taken to exclude malignancy.

Pregnancy and Lactation

■ Histology

During pregnancy, proliferative changes occur, with lobular hyperplasia, hyperemia, and fluid retention in breast tissue. Lactogenesis, the milk synthesis in the glandular cell, begins in the second half of pregnancy. Toward the end of pregnancy, the alveoli begin to secrete and parenchyma largely displaces the stromal tissue.

■ Clinical Examination

During pregnancy, the breast increases in size and acquires a firmer consistency, accompanied by hyperpigmentation of the areola and nipple and by prominent veins. The firmer consistency of the breast makes palpation more difficult.

The proliferative stimulation can cause existing fibroadenomas to increase rapidly in size, typically leading to smooth-contoured, mobile, and round or oval palpable findings with a firmer consistency than that of the surrounding glandular tissue (see p. 211). Nevertheless malignancy, which can occur during pregnancy, needs to be excluded with great care.

Milk retention can develop during lactation. This can lead to focal thickening, inflammation, or formation of a galactocele (see pp. 205–6).

■ Mammography

(Fig. 9.**10 a**)

Mammographically, the body of the gland appears very dense with heterogeneously coarse,

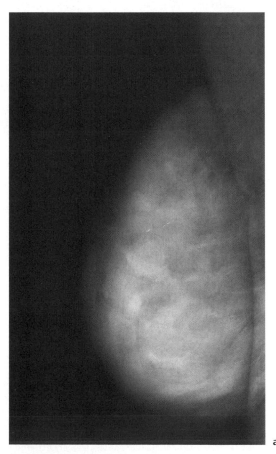

Fig. 9.**10 a–e** Lactating breast
a Mammography reveals an extremely dense, heterogeneous, coarse, nodular parenchymal structure. Mammographic evaluation is impaired

b A 34-year-old pregnant patient with a highly suspicious palpable finding in the left upper inner quadrant, which core biopsy confirmed as a carcinoma. Mammography on the second day after delivery: The mammogram reveals a second focal lesion with an irregular border and a highly suspicious cluster of microcalcifications in the upper outer quadrant. The microcalcifications are visible in greater detail on the magnification mammogram (**c**)

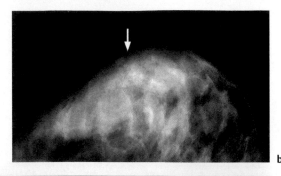

b

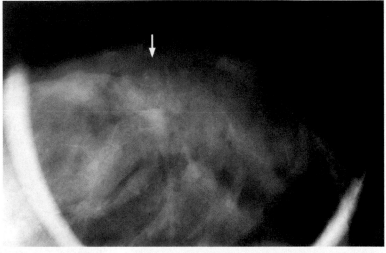

c

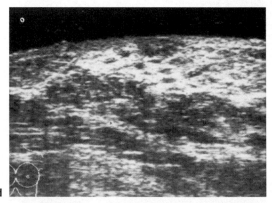

d

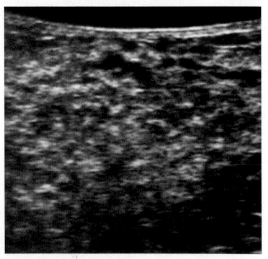

e

d Prepartum heterogeneous tissue changes in the glandular body (arrowheads) during late pregnancy (normal findings):
Whereas the peripheral glandular body appears extremely hypoechoic like fat, the tissue posterior to the nipple is primarily hyperechoic yet interspersed with hypoechoic tubular structures

e During lactation (different patient, normal findings), most of the glandular tissue shows a finely granular hypoechoic pattern. Individual expanded ducts are discernible

nodular, confluent densities and minimal fatty tissue. This severely limits the diagnostic value of mammography. If clinical examination and mammography become necessary during the nursing period, the examination should be performed after breast feeding or pumping since the breast then has a softer consistency and is less radiodense. Screening mammography is usually not performed during pregnancy or lactation. It should be delayed for 3 to 6 months after the cessation of lactation to allow the breast density to decrease. Diagnostic mammography may be indicated during pregnancy or lactation if clinical suspicion exists. Although mass lesions may not be discernible because of the increased radiodensity of the breast tissue, microcalcifications typical of malignancy can be detected even in extremely dense breasts (Figs. 9.**10 b, c**).

When mammography is performed during pregnancy, the abdomen should be shielded with lead aprons despite the fact that most of the extremely soft radiation will be absorbed in soft tissues of the abdomen and almost no radiation will reach the fetus.

■ Sonography
(Fig. 9.**10 c**)

In light of the limited diagnostic value of mammography during pregnancy and lactation, ultrasound is extremely helpful in evaluating palpable findings.

Normally, the echogenicity of the breast tissue decreases somewhat during pregnancy and lactation. The echo pattern generally appears homogeneous and finely granular. Particularly in late pregnancy and lactation, the distended lactiferous ducts are discernible as tubular, extremely hypoechoic or anechoic structures (Fig. 9.**10 d** and **e**).

■ Magnetic Resonance Imaging

MRI is not indicated during pregnancy and lactation since strong generalized contrast enhancement is expected in the engorged breast tissue and therefore identification of malignant processes would be difficult.

Breast Response with Hormone Replacement Therapy

The number of women receiving hormone replacement therapy, either for relief of menopausal symptoms or as prophylaxis against osteoporosis and cardiovascular disease* has increased within the past few years. Due to the hormonal proliferation stimulus, breast size increases in some of these women, occasionally accompanied by a sensation of fullness and breast pain.

Hormone replacement has an impact on the mammographic image[7-12]:

- A generalized increase in the extent and density of partially involuted parenchyma is possible.
- In older women, single or multiple cysts, fibroadenomas, and other benign breast changes can develop in one or both breasts.
- Cysts and fibroadenomas can enlarge and simulate a malignant process.
- After breast-conserving treatment of a mammary carcinoma, the extent and density of the parenchyma of the healthy breast can increase unilaterally since the irradiated fibrosed breast tissue generally does not respond to hormones.

* The value of HRT for this particular indication is debated.

The degree of increased density and appearance of masses appears to be more pronounced for hormone replacement therapy with estrogenprogesterone combinations than for estrogen alone.[11,12]

Discontinuing hormone replacement therapy generally leads to involution of the proliferative parenchymal effects.

Increasing evidence exists that hormone replacement therapy thus has a negative effect on the accuracy of mammography, at least in some patients.[13-15]

■ Mammography
(Figs. 9.**11 a–f**)

Where previous mammograms are available for comparison, the examiner may observe a unilateral or bilateral increase in the extent and density of the parenchyma due to hormone replacement therapy. This increase can be diffuse or patchy. Generally, the specific architecture will still be discernible.

The increase in density can be so profound that mammographic interpretation is impaired. Under hormone replacement therapy, new cysts and fi-

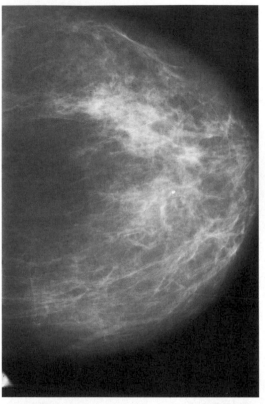

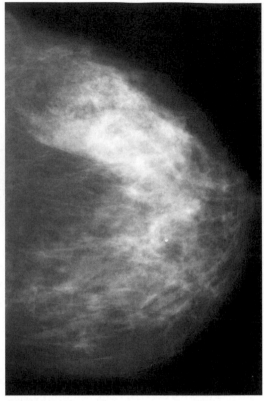

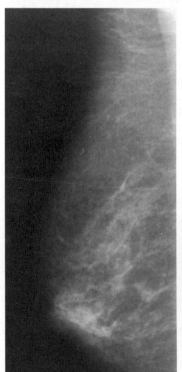

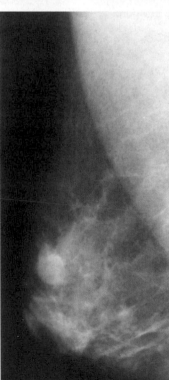

Fig. 9.**11 a** and **b** Changes under hormone replacement therapy
a Normal, partially involuted breast in a 59-year-old patient
b After 12 months of hormone replacement, the patient complained of a sensation of fullness and breast enlargement. Mammography reveals extensive generalized nodular proliferation of glandular tissue. Mammographic evaluation is impaired under hormone replacement therapy compared to before
c–d In some patients new masses may develop during hormone replacment therapy
c Baseline mammogram before hormone replacement therapy in a 66-year old patient
d Two years later. The patient has been on hormone replacement therapy for 6 months. Note that there is a proliferation of glandular tissue in the breast. The mass in the upper breast was shown to be a simple cyst on sonography

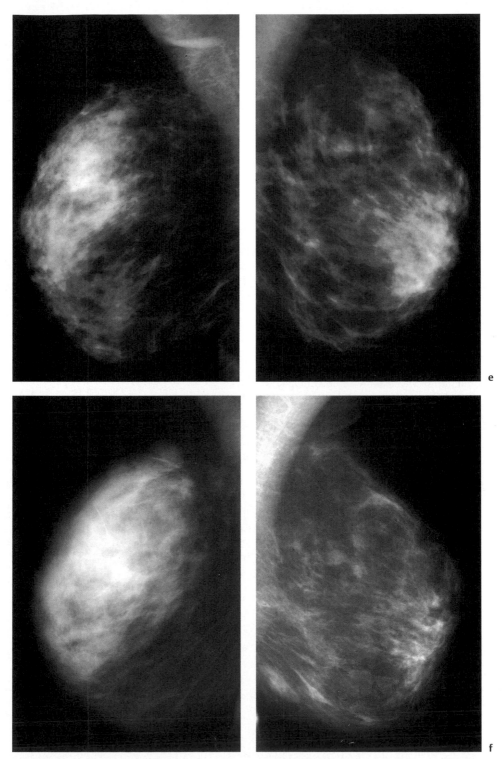

e

f

e–f Sometimes breast density may increase asymmetrically during hormone replacement therapy. Striking cases such as this one require further workup. (Diagnosis proven by vacuum biopsy and follow-up)

e Oblique mammograms before hormone replacement therapy
f Oblique mammograms 14 months later, 7 months after the onset of hormone replacement therapy

broadenomas can develop or existing ones can increase in size, representing an exception to the rule that any new occurrence or increase in size of a focal lesion in a postmenopausal patient represents a sign of malignancy. Thus, particular care is necessary in further diagnostic workup of increasing densities. Multiple or single cysts or fibroadenomas can develop bilaterally or unilaterally.

Sonography

Sonography is an important diagnostic procedure in assessing mammographically dense parenchyma and as an adjunct in diagnosing probably benign focal findings detected mammographically, especially those that have recently developed or increased in size. The glandular tissue under hormone stimulation will generally appear homogeneous and moderately hyperechoic. However, variations such as those seen in breast dysplasia are possible.

If a simple cyst is diagnosed sonographically, no further workup will be required. Upon consultation with the patient, solid focal lesions that are not definitely benign mammographically and sonographically usually require biopsy to assess for malignancy. If they are suspected to represent a process due to hormonal stimulation, the patient may be given the option of discontinuing hormones for 2 or 3 months, then reimaging the breast to determine if the lesion has regressed.

Magnetic Resonance Imaging

MRI is not indicated for diagnosing changes occuring under hormone replacement therapy. The resulting proliferative changes can be expected to enhance with MR contrast agents, impairing both detection and exclusion of malignancy.

Percutaneous Biopsy

This method can be used to diagnose uncertain focal findings developing during hormone placement therapy.

Summary

Knowledge of hormone replacement therapy is extremely important for interpreting diagnostic imaging studies. This underscores the value of taking a thorough history.
Hormone replacement therapy can produce significant parenchymal changes which can

include an increase in the amount and density of parenchymal tissue, and a new occurrence or an increase in the size of focal densities. Mammographic evaluation is limited instead of improved with increasing patient age and breast involution. The additional information from sonography may be helpful in older women undergoing hormone replacement therapy. Percutaneous or excisional biopsy may be indicated for further workup of focal findings during hormone replacement therapy.

References

1   Bässler R. Pathologie der Brustdrüse. Pathol Anat. 1978; 11
2   Beck R, Heywang-Köbrunner SH, Untch M et al. Contrast-enhancement of proliferative dysplasia in MRI of the breast due to the menstrual cycle. ECR '93. Book of Abstracts. Springer International; 1993:151
3   Kuhl CK, Seibert C, Kneft BP et al. Focal and diffuse contrast enhancement in dynamic MR mammography of healthy volunteers. Radiology. 1995;193(P):121
4   Vorherr H. The Breast. New York: Academic Press; 1974
5   Kopans DB, Swann CA, White G et al. Asymmetric breast tissue. Radiology. 1989;171:639
6   Heywang-Köbrunner SH, Beck R. Contrast-enhanced MRI of the breast. 2nd ed. Berlin, New York, Heidelberg: Springer 1996
7   Stomper PC, Van Vorrhis BJ, Ravnikar VA et al. Mammographic changes associated with postmenopausal hormone replacement therapy: a longitudinal study. Radiology. 1990;174:487
8   Laya MB, Gallagher JC, Schreiman JS et al. Effect of postmenopausal hormonal replacement therapy on mammographic density and parenchymal pattern. Radiology. 1995;196:433–7
9   Lundstrom E. Wilczek B, von Palffy Z et al. Mammographic breast density during hormone replacement therapy: differences according to treatment. Am J Obstet Gynecol. 1999;181:348–52
10 Sterns EE, Zee B. Mammographic density changes in perimenopausal and postmenopausal women: is effect of hormone replacement therapy predictable? Breast Cancer Res Treat. 2000;59:125–32
11 Greendale GA, Reboussin BA, Sie A et al. Effects of estrogen and estrogen-progestin on mammographic parenchymal density. Postmenopausal Estrogen/Progestin Interventions (PEPI) Investigators. Ann Intern Med. 1999;130:262–9
12 Marugg RC, van der Mooren MJ, Hendriks JH et al. Mammographic changes in postmenopausal women on hormonal replacement therapy. Eur Radiol. 1997;7:749–55
13 Laya MB, Larson EB, Taplin SH et al. Effect of estrogen replacement therapy on the specificity and sensitivity of screening mammography. J Natl Cancer Inst. 1996;88:643–9
14 Litherland JC, Stallard S, Hole D et al. The effect of hormone replacement therapy on the sensitivity of screening mammograms. Clin Radiol. 1999;54:285–8
15 Kavanagh AM, Mitchell H, Gilles GG et al. Hormone replacement therapy and accuracy of mammographic screening. Lancet 2000;355:270–4

10. Benign Breast Disorders

■ **Definition**

In contrast to the age-related physiologic changes in the mammary gland, benign breast disorders involve hormonally mediated, increased qualitative and quantitative tissue transformation prior to and during menopause. Approximately 30% of the time these changes involve ductal and lobular epithelial hyperplasia. Only these are significant for their relation to possible cancer in the future. Breast disorders characterized by epithelial hyperplasia belong to the group of proliferative or hyperplastic changes. Breast disorders without epithelial hyperplasia belong to the group of nonproliferative fibrocystic changes. The distinctions between normal findings, variations, and fibrocystic changes are blurred, as are the distinctions between individual types of this disorder.

■ **Pathogenesis**

The causes of benign breast disorders lie in hormonal imbalances and in the interactions of several substances (estrogens, progesterone, prolactin, thyroxin, and insulin), which trigger two important mechanisms:

1. Hormonally induced secretion (with retention of the secreted substance) and development of duct ectasia and cysts
2. Endocrine-stimulated proliferation of the ductal and lobular epithelium with development of various patterns and degrees of epithelial hyperplasia in the form of adenosis, epitheliosis, or atypical hyperplasia

■ **Incidence**

Data on the frequency of benign breast disorders vary considerably and depend on the study group. According to statistics, the frequency of benign disorders lies between 50% and 70% for all types and 30% for types with epithelial proliferation.

A diagnosis of a benign breast disorder is significant for three reasons:

1. Even a benign disorder can be accompanied by clinical *symptoms* (such as pain or palpable findings) that frighten patients and can arouse clinical suspicion of malignancy.
2. Benign disorders are generally characterized by increased radiodensity, occasionally microcalcifications, and often nodular or firm palpable findings. Therefore mammographic *visualization* is *limited* in comparison with fatty breasts. Locally pronounced benign changes may mimic a focal lesion suggestive of a malignant process.
3. Most cases of benign breast disorder (approximately 70%) *do not have an increased risk of cancer* in comparison with the normal population. A portion of these cases (approximately 25%) show an increased risk of cancer (by a factor of 1.5–2). From 3 to 5% of cases of benign disorder are associated with an increased risk of cancer (by a factor of 4–5).

■ **Histopathology**

Benign breast disorders involve a variety of parenchymal and stromal changes thought to originate in the terminal ductal lobular segment. Small cysts containing secretion develop in the lobules. As these increase in size, they involve the immediately adjacent ductules (acini). The appearance of cysts, whose occurrence and growth is further conditioned by proliferative changes in the ducts and lobules as well as the presence of edema and fibrotic changes in the stroma lead to the clinical syndrome of benign breast disorder. Benign breast disorders can involve the entire mammary gland or may be focal. They can form a complex with numerous histologic components, or present as more limited entities such as sclerosing adenosis or a radial scar. The histopathologic diagnosis of a benign breast disorder involves the following components:

■ Cysts

The breasts can form *microcysts* measuring 1–2 mm diameter and *macrocysts* (which may be simple or multiloculated cysts), as well as multiple and solitary cysts (see Chapter 11).

■ Adenosis

This term refers to parallel arrangements of bundle-shaped nonneoplastic proliferations of terminal ductal segments. The most frequent forms include:

Blunt duct adenosis: Small cystic expansions of ductules containing secretion, lined with a flattened or slightly hyperplastic epithelium are typical of this frequent form of adenosis. The clustered arrangement of the ductules is suggestive of adenosis originating in the glandular lobules as opposed to the ductal segments.

Sclerosing adenosis: Sclerosing adenosis refers to focal, generalized, and tumor-like proliferations (i. e., adenosis tumor) of the epithelium and myoepithelium that originate in the glandular lobules and are accompanied by desmoplasia. Sclerosing adenosis is frequently, but not always, associated with other benign breast disorders. It can also occur in the stromal tissue of fibroadenomas, papillomas, or ductal adenomas. It can be associated with atypical lobular hyperplasia or a lobular carcinoma in situ. The relative risk of malignancy is increased by a factor of 1.5–2.

Microglandular adenosis: This rare benign form of adenosis is characterized by densely packed, isomorphic, small-diameter tubules that grow into the connective and fatty tissue either resembling a tumor or occasionally as a generalized process.

Radial scar: This term refers to single or multiple occurrences of nonneoplastic focal tubular proliferative adenosis developing around a fibrous elastoid center that radiate outward and are associated with areas of intraductal epithelial hyperplasia.

The radial scar is particularly significant as its spiculated form simulates an invasive carcinoma both macroscopically and in diagnostic imaging studies. Areas of atypical hyperplasia, and tubular, ductal, or lobular carcinomas can develop within radial scars.

■ Focal Fibrosis

Focal fibrosis is a proliferation of mammary stromal tissue in younger women (age from 25 to 40 years) that is associated with focal parenchymal atrophy and leads to induration. The mean focus size measures 1–3 cm in diameter. Mammography shows increased density without microcalcifications.

■ Forms of Epithelial Hyperplasia

● **Ductal hyperplasia (epitheliosis):** By definition, benign intraductal proliferations of the epithelium are seen in widespread or focal areas whose pattern and extent can vary.
Particularly in American medical literature, the term papillomatosis is used in the same sense as epitheliosis. In Europe the term papillomatosis is used to describe particular villous epithelial structures oriented along septa of connective tissue.

● **Lobular hyperplasia:** It is characterized by an enlargement of the lobule due to extensive acinar hyperplasia in the sense of adenosis but also due to hyperplasia of the epithelium similar to epitheliosis of the extralobular ducts.

● **Atypical hyperplasia (atypia):** Ductal atypical hyperplasia occurs in ducts, and lobular atypical hyperplasia in the lobules in approximately 3.6% of all biopsies. Histopathologically, these areas show some but not all of the histologic characteristics of carcinoma in situ. Histologic and cytologic assessment of these lesions is difficult even for experienced pathologists in comparative studies, and these lesions represent a gray area in diagnosis. The relative risk of degeneration into carcinoma is from 4 to 5 times higher than in the normal population and increases with age. The absolute risk with atypical hyperplasia is 8–10% in 10 years; with a history of cancer in the family, it will increase to about 25% in 10 years. Forms of atypical hyperplasia include:

– *Atypical ductal hyperplasia* is primarily observed in postmenopausal patients and corresponds to a lesion with some but not all of the characteristics of ductal carcinoma in situ.

– *Atypical lobular hyperplasia,* likewise, has some but not all of the characteristics of lobular carcinoma in situ. Here, the size of the lobule (in contrast to a fully developed carcinoma in situ) is not measurably enlarged.

To assess the risk of malignancy of benign breast disorders, the results of long-term studies of Prechtel[1, 2] and of studies by Dupont and Page[3, 4] have proven valuable. With similar goals, a consensus meeting of American pathologists[5] recommended a slightly modified classification system:

1. *Mild epithelial hyperplasia (ductal or lobular hyperplasia)* is defined as a proliferation of a layer 2–4 cells thick. There is no increased risk of malignancy. The disorder can occur as adenosis, cystic disease, or duct ectasia corresponding to Prechtel's Grade I benign disorder. Frequency is about 70%. It may also occur in fibroadenomas, adenomas, and in mastitis.
2. *Florid epithelial hyperplasia* is defined as hyperplasia exceeding 4 layers of cells without atypia. The risk of malignancy is slightly increased to 1.5–2. It occurs as solid or papillary hyperplasia (epitheliosis), corresponding to Prechtel's Grade II benign disorder. Frequency is about 25–30%, also as papilloma with a stromal component.
3. *Atypical epithelial hyperplasia (ductal and lobular hyperplasia)* is defined as cellular atypia with disturbance of regular epithelial layering, where the myoepithelial layer and basal membrane remain intact, corresponding to Prechtel's Grade III benign disorder. The relative risk of malignancy is increased by a factor of 4 or 5. Frequency is about 4%.

The risk of malignancy for Grade I and Grade II disorders clearly differs from that of Grade III. In light of this, the overriding clinical consideration is: does the benign disorder involve atypical hyperplasia or nonatypical hyperplasia, and is there a history of cancer in the family?

■ Clinical Findings

- Benign breast disorders can be completely *asymptomatic.*
- They can cause pain *(mastodynia).*
- Breast pain due to a benign disorder will typically be more pronounced in the premenstrual phase (i. e., premenstrual tension or sensitivity to touch).
- The pain usually is bilateral.
- Most often it will occur as generalized pain in the upper outer quadrants. Localized pain that is not due to a cyst is not typical of benign breast disease (see also p. 273).

- In some cases, *discharge* may accompany benign breast disease. This will usually occur *bilaterally* and involve several excretory ducts. The color of the discharge is usually clear or amber-colored, occasionally yellowish green or greenish black.
- The palpable findings in the presence of a benign breast disorder can vary greatly from patient to patient.

Typical findings in the presence of a benign breast disease include:

- The tissue has a *firmer consistency.*
- Palpation reveals *finely to coarsely nodular* changes.
- The firmer consistency and nodular transformation are most often *symmetrical* and particularly pronounced in the upper outer quadrants.
- *Cysts* are usually palpable as round, elastic lumps. Deeper-lying cysts or cysts that are not completely filled may not be palpable.

Some benign breast disorders can also be associated with *unilaterally firmer consistency* or *formation of focal lumps.* With focal findings, it can be difficult or even impossible to distinguish the disorder from a malignant process. Further diagnostic workup (diagnostic imaging, percutaneous biopsy, or perhaps excisional biopsy) is indicated.

■ Diagnostic Strategy and Objectives

Benign breast disorders can only be classified histologically. Palpation, mammography (structural changes, radiodensity, microcalcifications), or sonography (hyperechoic glandular tissue with or without cysts or dilated ductal structures) can be suggestive of a benign breast disease, but cannot prove it.

Since there is insufficient correlation among mammographic, sonographic, or MRI findings and cellular proliferations or the degree of cellular atypia present, it is *not possible to assess the risk of carcinoma based on diagnostic imaging studies.* However, it is a general rule that the *majority of benign breast disorders* (70–80%) are *associated with no risk or only a slight risk of carcinoma.*

The increased radiodensity and firmer nodular consistency associated with typical cases of benign breast disorders *limit diagnostic accuracy* in comparison to a fatty breast. Mammographic and clinical examination can, therefore, be more difficult in these women. Annual mammography is strongly recommended to improve detection of small carcinomas, which are more difficult to discern in dense tissue[6, 7].

Additional diagnostic methods are *not indicated* in the presence of typical findings of benign breast disease without an increased risk or without mammographically or clinically suggestive findings. Where *clinical examination reveals suspicious findings* (i. e., palpable findings, uncertain palpable asymmetry, or atypical discharge), *mammography* is indicated as the first step in additional workup.

Mammography can detect a carcinoma at the site of the palpable findings, or at another unexpected location, by revealing a typical density or typical microcalcifications. *The absence of microcalcifications or densities typical of malignancy* in radiodense tissue *does not exclude* a malignancy *suspected on the basis of clinical findings.*

Therefore in the presence of clinically suggestive findings or suspected cysts in radiodense tissue, *sonography* is indicated as an adjunctive modality to mammography. Ultrasound is particularly helpful when it can identify a simple cyst as the cause of uncertain palpable findings, uncertain mammographic densities, or asymmetry. Aside from this, most palpable carcinomas in radiodense tissue are also discernible as hypoechoic mases. For this reason, sonography is also used to confirm suspected malignant findings.

Some small carcinomas, and particularly carcinomas in situ, cannot be reliably identified by sonography. *Therefore the absence of ultrasound findings does not exclude a malignancy suspected on the basis of clinical or mammographic evidence.*

Percutaneous biopsy is the next most important diagnostic step and most valuable alternative to open biopsy in the diagnosis of probably benign palpable findings or changes detected at mammography.

Open biopsy is indicated as a diagnostic and therapeutic method when a malignancy is suspected, and as the diagnostic method if the finding is not readily accessible (i. e., a small deep lesion), if core biopsy yielded a borderline lesion (atypical hyperplasia), or if results of the existing diagnostic studies or of imaging versus percutaneous biopsy are contradictory.

■ Mammography

The mammographic appearance of benign breast disease (Figs. 10.1 a–e) is characterized by the following features:

- Structural changes and/or increased density in the parenchyma
- Calcifications

These changes can occur individually or in combination.

■ Structural Changes and/or Increased Density

These changes include:
- Coarsened structure.
- Finely to coarsely nodular densities, usually relatively uniform, often found along the tree-shaped structure of the mammary gland.
- Areas of increased density or generalized increased density.
- In some cases, the structures appear indistinct and not readily discernible. This is probably due to increased water retention.
- Fibrosis and/or secondary inflammatory processes can produce random and irregular densities.

Structural changes or densities are suggestive of a benign breast disorder, although they are not conclusive.

Benign changes are *typically generalized and symmetrical.* When this is the case, the findings are characteristic of benign breast disorders and cannot usually be confused with changes typical of malignancy. However, in the presence of generalized and symmetrical benign changes, detection or exclusion of carcinomas without microcalcifications is more difficult because they may easily be obscured by the surrounding dense tissue. Diagnostic problems occur with increased density, architectural distortion, or even a smooth or irregular mass:

- *Asymmetrically,* or
- *As a focal lesion* (Figs. 10.1 f–i).

Nodular, irregular, or spiculated masses can occur in certain benign breast diseases and characteristically also in the rare tumorous form of sclerosing adenosis.

Note:
- Irregular foci of benign breast disease and radial scars will often produce palpable findings smaller and less pronounced than the findings expected with a carcinoma of comparable size
- Radial scars may produce an architectural distortion with a „star-like" pattern. The center

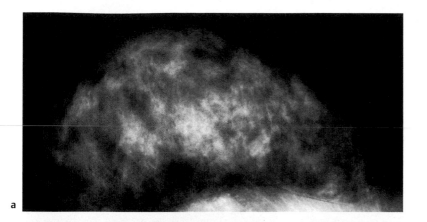

a

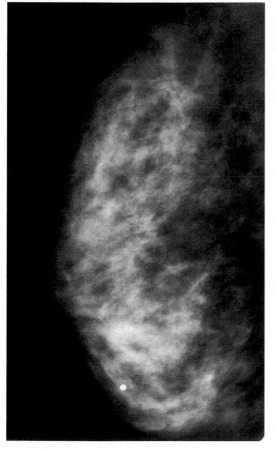

b

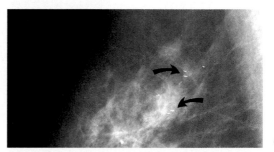

c

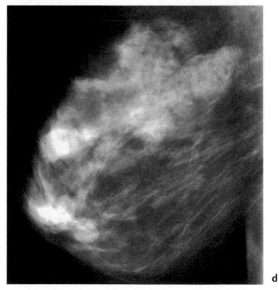

d

Fig. 10.**1 a–i**
a Relatively uniform, finely nodular benign breast parenchyma of increased density
b Nodular parenchymal pattern with multiple disseminated calcifications appearing as round or linear structures
c This breast tissue shows a coarsely nodular structure in the upper part. One coarse and some smaller calcifica-

tions are seen. The curved arrows point to calcifications with a typical „teacup" appearance, indicating benign microcystic changes
d This breast exhibits a coarsely nodular structure. The nodules partially correspond to cysts, partially to well-circumscribed hyperechoic lesions (e. g., fibroadenomas) on ultrasound

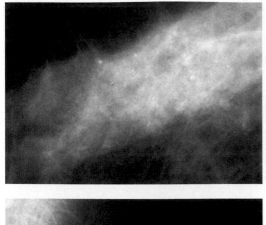

e

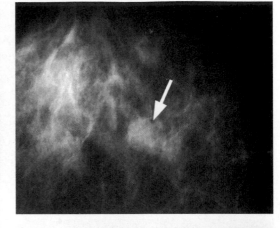

f

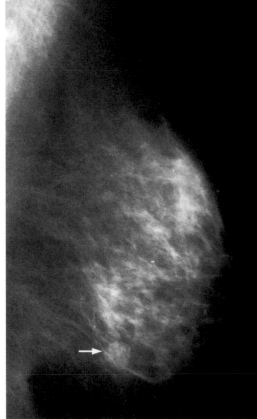

g

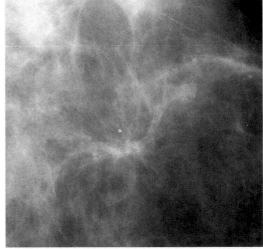

h

Fig. 10.1 e–h
e Dense breast tissue with various microcalcifications is shown. As this is frequently seen in benign changes these microcalcifications are not completely monomorphic
f and **g** Circumscribed nodular mass in the left inferior medial breast. The margin is partially smooth and partially indistinct. *Histology:* Nodular adenosis 10 mm in diameter
h An architectural distortion with radiating strands is typical for a radial scar. Typically, radial scars are imaged more clearly with spot compression views. If a radial scar is suspected, further work-up (biopsy) is indicated

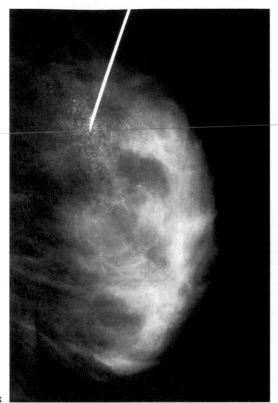

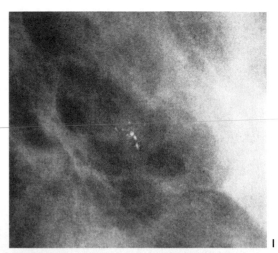

l

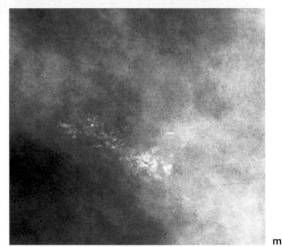

m

Fig. 10.**1 k–o** Some microcalcifications that occur with benign changes raise suspicion due to their regional, segmental, or even duct-like distribution. Even casting microcalcifications may occur in benign disease. If one of these patterns is seen or suspected, workup is indicated
k Mammary parenchyma has a coarsely nodular benign structure. There are multiple, uniformly distributed, relatively round, monomorphic and punctate microcalcifications. Histologic examination (performed because of a planned liver transplant) revealed simple fibrocystic benign breast disease with psammomatous calcifications. Even though morphology of the calcifications themselves appears benign, workup is justified by their regional (possibly even segmental) distribution
l Magnification mammography reveals a tiny cluster consisting of round and 2–3 linear microcalcifications arranged in a linear pattern. *Histology:*focal fibrous breast disease
m Magnification mammography shows a long cluster of round, linear, and polymorphic microcalcifications. *Histology:* focal fibrous breast disease
n Specimen radiography: One large and two adjacent smaller clusters of polymorphic microcalcifications. Fibrocystic benign breast disorder with focal sclerosing adenosis and intraductal papillomatosis

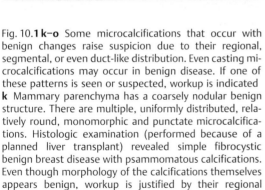

k

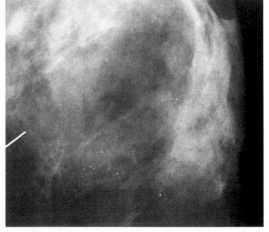

n

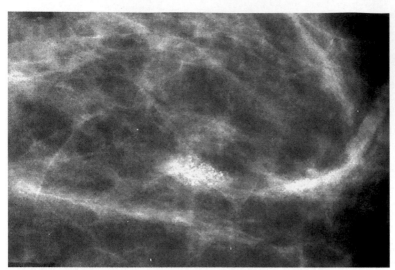

Fig. 10.**1 o** Sometimes fine granular calcifications may be strictly localized in a small nodular mass or dilated duct. These very fine microcalcifications with the described distribution often indicate a papillary lesion (papillomatosis, papilloma, papillary ductal carcinoma in situ, or rarely papillary carcinoma). Unless other signs (e. g., of malignancy) exist, their distinction is not possible radiologically. Therefore, further workup is indicated. Histology: papillomatosis

should be small. It may be dense („white star") or lucent („dark star"). Irrespective of the center, such changes cannot be distinguished from lobular or tubular carcinoma with sufficient reliability. Furthermore, a high percentage (up to 50%) of radial scars may be associated with or develop ductal carcinoma in situ or tubular carcinoma. Therefore, such changes require further workup

These characteristics can only be regarded as suggestive of a benign process and not as conclusive evidence.[8, 9, 10, 11] Since carcinomas can have a similar appearance, biopsy should be considered in the presence of these changes.

Cysts can produce sharply defined round shadows, semicircular discernible shadows, or poorly discernible densities (when obscured by superimposition). They may merely contribute to a nonspecific increase in density, or they may not be visible at all.

Diagnosing cysts and differentiating cysts from solid masses is a task for sonography (see also p. 88 and Chapter 11).

■ Significance of Changes in Structure and Density

Whereas focal and asymmetrical densities or structural changes can simulate a carcinoma at mammography and clinical examination, generalized changes can make detection of malignant processes difficult as a result of generally increased radiodensity.

There is no correlation between the extent of structural changes or increased radiodensity and

the degree of cellular proliferation or atypia. As a result, it is *not possible to correlate mammographically detected structural changes and changes in density with the possible risk of carcinoma.*

■ Calcifications

Microcalcifications frequently occur in benign breast disorders. They exhibit a broad range of variation with respect to their morphology and pattern of distribution. They can be the result of calcified secretions. Necrotic cells shed into intraductal or intralobular spaces can calcify, and calcifications can occur in the stroma. Accordingly, they may be found diffusely disseminated, arranged in a lobular pattern, or without any clear pattern of distribution.

Spectrometry has revealed these structures to consist primarily of calcium phosphates in addition to compounds involving other elements[9].

The following forms are *typical of benign breast disorders.*[12, 13, 14]

- *Isolated,* generally round *calcifications.*
- *Scattered punctate microcalcifications,* generally occurring *symmetrically.* These occur in many benign breast disorders and particularly often with sclerosing adenosis.
- *Milk of calcium in microcysts.* These correspond to the typical teacup-shaped calcifications described by Lanyi. They represent small "lakes" of milk of calcium in cystic distended lobules. The milk of calcium contains extremely fine suspended particles of calcium not resolved on the mammogram. This accu-

mulation of calcified milk in distended micro-cystic structure appears as one "calcification." In the craniocaudal view, these individual "calcifications" appear as lakes of calcified milk, generally round, sometimes faceted, and frequently of different size. Their margins are often indistinct or amorphous. They are non-specific and can vary in density. The lobular arrangement of these deposits can only be assessed when some of these calcifications lie close together in small flower-like or rosette-like clusters.

In the mediolateral 90° view, the characteristic sedimentation of extremely fine particles in the calcified milk produces a characteristic sign: The inferior border of the small lake that appears to be a calcification is arc-shaped and shows a horizontal surface produced by sedimentation. This surface corresponds to the fluid–fluid level of sedimented milk of calcium.

Intense compression can cause the calcium salt precipitates to well up so that the fluid–fluid level appears to form a superior dome. These so-called teacups generally occur bilaterally, but can also be observed unilaterally or asymmetrically. The typical teacup sign can usually only be demonstrated in some of the calcifications.

Where the *typical teacup sign can be demonstrated* and other changes typical of malignancy (casting or pleomorphic microcalcifications, or suggestive densities) are absent, the examiner can diagnose a *benign breast disorder.*

● *Clusters of microcalcifications following a lobular pattern.* These may be isolated or multifocal. The calcifications lie *closely clustered together* in a small area corresponding to the size of a normal or hypertrophic lobule (1–5 mm). At mammography, this will appear like a *morula or rosette.* Several lobules may be involved. Despite certain variations in the size of the individual calcifications, the individual calcifications within a cluster appear round and monomorphic. Such clusters occur primarily in the presence of *cystic and sclerosing adenosis.*

Unfortunately, aside from these typical benign calcifications, benign breast disorders can also involve *indeterminate and, occasionally, even suspicious calcifications.*

Indeterminate microcalcifications that can occur in benign breast disorders include the following forms.[12–14]

– Ill-defined and amorphous calcifications with slight to pronounced pleomorphism
– Microcalcifications appearing in an isolated area that are asymmetrical with the contralateral side and not clearly benign
– Clusters of microcalcifications that are not clearly arranged in a monomorphic lobular pattern.

Suspicious calcifications may rarely also occur in benign breast disorders. These appear as:

– Casting, rod-like, V-shaped, or Y-shaped
– Coarsely granular and pleomorphic
– They may even be arranged in a segmental configuration, and/or follow the ductal structures, indistinguishable from microcalcifications associated with malignancy and therefore necessitating biopsy

Indeterminate calcifications and, rarely, suspicious calcifications may be associated with benign breast disease as well. This is just an expression of the fact that benign transformation can affect both the lobules and the ductal system. Calcifications can occur in a typically benign "lobular" configuration but also in a ductal configuration simulating a malignant process, albeit less frequently. In sclerosing adenosis, myothelial and connective-tissue proliferation can lead to deformity of the lobules. This can explain the greater polymorphism of the individual calcifications detected in sclerosing adenosis as well as individual rod-like microcalcifications.

■ Importance of Microcalcifications in Benign Breast Disorders

On the whole, indeterminate and suspicious *microcalcifications occur more frequently in benign proliferative disorders* than in nonproliferative breast disorders. Microcalcifications associated with benign breast disorder nevertheless *do not permit an assessment of the risk of malignancy of the underlying breast disease* in a specific case.

In the presence of *calcifications typical of benign breast disorders,* routine follow-up is all that is needed. Biopsy should not be performed. The examiner should verify that these benign calcifications are not accompanied by additional microcalcifications or calcification clusters typical of malignancy.

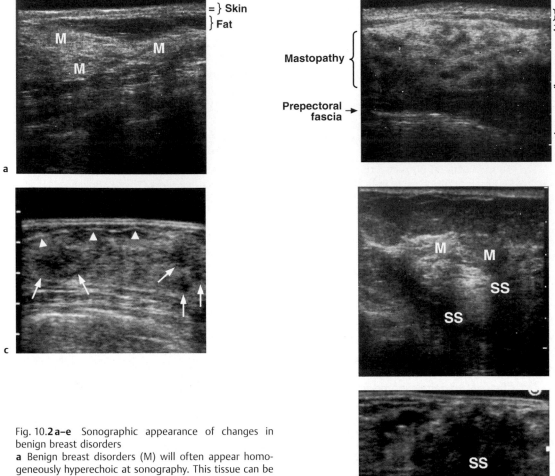

Fig. 10.**2 a–e** Sonographic appearance of changes in benign breast disorders

a Benign breast disorders (M) will often appear homogeneously hyperechoic at sonography. This tissue can be visualized well on sonography. However, even this image cannot exclude a carcinoma in situ or very small carcinoma if one is suspected (e. g. in the presence of mammographically suspicious microcalcifications)

b Less frequently, extremely regular hypoechoic tubular structures will be discernible within the hyperechoic benign tissue. These most likely correspond to ductal or lobular structures in the presence of periductal fibrosis or adenosis. This image is relatively characteristic of a benign breast disorder, but it can make it difficult to detect or exclude small carcinomas

c Sometimes single or multiple nodular hypoechoic structures (arrows) that do not correspond to fat lobules will appear within hyperechoic benign tissue (Fig. 9.**5 g**). These most likely represent focal areas of adenosis or fibroadenomas. These focal findings often render a differential diagnosis difficult and would, if biopsied, lead to an unacceptably high false positive rate. Therefore we tend to follow these lesions by sonography if they are small, do not clearly correlate with mammographic or clinical findings, and lack sonographic signs of malignancy (acoustic shadow, hyperechoic halo and so forth). The arrowheads indicate the subcutaneous fascia, which is clearly visible in this image

d In some cases, acoustic shadows (SS) can occur in benign tissue (M). These probably correspond to areas of increased fibrosis, whereas variable shadows are nonspecific, particularly when they disappear under compression or when the transducer is moved. Constant shadows, as shown here, may occur in the presence of extensive focal fibrous breast disease or proliferative disorders, but have also been reported with some carcinomas in situ. They reduce the diagnostic value of sonography

e Distinct acoustic shadows (SS) with extensive focal fibrous breast disease. The suspicious area corresponded to a suggestive palpable finding (in a radiodense breast), histologically confirmed to be extensive focal fibrous breast disease

Suspected microcalcifications require biopsy for histologic examination. Where *nonspecific microcalcifications* are present, the physician may elect follow-up imaging studies or further workup (i. e., needle core biopsy or excisional biopsy). This decision should be made on the basis of the analysis of the microcalcification, clinical examination, and patient history data (see also Chapter 22).

Isolated or multiple cysts can also occur frequently in benign breast disorders.

■ Sonography

At sonography (Figs. 10.2 a–e), *benign breast disorders* are typically characterized by the following features:[15–18]

- *Mammary gland is homogeneously hyperechoic* (a frequent finding).
- *Cysts* are frequently encountered. They may appear in various sizes and can be diagnosed beginning from a size of about 2 mm in diameter.
- *Ectatic ducts* (occasionally present).
- *Extremely regular hypoechoic structures (generally tubular, less frequently nodular)* extending throughout the mammary gland. These hypoechoic structures that follow the ductal system most likely correspond to periductal fibrosis or to foci of adenosis. Where such a regular overall structure is present, there is a high probability that these changes are benign.
- *Mammary gland* is partially or entirely homogeneously *hypoechoic*. This finding is rare. Differentiation between hypoechoic areas of breast disease and fat is significantly more difficult here, and the capability to discern hypoechoic tumors is greatly reduced.

The following *focal changes* may also be due to just benign breast disorders:

- *Hypoechoic foci.* These are generally irregular, less frequently round, and circumscribed. They can appear as isolated foci, in which case they are usually suspicious. They can also occur as multiple foci. Histologically, they may correspond to foci of adenosis, foci of benign proliferative disorders, or areas of focal fibrosis (this usually is accompanied by an acoustic shadow). The tumorous form of sclerosing adenosis can also appear as hypoechoic focus.

- *Acoustic shadows with or without hypoechoic focal findings.* Shadows can occur at multiple locations or in an isolated area. These changes may occur in the presence of diffusely proliferative fibrosis or focal fibrosis. Often, tumorous sclerosing adenosis or radial scar will appear as a hypoechoic focus with an acoustic shadow or as an isolated acoustic shadow[19].

Hypoechoic foci resulting from benign breast disorders usually do not show a typical hyperechoic halo and have a less pronounced acoustic shadow than "classic" carcinomas. However, carcinomas (and small carcinomas in particular) can vary considerably, and *a reliable differentiation of benign and malignant hypoechoic foci or acoustic shadows is not generally possible.*

■ Purpose

Identifying cysts as the cause of uncertain palpable findings or mammographically uncharacteristic densities allows sonography to *reduce the number of unnecessary biopsies.*

A malignant process in homogeneously hyperechoic benign tissue is improbable.[18] Since carcinomas are generally hypoechoic and are easily discernible in such tissue, sonography is often helpful as an adjunctive imaging modality in patients with homogeneously hyperechoic tissue. However, in the presence of clinical or mammographic suspicion (such as microcalcifications), *sonography alone cannot exclude malignancy* even in homogeneously hyperechoic tissue.[15, 17] This is because some carcinomas in situ and certain small carcinomas also appear hyperechoic and thus may escape detection by sonography.

The following applies in the presence of an heterogeneous or hypoechoic pattern:

- The capability of sonography to exclude a malignant process is reduced in the presence of a *hypoechoic mammary gland with a benign disorder* (rare).
- *Excluding a malignant process is not possible in the presence of sonographically heterogeneous breast tissue* (with hypoechoic foci and/or multiple acoustic shadows). Close correlation with clinical and mammographic findings is required.
- *Areas with acoustic shadows* or a *hypoechoic mass with and without acoustic shadows*—if reproducible—require further workup. Depending on the specific suspicion, mammo-

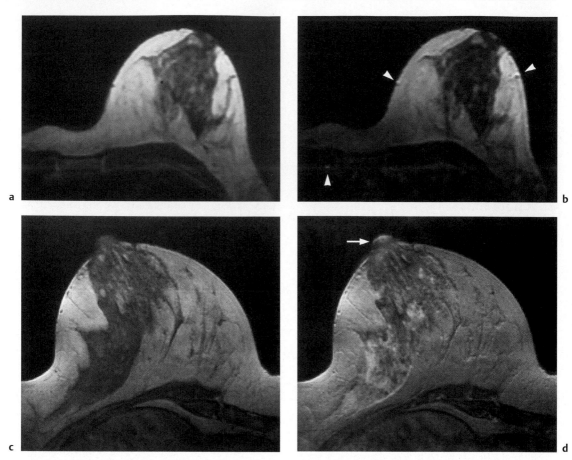

Fig. 10.**3 a–h** MRI appearance of benign breast disorders
a and **b** Most benign breast disorders (70–75%) only enhance slightly with Gd-DTPA
a Representative slice (FLASH 3D) before contrast administration
b The same slice after injection of Gd-DTPA:
Glandular tissue and fat show no significant changes in signal intensity; only vascular structures enhance (arrows).
MRI examination was performed as adjunct to mammography to verify the absence of a carcinoma in radiodense
tissue after a contralateral carcinoma was detected
c and **d** From 25 to 30% of all benign breast disorders demonstrate a diffuse milky to nodular pattern of enhancement (these disorders usually involve adenosis, proliferation, or atypia)

c Representative slice before injection of contrast medium. MRI was performed because of impaired mammographic assessment in the presence of radiodense breast
tissue, diffusely disseminated microcalcifications, and a
family history of malignancy
d The same slice after injection of Gd-DTPA. A confluent
patchy pattern of gradual contrast enhancement is demonstrated in the glandular tissue. This finding is compatible with a benign breast disease, but the capability to exclude a malignant process is considerably limited.
The nipple itself (arrow) enhances in approximately 50% of
all patients. In the absence of clinical suspicion this represents a normal finding

graphic findings, and clinical examination,
further workup may include excisional biopsy, ultrasound-guided core needle biopsy,
sonographic follow-up (in the case of benign-
appearing or very small hypechoic area).

■ Magnetic Resonance Imaging

Glandular tissue with benign breast changes has a
low signal intensity on MR images, as opposed to
fatty tissue (Figs. 10.**3 a–h**). After contrast injection:

● *Most benign breast disorders (70–75%) enhance
only slightly, if at all*

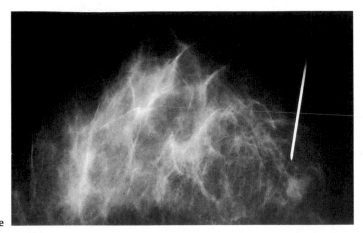

e

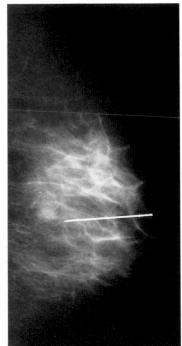

Fig. 10.**3e–h** Occasionally, mammography and MRI (sometimes only MRI) will reveal a benign focal breast disorder. Focal fibrous breast disease will not enhance (see Figs. 9.**8a–d**). In a benign proliferative breast disorder, the focus can enhance significantly, which represents a suggestive MRI finding
e and **f** Mammographically suspicious indistinct lesion on the craniocaudal and mediolateral preoperative localization images

f

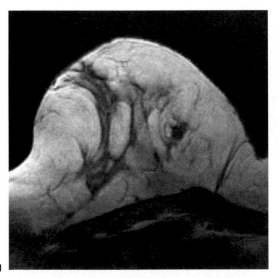

g

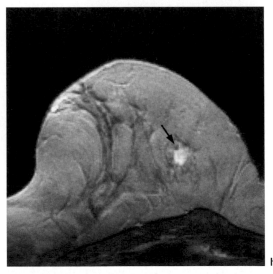

h

Fig. 10.**3g** Slice through the suspicious lesion before contrast injection (MR examination was part of a study protocol)
h After injection of Gd-DTPA, the indistinct focal lesion enhances rapidly and early, behaving in the same manner as a malignant process on MRI. Histologic examination revealed mildly proliferative benign focal breast disease accompanied by a pronounced but unspecific inflammatory reaction.

(Figs. 10.**3a** and **b** and Figs. 9.**8a–d**). Most of these cases involve nonproliferative disorders (fibrous or fibrosis benign breast disorders).
- Contrast enhancement occurs in 25–30% of benign breast disorders. The *pattern of en-* *hancement can vary greatly.* The following patterns can occur:
  - Diffuse milky enhancement. Diffuse enhancement is an enhancement over a wide area (for example, the entire breast or the upper outer

quadrant) without an abrupt transition from surrounding tissue.

- Diffuse nodular, confluent enhancement (Figs. 10.3 c and **d**).
- Focal enhancement with irregular contours, or focal nodular enhancement (Figs. 10.3 e and **f**).

Benign breast disorders without cellular hyperplasia or proliferation usually enhance slowly. Enhancement can occur infrequently in nonproliferative disorders where they involve inflammatory reactions (galactophoritis), when adenosis or significant hyperplastic changes are present, or sometimes under hormonal stimulation (see below). Proliferative breast disorders usually enhance.

■ **Effects of the Menstrual Cycle**

Enhancement due to breast disorders is often *inconstant* and *varies during the menstrual cycle*. Since enhancement due to breast disorders is often more pronounced in the second half of the cycle and since part of such enhancing areas disappears after menstruation, it is recommended that the *MRI examination be performed between the 6th and 17th day of the menstrual cycle* whenever possible.[20-22]

■ **Predictive Value**

Whether the degree of proliferation in breast disorders correlates with the extent or speed of contrast enhancement is controversial. Our experience has shown that, particularly with respect to the important distinction between proliferative breast disorders with and without atypia, *no reliable correlation with the extent or speed of contrast enhancement exists*.

■ **Advantages and Disadvantages**

Contrast-enhanced MRI has advantages and disadvantages for the differential diagnosis of changes due to benign breast disorders:

- Because of its high sensitivity for invasive carcinomas, lack of contrast enhancement (as occurs in approximately 70% of benign breast disorders) is a highly reliable sign of the absence of an invasive carcinoma. (Rare exceptions, however, have been encountered).
- In the presence of nonenhancing benign breast disorders, nonpalpable carcinomas (or focal carcinomas) can be detected even in radiodense or irregularly structured tissue. This may be of special interest when malignant foci need to be excluded within dense breast tissue, e. g., before conservative treatment of a small carcinoma.
- Presence of a generalized diffuse or patchy pattern of enhancement greatly limits the capability of MRI to detect or exclude a carcinoma.
- Focal enhancement resulting from benign breast disorders cannot reliably be distinguished from focal carcinomas and thus may lead to false positive results.
- MRI is not suitable for further differentiation between uncharacteristic microcalcifications. The sensitivity of contrast MRI for carcinomas in situ is not established. However, it probably does not lie much over 80–90%. Also, proliferative benign disorders with microcalcifications often lead to false positive results.

■ **Relevance for Differential Diagnosis**

Previously mentioned disadvantages pertain primarily to the impaired assessment of those benign breast disorders with generalized enhancement. Furthermore, focal areas of enhancement may cause false positive calls. In light of this, we *do not recommend using contrast-enhanced MRI for every form of benign breast disorder* or *unselectively* in radiodense tissue, but recommend *limiting its use to special cases*.

Contrast-enhanced MRI is not recommended in the following cases:

- Follow-up examination of known enhancing breast disorders (i. e., known from previous diagnostic studies).
- Differentiation between inflammatory and malignant changes. (Both enhance allowing no reliable distinction.)
- In patients undergoing hormone therapy (generally with preparations containing intermediate or high dosages of gestagen) who complain of tension (nonspecific enhancement will often impair diagnostic accuracy).
- In asymptomatic patients with dense breast tissue. The majority of these patients are below the age of 40. Here frequently occult fibroadenomas or areas of adenosis will be detected (nonspecific enhancement may be encountered in about 1 of 5 cases) leading to expensive workup, while the chance of detecting a malignancy is low since the prevalence

of malignancy (about 3 to 5 in 1000 patients or even fewer for patients below 40) is low in unselected patient populations.

Contrast-enhanced MRI, however, may be quite helpful for the following indications:

– In radiodense tissue to exclude *additional foci* or a *contralateral malignancy* where conservative treatment of a small breast carcinoma is planned.
– In radiodense tissue with a *high risk of malignancy,* such as locating a primary tumor. It has yet to be decided whether adjunctive contrast-enhanced MRI is cost-effective in monitoring high-risk patients.
– In selected cases with radiodense tissue with *uncharacteristic disturbed architecture or asymmetry, in patients with severe scarring.*
– In radiodense tissue in the presence of (multiple) *contradictory findings* (except for microcalcifications).

With these indications, the absence of enhancement during contrast MRI can help exclude a carcinoma. Focal enhancement on an MR image can provide an indication for percutaneous biopsy, and MRI can help guide the biopsy. MRI can thus aid in early detection of carcinomas or secondary foci in tissue that is difficult to assess by other imaging modalities.

■ Percutaneous Biopsy

There are three methods of obtaining biopsies of nonpalpable mammographic lesions for histopathologic or cytopathologic examination: excisional biopsy, fine-needle aspiration, and core needle biopsy. In an effort to minimize the number of excisional biopsies, percutaneous needle biopsies have become increasingly common practices.

Diagnostic accuracy correlates with the size and homogeneity of the focus, the amount of tissue obtained, and the examiner's experience.

The pathologist requires representative tissue specimens in sufficient quantity for examination. Such specimens cannot always be obtained.

For the workup of indeterminate findings and BI-RADS IV microcalcifications, vacuum biopsy has definite advantages over core needle biopsy.[23-29]

Heterogeneous changes in benign breast disorders and the occasional presence of atypical focal hyperplasia can limit the diagnostic accuracy of fine-needle aspiration or core needle biopsy. For these reasons diagnostic open biopsy is recommended in the following cases:

– In the presence of ductal atypia or radial scar, or where findings are insufficient for examination
– If there is a discrepancy between clinical and/ or imaging and/or needle biopsy findings

In the case of a malignancy proven by percutaneous biopsy, open surgery will be necessary for treatment.

■ Summary

Histologically, benign breast disorders encompass a broad spectrum of tissue changes. We differentiate the following types according to their prognosis:

– Benign nonproliferative breast disorders (70% of all benign disorders) without an increased risk of carcinoma
– Benign proliferative breast disorders without cellular atypia (approximately 25% of all benign disorders) with a slightly increased risk of carcinoma (by a factor of 1.5–2)
– Benign proliferative breast disorders with cellular atypia (4–5% of all benign disorders) with an increased risk of carcinoma (by a factor of 5)

Diagnostic imaging studies do not permit reliable assessment of risk. *Above all, diagnostic imaging cannot reliably identify the benign breast disorders that entail a genuinely increased risk* (by a factor of 5). *Clinical signs* of benign breast disorders can include pain, palpable findings, and, rarely, discharge.

The primary *mammographic signs* are increased density and microcalcifications.

Sonography may reveal hyperechoic tissue texture. Often cysts can be identified. Hypoechoic structures or acoustic shadows may also be found.

On MRI examination, nonproliferative disorders usually enhance only slightly, while contrast enhancement can vary greatly in adenosis and proliferative benign disorders (uptake can vary equally in proliferative changes with and without atypia).

Depending on the extent of the benign changes, findings in all modalities will *overlap* with changes associated with preinvasive and early invasive carcinomas.

Diffuse benign changes are usually recognizable as such but can often *limit visualization of malignancy. Focal changes* usually differ qualitatively and quantitatively from surrounding benign tissue. Such changes require particularly careful workup. In general diagnostic imaging studies are unable to reliably distinguish these changes from malignant processes. Therefore focal changes frequently lead to *false positive findings* and necessitate percutaneous or open biopsy of benign changes.

Clinical examination and mammography are the methods of choice for assessing benign breast disorders detected by *screening,* and they are fully adequate for this purpose. In the presence of *questionable or suggestive mammographic or clinical findings, adjunctive procedures* are indicated for the following reasons:

– To minimize the number of excisional biopsies of benign findings
– To improve early detection of malignancy where the risk of malignancy is high and visualization is limited

In the presence of indeterminate focal findings, adjunctive sonography is recommended as a first step of the workup. Biopsy should follow in all cases where carcinoma is not excluded with reasonable certainty.

Contrast-enhanced MRI may be helpful in selected cases with breast tissue that is difficult to assess by other methods (e. g., due to severe scarring or pronounced asymmetry), if a high risk of malignancy exists.

Open biopsy remains the most reliable method for assessing borderline lesions (e. g., benign breast changes with atypias), or contradictory findings. In the case of malignancy, it will constitute the first therapeutic measure as well.

■ References

1   Prechtel K. Mastopathie. Histologische Formen und Langzeitbeobachtungen. Zentralbl Pathol. 1991; 137:210
2   Prechtel K, Gehm O, Geiger G, Prechtel P. Die Histologie der Mastopathie und die kumulative ipsilaterale Mammakarzinomsequenz. Pathologe. 1994;15:158
3   Dupont WD, Page DL. Risk factors for breast cancer in women with proliferative disease. N Engl J Med. 1985;312:146
4   Dupont WD, Page DL. Relative risk of breast cancer varies with the time since diagnosis of atypical hyperplasia. Hum Pathol. 1989;20:723
5   Consensus Meeting: Is fibrocystic disease of the breast precancerous? Arch Pathol Lab Med. 1986;110:171
6   van Gils CH, Otten JD, Verbeck AL et al. Effect of mammographic breast density on breast cancer screening performance: a Study in Nijmegen, The Netherlands. J Epidemiol Community Health 1998;52:267–71
7   Young KC, Wallis MG, Blanks RG, Moss SM. Influence of number of views and mammographic film density on the detection of invasive cancers: results from the NHS Breast Screening Programme. Br J Radiol. 1997;70:482–8
8   Adler DO, Helvie MA, Obermann HA. Radial sclerosing lesion of the breast: mammographic features. Radiology. 1990;176:737
9   Dessole S, Meloni GB, Capobianco G et al. Radial scar of the breast: mammographic enigma in pre- and postmenopausal women. Maturitas. 2000;34:227–31
10 Orel SG, Evers K, Yeh IT, Troupin RH. Radial scar with microcalcifications: radiologic–pathologic correlation. Radiology. 1992;183:479
11 Alleva DQ, Smetherman DH, Farr GH, Cederbom GJ. Radial scar of the breast: radiologic-pathologic correlation in 22 cases. Radiographics 1999;19:S27–35
12 Lanyi M. Diagnostik und Differentialdiagnostik der Mammaverkalkung. Berlin: Springer; 1986
13 Linden SS, Sickles EA. Sedimented calcium in benign breast cysts: the full spectrum of mammographic presentations. AJR. 1989;152:967
14 American College of Radiology: Breast imaging reporting and data system (BI-RADS™) 3rd ed. Reston, Va: 1998
15 Bassett LW, Kimme-Smith C. Breast sonography. AJR. 1991;156:449
16 Jackson VP, Hendrick RE, Feig FA. Imaging of the radiographically dense breast. Radiology. 1993;188:297
17 Pamilo M, Soiva M, Anttinen I et al. Ultrasonography of breast lesions detected in mammography screening. Acta Radiol. 1991;32:220
18 Stavros AT, Thickman D, Rapp CL et al. Soled breast nodules: use of sonography to distinguish between benign and malignant lesions. Radiology 1995;196:123–134
19 Cohen MA, Sferlazza SJ. Role of sonography in evaluation of radial scars of the breast. AJR. 2000;174:1075–8
20 Heywang-Köbrunner SH. Contrast-enhanced MRI of the Breast. Heidelberg, New York: Springer; 1996
21 Kuhl C et al. Fokale und diffuse KM-anreichernde Läsionen im der MR-Mammographie bei gesunden Probandinnen: Bandbreite des Normalverhaltens und Zyklusphasenabhängigkeit. Radiologe. 1995;35:86
22 Müller-Schimpfle M, Ohmenhäuser K, Stoll P. Menstrual cycle and age. Radiology. 1997;203:145–9
23 Brenner RJ, Fajardo L, Fisher PR, Dershaw DD et al. Percutaneous core biopsy of the breast: effect of operator experience and number of samples or diagnostic accuracy. AJR. 1996;166:341–6
24 Liberman L, Dershaw DD, Glassman JR et al. Analysis of cancers not diagnosed at stereotactic core breast biopsy. Radiology. 1997;203:151–7
25 Mainiero MB, Philpotts LE, Lee CH et al. Stereotaxic core needle biopsy of breast microcalcifications: correlation of target accuracy and diagnosis with lesion size. Radiology. 1996;198:665–9
26 Brenner RJ, Fajardo L, Fisher PR et al. Percutaneous core biopsy of the breast: effect of operator experience and number of samples on diagnostic accuracy. AJR. 1996;166:341–6
27 Meyer JE, Smith DN, Dipiro PJ et al. Stereotactic breast biopsy of clustered microcalcifications with a directional, vacuum-assisted device. Radiology. 1997;204:575–6
28 Jackmann RJ, Marzoni FA, Nowels KW. Percutaneous removal of benign mammographic lesions: comparison of automated large-core and directional vacuum-assisted biopsy techniques. AJR. 1998;171:1325–30
29 Heywang-Köbrunner SH, Schaumlöffel U, Viehweg P et al. Minimally invasive stereotactic vacuum core breast biopsy. Eur Radiol. 1998;8:377–85

11. Cysts

Cysts are by far the most common mass in the female breast. Approximately half of all women 30 to 40 years and older develop fibrocystic changes in the breast that manifest themselves in single or multiple cysts of varying sizes. Larger cysts occur in 20–25% of all women.[1, 2] Simple cysts are benign lesions.

Cysts become clinically important when the patient presents with pain, or when palpable findings require further diagnostic studies to determine if they are benign or malignant. Asymptomatic cysts may also be initially detected by mammography or sonography.

Cysts can simulate tumors and conceal malignancy.

■ Histology

Cysts are locally distended peripheral ductal segments filled with fluid. They usually occur in the terminal ductal lobular units and are associated with fibrocystic changes in the breast. While simple cysts are always benign, "complicated cysts" can sometimes harbour malignancy.

■ Definition

Simple cysts consist of two layers of cells, an inner layer of epithelial cells and an outer layer of myoepithelial cells. They are benign processes that are not associated with an increased risk of cancer.

The term "complicated cysts" refers collectively to cysts or conglomerate cysts detected in imaging studies or by clinical examination that are "complicated" by inflammation or bleeding or contain neoplastic tissue changes in their wall or lumen. In the widest sense of the term, these include cavities containing hemorrhage and necrotic carcinomas.

Simple cysts are usually lined with linear epithelium surrounded by a layer of compressed connective tissue. Like the surrounding fibrocystic disease, the cyst wall can exhibit various forms of epithelial hyperplasia, sometimes even atypia. The risk of malignant degeneration only depends on the cellular changes of the underlying fibrocystic alterations. Simple cysts themselves are not premalignant lesions.

Complicated cysts have a heterogeneous origin, occuring in either preformed cavities (lactiferous ducts or cysts) or in cavities resulting from necrosis or bleeding.[3, 4]

Inflammatory changes in cysts occur in retention cysts or in the presence of chronic mastitis. Cystic cavities can also develop in centrally necrotic tumors, or they can occur as a result of secretion and recurrent bleeding, as in intraductal papillomas and papillary carcinomas.

■ Medical History and Clinical Findings

Cysts can be totally asymptomatic. As they become larger, they manifest themselves as palpable findings, sometimes associated with breast pain.

Cysts are typically seen to develop acutely. They may wax and wane. However, based on the history, it is mostly impossible to distinguish a suddenly developed cyst from a slowly developed lesion (e.g., carcinoma) that has just been noticed by the patient.

Generally, cysts will first appear after the age of 30 or 40, occurring with peak frequency in premenopausal and perimenopausal women between the ages of 40 and 45.

In women under 40 and especially under 30, fibroadenomas tend to occur more frequently than cysts; after 40, the opposite is true. Since the risk of cancer is also higher in this age group, special care should be taken to exclude the possibility of breast cancer in these patients.

■ Breast Examination

Cysts are generally palpable as smooth-contoured, mobile masses. Most frequently, they are firm and somewhat compressible. However, they can also manifest themselves as hard masses. Particularly in the presence of conglomerate cysts and surrounding inflammation, distinguishing a cyst from a malignant growth can be difficult.[3, 4] Since some malignancies are relatively smooth-contoured and mobile, further diagnostic studies are always indicated in the presence of a clinical diagnosis of suspected breast cysts.

■ Objectives of Diagnostic Studies

1. To differentiate between simple cysts and noncystic changes, such as benign tumors or breast cancer (most important diagnosis to be excluded).
2. To distinguish simple cysts from other cystic masses. These include complicated cysts accompanied by inflammation, papilloma, or proliferative changes as well as cystic carcinomas (mural cancer growing into a cyst and carcinomas with central necrosis that can have the appearance of a cystic mass) (see also Fig. 11.3).

If a simple cyst is confirmed, further diagnostic studies will not be necessary. In the presence of complicated cysts or solid masses, further studies are essential, and if necessary the mass should be biopsied.

■ Diagnostic Strategy

Sonography is the method of choice for diagnosing cysts.[5, 6, 7]

In women under 35, sonography should be the initial imaging study in the workup of a palpable lump. If it confirms that the mass is a cyst, the workup is completed. If the cyst is painful, aspiration may be performed for symptomatic relief.

In women over 35 years of age and in particular in women over 40, both mammography and sonography must be performed due to the increasing risk of carcinoma. Mammography may, for example, reveal a carcinoma close to (or even remote from) the cyst, which—when small or preinvasive—may go undetected sonographically. Therefore mammography should be used liberally.

If the diagnosis of a cyst is equivocal sonographically, aspiration should be attempted. In patients with frequently recurring masses, a repeat mammogram is not necessary if a recent mammogram exists and the new lump is proven to be a cyst based on the sonogram.

When mammographic and sonographic findings are consistent with a cyst, and malignancy is excluded in the remaining breast tissue as well, the workup is done. If the lesion is solid, the diagnostic workup of solid masses is followed (see p. 397). If the diagnosis of a cyst is equivocal and aspiration is attempted, the further workup will depend on the result of aspiration (see pp. 201–2).

■ Sonography

■ Unit Settings/Examination Technique

Optimum unit settings are particularly important in diagnosing cysts. If the gain is set too low, solid hypoechoic processes can appear anechoic, which can lead to serious diagnostic errors.

In case of doubt, the following simple technique can be helpful (Figs. 11.1 e–g). Gradually increase the gain on the unit until the echoes in the lesion begin to appear:

- Typically, cysts will fill with echoes from the periphery, whereas echoes in solid structures will simultaneously increase at different places within the mass.
- Occasionally, reverberation echoes will also be visible in cysts. They are more prominent in the upper part of the cyst adjacent to its leading wall and are parallel to the transducer. (Reverberation echoes are artifacts and do not represent tissue in the cyst.)

Turning and tilting the transducer can visualize the entire length of septa, making it possible to distinguish them from intracystic processes (Fig. 11.1 h). Changing the patient's position and repeating the examination can be helpful in identifying sedimentation, which layers in the dependent portion of the cyst appears as hypoechoic material on its floor.

■ Typical Appearance
(Figs. 11.1 a–k)

The simple cyst is characterized by its smooth thin wall, absence of internal echoes, and distal enhancement. The walls of the cyst are smooth. Fine acoustic shadowing can extend from the lateral walls. If a wide shadow that is not explained by a mammographically visible large calcification appears on the wall of the cyst, the possibility of malignancy in or directly adjacent to the wall of the cyst must be considered (Fig. 11.3 e). If the contents of the cyst are not

Fig. 11.**1 a–k** Sonographic appearance of cysts
a Schematic drawing of a typical cyst:
The typical cyst is anechoic with pronounced distal enhancement. Fine lateral acoustic shadowing can occur at the margins
b Sonographic image of a small cyst that mammography was unable to detect in dense tissue (see Figs. 11.**2 a–d**)
c Sonographic image of a large cyst (black arrow) and a partly imaged cyst beneath it (outlined arrow). Another extremely small cyst, only partially visible in this imaging plane, is suspected (tip of arrow)

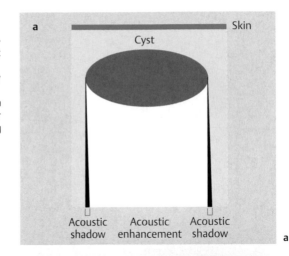

d Reverberation echo occurring at the wall of the cyst: Echoes are repeatedly reflected between the transducer and the anterior wall of the cyst. The ultrasound system registers echoes that are reflected twice (or several times) as if they came from twice (or several times) as deep in the tissue

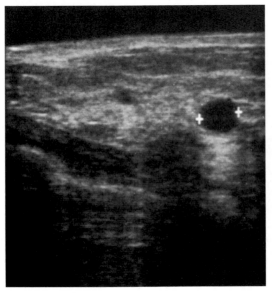

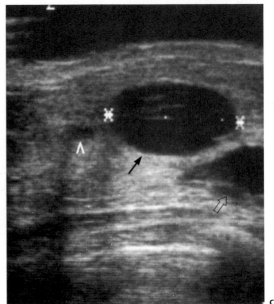

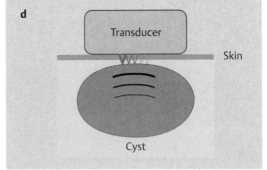

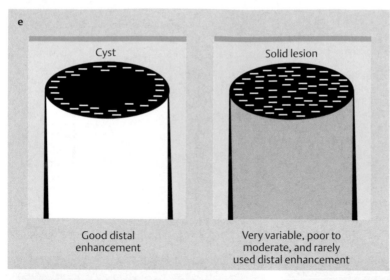

e In genuine cysts, increasing the gain produces additional echoes beginning at the periphery, i. e., the cyst appears to "fill in" from the periphery

Good distal enhancement

Very variable, poor to moderate, and rarely used distal enhancement

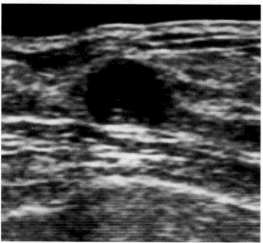

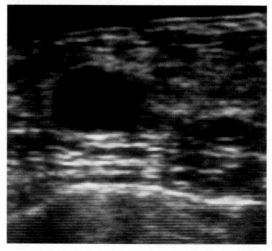

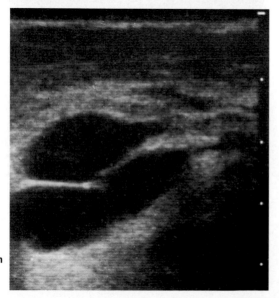

f Cyst visualized with increased gain. The echoes fill in from the periphery of the cyst, but a few reverberation echoes are visible in the cyst near the transducer as well. The echoes that fill in from the periphery of the cyst make it appear to shrink (compare **g**)

g The same cyst with reduced gain. No echoes are seen in the cyst. However, distal enhancement remains readily visible

h Septa in the cyst can be visualized by rotating and angling the transducer accordingly

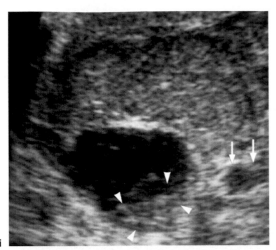

i

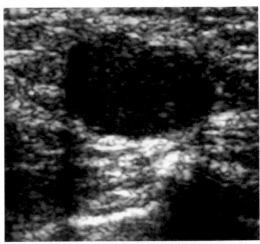

k

Fig. 11.**1 i**   Cystic mass (imaged with 13 MHz) containing echoes at the floor of the cyst. Slight distal enhancement. A hypoechoic duct is also present (arrows). Suspected cyst with sedimentation, later confirmed by aspiration

k This oval mass has well-defined margins and some posterior enhancement of the sound beam. The low-level internal echoes throughout most of the mass suggest that it is solid. Histology: medullary carcinoma

completely anechoic or if adequate enhancement is not present behind the cyst, it does not meet the criteria of a simple cyst. Some simple cyst of the breast may not appear as such on ultrasound.

If echoes are detected within the cyst, the examiner should above all consider the following questions:

● Can sedimentation, blood clots, or septa be identified?
● Does the cyst contain a tumorous process?
● Does the image not show a cyst at all, but a solid process?

In such cases the major differential diagnostic considerations include:

● High-protein, inflamed, or blood-filled cysts (Figs. 11.**2 c** and **d**)
● Intracystic papillomas (see also Figs. 12.**7 a–d**) or malignancies that partially or completely fill the cyst
● Extremely hypoechoic benign tumors such as fibroadenomas
● Some malignancies, particularly a medullary carcinoma, which can occasionally appear very hypoechoic (Figs. 11.**1 k**, 11.**3 a–e**, and 17.**5 b**).[8]

■ **Diagnostic Accuracy**

When due care is exercised, sonography is highly accurate in diagnosing cysts. Depending on the

sonography unit and transducer, even very small cysts measuring 1–2 mm in diameter can be identified and diagnosed. However, only typical findings should be classified as cysts. If any doubt remains, further diagnostic studies are indicated.

■ **Aspiration of the Cyst**

Aspirating the cyst is the next step if sonography fails to reveal typical cyst findings or if the cyst is to be decompressed to relieve symptoms.

If sonographically the needle tip proves to be within the lesion and aspiration is unsuccessful, a solid tumor must be suspected (differential diagnosis, see p. 223).

Cysts may contain clear, yellowish, greenish, brownish or even black-tainted fluid, sometimes with increased protein content or with hemoglobin breakdown products. There is some controversy as to whether all aspirated fluids need to be submitted to cytology. The reason is that the vast majority of the findings from these cytologic examinations are negative, while numerous indeterminate findings due to necrotic material may cause unnecessary further workup. Furthermore, the cytologic examination of cysts with wall carcinoma or necrotic decaying tumor is frequently unreliable because the contents of such cystic lesions often just contain necrotic cells from which malignancy cannot be diagnosed.

If the clinical imaging findings or the fluid itself are not consistent with a simple cyst (green or yellow fluid), cytologic examination must be performed. The usual cytology of a cyst is apocrine metaplasia.

However, when imaging findings show a solid lesion in a cyst or suggest that it corresponds to a necrotic mass, a negative cytology should never dissuade the physician from a biopsy.

If blood is present in the contents of the cyst, then the possibility of an intracystic papilloma or cancer should be considered in addition to possible iatrogenic introduction of blood. In the presence of inconclusive sonographic findings, or findings suggesting malignancy, a biopsy is indicated to verify the diagnosis.

If cytologic examination reveals atypical cells or groups of papillary cells, further workup of the cyst (which will usually fill up again) is necessary. The same applies if an intracystic tumor has been verified sonographically.

For some pathologists the differentiation of various papillary lesions may be difficult, with the small volume of tissue obtained with percutaneous biopsy procedures. In this setting, surgical excision of these lesions is desirable because papillary lesions represent the majority of intracystic masses. If these diagnoses are readily made by consulting pathologists on the basis of percutaneous biopsy procedures, they should be performed when histologic assessment of these lesions is needed.

■ Pneumocystography

Pneumocystography (Fig. 3.41) can be performed through the aspiration needle following aspiration of the cyst (see Chapter 3, pp. 81–3 for examination technique).

■ Typical Appearance

Typically, a simple cyst is oval or round, with a smooth thin wall. In the presence of inflammation, the wall may appear thickened but the inner wall will not usually show any irregularities. Papillomas, carcinomas of the wall of the cyst, and decaying carcinomas can be identified as solid irregularities in the wall (Figs. 11.2d and 11.3c[3, 9]).

■ Indications

The high accuracy of sonography has largely eliminated the use of pneumocystography.

The diagnostic value or indication for pneumocystography is a matter of controversy.[3,

[10] While some authors appreciate this method for assessing wall thickness and absence of a hidden solid lesion, others feel that complete aspiration under sonographic guidance can replace pneumocystography.

In addition, some investigators use it therapeutically, believing that it has a favorable effect on involution of the cyst (prevents refilling and improves adhesion due to the pressure exerted by the air, which is gradually resorbed). This effect is controversial.

■ Mammography

(Figs. 11.2a–d)

Cysts surrounded by fatty tissue usually appear as round or oval, well-circumscribed masses on the mammogram.

If they are partially or completely surrounded by breast parenchyma, the cysts can appear as a nonspecific mass, as a smooth-contoured, or partially obscured mass. They may also be invisible when completely surrounded by dense parenchyma. Due to compression of adjacent fat, cysts can sometimes have a partial or complete halo sign (see also p. 211). When a mass that may be a cyst is palpable, it is helpful to place a radiographic skin marker over the mass to help to identify it on the mammogram.

A thin, semicircular calcification may appear in the wall of a cystic process (such as a calcified oil cyst, calcified sebaceous cyst or calcified simple cyst) or along the periphery (semicircular-appearing level of milk of calcium). In rare cases, calcification of the wall can be due to bleeding into cysts. Particular care should be taken to exclude a small intracystic tumor via sonography.

■ Magnetic Resonance Imaging

■ Indication and Diagnostic Accuracy

Diagnosis or exclusion of cysts is not an indication for breast MRI. However, if a contrast-enhanced MRI study conducted for other reasons reveals cysts, malignant growths in simple cysts can be easily excluded by the absence of enhancement.

■ Examination Technique

In contrast to what some regard as standard practice, we see hardly any need for using T2-weighted images. On these images, cysts typically

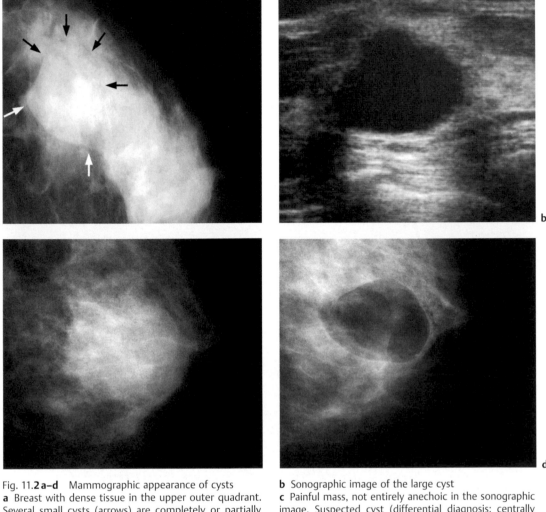

Fig. 11.**2 a–d** Mammographic appearance of cysts
a Breast with dense tissue in the upper outer quadrant. Several small cysts (arrows) are completely or partially surrounded by fat, making them readily discernible. A large cyst with a halo sign is shown. Further small cysts are only visualized sonographically (**b** and **c**) but cannot be distinguished from the dense tissue in the mammogram

b Sonographic image of the large cyst
c Painful mass, not entirely anechoic in the sonographic image. Suspected cyst (differential diagnosis: centrally necrotic tumor), ill defined on the mammogram
d Pneumocystography reveals smooth inner contour of the wall
Surgery followed aggravation of symptoms. *Histology:* inflamed cysts

exhibit an extremely high and homogeneous signal intensity. To exclude safely other smooth-contoured lesions with high water content (such as mucinous carcinoma or a phyllodes tumor) that can have a similar appearance, a T2-weighted multiecho sequence or the usual T1-weighted pulse sequence before and after intravenous injection of a contrast medium will be required anyway and is more important.

■ **Typical Appearance**

In the customary T1-weighted pulse sequence before and after intravenous contrast-medium injection, simple cysts have the following MRI appearance: in the precontrast T1-weighted image, they typically exhibit a smooth contour and an extremely low signal intensity. If the cyst contains old blood products (especially methemoglobin), the contents of the cyst can have a high signal intensity or a fluid level. The decisive criterion is the

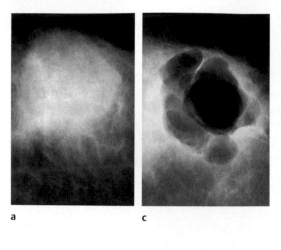

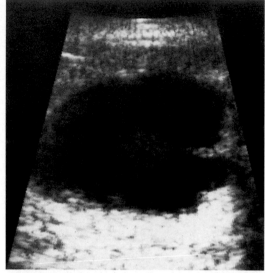

a c

b

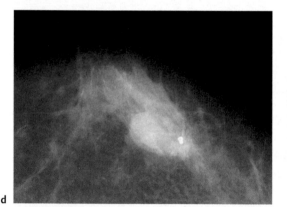

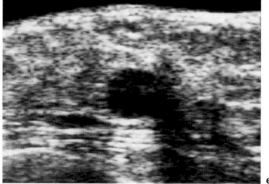

d

e

Fig. 11.**3 a–e** Differential diagnosis of cystic processes
a Round, posteriorly ill defined mass
b Sonographic image reveals echoes and septum-like structures in the center. The sonographic findings themselves suggest a malignancy
c Pneumocystography does not provide any additional information to the sonographic findings. The image reveals several chambers in the mass: *Histology:* necrotic decaying medullary carcinoma

d Mammography shows a partially smooth-contoured mass with a partial halo sign. Dystrophic calcification and a spiculated mass are visible posteriorly. Suspected malignancy
e Sonography shows hypoechoic, smooth-contoured mass with very good posterior enhancement. The presence of echoes throughout the mass suggests a solid process. A conspicuous lateral acoustic shadow is present. Histologically, this shadow corresponds to a small spiculated carcinoma that probably led to congestion of the blood-filled cyst

enhancement behavior. If the lesion enhances, it is not compatible with a cyst but must represent a solid mass. Enhancement of walls without focal thickening is a sign of inflammation or mastopathic changes.

Papillomas and carcinomas in the wall of the cyst generally appear as an irregularity in the contour of the wall with moderate to intense contrast enhancement.[15]

■ **Summary**

Sonography ist the method of choice for the diagnosis of cysts. This method usually permits differentiation between simple and complicated cysts, which is crucial for further management.

Simple cysts appear as smooth-contoured, thin-walled anechoic masses with distal enhancement.

If the sonographic findings cannot be definitively categorized as simple cysts, the next step is aspiration of the cyst. Mammography is performed to further characterize the mass, if it is not a cyst, and to exclude malignancy in the cyst or in the rest of the breast. Mammography is therefore indicated as the initial workup for a palpable mass in all symptomatic patients over the age of 35. In patients under 35 years of age, the workup should begin with sonography and needs to be complemented by mammography, unless sonography proves, for example, that the palpable mass is a simple cyst.

Indications for biopsy include:

– Malignancy is suspected or cannot safely be excluded, as is the case when solid findings remain after aspiration, or when suspicious microcalcifications or other suspicious findings are detected close to the cyst or at another site
– Sonographic or cytologic studies demonstrate or suggest the presence of intracystic proliferation
– Blood is present in the contents of the cyst, unless it is felt to be iatrogenic

Appendix: Galactoceles and Oil Cysts

Definition: A galactocele is a single or multichambered, milk-filled retention cyst. Galactoceles develop during pregnancy or lactation, and in newborns and infants, due to disturbed absorption of the so-called witch's milk (infantile galactoceles).

In mammography, galactoceles appear as follows (Fig. 11.**4 a**):

– They can be hidden in dense glandular tissue, or can appear as round or oval masses (similar to a cyst). They may be of fatty rather than water density.
– A typical but infrequent sign is an oil-fluid level in the 90° lateral mammogram.[11–14] The fluid surface appears as a horizontal border between the transparent fatty and non-fatty fluid.

In sonography, galactoceles appear as follows:

– Like cysts, they are single or multichambered masses that are easily compressed (Fig. 11.**4 b**)
– Depending on the consistency of the milk in the galactocele, the contents can be anechoic or hypoechoic. Good distal enhancement can be present, as can attenuation.

Definition: An oil cyst is a cystic mass that contains oily necrotic material. Oil cysts are usually associated with a history of previous trauma or operation. Some galactoceles may turn into oil cysts. Clinically oil cysts are usually palpable as non-mobile masses mostly located within tissue thickening. They are, therefore, often a reason for concern.

On mammography[16–19] oil cysts appear as follows (Fig. 11.**5 a, b**):

– They are visible as a radiolucent mass with smooth internal margins
– The mass is surrounded by a capsule, which is always smooth, may be thickened, and may blend with the surrounding tissues
– Typical eggshell-like calcifications may develop in the capsule

The above-described appearance is typical and requires no further workup, even if clinical findings may appear suspicious or if ultrasound classified it as an interdeterminate mass. Sometimes newly emerging calcifications may appear indeterminate to suspicious until they assume their characteristic eggshell-like appearance.

On sonography[20, 21] oil cysts may appear as follows (Figs. 11.**5 c, d**):

– Relatively smoothly outlined hypoechoic lesions.
– Rarely as echogenic lesions (Figs. 11.**5 c** and **d**).
– Sometimes they can contain echogenic material mimicking an intracystic tumor. This sonographic appearance can be due to the necrotic material and fibrin.
– The transmitted sound distal to the oil cyst can be unchanged, enhanced, or attenuated. Distal acoustic shadowing can be caused by sound-absorbing components within the necrotic contents, such as blood, or by calcifications in the wall of the oil cyst (Fig. 11.**5 c** and **d**).

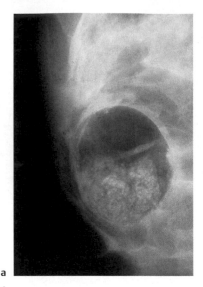

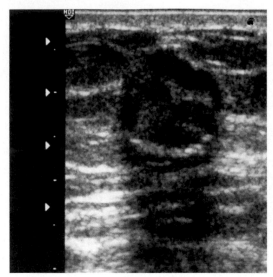

a

b

Fig. 11.4a and b
a Clinically smooth-contoured mass 4 months after nursing. Mammography reveals a large, oval, smooth-contoured radiolucent area about 3 cm in diameter. The lucent area is probably air that has entered the galactocele via the lactiferous ducts. The contents of the galactocele is coarsely granular and partly calcified, compatible with a saponifying galactocele

b This galactocele in a different patient was inapparent on the mammogram. Sonographically it has the appearance of a complex mass.

Even though at least some of the sonographic features by themselves could be considered worrisome, no further workup is necessary whenever mammography shows a typical appearance.

On MRI[15] (Figs. 11.5e,f) the oily content is identified by its high signal intensity on all pulse sequences (except fat-saturated pulse sequences). The internal wall is smooth. The capsule may enhance moderately with contrast agent. In the presence of a typical mammographic appearance this should not be interpreted as a sign of malignancy unless a definite nodule or mass is visualized within or beside the capsule.

In summary, mammography has to be considered the leading method for the diagnosis of oil cysts.

Fig. 11.5 a–d   Mammographic (**a** and **b**) and sonographic ▷ (**c** and **d**) delineation of oil cysts
a Mammography.
Status 1 year post reduction mammoplasty. Two oil cysts are visualized as sharply outlined, radiolucent lesion in the scar region (arrows)
b Mammography 12 months later. Both oil cysts are now surrounded by pleomorphic, linear, or ring-like calcifications, partially forming an eggshell-like pattern. Despite the pleomorphism of some of the individual calcifications, the finding itself is characteristic
c Sonographically, the subcutaneous oil cyst is delineated as a round and poorly compressible anechoic lesion within the hyperechoic scar tissue
d This slightly more deeply situated oil cyst is visualized as an isoechoic oval lesion (echogenicity comparable to that of the subcutaneous fat), with no acoustic shadowing behind the left and definite acoustic shadowing behind the right aspect of the lesion. Hyperechoic scar tissue surrounds it like a capsule. Both sonographic findings are compatible with oil cysts, that are only identified as such in conjunction with mammography. Reduced elasticity and moveability are characteristic of an oil cyst but can be mistaken for a carcinoma if only sonography is performed

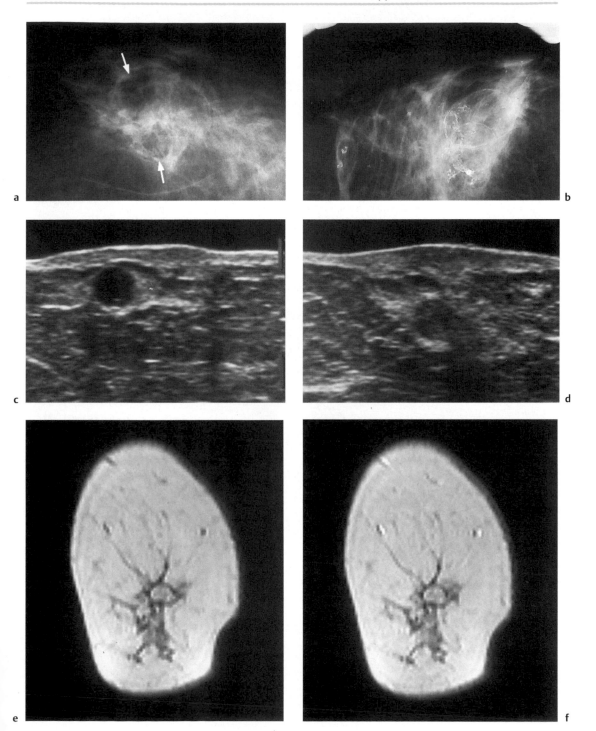

■ References

1   Bässler R. Pathologie der Brüste. In: Doerr W, Seifert G, Uehlinger E. Spezielle pathologische Anatomie. Berlin: Springer; 1978

2   Hughes LE, Mansel RE, Webster DJT. Benign disorders and diseases of the breast: concepts and clinical management. London: Baillière Tindall; 1989

3   Barth U, Prechtel K. Atlas der Brustdrüse und ihrer Erkrankungen. Stuttgart: Enke; 1990

4   Haagensen CD. Diseases of the breast. 2nd ed. Philadelphia: Saunders; 1986

5   Jackson VP. The role of ultrasound in breast imaging. Radiology. 1990;177:305–11

6   Pamilo M, Soiva M, Anttinen I et al. Ultrasonography of breast lesions detected im mammography screening. Acta Radiol. 1991;32:22

7   Venta LA, Dudiak CM, Salomon CG et al. Sonographic evaluation of the breast. Radiographics. 1994;14:29

8   Khalegian R. Breast cysts; pitfalls in sonographic diagnosis. Australas Radiol. 1993;37:192

9   Dyreborg U, Blichert-Toft M, Boeght M, Kiaer H. Needle puncture followed by pneumocytography of palpable breast cysts: a clinical trial. Acta Radiol Diagn. 1985; 26:277

10 Ikeda D, Helvie M, Adler D et al. The role of fine needle aspiration and pneumocystography in the treatment of inpalpable breast cysts. AJR. 1992;158:1239–41

11 Gomez A, Mata JM, Donoso L et al. Galactocele: three distinctive radiographic appearances. Radiology. 1986; 126:95

12 Salvador R, Salvador M, Jimenez JA et al. Galactocele of the breast: radiologic and ultrasonographic findings. Br J Radiol. 1990;63:140

13 Sickles EA, Vogelaar PW. Fluid level in a galactocele seen on lateral projection mammogram with horizontal beam. Breast Dis. 1981;7:32

14 Heywang SH, Lipsit ER, Glassman LM, Thomas MA. Specificity of ultrasound in the diagnosis of benign breast masses. J Ultrasound Med. 1984;3:453

15 Heywang-Köbrunner SH, Beck R. Contrast-enhanced MRI of the breast. Heidelberg, New York: Springer; 1996

16 Eidelman Y, Liebling RW, Buchbinder S et al. Mammography in the evaluation of masses in breasts reconstructed with TRAM flaps. Ann Plast Surg.1998;41:229–33

17 Hogge JP, Zuurbier RA, de Paredes ES. Mammography of autologous myocutaneous flaps. Radiographics 1999;19(Spec. No):63–72

18 Beer GM, Kompatscher P, Hergan K. Diagnosis of breast tumors after breast reduction. Aesthetic Plast Surg. 1996;20:391–7

19 Mandrekas AD, Assimakopoulos GJ, Mastorakos DP, Pantzalis K. Fat necrosis following breast reduction. Br J Plast Surg. 1994;47:560–2

20 Soo MS, Kornguth PJ, Hertzberg BS. Fat necrosis in the breast: sonographic features. Radiology. 1998;206:261–9

21 Harvey JA, Moran RE, Maurer EJ, De Angelis GA. Sonographic features of mammary oil cysts. J Ultrasound Med. 1997;16:719–24

12. Benign Tumors

Hamartoma or Adenofibrolipoma

The hamartoma of the breast is an abnormal collection of tissues that are normally found within the breast. It is surrounded by a pseudocapsule.

■ Histology

Hamartomas are demarcated from the surrounding tissue by a pseudocapsule and not by a connective tissue capsule. They are composed of the same elements as normal breast parenchyma. Hamartomas present as collections of parenchymal tissue (adenolipomas) and rarely as myoid hamartomas with smooth muscles, parenchyma, and fatty tissue. Hamartomas are not premalignant, and only rarely have malignant neoplastic changes been observed within them. Neoplasms are found no more frequently in hamartomas than in the respective mammary parenchyma.

■ Clinical Findings

Hamartomas are usually nonpalpable, but like lipomas can present as soft, smoothly delineated tumors. They are often only found mammographically. When the mammographic pattern corresponds to a firm, palpable mass, the diagnosis of hamartoma should be questioned.

■ Diagnostic Strategy

The diagnosis is usually made on mammography. A mammographically pathognomonic image, which is to be expected in the majority of the hamartomas, does not require further evaluation.

A mammographically atypical manifestation may undergo further evaluation by sonography.

A needle biopsy cannot establish the diagnosis of a hamartoma since it will only demonstrate normal breast tissue.

■ Mammography

Most hamartomas are definitively diagnosed by mammography (Fig. 12.**1a**). The following mammographic findings are pathognomonic:

- A smoothly demarcated mass that contains fat and soft tissue density comingled in varying amounts,
- Smooth demarcation of the mass and a thin pseudocapsule seen in its entirety or in part

The classic description of the pattern is that of a piece of "cut sausage." If these findings are present, no further evaluation is indicated. Suspicious findings, such as microcalcifications, within a mammographically diagnosed hamartoma of course need clarification.

The mammographic finding is atypical if fat lobules cannot be identified due to inadequate fat content or if the nodule is not well demarcated. Features not distinctive enough to allow the diagnosis of a hamartoma must be differentiated from other causes of asymmetric glandular tissue, occasionally also from irregularly outlined densities.[1]

■ Sonography

The mammographically unequivocal finding does not require sonography. If a mammographically suspected hamartoma is partially obscured by dense tissue, supplementary sonography might be helpful.

The sonographic diagnosis of a hamartoma (Fig. 12.**1b**), which should be made together with mammography, is based on the following findings:

- A smooth margin of the entire nodule with or without delicate shadows at the lateral wall

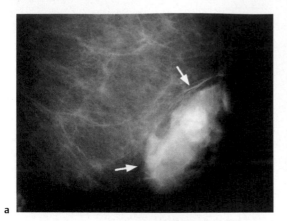

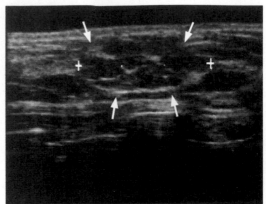

a

b

Fig. 12.**1a** and **b**   Hamartoma
a Mammography. The density of the hamartoma is variable, incorporating areas of fatty and soft tissue, surrounded by a thin pseudocapsule
b Fat-containing lobules are sonographically hypoechoic. They are separated by hyperechoic septa of connective tissue and surrounded by a pseudocapsule, which is best seen distally. Good compressibility supports the diagnosis. The characteristic image shown here is sonographically not always as impressive. If the mammographic finding is typical, sonography is not necessary

- Hypoechoic, smoothly marginated fat islands can be identified within the nodule
- The nodule must be compressible and easily moveable

■ Percutaneous Biopsy

It supports the exclusion of malignancy, but cannot diagnose a hamartoma, since its components are that of normal breast tissue. The histologic diagnosis of a "hamartoma" can only be established by excisional biopsy.

■ Magnetic Resonance Imaging

MRI is not needed for diagnosing a hamartoma.

Fibroepithelial Mixed Tumors

Fibroadenoma, Adenofibroma, Juvenile or Giant Fibroadenoma

The fibroadenoma is by far the most common tumor of the breast. It is important to know that the fibroadenoma occurs in all age groups, but that it is predominantly a lesion found in young women, even during puberty and adolescence. Fibroadenomas are hormone-induced hyperplastic tumors of the lobular connective tissue with the highest incidence between the ages of 25 and 35 years.

Because the incidence of fibroadenomas decreases after the age of 40 years, while that of carcinomas increases, a well-circumscribed malignancy, which is always a possibility, should be even more strongly considered if a smoothly marginated, solid lesion is newly discovered in a woman above the age of 40 years.[2, 3]

The fibroadenoma is a benign tumor. Only in rare instances (0.1–0.3%) are carcinomas, which are predominantly in situ, located within a fibroadenoma—as in any otherwise normal mammary tissue.[4]

Most fibroadenomas (about 80%) show a smooth, round or oval contour. Variations of the pattern, however, are not unusual. Certain malignancies can present as lesions that are similar in appearance.

The diagnostic relevance of the fibroadenoma rests on differentiating it from smoothly margi- nated malignant tumors.

■ Histology

■ Fibroadenoma

The fibroadenoma is a benign fibroepithelial mixed tumor, surrounded by a pseudocapsule and generally exhibiting an oval, round, or lobulated shape with a smooth surface.

1. **Adult fibroadenomas** are usually found in young women as solitary tumors about 1–3 cm in size.
   Depending on the arrangement of the stromal and epithelial components, they are histologi- cally divided into intracanalicular and peri- canalicular tumors. This differentiation is clinically and prognostically irrelevant and also plays a secondary role in determining its presentation on imaging. Only minor differ- ences in its calcification pattern have been de- scribed.
   Types characterized by edematous stroma correspond radiographically to *"young" fi- broadenomas.*
   They predominantly occur in young women and under hormonal stimulation, correspond- ing to fibroadenomas in the growth phase. They frequently show a high proportion of loose, edematous and mucopolysaccharide- containing stroma and generally are well vascularized. The edematous stroma can com- press the epithelial components. In addition, there are fibroadenomas with hypercellular, adenomatous components. The "young" fi- broadenoma is usually soft and easily com- pressible.
   Focal or total sclerosis of the stroma occurs in *"older fibroadenomas,"* which are predomi- nantly diagnosed in older patients during or after menopause.
2. **The juvenile fibroadenoma** of puberty and adolescence frequently occurs as the so-called giant fibroadenoma, generally before the age of 20 years. It has a strong growth tendency and must be differentiated histologically from a phyllodes tumor. The juvenile fibroadenoma is a benign tumor. Even juvenile fibroade- nomas with florid cellular hyperplasia have a good prognosis and are adequately treated with simple excision.

■ Adenoma

Adenomas of the breast[5, 6] are rare, benign, usu- ally solitary, and well-differentiated neoplasms characterized by a dominant ductulolobular com- ponent. Adenomas are subject to hormonal regu- lation during pregnancy and lactation, and are further subclassified into tubular, lactating, ductal adenomas, and a few unusual types. Adenomas are mammographically indistinguishable from fi- broadenomas. Their imaging aspect will be pre- sented together with the fibroadenomas.

■ History

Fibroadenomas are often detected as a palpable finding but are also found mammographically. They rarely cause secretion. They can grow, decrease in size, or remain stationary through hormonal interaction.

■ Clinical Findings

Like the juvenile fibroadenoma, the "young" adult fibroadenoma feels smoothly marginated, elastic, and easily moveable on palpation. "Old" fibroade- nomas can be very firm on palpation. Since a few smoothly marginated malignant lesions can be soft on palpation, diagnostic clarification is nec- essary for all noncystic nodules.

■ Mammography

■ Image Presentation—Soft Tissue Density

The mammographic manifestations of the fi- broadenoma are as follows (Figs. 12.**2 a–h**):

- It usually presents as circumscribed, oval, lobulated, or round mass (Figs. 12.**2 a–h**)
- *Characteristically, it is sharply demarcated from the surrounding structures or accom- panied by a halo* (Fig. 12.**2b**)

The halo is a radiolucent border frequently seen around smoothly marginated lesions.

According to Sickles,[7] a round or oval nodule is called "circumscribed" if it is sharply outlined and more than 75% of its circumference is not ob- scured by adjacent isodense fibroglandular tissue.

If a round or oval nodule is well circum- scribed, with or without a halo, it can be assumed to represent a benign tumor, generally a fibroade- noma, with a probability exceeding 98%.

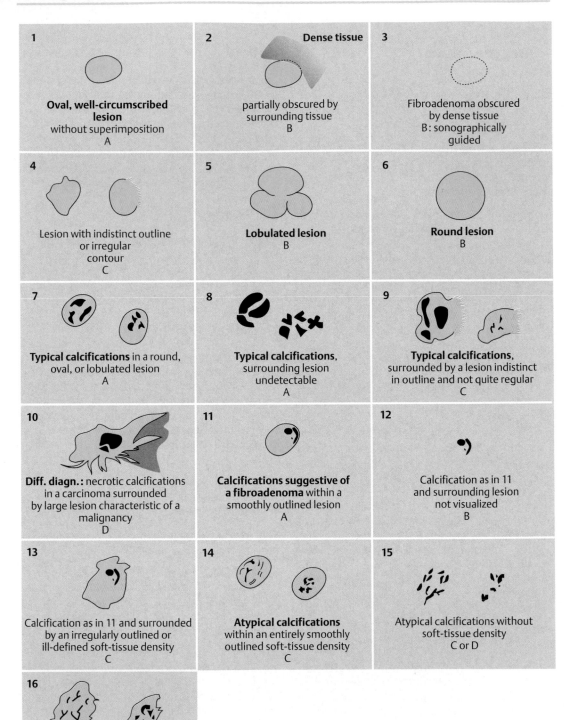

1

Oval, well-circumscribed lesion
without superimposition
A

2 Dense tissue

partially obscured by
surrounding tissue
B

3

Fibroadenoma obscured
by dense tissue
B: sonographically
guided

4

Lesion with indistinct outline
or irregular
contour
C

5

Lobulated lesion
B

6

Round lesion
B

7

Typical calcifications in a round,
oval, or lobulated lesion
A

8

Typical calcifications,
surrounding lesion
undetectable
A

9

Typical calcifications,
surrounded by a lesion indistinct
in outline and not quite regular
C

10

Diff. diagn.: necrotic calcifications
in a carcinoma surrounded
by large lesion characteristic of a
malignancy
D

11

Calcifications suggestive of
a fibroadenoma within a
smoothly outlined lesion
A

12

Calcification as in 11
and surrounding lesion
not visualized
B

13

Calcification as in 11 and surrounded
by an irregularly outlined or
ill-defined soft-tissue density
C

14

Atypical calcifications
within an entirely smoothly
outlined soft-tissue density
C

15

Atypical calcifications without
soft-tissue density
C or D

16

Atypical calcifications within a
not entirely smoothly
outlined soft-tissue density
C

Fig. 12.**2a–h a** After a complete mammographic workup, mammographic appearance of fibroadenomas with the conventional therapeutic recommendation:
A = Follow-up adequate
B = Follow-up or biopsy
C = Biopsy

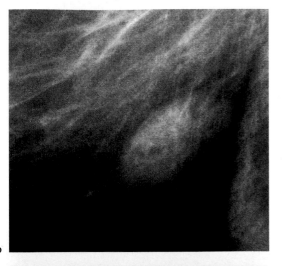

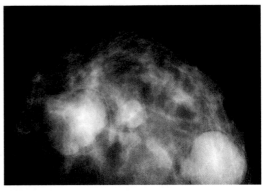

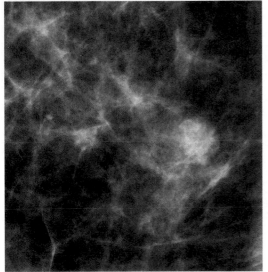

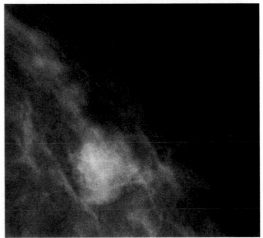

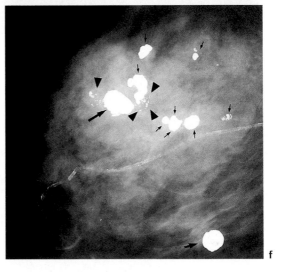

Fig. 12.**2b** Mammographically entirely smoothly outlined lesion (removed upon patient's request). *Histology:* myxoid fibroadenoma

c Young patient with multiple, smoothly outlined lesions with typical gentle lobulations

d Round mass. About 60 % of its margin is smoothly outlined. 40 % of its margin is obscured by overlying and adjacent breast tissue
(Sonography, see Fig. 12.**4e**)

e Nodular lesion, not entirely smoothly outlined, detected by screening mammography. *Histology:* predominantly fibrotic fibroadenoma

f In addition to fibroadenomas with typical coarse calcifications (arrows), fibroadenomas with small and partially bizarre calcifications (arrow heads) are present. The corresponding (and, because of fibrotic changes, indistinctly outlined) soft-tissue densities are only partially seen in the surrounding soft tissues

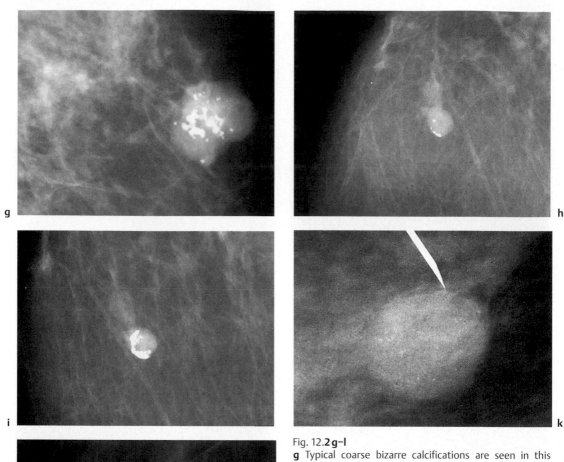

g

h

i

k

l

Fig. 12.**2 g–l**

g Typical coarse bizarre calcifications are seen in this lobulated fibroadenoma

h and **i** Often calcifications of the fibroadenomatous stroma begin along the periphery. Such eggshell-type calcifications are characteristic. They may increase with time. The second nodular lesion probably corresponds to a fibrosed fibroadenoma with somewhat irregular contours. It did not change for years

k Round to oval localized density with many delicate, punctate calcifications. Even though fine microcalcifications may occur in fibroadenomas, further workup is considered necessary to rule out other causes such as low-grade ductal carcinoma in situ. *Histology:* intracanalicular fibroadenoma

l Lobulated but sharply outlined localized density (arrows) with multiple most delicate, occasionally also linearly arranged, calcifications (as well as coarse calcifications) requiring further work-up. *Histology:* pericanalicular fibroadenoma

Fig. 12.**2m** In some fibroadenomas the mass itself may be obscured by dense tissue. In some old fibroadenomas the mass may disappear and only the calcifications persist. Only if these calcifications are characteristic (see Figs. 12.**2f–i**), the diagnosis of a fibroadenoma is obvious. In this case biopsy was recommended because of indeterminate microcalcifications, which also included some elongated shapes

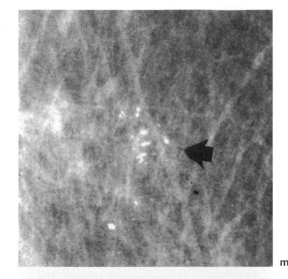

m

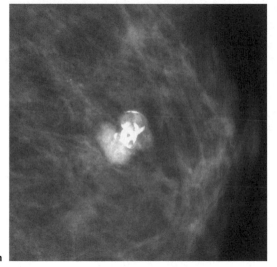

n

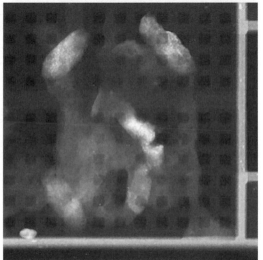

o

Fig. 12.**2n** and **o** Adjacent to a typical fibroadenoma there is an oval well-circumscribed mass (**n**). Its increased density is due to numerous very fine microcalcifications, which are better visualized on the specimen radiograph of the vacuum biopsy cores (**o**). In spite of its smooth margin and the halo, biopsy was performed because of the very fine microcalcifications. Histology: non-high-grade ductal carcinoma in situ

If a distinct margin is not observed on the standard mammographic views, a magnification view may be helpful to improve visualization of the lesion's contour (Fig. 3.**27**).

However, not all fibroadenomas are well-defined (Figs. 12.**2d** and **e**, Figs. 12.**5a–d**, and Figs. 12.**6a–d**):

● If a fibroadenoma is partially surrounded or obscured by dense parenchyma, its presence might only be suggested by a semiconvex density. If a fibroadenoma is completely surrounded by dense parenchyma, it may be totally obscured.

● Older fibroadenomas can shrink and become irregular or indistinct, causing differential diagnostic problems (Fig. 12.**2e**).

● The *juvenile or giant fibroadenoma* is mammographically indistinguishable from other hypercellular fibroadenomas. Since it is mainly found in juvenile patients, it is often obscured by dense parenchyma. Because of its rapid growth, it can be rather large at the time of presentation (Figs. 12.**3a–c**).

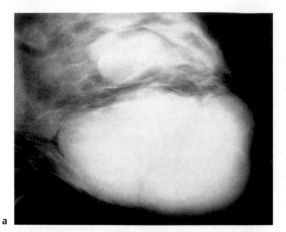

a

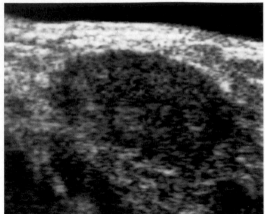

b

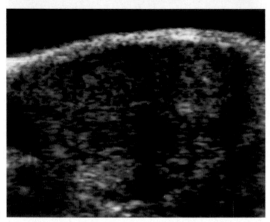

c

Fig. 12.**3a–c** Specific manifestations of fibroadenomas. Juvenile fibroadenoma of a 19-year-old patient

a A larger and a "smaller" macrolobulated fibroadenoma with smooth outline. The outline of the smaller fibroadenoma is partially obscured by dense parenchyma. The rapidly growing juvenile fibroadenomas characteristically do not contain any calcifications

b and **c** Sonographically, the juvenile fibroadenomas characteristically exhibit a homogeneous internal structure but can be heterogeneous. They are characteristically smooth in outline, show good sound transmission and are easily compressible. The sound transmission of both juvenile fibroadenomas shown here is moderate. The large one (**c**) also shows heterogeneity

- The adenoma may present on mammography like a typical fibroadenoma. Some adenomas (predominantly those in older patients) may be ill-defined, similar to a malignancy.

■ Image Presentation—Calcifications

Old fibroadenomas may partially calcify. The following types of dystrophic calcifications can be seen in fibroadenomas:[8, 9]

- A calcification completely or almost completely occupying the fibroadenoma is pathognomonic. A surrounding soft tissue density can be, but is not always, present (Figs. 12.**2a** and **f**).
- Coarse, popcorn-like, or bizarre calcifications (>2 mm!) are also pathognomonic (Figs. 12.**2a** and **f**).
- Evolving calcifications in a fibroadenoma can be rather indeterminate and include (Figs. 12.**2g** and **h**):

- Punctate calcifications
- Linear calcifications
- Granular, pleomorphic calcifications <2 mm

Only if such evolving calcifications are found within a circumscribed (see definition) soft tissue density, or if at least one additional shell-like calcification is present, is the finding mammographically highly consistent with a fibroadenoma. (Calcifications of the fibroadenomatous stroma characteristically begin along the periphery). Otherwise, the evolving and usually uncharacteristic calcifications may require biopsy for diagnosis.

Calcification Pattern in Various Subtypes

There seem to be minor differences in the calcification pattern of the *pericanalicular and intracanalicular fibroadenomas,* according to their different histologic compositions (Figs. 12.**2g** and **h**).[8, 9]

Evolving calcifications in the pericanalicular fibroadenoma begin frequently in the lactiferous ducts, and consequently can be linear, Y-shaped, or V-shaped like the branching calcifications observed in comedo carcinomas.

In contrast, the calcifications in the intracanalicular fibroadenoma, which has its epithelium usually compressed and atrophied by the myxoid stroma, are more often round or punctate.

While both calcification patterns can be explained by the histologic findings, they are by no means specific. Unless additional mammographic findings characteristic of a fibroadenoma are present (circumscribed and smoothly outlined soft tissue density or additional characteristic coarse calcifications), a reliable differentiation from calcifications of malignancy may be impossible.

Adenomas, too, may develop microcalcifications. These appear to be mostly punctate, densely packed, and sometimes irregular.[10]

■ Accuracy

- If mammographically characteristic calcifications are found, the diagnosis of a fibroadenoma can be established with a high degree of certainty. Further evaluation is unnecessary.
- In the presence of a mammographically smooth border (circumscribed nodule, see definition on p. 169), a benign mass can be assumed with a 98% certainty, usually a fibroadenoma.[7] Follow-up mammography is indicated at 6, 12, 24, and 36 months to assess stability.
- For the remaining variants, the accuracy is less. Depending on the imaging features, history, and clinical findings, follow-up mammography may be adequate. Otherwise, the evaluation should continue with percutaneous biopsy or, if multiple nodular densities are present, possibly with MRI.
- Because of the higher risk of malignancy, biopsy in the case of equivocal findings should be generously used in women above the age of 40 years.[11] Percutaneous biopsy is always appropriate if the lesion has an indistinct border, contains suspicious calcifications, or has enlarged on serial mammography.
- Excisional biopsy is recommended if the lesion has increased in size after core biopsy.

■ Sonography

■ Indications

Sonography is indicated in the diagnostic evaluation of presumed fibroadenomas if a cyst needs to be distinguished from a noncystic, i.e., solid, lesion or if a questionable palpable finding in a mammographically dense breast requires further evaluation.

Sonography is not indicated for differentiating between benign and malignant tumors if the mammographic or clinical findings are inconclusive. It is also inappropriate if the mass contains calcifications, excluding a cyst. It may, however, be useful in biopsy guidance.

■ Image Presentation

The following sonographic features are characteristic of a fibroadenoma
(Figs. 12.**4a, b**):[11, 12]

- Oval nodule whose long axis is oriented parallel to the transducer and whose horizontal diameter exceeds the vertical diameter by a factor of at least 1.5
- A completely smooth contour with or without delicate lateral boundary echo
- Uniform internal echoes
- Good moveability
- Delicate hyperechoic capsule

In addition, good sound transmission further supports the diagnosis of a fibroadenoma, but it is not an indispensable prerequisite for this diagnosis. Good compressibility has been mentioned by some investigators. However, this is not a widely accepted criterion.[40]

In contrast to these typical sonographic features, which are primarily found in young fibroadenomas with a high water content, two-thirds of fibroadenomas show the *following variations* (Figs. 12.**4c–g**, 12.**5b**, 12.**6b**):

- A macrolobulated nodule is suggestive but not diagnostic of a fibroadenoma
- A round configuration can be primarily found in small fibroadenomas (Fig. 12.**6b**), but other lesions, including malignant lesions, can have an identical pattern
- Some fibroadenomas are not sonographically detectable. They are isoechoic with the surrounding tissue

Fibroadenomas are characteristically seen as oval, smoothly outlined lesions with homogeneous internal structure and good to moderate acoustic enhancement:

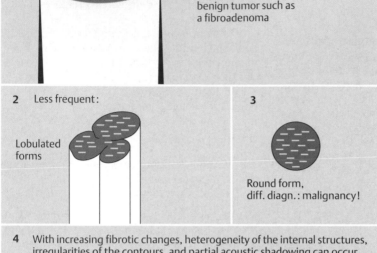

1

A delicate hyperechoic capsule is another important sign of a benign tumor such as a fibroadenoma

2   Less frequent:

Lobulated forms

3

Round form, diff. diagn.: malignancy!

4   With increasing fibrotic changes, heterogeneity of the internal structures, irregularities of the contours, and partial acoustic shadowing can occur. The compressibility of these fibroadenomas is generally poor:

5   Within calcified fibroadenomas, large acoustic shadows can be seen, sometimes arising behind hyperechoic structures:

Fig. 12.**4a–h** Sonographically characteristic appearance
a Diagrammatic scheme

Fig. 12.**4b** A typical fibroadenoma is shown: smooth margins; faint, very delicate capsule, homogenous echo texture. The ratio of the longitudinal and transverse diameters exceeds 1.5, and the long axis is parallel to the transducer. At the left lower margin a small cyst is imaged.
c Smoothly outlined fibroadenoma. The heterogeneous internal echo structures and the variable sound transmission are uncharacteristic. On the left, better distal acoustic enhancement (l) than right (r)
d Atypical fibroadenoma: Even though a hyperechoic capsule is shown, it appears somewhat irregular. The echo texture is not homogenous throughout the lesion.

(Furthermore, some posterior shadowing is seen.) Histology: fibrosed fibroadenoma.
e Fibroadenoma with irregular outline and heterogeneous internal structure. This finding is sonographically not distinguishable from a malignancy
f Fibrosed fibroadenoma. The fibrosed fibroadenoma (arrows) is markedly sound-absorbing. Consequently, it has a strong acoustic shadow and cannot be sonographically distinguished from a malignancy
g This fibroadenoma with shell-like calcifications mammographically exhibits hyperechoic structures (arrows) with dorsal acoustic shadowing. More delicate calcifications are not resolved sonographically

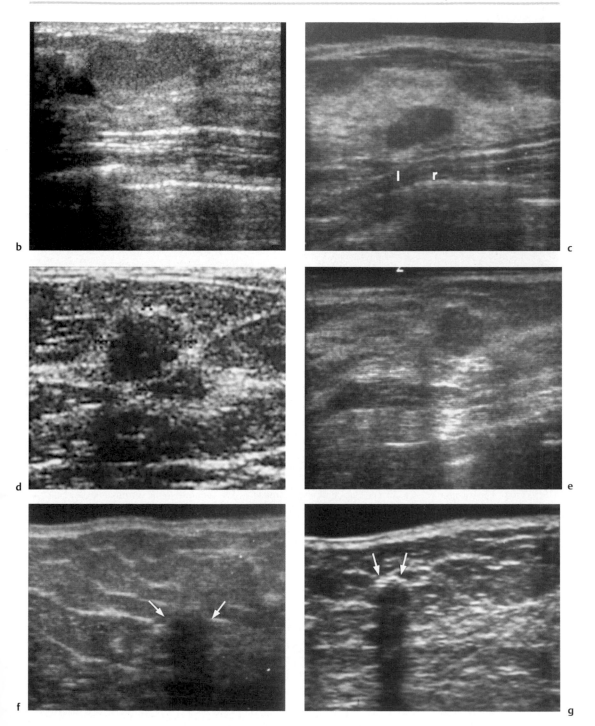

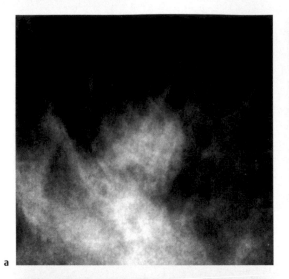

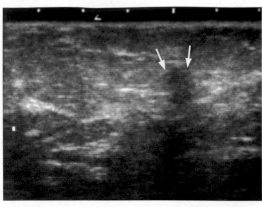

a

b

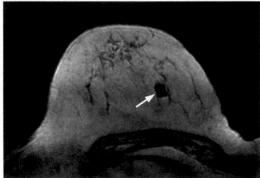

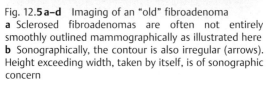

c

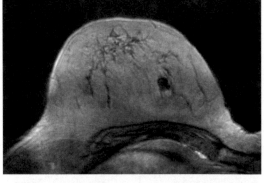

d

Fig. 12.**5 a–d** Imaging of an "old" fibroadenoma
a Sclerosed fibroadenomas are often not entirely smoothly outlined mammographically as illustrated here **b** Sonographically, the contour is also irregular (arrows). Height exceeding width, taken by itself, is of sonographic concern

c MRI (FLASH-3D) before contrast enhancement. The fibroadenoma is seen within the surrounding fat as nodular, not entirely smoothly outlined, low signal-intensity lesion (arrow)
d There is very little contrast enhancement of the tumor, which excludes a malignancy with a high degree of certainly (this is confirmed by stable mammographic and clinical findings over a 3-year period)

The following findings develop with increasing fibrosis within a fibroadenoma:

- Contour irregularities
- Heterogeneous internal echoes
- Formation of a complete or partial acoustic shadow behind the lesion
- Impaired compressiblity

Fibroadenomas with the above-mentioned sonographic features cannot be differentiated from malignancies.

- Calcifications in a fibroadenoma often cause acoustic shadowing. With increasing size of

the calcification, the acoustic shadowing often arises from a well-recognized echogenic structure (Fig. 12.4g). Though shadowing is in general atypical for a benign tumor, it is not significant when mammographically the mass contains calcifications that are typical of a fibroadenoma.

■ **Accuracy**

If all features above mentioned as sonographically typical are present, which is the case in only 20–30% of fibroadenomas, the diagnosis of a fibroadenoma can be made with reasonable cer-

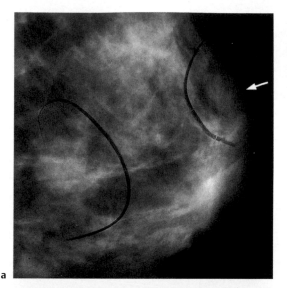

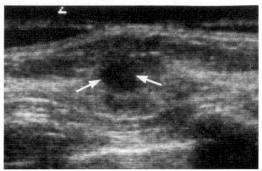

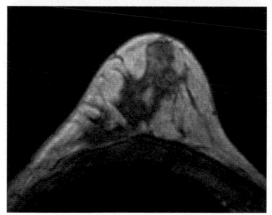

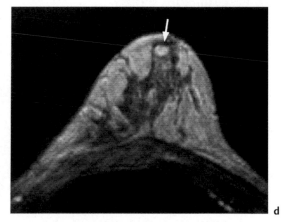

Fig. 12.**6a–d** Imaging of the nonfibrosed fibroadenoma. Since most nonfibrosed fibroadenomas show definite contrast enhancement and are consequently not distinguishable from a smoothly outlined fibroadenoma, core biopsy should be preferred rather than MRI as the most cost-effective method to evaluate a suspected fibroadenoma (young woman, soft to palpation and sonographically without acoustic shadowing)

a A palpable moveable tumor that is mammographically smoothly outlined anteriorly and not quite smoothly outlined posteriorly, located about 8 mm behind the nipple (as well as an additional lesion located centrally)

b Sonographically noncystic round hypoechoic lesion (arrow) with moderate sound transmission, not quite smoothly outlined

c and **d** MRI before (**c**) and after (**d**) intravenous injection of contrast medium. The nodule exhibits—as typical, but not diagnostic, of a "young" fibroadenoma—a smoot outline and intense enhancement. *Histology:* nonfibrosed intracanalicular fibroadenoma

tainty. (Reliable percentages of the accuracy, as available for mammographically circumscribed lesions, cannot be found in the sonographic literature.)

The following approach is recommended:

– Follow-up examinations (at intervals of 6 months) are justified if the sonographic features are characteristic of a fibroadenoma (compressible, easily moveable nodule with a smooth contour and homogeneous internal structure, as well as acoustic enhancement or unchanged dorsal acoustic intensity) and if there is no clinical or mammographic evidence of malignancy in a young woman (under the age of 35 years).

– Newly discovered findings should be evaluated by needle biopsy for further confirmation.

- Since malignancies may occasionally have findings resembling those of a fibroadenoma, a sonographic presentation typical of a fibroadenoma does not eliminate the possibility of a malignancy.

For *deviations from the typical image presentation,* the following applies:

- Even if the sonographic features are atypical, follow-up examinations are adequate as long as the mammographic diagnosis is unequivocal on the basis of typical calcifications or the nodule is known not to have changed for several years. This implies a fibroadenoma with a high degree of certainty.
- If mammographic and sonographic findings are atypical, biopsy should be considered.

■ Percutaneous Biopsy

Percutaneous biopsy is a proven and cost-effective method of establishing the diagnosis of a fibroadenoma if an adequate amount of tissue has been obtained. Hypercellular and edematous fibroadenomas are, in general, reliably diagnosed by percutaneous biopsy.

The diagnosis of sclerosed fibroadenomas is more difficult. Because of the generally decreased cellular content, they cannot always be diagnosed with certainty by conventional biopsy. However, vacuum biopsy will in doubtful cases usually allow a definite diagnosis.

■ Magnetic Resonance Imaging

■ Image Presentation

The MRI appearance depends on the composition of the fibroadenoma:[13, 14, 15]

- *Sclerosed fibroadenomas* (Fig. 12.**5a–d**) do not enhance, or enhance only minimally following injection of Gd-DTPA. Since some mucinous carcinomas can also show faint enhancement (most mucinous carcinomas show very intense enhancement), additional T2-weighted images are indicated for a nonenhancing solid lesion. A nonenhancing, sharply outlined nodule (which can have subtle contour irregularities) with *low signal intensity on the T2-weighted images can be excluded as being malignant with a high degree of certainty* and assumed to be a sclerosed fibroadenoma. Because of their high water content,

mucinous carcinomas have a high signal intensity on T2-weighted images.

- *Edematous and hypercellular young fibroadenomas,* however, show good and often also rapid enhancement of Gd-DTPA (Figs. 12.**6a–d**). The only features which appear to allow a quite reliable diagnosis concern smooth contours, oval shape, or gentle lobulations combined with visualization of low signal intensity septations. Though slow enhancement, as well as a smooth contour, are indicative of a fibroadenoma, a malignancy cannot be excluded with certainty. The reason is that part of the well-circumscribed malignancies also exhibit delayed enhancement (papillary, medullary carcinoma, some ductal carcinomas, and ductal carcinomas in situ). This is, in fact, usually compatible with a typically slow growth rate.

Since on the one hand MRI is very sensitive in the detection of *enhancing, sometimes tiny, fibroadenomas,* and on the other the workup of the numerous MRI-detected nodules is quite difficult yielding a very low number of malignancies, the following approach to well-circumscribed enhancing lesions is suggested:

- If the lesion is also visualized with other methods (mammography, sonography, physical examination) and not clearly classified as benign, it needs further evaluation by *percutaneous or excisional biopsy.*
- If the lesion is only detected by MRI in an asymptomatic patient, it should be *followed by MRI* (e.g., repeat MRI after 4 and 12 months, or after 6 and 18 months). If there are any doubts or if the patient is at high risk, MR-guided biopsy of the lesion, which is only visible on MRI, should be considered.

It should be pointed out that a ring-like enhancement or an early washout of contrast agent, if present, would speak against a fibroadenoma. This finding should lead to further workup (biopsy).

■ Accuracy

Because of the recognized high sensitivity of MRI in detecting malignancies, and the resultant high reliability of negative MRI findings in sclerosed fibroadenomas (contrast-enhanced MRI combined with a T2-weighted pulse sequence), MRI appears to the suitable for the diagnosis of the sclerosed fibroadenoma. The high sensitivity of MRI in the detection of young enhancing fibroadenomas and the inadequate specificity in differentiating them from circumscribed malignancies is problematic.

Therefore percutaneous biopsy is most appropriate for evaluating clinically, mammographically, or sonographically suspected fibroadenomas.

For the evaluation of suspected fibrous fibroadenomas (older woman, mammographically detected contour irregularity without direct signs of malignancy, sonographically diminished elasticity, moderate sound transmission or even attenuation), MRI appears appropriate. It appears to be particularly advantageous if the lesions are small, deep, and multiple.

■ Diagnostic Goals

The most important role of imaging in the diagnosis of fibroadenoma consists of differentiating it from well-circumscribed malignancies with similar findings. In addition to the well-circumscribed ductal carcinoma, this includes medullary and papillary carcinomas, lymphomas, sarcomas, and metastases. The phyllodes tumors can also have a similar pattern. All these tumors can occasionally be completely well circumscribed, even surrounded by a mammographically detectable halo (see p. 211 for significance of the halo).

An excision of all circumscribed or round lesions, performed as a safety measure to find all rare circumscribed malignancy, does not appear in the best interest of the patient and cannot be justified for economic reasons. Even if only lesions deemed benign with a probability of benignity lower than 98% were all biopsied, a biopsy rate of over 1:10, or worse, would result. (This means that less than 1 carcinoma will be found in 10 recommended biopsies). It is for this reason that imaging methods should be used as much as possible to avoid unnecessary biopsies.

■ Overview of the Diagnostic Strategy

- The typically calcified fibroadenoma is mammographically pathognomonic. Additional evaluation or follow-up examinations are not necessary.
- Mammographically well-circumscribed solid masses (definition see p. 211), which are primarily fibroadenomas, are benign in 98% of the cases. In this situation follow-up mammo-

graphy at intervals of 6, 12, 24, and 36 months is appropriate.
- The remaining solitary, circumscribed non-palpable, and most likely benign lesions that do not entirely fulfill the above-mentioned criteria may be subjected to percutaneous or excisional biopsy.

Because of the characteristic doubling rates of breast carcinomas and the rather slow growth rates of some circumscribed malignancies, the intervals of follow-up examinations should not be less than 6 months. The follow-up period should not be less than 3 years, and the current examination should be compared with the initial and not with the most recent examination.
- When masses do not contain calcifications, sonography should be used to differentiate between cyst and solid tumor, as well as to characterize palpable lesions that are hidden by mammographically dense tissue.
- Sonography cannot achieve a definitive differentiation of mammographically indeterminate noncystic masses from malignancy.
- A lesion seen only sonographically and exhibiting the typical features of a fibroadenoma (p. 217) may be followed at regular intervals or undergo a percutaneous biopsy if neither the patient's history nor clinical and mammographic findings reveal evidence of malignancy.
- For further evaluation of a suspected fibroadenoma that has been newly discovered and appears clinically and mammographically benign but does not fulfil all criteria of a benign lesion, percutaneous biopsy is appropriate. If biopsy reveals a fibroadenoma, an excisional biopsy is not necessary.
- If a small sclerosed fibroadenoma is not amenable to percutaneous needle biopsy, or if the lesions are multiple, MRI (contrast-enhanced MRI combined with T2-weighted pulse sequence) can be obtained.
- Increasing size of a circumscribed tumor or suspected malignancy (irregular contour, suspected calcifications) is an indication for biopsy.

■ Summary

The most important role of the diagnostic methods in diagnosing a fibroadenoma is the definitive differentiation, if possible, from the rare circumscribed malignancies and the avoidance of high rates of excisional biopsies exclusively performed for diagnostic purposes.

The mammographically pathognomonic finding of a calcified fibroadenoma unfortunately only makes up for a small proportion of the fibroadenomas. The typical mammographic finding is the well-circumscribed nodule (see definition, p. 211), with or without halo. Its risk of malignancy is less than 2%.

Sonography serves to separate fibroadenomas from cysts and to diagnose fibroadenomas that are mammographically obscured by dense tissue, but not to characterize unclear mammographic findings. If the sonographic lesion corresponds to a newly detected finding, confirmation of the presumed diagnosis by percutaneous biopsy is recommended.

Exceptions and variations of the typical mammographic and sonographic findings are common. They require further evaluation, which can be achieved by follow-up examinations, percutaneous biopsy, MRI, or excision. Percutaneous biopsy should be done first because of its cost-effectiveness. MRI should be considered for fibrosed fibroadenomas (very small lesions, multiple lesions, unfavorable location).

When a lesion is being followed, the follow-up examinations should be done initially at 6 months and then at intervals of 12 months for at least a total of 3 years. If any suspicion arises, e.g., if the lesion increases in size, excisional biopsy should be considered.

Papilloma

The papilloma is a benign fibroepithelial tumor of the breast. It represents 1–1.5% of the breast tumors. Even relatively small papillomas can become symptomatic by causing a clear or bloody nipple discharge. The role of clinical evaluation and diagnostic imaging (including galactography, see pp. 74–80) consists of determining the localization and extent of the papilloma or papillomas.

Occasionally a papilloma can be detected as a palpable finding or mammographic density and is then to be differentiated from other nodular-shaped masses.

It is important to know that certain types of papilloma can be associated with an increased risk of malignancy, depending on presentation (singular or multiple) and localization (subareolar versus peripheral).

Because of the difficult differentiation among papilloma, papillary carcinoma, or other nodular lesions, excision of papillomas is often diagnostically and therapeutically desirable.

■ Histopathology

They are classified as:[2, 16–19]

1. *Intraductal, subareolar, solitary papilloma:* It generally extends over a length of 0.5 to 3.5 cm and is subject to involutional changes. These tumors are benign. Related to the occasional coexistance of atypical hyperplasia or foci of in situ carcinoma, they are followed by papillary or other carcinomas after excision in 4%.

2. *Small peripheral intraductal papillomas:* They are situated in the peripheral ductal segments and generally are coexistent finding of proliferative changes seen in fibrocystic breasts. They are associated with an increased recurrence rate and cancer incidence of 12%.

3. *Papillary adenoma of the nipple:* It is a benign tumor, frequently leading to erosions and occurring unilaterally and bilaterally. In 12% of the cases, concurrent or subsequent ipsilateral and contralateral carcinomas are found.

4. *Juvenile papillomatosis:* It is a disease of puberty and adolescence, featuring atypical papillary duct hyperplasia, which has been observed in families with an increased incidence of cancer. An increased risk of breast cancer has not yet been found in these patients.

■ Properties

Papillomas usually show evidence of secretory activity (watery to yellowish discharge). They are very friable and bleed easily (brownish or bloody discharge). Papillomas have the tendency to infarct. Old papillomas can become completely fibrosed and can contain calcifications.

Because of their intraductal location and high vulnerability, they can

- Lead to watery or bloody discharge
- Distend ducts
- Distend cysts
- Be surrounded by a blood-containing cavity

■ Differentiation

The histologic differentiation from a papillary carcinoma is not always easy. Singular or multiple papillomas must be differentiated from papillomatosis. In contrast to singular and multiple papillomas, which are spatially separate tumors, papillomatosis manifests itself as regional epithelial hyperplasia and can be part of proliferative changes in fibrocystic breasts. In papillomatosis the risk of malignancy is increased—as in other proliferative changes—depending on degree and extent of cellular atypia.

■ Clinical Findings

Discharge can be found in 80% of the papillomas and can be watery, yellowish, brownish, or bloody, whereby a bloody discharge strongly suggests a papilloma. Carcinomas can also cause a bloody discharge (in up to 25% of the cases) and rarely a watery discharge, occurring in only 2–3% of carcinomas with discharge. A thorough diagnostic evaluation is therefore indicated.

Not infrequently, the localization of one or multiple papillomas can be suspected clinically if nipple discharge can be elicited by pressure on the so-called *trigger points.*

Only a few papillomas are primarily detected by palpation, mammography, or sonography. These papillomas are usually large, superficial, or have caused a retention cyst or "hemorrhagic cyst" through ductal obstruction.

■ Cytology of Nipple Discharge

The cytologic evaluation of nipple discharge can be easily performed and does not put any demand on the patient. A positive finding (cords of papillary cells, suspected cells, blood) should be an indication for further evaluation.

Cytology of the nipple discharge, which is based on the necrotic changes of the shed cells found in the discharge, is only of moderate sensitivity. A negative finding does not exclude a carcinoma. Furthermore, a reliable differentiation between carcinoma and papilloma cannot be expected from the cytologic assessment of the nipple discharge.

■ Diagnostic Strategy and Goals

Since most papillomas are detected by their secretory activity, the diagnostic questions to be answered are:

- *Confirmation of a papillary lesion.* In addition to papillary tumors, there are other causes of nipple discharge (as to the differential diagnosis of pathologic nipple discharge, see Chapter 22)
- *Localization* (search for the point of origin of the secretion)
- *Extent* (one papilloma or multiple papillomas)

Initially, noninvasive methods like mammography, sonography, and a careful clinical examination are utilized.

Clinical examination (trigger point) as well as *mammography* (for large papillomas in a fatty breast) can point to the correct localization in some cases. The full extent is rarely appreciated mammographically or clinically.

In selected cases (intracystic or large papillomas, very rare small papillomas located in the subareolar ducts), a papilloma can be detected *sonographically.*

In many instances, localization and extent cannot be adequately evaluated with noninvasive methods. Above all, this applies to small papillomas surrounded by nonfatty tissue. In these cases, galactography is indicated as a supplemental examination. By showing filling defects or, less frequently, truncated ducts, it can detect papillomas and allows an assessment of their extent. Absence of any filling defects or truncated ducts—together with cytologic absence of suspected cells or cords of papillary cells—excludes an intraductal lesion with a high degree of certainty.

Thus the imaging methods can suggest or exclude a papillary lesion in the majority of cases.

The important differentiation between papilloma and carcinoma is radiologically not possible. Consequentially, *imaging is not adequate for determining the histology of suspected papillary lesions,* and should primarily support the planning of the inevitable diagnostic excision.

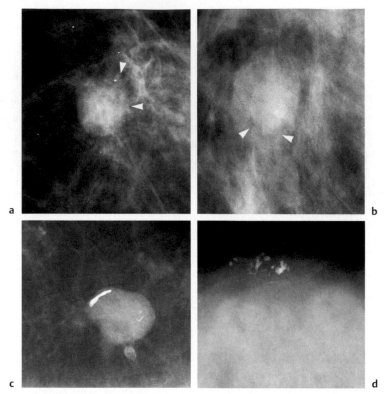

Fig. 12.**7a–d**   Papilloma. Mammographic presentation

a As in this case, the papilloma is often visualized as mass that frequently is incompletely outlined or even shows irregularities of contour (arrows).
A papilloma can occasionally be suspected on the basis of the lesion's location in the region of the retromamillary ducts
b Intracystic papillomas are often visualized—caused by the smooth wall of the surrounding cyst—as smoothly outlined lesions. In this case, the distal aspect of the cyst (arrow heads) is superimposed by dense surrounding tissue (sonography of this lesion, see Fig. 12.**9a**).
The cyst surrounding the papilloma can be a true cyst or a hemorrhagic cavity around the papilloma

c Nodular lesion with a shell-like calcification. A few uncharacteristic and v-shaped microcalcifications are visible. Although malignancy is possible because of the indistinct posterior border as well as the v-shaped microcalcifications, the shell-like calcification is consistent with a calcified wall of the cyst, as observed in a hemorrhagic cyst. By itself, such a marginal calcification could also be typical for a fibroadenoma. *Histology:* benign intracystic papilloma with occasional calcifications and partially calcified hemorrhagic cyst
d Some papillomas may contain characteristic calcifications. In this case, typical coarse calcifications as well as occasional elongated, delicate, suspicious calcifications in the retroareolar ducts are shown. Because of the latter calcifications, an excisional biopsy was obtained. *Histology:* benign largely calcified retroareolar papilloma

■ Mammography
(Fig. 12.**7a–d**)

Conventional mammography[23, 21] generally does not reveal small papillomas surrounded by dense tissue. If papillomas are suspected because of nipple discharge, magnification and compression views might delineate them in the subareolar region as a small mass or as isolated ductal dilatation. Sometimes high-resolution ultrasound can show an intraductal abnormality. If the cause of

secretion or the exact extent of the pathologic intraductal changes cannot be determined with certainty, galactography can be performed.

If papillomas—as is often the case in older patients—are surrounded by fatty tissue, they appear as nodular, round, or oval masses, ranging from a few millimeters to, though rarely, 2–3 cm in size. They are—in particular, if large—not as sharply outlined as fibroadenomas, and are then not reliably distinguishable from a carcinoma.

Papillomas that cause cystic dilatation of a ductal segment or a hemorrhagic cyst might be seen as a smoothly outlined, well-circumscribed mass, with or without halo. The smooth contour corresponds to the wall of the cyst.

If solitary papillomas appear as a round or oval mass in the subareolar area, the correct diagnosis can be presumed on the basis of their location. Only a few papillomas develop sclerotic changes and can subsequently calcify. Typical calcifications appear intraductally following a duct that may be dilated. They can be—resembling fibroadenoma-type calcifications—coarse or shell-like, but also punctate and densely aggregated in a round group (Fig. 22.**47a**). Only this typical manifestation allows the mammographic assumption of a papillary tumor.

■ Galactography
(Fig. 12.**8**)

Galactographically,[21, 22] papillomas appear as filling defects or truncated ducts. While small blood clots or debris can cause similar defects, multiple irregular filling defects and obstructed ducts strongly suggest the presence of intraductal papillary tumors. Uncertain findings can be differentiated from blood clots, debris, or even small air bubbles by emptying the ductal system, followed by a repeat instillation of contrast medium. Only true intraductal lesions reappear at the same site (see also Chapter 3, pp. 74–80).

Galactography can confirm the presence of an intraductal lesion and determine its exact location and extent. *Differentiation of a benign lesion from an intraductal carcinoma* is galactographically *not possible,* and excision of the suspicious ductal segment is always necessary.

■ Sonography
(Fig. 12.**9a–f**)

Sonographically,[23–25] intraductal papillomas can occasionally be identified in the subareolar ducts. Because of the unreliable detection of smaller and peripherally located papillomas, sonography cannot replace galactography.

Sonography can reliably detect intracystic papillomas. They are recognized as hypoechoic lesions surrounded by echo-free cystic fluid. In contrast to intracystic sediment, their appearance remains constant with positional changes. If the papilloma occupies the cyst entirely or almost entirely, or if the cystic fluid has become echogenic

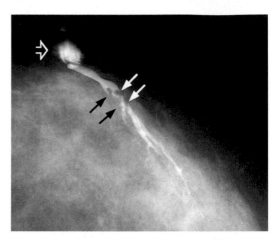

Fig. 12.**8** Papilloma: galactography. The galactographic delineation of a slightly dilated retroareolar duct reveals several small filling defects (arrows) caused by a benign papilloma growing along the duct (small retroareolar extravasation [open arrow])

due to hemorrhage, the hypoechoic to hyperechoic lesion cannot always be differentiated from other solid lesions.

Furthermore. benign papillomas may be imaged as a solid, smooth, well-defined nodule, compatible with a benign tumor. Sometimes contours may not be completely well-circumscribed. If calcifications are present in the papilloma, shadowing will be seen. Differentiating a benign papilloma from a papillary carcinoma cannot be achieved by any imaging method, even sonography.

■ Magnetic Resonance Imaging
(Figs. 12.**10a–d**)

The MR characteristics of papillomas are similar to those described for fibroadenomas.[13]

Sclerosing papillomas do not or only minimally enhance, and nonsclerosing papillomas, even if small, demonstrate marked enhancement. Differentiation of a small enhancing, nonsclerosing papilloma from enhancement of other benign proliferations, or from malignancies, is not possible.

Furthermore, discharge can be associated with diffuse or patchy enhancement in the entire breast parenchyma (probably secondary to concurrent inflammatory changes). Since this can cause differential diagnostic problems, MRI cannot be recommended as the first method for evaluating the breast with nipple discharge.

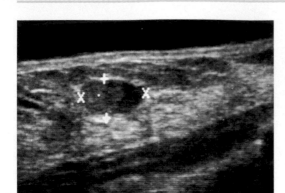

a

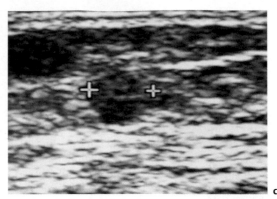

c

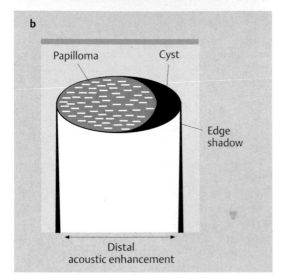

b

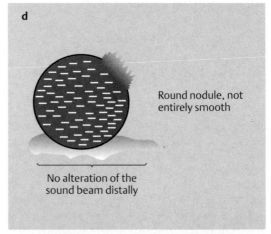

d

Fig. 12.9 a–f Papilloma: sonography
a The intracystic papilloma is characteristically seen as a hypoechoic to hyperechoic (as observed here) lesion within a mostly hypoechoic, smoothly outlined hemorrhagic "cyst"
b Diagram
c A hypoechoic, not quite smoothly outlined lesion is found if the content of the cyst becomes thickened. In this case, a distinction of the papilloma itself and the surrounding echogenic fluid is no longer possible, and the complete complex lesion is only visible as a hypoechoic mass
d Diagram
e This oval solid mass distends the surrounding duct. Biopsy demonstrates it to be a papilloma

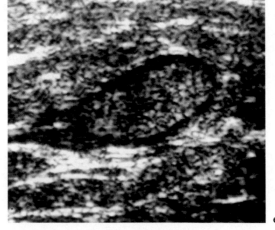

e

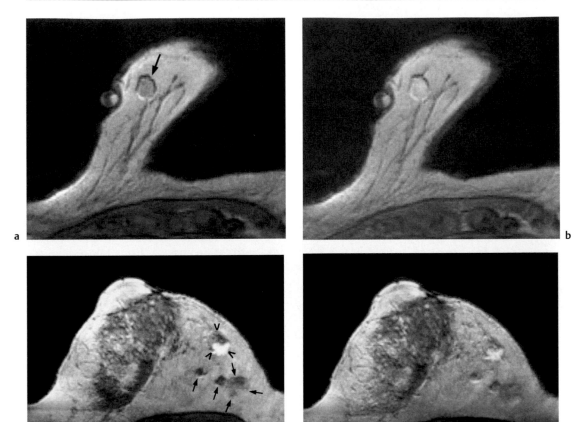

Fig. 12.**10 a–d**   Papilloma: MRI

a and **b** MRI of a nonsclerosing large papilloma. The papilloma (arrow), which was palpable, shows contrast enhancement and consequently is not distinguishable from an enhancing fibroadenoma or a smoothly outlined malignancy

c and **d** In this patient with multiple, not quite smoothly outlined lesions, the T1-weighted image shows a moderately decreased signal intensity in three of the lesions (arrows) that is compatible with solid tumors. The fourth nodule (arrow head) is seen as a complex lesion. The very high signal intensity, already seen in the unenhanced image (**c**), is characteristic of a hemorrhagic cyst. The anterior wall, which exhibits a low signal, is thickened and nodular. This finding of an MRI already suggests a cystic papilloma before Gd-DTPA application.

All papillomas show only slight and delayed enhancement. Since papillary carcinomas often show the same enhancement pattern, an excisional biopsy was advised. *Histology:* fibrosed, nodular growing, and partially intracystic papillomas

■ Percutaneous Biopsy

The differentiation between papilloma and papillary carcinoma is difficult, and many pathologists cannot differentiate between these with satisfactory certainty on the basis of a core biopsy. Therefore, if a papilloma is suspected, it may be desirable to perform excisional biopsy.

If a core needle biopsy yielded a papillary tumor, correlation with imaging is important.[26] In case of any discrepancy or in case—based on the available material—the pathologist requires further workup, surgical biopsy should be performed.

■ Summary

Standard mammography generally shows the somewhat larger papillomas surrounded by fat. A definitive diagnosis is only rarely possible. In a few cases, typical calcifications are found in sclerosing papillomas.

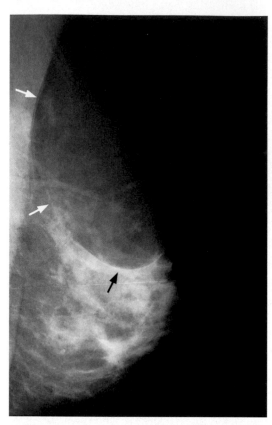

Fig. 12.**11** Lipoma. It is visualized as a smoothly outlined nodule of fat density and a delicate capsule of fibrous tissue. (The subtle densities observed in a pure lipoma should correspond to superimposed parenchyma.) This unequivocally benign finding is not an indication for a biopsy

Galactography is the examination of choice for detecting or excluding intraductal papillomas that are symptomatic because of secretion. It confirms an intraductal process and demonstrates the exact location and extent, as well as any possible additional papillomas.

Intracystic papillomas may be detected and diagnosed sonographically if they do not occupy the entire cyst. Otherwise, they are not distinguishable from other solid masses.

Since reliable differentiation of a benign papilloma from a carcinoma is not possible with any imaging modality, and since some papillomas are at risk of malignant degeneration, surgical biopsy should be applied generously on diagnostic and therapeutic grounds whenever a papillary lesion is suspected.

Lipoma

Lipomas are benign tumors composed of fat. They may be palpable lesions or a dominant area of fat within the breast, usually surrounded by a thin capsule.

Differentiation: Lipomatous metaplasias of the connective tissue may appear with advancing age. They are a manifestation of lipomatous atrophy of the breast parenchyma. Occasionally, these lipomatous structures are incorrectly termed lipomas but do not correspond to real ones.

Tumors, which are largely but not completely composed of fat and surrounded by a pseudocapsule, may be found in the breast as well. These are adeno-(fibro)-lipomas or hamartomas and not true lipomas.

■ Clinical Findings

Clinically, lipomas appear as soft, smoothly outlined tumors, but can be firm, smoothly outlined, and moveable. They might only be seen mammographically.

■ Diagnostic Strategy

Mammography is the most important method for diagnosing the lipoma. Definitive diagnosis and reliable exclusion of a malignancy can be achieved for all lipomas by mammography.

■ Mammography
(Fig. 12.**11**)

Lipomas are positively diagnosed mammographically:

- Pathognomonic is the fat density of the nodule, exclusively comprising fat lobules, which are traversed by thin connective tissue septa.
- The delicate connective tissue capsule is seen completely or partially around the nodule. This mammographic appearance is so characteristic that further evaluation is superfluous.

■ Sonography, Magnetic Resonance Imaging, or Needle Biopsy

These methods are not indicated in the diagnostic investigation of the lipoma.

Rare Benign Tumors

The following rare benign tumors of the breast are briefly discussed:

1. Leiomyoma, neurofibroma, neurilemmoma, benign spindle cell tumor, chondroma, osteoma
2. Angioma
3. Granulosa cell tumor

Leiomyoma, Neurofibroma, Neurilemmoma, Benign Spindle Cell Tumor, Chondroma, Osteoma

(Fig. 12.**12**)

These benign tumors are very rare.[27–29]

The leiomyoma[27] arises from the smooth muscles of the vessels, nipple region, and ductal structures.

The neurofibroma, as well as the rarer neurilemmoma, derives from the sheath of the peripheral nerves. It usually is located intracutaneously (see Chapter 19), less frequently subcutaneously.[28]

The extremely rare benign spindle cell tumor originates from the mesenchymal cells,[29] similar to the mesenchymal origin of the metaplastic chondroma and osteoma.

Epithelial and dermoid cysts are found more frequently in the cutaneous or subcutaneous connective and lipomatous tissues.

In accordance with their histologic growth pattern, these tumors are seen as smoothly outlined, oval to round structures. Except for their frequent subcutaneous location, there are no further criteria that distinguish these tumors from fibroadenomas or other smoothly outlined lesions. Only chondromas and osteomas can have characterizing matrix calcifications that might resemble bizarre fibroadenomatous calcifications.

Because of the nonspecific appearance, the final diagnosis cannot be made by diagnostic imaging. The diagnostic approach is the same as applied to other masses with a nodular pattern (e.g., fibroadenoma). The diagnosis of benignity is possible for those rare benign tumors that are well circumscribed or fat-containing (definition, see p. 211). The specific diagnosis is only possible histologically.

Angiomas

Intramammary angiomas that are not in the skin or in the subcutaneous tissues are rare. They encompass:[2, 30–32]

– Various forms of hemangiomas
– The angiolipoma, the lymphangioma, and
– The Angiomatosis

These tumors are benign. Hemangioma, angiolipoma, and angiomatosis are well vascularized. *Clinically,* they are inconspicuous, unless intracutaneous or subcutaneous. They can cause the sensation of tension or pain, grow slowly or thrombose, and then become painful. Subcutaneous angiomas may appear bluish through the overlying skin and can even grow into the skin. If they are palpable, they feel soft and sponge-like.

Most hemangiomas are smoothly marginated and oval to lobulated. An indistinct outline is rare. Lymphangiomas, angiolipomas—which always contain lipomatous inclusions—and angiomatoses often grow in lobulated and permeative fashion,

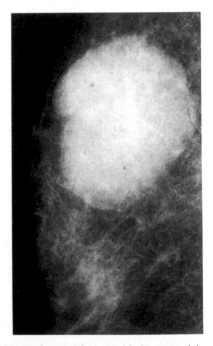

Fig. 12.**12** This painless, easily moveable breast nodule in a 58-year-old man was found to be a leiomyoma (from Barth[27]). The mammographic pattern is nonspecific

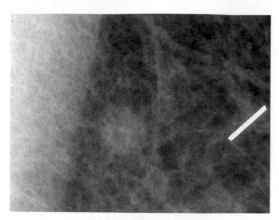

Fig. 12.**13** Mammographically indistinctly outlined nodular lesion, right upper quadrant. This indistinctness prompted a diagnostic excision. *Histology:* granular cell tumor

with corresponding image presentation. Rarely, round calcifications can occur in angiomas.

The sonographic pattern is variable. An echogenic pattern can be expected because of their vascularity.

A typical clinical presentation of an intracutaneous or subcutaneous hemangioma obviates the diagnostic biopsy.

For nodules situated in deeper structures, the histologic diagnosis after excision is decisive. Increasing size is always an indication for an excision, since the differentiation from an angiosarcoma can only be settled histologically.

Granular Cell Tumor (Myoblastoma)

(Fig. 12.**13**)

The granular cell tumor is a rare benign neurogenic tumor, derived from Schwann cells and histologically recognized by an eosinophilic granular cytoplasm.[4] It is distinguishable from other benign tumors by its ill-defined, sometimes spiculated margins.

Mammographically and sonographically, it exhibits features of a spiculated mass and resembles a scirrhous carcinoma macroscopically.[33–35]

A single case of granular cell tumor know to us was examined by contrast-enhanced MRI[36] and found to be indistinguishable from a scirrhous carcinoma due to its irregular margin and enhancement pattern.

Benign Fibroses

The benign fibroses include diabetic mastopathy and focal fibrosis.

Diabetic Mastopathy or Fibrosis

Diabetic mastopathy is a relatively rare disease, found in one study in 13% of insulin-dependent diabetics, with all patients under the age of 40 years.[37] Presenting as palpable breast masses and asymmetric mammographic densities, it can mimic a malignancy and poses a diagnostic problem. Such palpable masses can recur in different regions of the breast.

■ Histology

Microscopically, it is a unifocal or multifocal fibrosis associated with lymphoid lobulitis or perivasculitis. These changes are attributed to autoimmune reaction to diabetogenic abnormal matrix accumulation.

■ Clinical Findings

Clinically, newly developed palpable breast masses and indurations that cannot be distinguished from malignancies are noticed.

■ Diagnostic Strategy

Imaging cannot be expected to provide definite differentiation between diabetic mastopathy and carcinoma. Suspected calcifications, however, would speak against a diabetic mastopathy. In insulin-dependent diabetics with recurrent suspected nodules, the possibility of a diabetic mastopathy should be considered.

■ Mammography
(Fig. 12.**14a**)

Based on current knowledge, the mammographic spectrum encompasses radiodense tissue as seen with mastopathy, indeterminate masses, or asym-

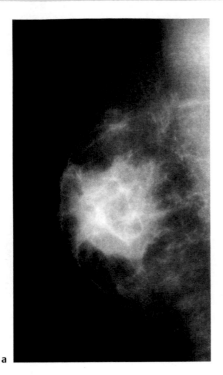

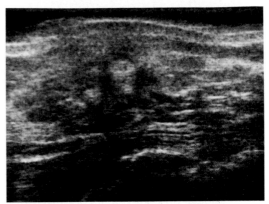

Fig. 12.**14a** and **b**   Diabetic mastopathy, 39-year-old patient with juvenile diabetes
a Mammographically and clinically very suspicious spiculated central mass
b Sonographically, the lesion is hypoechoic with moderate sound attenuation and ill-defined margins.
Histology: fibrosis with signs of inflammation. Follow-up visit a year later because of similar finding in the contralateral breast. MRI shows intense enhancement. Suspecting a diabetic mastopathy, a core biopsy was obtained and the patient observed. Resolution of the mammographic and clinical findings and of the MRI contrast enhancement within 1 year

metries and ill-defined nodules with spiculation. A mammographic differentiation from a carcinoma is generally not possible.[38–40]

■ Sonography
(Fig. 12.**14b**)

Sonographically, dense acoustic shadowing is observed posterior to the region of concern.[38, 41,42]

■ Magnetic Resonance Imaging

In a single patient,[40] early and intense enhancement was found in an irregularly outlined area corresponding to a suggestive palpatory finding. This regressed within a year. The strong enhancement can be explained on the basis of an inflammatory process.

In the acute stage, therefore, MRI does not offer any distinguishing feature from a malignancy.

■ Percutaneous Biopsy

In suspected diabetic mastopathy, the percutaneous biopsy appears to offer an approach that avoids the otherwise necessary repeated diagnos-

tic excisional biopsies of recurrences (usually appearing at a different site).

■ Summary

Diabetic mastopathy induces the formation of palpable nodules and asymmetries that correspond histologically to inflammatory infiltrative fibrosis.
The mammographic image shows dense tissue with or without focal thickening or formation of masses, possibly with retraction and spiculation. The sonographic findings include marked shadowing and MRI shows intense enhancement. Thus, no reliable differentiation from or exclusion of a carcinoma is possible.

Focal Fibrous Disease or Fibrosis Mammae

Focal fibrous disease is found in young women. It is a circumscribed fibrous proliferation of the mammary stroma associated with regional atrophy of the surrounding parenchyma. The average size is 1–3 cm and is observed in biopsies with an incidence of 4–8%.

Mammographically, focal fibrous disease can appear as a sharply outlined nodule or as an irregularly outlined mass.[43]

Sonographically, acoustic shadowing should be expected behind an echo-poor irregular mass.

MRI shows no enhancement and excellent differentiation from a carcinoma can be expected.

Percutaneous biopsy shows the presence of abundant fibrosis, which is an unspecific finding. (With larger sample, confidence in the diagnosis will increase.)

In summary, the focal fibrous disease is mammographically visualized as a single, smoothly or irregularly outlined mass. To distinguish it from a carcinoma, percutaneous biopsy, MRI, or excisional biopsy is necessary.

Intramammary Lymph Nodes

■ Definition

Intramammary lymph nodes are lymph nodes that are located within the breast, i.e., between the parenchyma and connective tissue of the breast. Lymph nodes in the axillary extension of the breast are still considered intramammary if they are in regions surrounded by parenchyma. Outside these regions they are assigned to the axilla.

■ Prevalence

Intramammary lymph nodes are frequently seen by mammography. Small intramammary lymph nodes are often not visualized because of their small size and insufficient density, particularly within mammographically dense parenchyma.

■ Purpose

In the *asymptomatic patient,* the intramammary lymph node is considered a *normal structure.* The correct diagnostic identification—often achievable on the basis of the image presentation—is important, to avoid unnecessary biopsies.

If an underlying malignant condition is present, the intramammary lymph nodes may contain metastatic deposits. Macroscopic metastatic involvement causes the mammographically typical nodal morphology to disappear. Microscopic involvement is undetectable by imaging.

■ Histology

Histologically, intramammary are not different from other lymph nodes.

■ Clinical Findings

Clinically, the intramammary lymph node is generally not noticed. On occasion, these can be palpable.

■ Diagnostic Strategy and Goals

The goal of the diagnostic workup should be:

- The correct recognition of a lymph node in asymptomatic patients, to avoid unnecessary biopsies
- The detection of macroscopically involved intramammary lymph nodes (contour, density, hilus) in patients with a known carcinoma

■ Imaging

The imaging morphology of normal lymph nodes and of lymph nodes with benign and malignant changes is described in Chapter 16. Imaging morphology of intramammary lymph nodes is identical to that of axillary lymph nodes.

■ Percutaneous Biopsy

If a mass suspected to be a lymph node by imaging does not show the typical characteristics of a benign or normal lymph node, further workup is required. If microscopic involvement needs to be excluded (e.g., staging of a known carcinoma), histopathologic evaluation of the complete mass is needed. Excisional biopsy may be necessary to accomplish this.

■ Summary

Intramammary lymph nodes are a frequent normal findings and only some are detected by imaging methods. If the findings are typical, the correct diagnosis can be made in the majority of intramammary lymph nodes. Sonography and MRI are generally not indicated for further evaluation of intramammary lymph nodes.

■ References

1 Helvie MA, Adler DD. Rebner et al. Breast hamartomas: variable mammographic appearance. Radiology. 1989;170:417

2 Bässler R. Pathologie der Brustdrüse. In: Doerr W, Seifert G, Uehlinger E. Spezielle pathologische Anatomie. Berlin, Heidelberg, New York: Springer; 1995

3 Bauer BS, Jones KM, Talbot CW. Mammary masses in the adolescent female. Surg Gynecol Obstet. 1987;165:63

4 Dupont WD, Page DL, Parl FF et al. Long-term risk of breast cancer in women with fibroadenoma. N Engl J Med. 1994;331:10

5 Azzopardi JG, Salm R. Ductal adenoma of the breast: a lesion which can mimic carcinoma. J Pathol. 1984;144:15

6 Hertel BG, Zaloudek C, Kempson RL. Breast adenomas. Cancer. 1976;37:2891

7 Sickles EA. Nonpalpable, circumscribed, noncalcified solid breast masses: likelihood of malignancy based on lesion size and age of patient. Radiology. 1994;192:439

8 Lanyi M. Diagnostik und Differentialdiagnostik der Mammaverkalkungen. Berlin: Springer; 1986

9 Travade A, Isnard A, Gimbergues H. Imagerie de la pathologie mammaire. Paris: Masson; 1995

10 Soo MS, Dash N, Bentley R et al. Tubular adenomas of the breast. AJR. 2000;174:757–61

11 Jackson VP, Rothschild PA, Kreipke DL et al. The spectrum of sonographic findings of fibroadenoma of the breast. Invest Radiol. 1986;21:34

12 Stavros AT, Thickman D, Rapp CL at al. Solid breast nodules: use of sonography to distinguish between benign and malignant lesions. Radiology. 1995;196:123–34

13 Heywang-Köbrunner SH, Beck R. Contrast-enhanced MRI of the breast. Heidelberg, New York: Springer; 1996

14 Hochman MG, Orel SG, Powell CM et al. Fibroadenomas: MR imaging appearances with radiologic-histopathologic correlation. Radiology. 1997;204:123–9

15 Brinck U, Fischer U, Korabiowska M et al. The variability of fibroadenoma in contrast-enhanced dynamic MR mammography. AJR. 1997;168:1331–4

16 Murad T, Contesso G, Mouriesse H. Papillary tumors of large lactiferous ducts. Cancer. 1981;48:122

17 Ohuchi N, Abe R, Kasai M. Possible cancerous change in intraductal papillomas of the breast: a 3D reconstruction study of 25 cases. Cancer. 1984;54:605

18 Rosen PP, Caicco J. Florid papillomatosis of the nipple: a study of 51 patients, including nine with mammary carcinoma. Am J Surg Pathol 1986;10:87

19 Rosen PP, Holmes G, Lesser M et al. Juvenile papillomatosis and breast carcinoma. Cancer. 1985;55:1345

20 Cardenosa G, Eklund GW. Benign papillary neoplasms of the breast: mammographic findings. Radiology. 1991;181:751

21 Woods ER, Helvie MA, Ikeda DM et al. Solitary breast papilloma: comparison of mammographic, galactographic and pathologic findings. AJR. 1992;159:48

22 Gregel A. Color atlas of galactography. Stuttgart: Schattauer; 1980

23 Hackelöer BJ, Duda V, Hüneke P et al. Ultraschallmammographie: Entwicklung, Stand und Grenzen. Ultraschall. 1982;3:94

24 Reuter R, D'Orsi CJ, Reale F. Intracystic carcinoma of the breast: the role of ultrasonography. Radiology. 1984;26:277

25 Yang WT, Suen M, Metreweli C. Sonographic features of benign papillary neoplasms of the breast: review of 22 patients. J Ultrasound Med. 1997;16:161–8

26 Liberman L, Bracero N, Vuolo MA et al. Percutaneous large core biopsy of papillary breast lesions. AJR. 1999;172:331–7

27 Barth V. Mammographie: Intensivkurs für Fortgeschrittene. Stuttgart: Enke. 1994

28 Krishan MM, Krishnan SR. An unusual breast lump: neurilemnoma. Aust N Z J Surg. 1982;52:612

29 Toker C, Tang CK, Whitely JF et al. Benign spindle cell breast tumor. Cancer. 1981;48:1615

30 Brown RW, Bhathal PS, Scott Pr. Multiple bilateral angiolipomas of the breast: a case report. Aust N Z J Surg. 1982;5:614

31 Josefcyk MA, Rosen PP. Vascular tumors of the breast. II. Perilobular hemangiomas and hemangiomas. Am J Surg Pathol. 1985;9:491

32 Rosen PP. Vascular tumors of the breast. III. Angiomatosis. Am J Surg Pathol. 1985;9:652

33 Bassett LW, Cove HC. Myoblastoma of the breast. AJR. 1979;132:122

34 D'Orsi CJ. Zebras of the breast. Contemp Diagn Radiol. 1987;10:1

35 Durante E. Benign disease assessment. In: Jellins J, Madjar H, eds. International breast ultrasound seminar. Basel: IBUS Publ; 1994

36 Allgayer B. Personal communication, Jan. 1995

37 Tomaszewski JE, Brooks JS, Hicks D et al. Diabetic mastopathy: a distinctive clinicopathologic entity. Hum Pathol. 1992;23:780

38 Garstin WIH, Kaufmann Z, Michell MJ et al. Fibrous mastopathy in insulin dependent diabetes. Clin Radiol. 1991;44:89

39 Logan WW, Hofmann NY. Diabetic fibrous breast disease. Radiology. 1989;172:667

40 Viehweg P, Heywang-Köbrunner SH, Bayer U, Friedrich T, Spielmann, RP. Simulation of breast carcinoma by diabetic mastopathy. Rofo 1996;164:519

41 Tohno E, Cosgrove DO, Sloane JP. Ultrasound Diagnosis of Breast Diseases. Edinburgh: Churchill Livingstone; 1994

42 Engin G, Acunas G, Acunas B. Granulomatous mastitis: gray scale and color Doppler sonographic findings. J Clin Ultrasound. 1999;27:101–6

43 Hermann G, Schwartz IS. Focal fibrous disease of the breast: mammographic detection of an unappreciated condition. AJR. 1983;140:1245

13. Inflammatory Conditions

In the last decades, the etiologic and pathologic spectrum of the various inflammatory breast conditions has changed: With the decreasing incidence of bacterial puerperal mastitis. Today, chronic inflammatory conditions that are unrelated to gravidity or delivery are in the foreground of the clinical and radiological diagnostic evaluation of these conditions.

Mastitis is frequently associated with an inflammatory pseudotumor (infiltration, abscess, granuloma). This can imitate malignancy, particularly an inflammatory carcinoma.

Pathogenetic and clinical criteria distinguish:

- Puerperal mastitis
- Nonpuerperal mastitis (bacterial, purulent and granulomatous types)
- Specific granulomatous mastitis
- Mycoses and parasitic infestations

Mastitis

■ Etiology

Acute puerperal mastitis occurs during pregnancy and lactation. It is bacterial in origin and develops through infection of the lactiferous ducts and lymphatic clefts during nursing, primarily in the presence of galactostasis.

If the therapy is inadequate, the acute mastitis can change into a subacute or chronic mastitis, causing abscesses or fistulous tracts.

■ Acute Nonspecific Mastitis

Outside lactation and the post-operative period, acute mastitides are rare. They can be caused by:[1]

- Infection of distended subareolar lactiferous ducts = *subareolar abscess formation*. This can be precipitated by squamous metaplasia and hyperplasia of the subareolar lactiferous ducts, resulting in obstruction, secretory retention, and infection.
- Infection in the presence of secretion and/or ductectasia.
- Hematogenous bacterial (or mycotic) spread, a rare occurrence.
- Other rare causes.

■ Subacute and Chronic Mastitis

Any acute mastitis can evolve into a subacute or chronic mastitis, usually after inadequate therapy. In some cases, abscesses or fistulas may occur. They can be quite resistant to therapy and might persist or recur.

Chronic nonbacterial mastitis is often incorrectly called "plasma cell mastitis," though plasma cells are found neither frequently nor invariably. Actually, it is a chronic granulomatous mastitis. It usually occurs in older women and is mostly bilateral. It is caused by secretory retention due to duct ectasia, leading to pressure atrophy of the epithelium and diffusion of the secretion into the periductal connective tissue. It progresses to galactophoritis and to total ductal obliteration. Fibrosis and retraction of the parenchyma and nipple may develop.[1, 2]

■ Prevalence and Purpose

Aside from puerperal mastitis, acute and subacute mastitides are rare. Consequently, the *diagnosis of a nonpuerperal acute or subacute mastitis* must be *carefully assessed*. In particular, inflammatory carcinoma must be excluded. If nipple or parenchymal retraction develops or parenchymal thickening is palpable, *differentiation* from a *diffusely growing carcinoma* is necessary.

■ Clinical Findings

■ Acute Mastitis

Acute mastitis presents as:

- Pain
- Erythema
- Swelling, and
- Hyperthermia of the breast

The thickened skin can resemble a peau d'orange and might be fixed. In addition, the axillary lymph nodes may be swollen and painful. Together with an elevated sedimentation rate, leukocytosis, and systemic symptoms, the *diagnosis of the typical acute mastitis* can be made on the basis of these findings, without further diagnostic tests, and the appropriate therapy (antibiotics, incision, and drainage) can be instituted.

It is important to monitor therapy. Atypical findings, no association with pregnancy, lactation, or surgery, and inadequate resolution are an indication to proceed with diagnostic tests to exclude an *inflammatory carcinoma.*

■ Subacute and Chronic Mastitides

Depending on their manifestation, they can be:

- Unnoticed or associated with minimal inflammatory changes.
- Lead to chronic retracting changes such as nipple retraction or diffuse density. Symmetric presentation supports a "plasma cell mastitis" and speaks generally against a malignancy.
- Thickening and erythema of the skin.
- Progression to a more or less circumscribed palpable finding with or without erythema and/or hyperthermia.
- Chronic fistulous tracts and abscess formation.

It is important to exclude an *inflammatory or diffusely spreading* carcinoma by observing the clinical course and by proceeding with supplemental diagnostic evaluation.

■ Diagnostic Strategy and Goals

■ Acute Mastitis

- Imaging (usually sonography) can detect *abscesses* that need surgical intervention. This not only allows early intervention but also informs the surgeon of the extent of the abscess cavity.
- Through *follow-up examinations* (usually *sonography*) obtained at short intervals, *the therapeutic response* can be evaluated objectively and therapeutic failure recognized early.
- Mammography and further evaluation (above all, *skin biopsy*) is absolutely necessary if the therapeutic response is inadequate, to rule out an inflammatory carcinoma.

■ Subacute or Chronic Mastitis

- Imaging can be used to determine preoperatively the extent of fistulae and abscesses.
- Imaging and histologic evaluation is absolutely necessary to exclude diffusely spreading or inflammatory carcinoma.

■ Mammography

Mammography should be used in cases of *acute mastitis* that show no therapeutic response or have equivocal sonographic findings.

Mammographically, acute mastitis is characterized by (Figs. 13.**1 a–c**):[1]

- Skin thickening, which is often pronounced in the caudal region of the breast and around the areola.
- Diffusely increased density and edema-related impaired structural delineation. It is characteristically pronounced around and beneath the areola.
- Edema-related linear to reticular thickening of the entire connective tissue, including Cooper ligaments.
- Possible formation of abscesses, mostly seen as ill-defined masses.

Despite the characteristic periareolar and subareolar increased density seen in acute mastitis, there are *no findings pathognomonic of acute mastitis* that exclude a malignancy in the absence of any therapeutic response.

Mammography is important for detecting or excluding any *microcalcifications* suggestive of

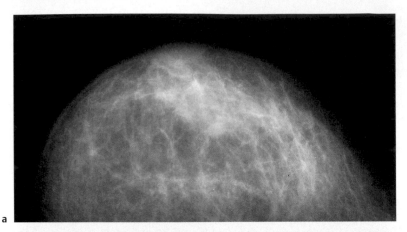

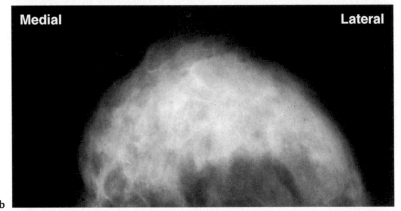

Medial   Lateral

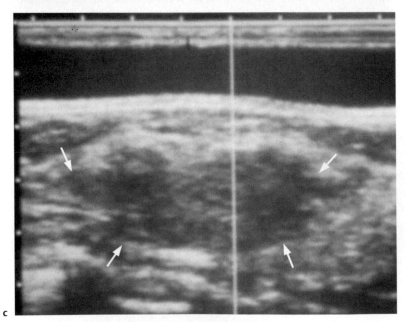

Fig. 13.**1a–c** Acute mastitis
a Mammographically, acute mastitis presents with diffuse skin thickening, coarsened septa, indistinct structures, most pronounced in the retroareolar region
b This focal mastitis was detected as palpable density. Mammographically, the medially located inflamed region is not separable from the adjacent dense parenchyma. The only finding is an unusually radiodense upper inner quadrant (in comparison to the usual distribution of more radiodense tissue in the upper outer quadrant)
c Sonographically (arrows), the inflamed region is swollen and hypoechoic. The narrowed subcutaneous space shows increased echogenicity. Skin thickening is not yet apparent. *Histology:* focal mastitis

malignancy. If such calcifications are present, an *inflammatory carcinoma* should be strongly suspected. *Absent mammographic microcalcifications do not exclude* a malignancy, since no reliable differentiating findings exist between inflammatory carcinoma without microcalcifications and mastitis.

The *subacute* or *chronic* mastitis (Fig. 13.**2a–e**) can be present mammographically as follows:

– Skin thickening.
– Reticular densities in the subcutaneous or prepectoral.

– Diffuse or localized increase in density—unilateral increased breast density.
– Retraction of ligaments and/or nipple.
– Obvious scar formation and fistulous tracts (elongated structures of increased density).
– It may also be barely or not visualized at all in dense parenchyma.[1, 2]

Chronic mastitis can cause mammographically characteristic calcifications (Fig. 13.**2e**) (so-called "plasma cell mastitis").[3, 4] These calcifications are *intraductal, in the wall of the lactiferous duct* (intramural) and *periductal.*

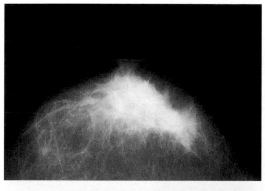

a

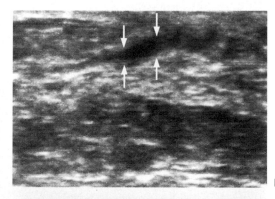

b

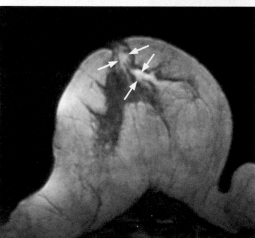

c

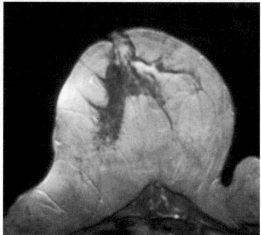

d

Fig. 13.**2a–e**   Chronic mastitis
a–d Patient with mammographically indeterminate density detected by screening mammography. No signs of acute inflammation
a With chronic mastitis, architectural distortion and masses can develop secondary to increasing fibrosis. Mammographically, differentiation from a diffusely growing carcinoma is extremely difficult at this stage. The clinical changes (palpation) were discrete in comparison to the mammographic findings, speaking against a diffusely growing carcinoma

b Furthermore, the sonographically dilated ductal structures (arrows) suggest a so-called chronic comedomastitis caused by retained secretion
c The MRI image before administration of Gd-DTPA shows dilated ducts of high-signal intensity (arrows). The remaining low-signal parenchyma exhibits the same irregular structure that is apparent mammographically
d After administration of Gd-DTPA, the entire visualized parenchyma fails to show any appreciable enhancement. *Diagnosis:* "burnt-out" comedomastitis with fibrosis, no evidence of malignancy

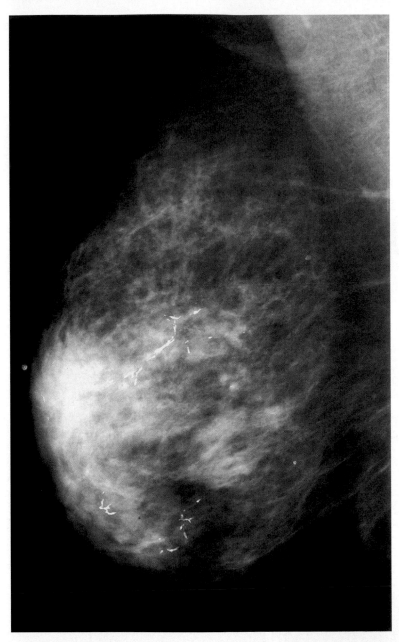

Fig. 13.**2e** Periductal calcifications that develop in context with a so-called "plasma-cell mastitis" generally have a characteristic pattern. The individual calcification is coarse and relatively large, needle-like, or round, occasionally with central radiolucency. Corresponding to their periductal and intraductal location, the typical calcifications of the so-called "plasma-cell mastitis" follow the orientation of the ductal structures

Pathognomonic are:

– Coarse, elongated (measuring several milli-meters) calcifications.
– Elongated calcifications with central radiolu-cency.
– Round calcifications with or without radiolu-cency.

– The orientation of the coarse elongated intra-ductal and periductal calcifications follows the ductal structures (as seen with malignant intraductal calcifications).

While these described calcifications are pathognomonic, *differentiation* from *intraductal carcinoma* may be uncertain if the calcifications are small and delicate. This happens only occasionally. Calcifications may also be absent. Moreover, chronic mastitis (so-called "plasma cell mastitis") can present as (Fig. 13.**2a**):[1, 2]

- Diffusely increased density.
- Linear or reticular accentuation in the lipomatous tissue (reactive fibrous strands).
- Retractions (in the parenchyma, thickening and shortening of Cooper's ligaments).
- Nipple retraction.

The presence of characteristic calcifications is pathognomonic.[3, 4] Since it is possible to have a carcinoma within a plasma cell mastitis, further evaluation is indicated, even in the presence of calcifications, if an additional *suspected mass, architectural distortion,* increasing nipple retraction, or *suspicious* microcalcifications exist. The distinction between malignant and chronic inflammatory masses and retractions can be extremely difficult.

■ Sonography

Acute mastitis is sonographically characterized (Fig. 13.**1c**) by:

- Skin thickening.
- Increased echogenicity in the subcutaneous space and poor separation between subcutaneous space and parenchyma.
- Decreased echogenicity in the parenchyma (sometimes).
- Acoustic shadowing in the parenchyma (minimal to moderate in degree).
- Detection of dilated ducts (anechoic to hypoechoic) in cases of retained secretion. They are often indistinct in outline because of inflammatory reaction. Echoes might be seen within the ducts because of the high protein content of the inflammatory exudate.
- Possible detection of confluent hypoechoic cavities.
- Possible detection of large hypoechoic abscesses.

For acute mastitis, sonography is used to evaluate the therapeutic success, above all in the detection or exclusion of large abscesses that usually have to undergo surgical therapy, as well as for preoperative assessment of the extent of the inflammatory process.[5, 6]

For *subacute and chronic mastitis,* sonography (Fig. 13.**2b**) can:

- Detect dilated ducts (which, however, can also be present as a manifestation of mastopathy)
- Visualize fistulae and abscesses as hypoechoic or anechoic cavities or interconnected cavities

Subacute and chronic mastitis can—depending on stage and extension—cause[5, 6]

- Skin thickening (usually slight and sometimes absent)
- Structural changes in the parenchyma
- Dilated ductal structures with hypoechoic (rarely anechoic) content
- Acoustic shadowing (with increasing fibrosis)
- Hypoechoic structures (through local fibrosis or granulomas)
- Possible fistulae or abscesses (rare)

The *sonographic exclusion of a malignancy* is generally *not possible.*

■ Magnetic Resonance Imaging

Inflammatory changes show (depending on the activity) contrast enhancement:

- Moderate to strong, but sometimes rapid or delayed (during the acute stage)
- Mostly delayed and moderate (subacute to chronic)
- Minimal to negligible (chronic stage with minimal activity) (Fig. 13.**2c** and **a**)

Abscesses are imaged as nonenhancing cavities surrounded by an enhancing wall.[7]

Diffuse mastitic changes generally cause a diffuse enhancement of the entire parenchyma, often most pronounced in the subareolar region.

Since the enhancement in inflammatory processes, even when considering degree and rate of enhancement, is no different from the variable enhancement in malignancies, MRI is not suitable for the differential diagnosis between inflammatory and malignant changes.

■ Biopsy Methods

The response to antibiotic therapy determines the further approach to inflammatory processes.

If inadequate response of inflammatory changes to antibiotic therapy suggests a malignancy, excisional biopsy with sampling of the skin overlying the suspicious region is indicated. This should exclude a malignancy (inflammatory carcinoma, lymphoma, leukemia) as the cause of diffuse changes.

Abscesses and Fistulae

Abscesses can be formed:

- On the basis of an acute or chronic mastitis, also following a galactophoritis
- From a local infection, e.g., also following infections of the Montgomery glands, sweat glands, and so forth
- Through direct extension (arising from pleural or chest wall abscesses)

The causes to be considered are:[1, 8, 9, 10]

- Bacterial infections
- Tuberculosis (actinomycosis, syphilis)
- Fungal infections
- Parasitoses, such as echinococcal cysts, which are mentioned here as extreme rarity

■ Histology

An abscess is a pus-filled uniloculated or multiloculated cavity surrounded by a so-called abscess capsule, consisting of granulation tissue with inflammatory cells and fibroblasts. Abscess cavities are usually round or oval, ill-defined, and often surrounded by inflammatory edema.

Inflammatory processes with a subacute or chronic course can develop fistulae. The fistulous system consists of necrotic, often branching tracts containing pus and necrotic material, which are surrounded by granulation tissue.

■ Clinical Findings

Most abscesses are:

- Palpable as localized, often fixed mass sometimes with fluctuation
- Can have thickening and fixation of the overlying skin

The typical inflammatory changes are:

- Skin discoloration over the abscess (bluish-red)
- Hyperthermia
- Pain

Rarely:

- These typical inflammatory changes can be absent or minimally present (e.g., tuberculous "cold abscess")

- Such inflammatory changes can be imitated by a carcinoma with inflammatory component

Fistulae are generally diagnosed as:

- Tracts with openings on the skin or nipple
- With transient (or constant) purulent drainage
- The tissue surrounding the fistulous tracts is generally diffusely indurated and may—depending on the activity of the inflammation—exhibit inflammatory changes (skin discoloration, erythema, pain)

■ Diagnostic Strategy

A *clinically obvious diagnosis* does not require mammography.

- During the acute phase of a clinically evident abscess, mammography should be avoided because of the associated discomfort
- Sonography is appropriate to determine:
- Whether the abscess has one or several loculations
- Whether the abscess has an even larger solid component, and
- The extent of fistulization

Depending on the clinical findings, sonographic finding and size of the abscess, the clinician will select:

- Antibiotic therapy (e.g., multiple small abscesses)
- Aspiration
- Sonographically guided percutaneous drainage
- Incision and drainage
- Excision

Conservative therapy is *monitored* by:

- Sonography as the method of choice
- Mammography for clarifying remaining uncertainty in clinically confusing situations where the possibility of malignancy is suspected.

Diagnostic uncertainties, which may occur in the subacute or chronic stage and recurrent abscesses and fistulae, should be further evaluated by:

- Mammography to detect malignancy, when present

- Mammography and sonography to assist the preoperative assessment of the extent of the process

Since imaging generally cannot exclude a malignancy, in the presence of uncharacteristic inflammatory processes, excision is unavoidable for diagnostic—and often also for therapeutic—reasons in most cases.

■ Sonography

Sonographically, an abscess appears as (Fig. 13.3 b):[5, 6]

- Hypoechoic, generally round to oval lesion.
- The outline is smooth or irregular.
- The sound transmission is good to moderate.
- The central internal echoes found in the mature abscess are generally regular, but sedimentations—moveable echoes—or septations can occur. Individual, very strong echoes that rise with positional changes are suggestive of gas bubbles.
- Most abscesses are surrounded by edematous, hypoechoic tissue.

Fistulous tracts can be followed as hypoechoic, serpiginous tubular structure within an indurated area.

■ Value

Sonography is the method of choice for evaluating extent and morphology of abscesses and fistulae and to monitor the therapeutic response. It can be used to guide percutaneous drainage.

■ Mammography

An abscess is seen as (Fig. 13.3a):[1]
- Generally round, not entirely smoothly outlined, space-occupying lesion.
- Characteristically, it exhibits an ill-defined, indistinct demarcation caused by the surrounding edema. Also characteristically, but not always present, an edematous, ill-defined increased overall density that is most pronounced around the lesion extending to the subareolar region.
- In dense parenchyma, an abscess may only be seen as a nonspecific increase in density, or may not be noted at all.
- In addition, increased reticular markings and skin thickening may be observed.

- Occasionally, air collections or air–fluid levels are present, with the latter only seen in the mediolateral projection.

Fistulae are not mammographically visualized unless they contain air or are injected with contrast material. The fistulous segments that contain air (rarely observed with compression) can be seen as hypodense serpiginous structures.

Most fistulous inflammatory conditions are only revealed through ill-defined densities caused by thickening of the surrounding tissues. In dense parenchyma, this might only be seen as asymmetry or not at all.

Depending on the activity and extent of the inflammation, the same findings observed with an abscess, such as edematous changes, thickened Cooper ligaments, and skin thickening, might suggest the presence of a neoplastic process.

■ Value

If the diagnosis is unclear, mammography can be used as supplemental examination. Indistinct demarcation from the surrounding tissue due to edema as well as subareolar extension of the edema due to inflammation suggests an inflammatory process. There are no criteria that can reliably exclude a malignancy.

If suspicious calcifications are seen in the area in question or elsewhere in the breast, a malignancy must be considered.

■ Magnetic Resonance Imaging

Contrast-enhanced MRI can be used in selected cases with findings difficult to evaluate mammographically and sonographically (e.g., after multiple injections of silicone and wax), for the preoperative evaluation of the extent of the abscess and fistulous formation.

- MRI visualizes abscesses (Figs. 13.3c and d) as round or irregularly outlined fluid-filled cavities, with variable signal intensity and without enhancement
- They are generally surrounded by a thin, internally smooth capsule, which shows intense and early enhancement
- The inflammatory edematous tissue around the abscess usually accumulates Gd-DTPA, delayed and of moderate intensity

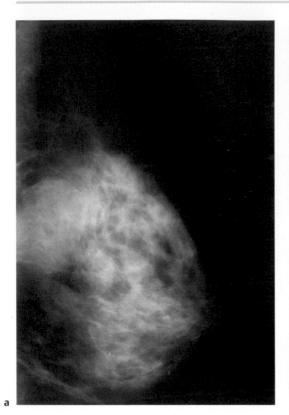

a

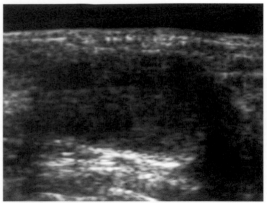

b

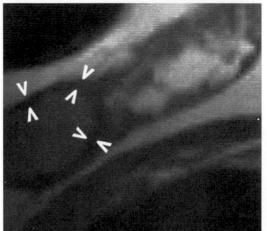

c

Fig. 13.**3 a–d** Abscess
a Mammographically (mediolateral view), the abscess is visualized as an oval, indistinctly outlined mass
b Sonographically, it is an oval, hypoechoic mass with a variable sound absorption pattern (insignificant enhancement on the left, slight enhancement in the middle, broad edge-shadow on the right). Its good compressibility is characteristic of a fluid-containing lesion
c On the unenhanced T1-weighted image, the signal intensity of the capsule of the abscess (arrowheads) is very low and that of its content somewhat higher
d After administration of Gd-DTPA, the capsule (arrowheads) and surrounding tissue show slight enhancement. There is no enhancement of the content of the abscess

d

■ Percutaneous Biopsy

If the therapy is successful, it is unnecessary, and if it is unsuccessful, it is superfluous since these cases require surgical intervention.

■ Percutaneous Drainage

This can be performed under sonographic guidance. In multiloculated abscesses, surgical drainage may be preferable.

■ Summary

Most abscesses and fistulae can be correctly diagnosed clinically. Sonography is the method of choice for the morphologic evaluation of the degree of liquefication and extent, and for monitoring the therapeutic response. Mammography is indicated in diagnostically unclear cases. Ill-defined, indistinct transition to the surrounding tissue and ill-defined subareolar densities mammographically favor the diagnosis of inflammation. Suspected calcifications can reveal a coexistent carcinoma, a centrally necrotic or inflammatory carcinoma, which may mimic an inflammation or abscess. In general, a clinically suspected malignancy cannot be reliably excluded. If the therapeutic response is inadequate, an excision is diagnostically and therapeutically indicated.

Granulomatous Conditions

Granulomas are an additional manifestation of inflammatory processes and can be seen in a variety of diseases. The most important granulomatous conditions encountered in the breast are:

- The chronic granulomatous mastitis and lobulitis, already presented in Chapter 12.
- Foreign body granulomas (including granulomas around deposits of wax and silicone)[7, 8, 11]
- Tuberculosis[12]
- Rare fungal infections (histoplasmosis)[1, 9]
- Sarcoidosis[12–14]
- Autoimmune diseases (Wegener granulomatosis, giant cell arteritis, polyarteritis nodosa)[15, 16]
- Rare parasitic infestations (cysticercosis)[12]

The diagnosis of foreign body granulomas may be suspected on the basis of the history, palpatory findings, and clinical course. A rare involvement of the breast should be considered in patients afflicted with one of the generalized granulomatous conditions. Since no distinguishing criteria exist, a malignancy (carcinoma, lymphoma) should be excluded first because of its considerably higher incidence.

■ Histologic and Microbiologic Confirmation

Foreign body granulomas are histologically diagnosed. Their underlying causes range from talcum and sutures to deposits of wax and silicone and can be recognized histologically.

Histologically, foreign body granulomas have a lobulated contour. In their first stage, they consist of highly vascularized granulomatous tissue with round cellular infiltrates and giant cells. The inflammatory process may resolve, replacing the granulation tissue with dense scar tissues containing inclusions of foreign body material.

The diagnosis of an *autoimmune disease* of the breast, such as Wegener granulomatosis, giant cell arteritis, or polyarteritis nodosa, has to be made histologically, supported by the clinical presentation (in the case of multiorgan involvement) and specific laboratory tests.[12–16]

The diagnosis of *tuberculosis* or another infectious granulomatous disease, such as a *fungal infection* or *parasitosis*, is made histologically. The causative agent can only be positively identified by microbiologic examination. *Sarcoidosis* is diagnosed histopathologically on the basis of characteristic granulomas. Infections with similar granulomas should be included in the differential diagnosis. A positive Kveim test supports the diagnosis of sarcoidosis.

■ Clinical Findings

Foreign body granulomas are characteristically found in scars. They are seen as small, barely moveable nodules, without erythema or pain. They are often indistinguishable from small recurrences within scars.

Foreign body granulomas around large silicone and wax deposits (following injection for breast augmentation or after rupture of a prothesis) are palpable as barely moveable nodules.

A sterile inflammation or a secondary infection with formation of abscesses and fistulae can develop many years after silicone or wax injection.

The findings of tuberculous mastitis include:
1. A so-called cold abscess formation: fluctuating nodule, with or without skin thickening, characteristically without erythema or hyperthermia
2. Mastitis through extension of a pleuritis
3. Involvement of the breast with one or multiple large and small granulomatous foci

Granulomatous lesions are palpable as barely moveable nodule or nodules, with or without fixation of the overlying skin. Rarely, such a mass may arise from an involved (tuberculous) intramammary lymph node.

Diffuse extension leads to a poorly outlined induration, with or without skin thickening or fixation, as seen with a diffusely spreading carcinoma. Furthermore, the few described cases of *sarcoidosis* or *autoimmune diseases*[12–16] of the breast had findings resembling those seen in tuberculosis. Overall, singular and multiple lesions, as well as diffuse spreading, cannot be clinically differentiated from a carcinoma.

■ Diagnostic Strategy

Foreign body granulomas in scars may be clinically suspected on the basis of their localization, postoperative development, and stable size. In cases that are difficult to differentiate from malignancy, the following should be considered:

- Imaging, primarily mammography, is indicated to exclude microcalcifications as a sign of malignancy within the area of question or at another site
- Differentiation between scar granuloma and recurrence is possible by contrast-enhanced MRI for those granulomas that are completely fibrosed

- In the remaining cases, the differentiation of a granuloma from a carcinoma or recurrence within the scar is difficult with any imaging modality, including MRI

  - Increasing size or clinical suspicion makes a diagnostic excision obligatory
  - Stable small size or a clinically suspected granuloma justify short-term follow-up examinations

Infectious granulomas as well as *granulomas caused by sarcoidosis and autoimmune disease* are generally indistinguishable from malignancy by clinical or imaging criteria. Even a palpable breast nodule that develops in a patient with known tuberculosis, sarcoidosis, and so forth, must first be assumed to be a carcinoma rather than a rare manifestation of the underlying disease.

The diagnosis can be established by percutaneous biopsy, supplemented by additional evaluation (microbiology, clinical findings). Often, an excisional biopsy is performed because of the strong suspicion of malignancy.

■ Mammography

Granulomas within scarring:

- Might not be visualized within the increased density of the scar
- Might be apparent as more or less sharply delineated nodular density (Figs. 13.**4a** and **b**)
- Dystrophic calcifications might develop as part of the scar formation but are rarely seen in granulomas
- Characteristic shell-like calcifications often form around silicone and wax deposits

Neither lack of visualization nor evidence of well-defined borders allows the *mammographic differentiation from a carcinoma with sufficient certainty.* It is therefore necessary to proceed with the diagnostic excision of a clinically suggestive abnormality regardless of the mammographic appearance.

The most important tasks of mammography are the detection of a possible carcinoma within the scar (e.g., microcalcification) and the preoperative exclusion of a carcinoma at a separate site.

Old granulomas around silicone and wax deposits are positively identified by their shell-like calcifications. The superimposition of masses and calcifications can interfere with mammographic evaluation and, consequently, limit the ability to detect *carcinoma in breasts with multiple silicone or*

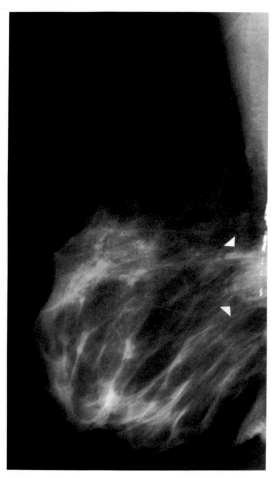

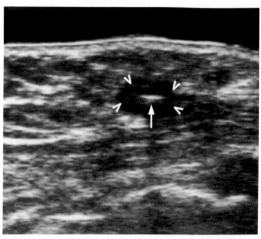

Fig. 13.**4a** and **b** Scar granuloma due to a long-standing ventriculoperitoneal shunt, situated subcutaneously and medially in the breast
a Mammographically, an indistinctly outlined density (arrow heads) is seen, traversed by calcified shunt material. Its mammographic size corresponds to the palpable finding
b Sonographically, the palpable lesion (arrow heads) is hypoechoic, traversed by the shunt material that appears as echogenic structure (arrow). *Histology:* scar granuloma

wax injections. Inflammatory granulomas and granulomas caused by autoimmune disease (Fig. 13.**6a** and **b**) *or sarcoidosis* can be visualized as:

– One or more indistinctly outlined focal densities.
– Diffusely increased density.
– Round or oval masses (rarely), e.g., originating from an involved lymph node.
– They might not be identified in dense parenchyma.
– Associated skin thickening might be present.
– Calcifications are rare. Microcalcifications are not part of the features of an inflammatory granuloma.

These granulomas produce mammographic and clinical findings resembling those found with malignancies, generally necessitating their surgical excision.

■ Sonography

Scar granulomas (Fig. 13.**4b**) are sonographically visualized as irregular small nodules that are hypoechoic and with or without distal acoustic shadowing. They cannot be reliably differentiated from a small carcinoma within the scar.

Silicone granulomas (Fig. 13.**5b**) are visualized as:

– Hyperechoic mass with marked acoustic attenuation. A thin, crescentic hyperechoic rim may appear on the side close to the transducer if the granuloma is calcified.
– Characteristically, the acoustic shadow within and distal to the lesion contains clearly identifiable echoes that decrease with increasing distance from the transducer (so-called snowstorm pattern).

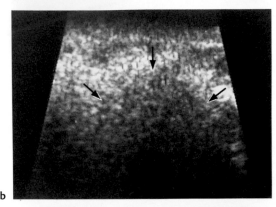

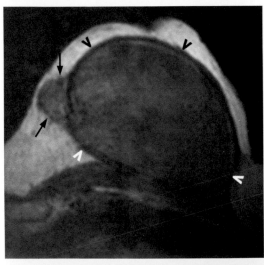

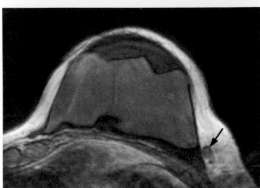

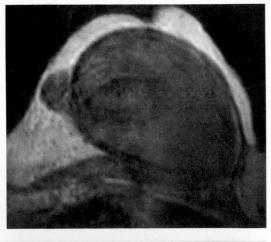

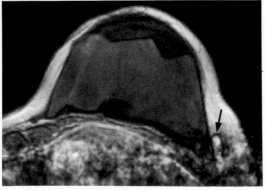

Fig. 13.**5 a–f**   Silicone granuloma
a–d   Fifty-year-old patient, 10 years after augmentation mammoplasty. For 6 months, palpable finding adjacent to the prosthesis
a   Mammographically, very dense lesion medial to the silicone prosthesis. The high density suggests a silicone granuloma (arrows)
b   Sonographically, the palpable lesion is hypoechoic with acoustic shadowing. Echoes that decrease distally (so-called snow storm) are seen in the proximal aspect of the acoustic shadow, supporting the presence of a silicone granuloma
c   MRI delineates a fairly well-circumscribed mass of low signal intensity medial to the prosthesis (arrow heads) in the region of the palpable finding (arrows)
d   After administration of Gd-DTPA, the palpable lesion fails to show any appreciable enhancement. (Special pulse sequence for the detection of silicone outside the prosthesis was not employed at that time). *Histology:* fibrosed granuloma with silicone inclusion
e–f   Fifty-four-year-old patient. Two years status post reconstruction mammoplasty.
e   A small low signal mass was discovered adjacent to the double-lumen prosthesis
f   The small nodule shows strong and early enhancement after administration of Gd-DTPA. This nodule discovered by MRI was followed after 3 months and thereafter every 6 months, without evidence of any growth. Subsequent follow-up confirmed the diagnosis

Despite these characteristic features, the differentiation from a carcinoma can be difficult in the individual case. Multiple silicone or wax deposits may considerably compromise the evaluation because of marked attenuation phenomena.

The remaining inflammatory granulomatous diseases, such as *tuberculosis, fungal infections, parasitosis, sarcoidosis, and autoimmune diseases,* have only be reported anecdotally. A sonographic separation from a carcinoma cannot be expected.

■ Magnetic Resonance Imaging

Scar granulomas as well as granulomas around small silicone leaks[7, 17] (Figs. 13.**5**c–f) show:

– An intense and early contrast enhancement in the early and inflammatory–granulating stage
– A moderate and delayed contrast enhancement, with increasing fibrosis
– No contrast enhancement, with complete fibrosis
– The MRI-demonstrated contour is generally round and nodular, with a more or less sharp outline

Due to absence of enhancement, a fibrotic granuloma can be easily distinguished from a carcinoma or scar recurrence. This is not applicable to the nonfibrotic granulomas.

Silicone and wax granulomas after injection of contrast medium:

– Can enhance peripherally or throughout due to a chronic granulating inflammation and are then indistinguishable from abscesses or malignancies
– Do not enhance in the fibrotic stage

Since no contrast enhancement can be expected in about two-thirds of the cases[18], contrast-enhanced MRI is advantageous as a supplemental examination to exclude a malignancy, especially in view of the limited evaluation after silicone and wax injections by other methods.

Granulomas along silicone protheses are induced by silicone that escaped in small amounts through leakage or frank rupture (silicone granulomas), but can also be caused by suture material or talcum.

Except for the few granulomas with only negligible enhancement, most show enhancement:[9, 19]

– In cases that arouse clinical or mammographic suspicion, the excision of enhancing granulomas is unavoidable.
– In our experience, follow-up examinations of nonenhancing granulomas can be justified.
– A small but otherwise inconspicuous, smoothly marginated, enhancing mass adja-

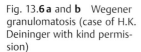

Fig. 13.**6a** and **b** Wegener granulomatosis (case of H.K. Deininger with kind permission)
a Craniocaudal mammographic view of a patient with known Wegener granulomatosis. The diagnosis was confirmed by fine needle aspiration
b The patient underwent immunosuppressive therapy. The follow-up examination three years later is unremarkable

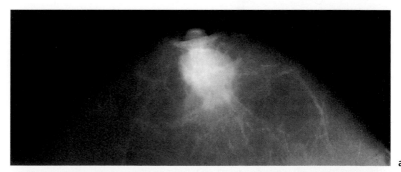

a

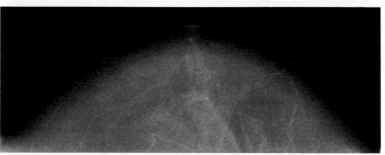

b

cent to a prothesis and only discovered by MRI can be, in our judgment, observed with short-term follow-up examinations (at 3, 6, and 12 months), to refrain from unnecessary biopsies of diminutive granulomas. We find that granulomas, contrary to carcinomas, do *not* increase in size.

The MRI features of the rare granulomatous conditions, such as *tuberculosis, fungal infections, parasitosis, sarcoidosis, and autoimmune disease,* have not yet been reported. It can be expected that these conditions enhance, precluding a differentiation from carcinomas by contrast-enhanced MRI.

■ Percutaneous Biopsy

Occasionaly, the diagnosis of a *scar granuloma* may be hampered by severe fibrosis and the resultant difficulty of obtaining an adequate amount of material. However, in most cases percutaneous needle biopsy, sometime even fine needle aspiration, will be valuable in differentiating a scar from a carcinoma.

The cytologic diagnosis of a *granulomatous inflammation* is difficult. The diagnosis can be made from a needle biopsy, but excisional biopsy is recommended for the differential diagnosis of a granulomatous inflammation.

■ Summary

Scar granulomas appear clinically as small nodules in the region of the scar and can be suspected by history and clinical course. Mammographically (nodular density) and sonographically (hypoechoic nodule, with or without acoustic shadowing), a differentiation from a malignancy cannot be achieved. In cases of clinical suspicion, biopsy of the usually superficially located lesions is therefore the method of choice. A suspected scar granuloma following multiple surgeries can be further evaluated by contrast-enhanced MRI to avoid further surgical interventions for diagnostic purposes. Granulomas that are fibrosed and do not enhance can be distinguished from malignancies and can be safely observed.

Granulomas around silicone or wax deposits, usually after cosmetic injections, can calcify.

Because of the increased density and the multiple superimposed calcifications, the mammographic evaluation of these breasts is compromised. The same applies to the sonographic evaluation. Since contrast-enhanced MRI shows no enhancement in two-thirds of the patients, MRI appears to be suitable as supplemental method for excluding and detecting malignancies.

Large silicone granulomas are sonographically characterized as hyperechoic to hypoechoic masses with acoustic shadowing that exhibit a snowstorm pattern.

MRI is highly sensitive in detecting diminutive silicone granulomas around breast prostheses. These granulomas often can be differentiated from small malignancies solely by absent growth over time. Only absent enhancement justifies the differentiation from a carcinoma. *Granulomatous diseases of the breast* can be found as extremely rare manifestations of tuberculosis, fungal infections, parasitosis, sarcoidosis, or autoimmune diseases.

■ References

1   Barth VK, Prechtel K. Atlas der Brustdrüse und ihrer Erkrankungen. Stuttgart: Enke; 1990
2   Rees BI, Gravelle IH, Hughes LE. Nipple retraction in ductectasia. Br J Surg. 1977;64:577
3   Lanyi M. Diagnostik und Differentialdiagnostik der Mammaverkalkungen. Berlin: Springer; 1986
4   Sickles EA. Breast calcifications: mammographic evaluation. Radiology. 1986;160:289
5   Blohmer JU, Bollmann R, Chaoui R et al. Die Mastitis nonpuerperalis in der Realtime- und Farbdopplersonographie. Geburtshilfe Frauenheilk. 1994;54:161
6   Harris VJ, Jackson VP. Indications for breast imaging in women under age 35 years. Radiology. 1989;172:445
7   Heywang-Köbrunner SH, Beck R. Contrast-Enhanced MRI of the Breast. Heidelberg; New York: Springer; 1996
8   Miller CL, Feig SA, Fox JW. Mammographic changes after reduction mammoplasty. AJR. 1987;149:35
9   Seymour EQ. Blastomycosis of the breast. AJR. 1982;139:822
10 Tabar L, Kett K, Nemeth A. Tuberculosis of the breast. Radiology. 1976;118:587
11 Stigers KB, King JG, Davey DD, Stelling CB. Abnormalities of the breast caused by biopsy: spectrum of mammographic findings. AJR. 1991;156:287
12 D'Orsi CJ. Zebras of the breast. Contemp Diagn Radiol. 1987;10:1
13 Gansler TS, Wheeler JE. Mammary sarcoidosis: two cases and literature review. Arch Pathol Lab Med. 1984;108:673
14 Ross MJ, Merino MJ. Sarcoidosis of the breast. Hum Pathol. 1985;16:185
15 Deininger, HK. Wegener's granulomatosis of the breast. Radiology. 1985;154:59

16 Jordan JM, Rowe WT, Allen NB. Wegener's granulomatosis involving the breast: report of three cases and review of the literature. Am J Med. 1987;83:159

17 Heinig A, Heywang-Köbrunner SH, Viehweg P et al. Value of contrast-enhanced MRI of the breast in patients after breast reconstruction with silicon implant. Radiologe. 1997;37:710–7

18 Yang WT, Suen M, Ho WS, Metreweli C. Paraffinomas of the breast: mammographic, ultrasonographic and radiographic appearances with clinical and histopathologic correlation. Clin Radiol. 1996;51:130–3

14. Carcinoma in situ

■ **Definition**

Carcinomas in situ are lesions with cells displaying the characteristic features of a carcinoma without any extension across the basement membrane. Carcinomas in situ can therefore not metastasize.

It is generally assumed that a large proportion of invasive carcinomas arise from carcinomas in situ. However, carcinomas in situ are not a required precursor of an invasive carcinoma. They are rather a marker of an increased risk for the development of an invasive carcinoma.

Lobular carcinoma in situ is distinguished from a ductal carcinoma in situ. Mixed types are rare.

Lobular Carcinoma in Situ (LCIS)

Unlike DCIS, LCIS is, according to the present classification, not considered to be a true carcinoma but a rather severe lobular atypia.

■ **Incidence**

The reported incidence of a lobular carcinoma in situ is 0.8–6%. Its diagnosis is clinically and mammographically occult, since there are no criteria differentiating it from benign changes or even normal parenchyma. It is generally an incidental histologic finding observed in a biopsy performed for another reason. It is frequently multicentric (up to 50%) and bilateral (30%).[1–4]

■ **Importance**

Risk estimates following biopsy for LCIS have revealed the lobular carcinoma in situ to represent a neoplastic proliferation process of the ductulolobular epithelium that develops slowly, expands, and persists unchanged for many years. The relative risk of developing an invasive carcinoma within the first 15 years after the biopsy is increased by a factor of 10. The risk is slightly decreased if the diagnosis is made above the age of 45 years and is increased in women with a family history of breast cancer.

In patients with a biopsy diagnosis of LCIS, the ipsilateral cumulative risk after 5 years is 10%, and after 10 years 15%. In a follow-up period of 15 years, invasive ductal or lobular carcinomas can be expected in 15–23% ipsilaterally and 9.5–20% contralaterally, i.e., the uninvolved contralateral breast shares the risk. Subsequent invasive cancers can be either lobular or ductal.

■ **Histology**

LCIS is a solid neoplasm of small isomorphic cells occupying the ductulolobular units, with frequent involvement of extralobular ductal segments as well as groups of lobules as manifestations of a multifocal or multicentric growth. According to Haagensen, a monomorphic cellular type A can be distinguished from a pleomorphic (hyperdiploid) cellular type B, with the latter variant presumably harboring an increased malignant potential (quoted after Stegner).[1–4]

Multicentric manifestations were found in more than 45% of mastectomy specimens (LCIS in 90% and invasive carcinoma in 4–10%). *Bilateral manifestations* were found in about 30%.

Atypical lobular hyperplasias contain the same but fewer abnormal cells, with less deformity and enlargement of the parenchymal lobules as found in LCIS.

Fig. 14.**1** In this patient vacuum biopsy was performed because of two adjacent foci of indeterminate microcalcifications that had newly developed. Both groups of microcalcifications were removed during vacuum biopsy. Histology revealed secretory calcifications located within proliferative changes. In addition, lobular carcinoma in situ was diagnosed in some of the 25 removed cores. Based on correlation of imaging and histopathology, lobular carcinoma in situ was an incidental finding. No further workup is necessary.

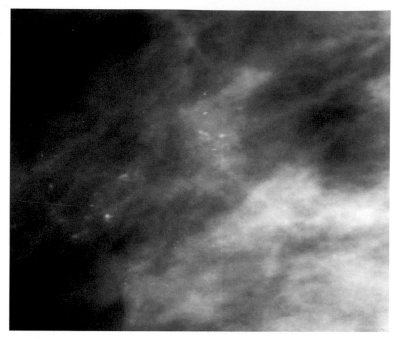

■ Clinical Presentation and History

Clinically, there is no characteristic finding.

Some lesions of LCIS are diagnosed in excisional biopsies performed because of a worrisome palpable finding or asymmetry. Others are incidental histologic discoveries in biopsies performed for fibroadenomas or adjacent microcalcifications.

■ Mammography
(Fig. 14.**1**)

There are also no mammographic findings characteristic of LCIS. This implies that LCIS generally cannot be distinguished from benign changes or normal breast parenchyma. Rarely is an asymmetry found mammographically. Microcalcifications—which are generally uncharacteristic in morphology and distribution—are only found in a few cases of LCIS (Fig. 14.**1**).

■ Sonography

Sonographically, LCIS is not recognizable.

■ Magnetic Resonance Imaging

Only limited experience is available so far. In the few examined cases, a mostly moderately diffuse enhancement was observed, and in our own patients, a focal enhancement was seen twice, similar to the enhancement found in proliferative benign changes.

■ Percutaneous Biopsy

The percutaneous biopsy diagnosis of a lobular carcinoma in situ is usually an incidental finding, which was obtained during percutaneous biopsy of another abnormality (mass, microcalcifications). Based on correlation of the histopathologic and the imaging findings it must be checked whether a definitive diagnosis of the lesion undergoing biopsy can be made with the material obtained. If this is the case, the percutaneous biopsy diagnosis of LCIS does not warrant a wider surgical excision.

■ Therapeutic Decisions after Documented LCIS, Goals and Value of Diagnostic Methods

Utilizing diagnostic methods with the goal of disclosing or excluding LCIS is at the present infeasible because of absence of characteristic features. Therefore utilizing diagnostic methods is restricted to the possible early detection of an invasive carcinoma. Presently, mammographic and clinical follow-up, supplemented by sonography in case of indeterminate findings, is recommended.

Whether other modalities, such as MRI and percutaneous biopsy, can be cost-effectively applied to the early detection of an invasive carci-

noma in these patients at increased risk needs to be confirmed by well-designed clinical trials.

Because of the uncertain clinical significance and prognosis of LCIS, therapeutic recommendations vary.

The current therapy consists of simple excision and regular clinical and mammographic follow-up examinations, for early diagnosis of an invasive carcinoma, should one develop.

Ductal Carcinoma in Situ (DCIS) (Intraductal Carcinoma)

■ **Definition**

Histopathologically, as well as clinically and prognostically, DCIS comprises a heterogenous group of carcinomas. As a result of mammography and screening, the incidence of DCIS detected in biopsies has increased from 2–4% to 10–29%.

According to the definition of these tumors, malignant cells are exclusively found within the lactiferous ductal system, i.e., intraductal, without destruction of the basement membrane.

They extend contiguously or noncontiguously through the ductal system, explaining the frequent multifocal and multicentric tumor manifestations found on average in 30% of all DCIS and in over 60% of the DCIS of large extent.

■ Incidence

The peak incidence of DCIS occurs between the ages of 40 and 60 years. Since most cases of imaging detectable DCIS contain microcalcifications, the detection rate has markedly increased with the expanding use of mammography. While the proportion of DCIS of all discovered carcinomas in patients with clinical findings is only 3–5%, it has now reached 20–30% in the screening group.[5–9]

Some noncalcified DCIS are incidentally discovered histologically in biopsies performed for other reasons.

■ Histology

Histologically, five types based on their microscopic architecture have been described. These are lesions not only of different histologic pattern, but also of diverse clinical and prognostic properties. These can generally be separated into the

comedo DCIS in distinction to the remaining tumors that are grouped together as non-comedo DCIS (Table 14.1).

Mixed types with two or more components are encountered in 30–50% of cases, particularly in large lesions.

■ Comedo DCIS

This subtype of DCIS is characterized by a dominant solid intraductal tumor component with the formation of areas of central necrosis that form calcifications and can occupy 50% or more of the ductal diameter.

In comparison to the other subtypes, the comedo carcinoma has an increased malignant potential, characterized by an increased proliferation rate of the tumor cells with a high nuclear grading leading to the formation of pleomorphic hyperchromatic cell nuclei. It is histologically more anaplastic appearing than other subtypes of DCIS.

There is a relationship between tumor size and likelihood of microinvasion[10] as well as between tumor size and likelihood of ipsilateral residual tumor.[11] Foci of microinvasion are the origin of the axillary nodal metastases found in 1–3% of the cases.[7, 11–13]

Cytomorphologic criteria and the marked overexpression of the c-erb-B-2 oncogene encountered primarily in comedo DCIS are prognostically significant.

■ Non-comedo Carcinoma

The *solid subtype* and the *cribriform carcinoma* are predominantly confined to one quadrant and express a higher degree of differentiation. *Micro-papillary carcinomas* generally extend in several quadrants and exhibit a high percentage of multi-centric growth. The *papillary carcinoma in situ* is divided into the typical DCIS confined to the duct and the intracystic papillary DCIS.

■ Importance

Based on current knowledge, there seem to be important prognostic differences between the subgroups of DCIS. While up to 50% of comedo carcinomas can be expected to progress to inva-sive ductal carcinoma, the noncomedo carci-nomas seem to have a lower progression rate of about 20–30%.[10, 14–24]

■ New Classification

Though the traditional histopathological classifi-cation is generally accepted, there have been dis-cordances between the expected and actual clinical behavior and prognosis of the mentioned subtypes. Therefore, new classifications have been proposed. They part from evaluating histopathologic patterns and entities in favor of evaluating cytonuclear differentiation (nuclear grading), architecture, and the presence or absence of various forms of necro-sis. Increasing necrosis and higher nuclear grade correspond with more aggressive lesions.

1. The **Van Nuys classification**[25, 26] combines nu-clear grading and necrosis as the determining criteria. This classification divides:
    – **High-grade DCIS with comedo-type necrosis,** corresponding to the classic comedo carci-noma
    – **Non-high-grade DCIS without comedo-type necrosis** as a favorable histology (non-comedo carcinoma), encompassing solid, cri-briform, papillary and micropapillary sub-types, and
    – **Non-high-grade DCIS** with comedo-type necrosis, representing an intermediate type with an intermediate prognosis
2. The **classification** proposed by **Holland and coworkers**[19] completely abolishes the con-ventional terminology and replaces it with cy-tonuclear and architectural criteria. The authors define specific proliferation patterns with cellular polarization and three categories of cytonuclear differentiation, associated with characteristic calcifications:
    – **Poorly differentiated DCIS** with amorphous calcifications and a poor prognosis

Table 14.1 Subclassification and incidence of intraduc-tale carcinomas related to all intraductal carcinomas

Comedo carcinoma	30–50%
Solid carcinoma	9–22%
Cribriform carcinoma	20–28%
Micropapillary carcinoma	8–14%
Papillary carcinoma	4–7%

– **Intermediately differentiated DCIS** with amorphous, laminated, coarse and fine-granular calcifications, and intermediate prognosis
– **Well-differentiated DCIS** with laminated, psammomatous, and fine-granular calcifica-tions, associated with a good prognosis

■ Therapeutic Decisions

In view of questions as to the exact prognostic classification of the subtypes of DCIS and because of the uncertain efficiency of the available thera-pies, a standard treatment for DCIS does not exist. In some cases, DCIS is treated today with a simple mastectomy without axillary dissection. Only if the findings are extensive is sampling of the axillary lymph nodes recommended. Mas-tectomy is associated with a cure rate approach-ing 100%.

Several studies indicate that DCIS can be successfully treated by breast-conserving surgical intervention. Whether or not radiotherapy is nec-essary is controversial.

There is a connection between the extent at the time of the primary diagnosis and therapy and the likelihood of locally recurrent disease. Com-paring patients having DCIS <25 mm with patients having DCIS >25 mm, Lagios et al.[10] found an increase in multicentricity from 14% to 46%, in occult invasion from 0% to 46% and in axil-lary nodal involvement from 0% to 4%.

■ Clinical Findings and History

In population screening, only 10% of DCIS lesions are clinically apparent. The clinical findings mostly present as a palpable abnormality, rarely as a pathologic secretion or Paget disease of the nipple. DCIS very rarely becomes symptomatic through localized (unilateral and usually not re-lated to the menstrual cycle) pain.

■ Diagnostic Methods: Value and Goals

Mammography alone, usually all by demonstrating microcalcifications, makes it possible to detect DCIS even in asymptomatic patients. But this is associated with problems since:

● DCIS does not progress to invasive ductal carcinoma in all patients. If mastectomy is recommended as the therapy of choice, some patients will be overtreated.

● The microcalcifications found in DCIS (primarily microcalcifications in comedo DCIS) show a relatively characteristic pattern in some lesions. In other cases they are indistinguishable from calcifications found in benign conditions. Surgical removal of all calcifications that might represent DCIS (including the non-comedo type) could increase the sensitivity of detecting DCIS but would result in an unacceptable high biopsy rate (more than 10 excisions of benign findings for each detected DCIS).

On the basis of current knowledge, good sensitivity and acceptable specificity may only be achieved by:

● Thorough analysis of the mammographic calcifications.

● One should proceed to supplemental methods only after thorough analysis of microcalcifications, guided by critical appraisal of the limitations of the supplemental methods (see pp. 436–452).

Currently, sonography does not play an important role in the detection and diagnosis of DCIS. The potential role of MRI in the diagnosis of ductal carcinoma in situ is under investigation. The accuracy of conventional percutaneous biopsy is lower for ductal carcinoma in situ than for invasive carcinoma. Percutaneous biopsy methods, which allow sampling of larger amounts of tissue (such as vacuum biopsy) appear to reduce this problem (see p. 134).

■ Mammography

Microcalcifications are the *cardinal finding* of DCIS, but *microcalcifications* can be *absent* in DCIS. DCIS can mammographically appear as a density or an asymmetry, can be clinically symptomatic, or can be incidentally diagnosed histologically (in excisional biopsies performed for an unrelated reason).

■ Image Presentation

Mammographically, DCIS can become visible:[3, 27–32]

– Through microcalcifications. They are the only finding in about 80% of DCIS lesions detected by mammography, rarely surrounded by soft tissue density. (The surrounding soft tissue density, encountered in some of the DCIS without invasion, can be explained as reactive periductal fibrosis.)

– As a spiculated mass often without central density (10% of DCIS lesions).

– As an irregularly outlined mass (5% of DCIS lesions).

– As well-circumscribed nodular mass (<5% of DCIS lesions).

– As a filling defect or amputated duct visualized by galactography.

Importance of Microcalcifications

Mammographic microcalcifications are the most *important characterizing feature* of DCIS, but their presence should *by no means be equated with the presence of DCIS.*

Actually, up to 80% of excised microcalcifications—depending on the technical quality of the mammographic films and experience of the examiner—turn out to be benign. Therefore, it represents an important diagnostic challenge to analyze the microcalcifications and above all to differentiate malignant calcifications from calcifications occurring in context with benign conditions (mostly in mastopathy).

Image Presentation of Microcalcifications in DCIS

The following calcifications can be found in DCIS:

1. *In the comedo type,* the central cells undergoing necrosis calcify. These necrotic cylinders can be extruded under pressure from the macroscopic specimen like common cutaneous comedos, as implied in the name given in analogy with this condition. Since this necrotic cellular materials is always within the lactiferous ductal system, it leads to:

– Typical segmental arrangement of the so-called ductal calcifications following the ductal system (Figs. 14.**2a–c**). Depending on the location within the breast, a linear, branching arrangement, with or without segmental or triangular distribution with the apex oriented toward the nipple can be observed. Rectangu-

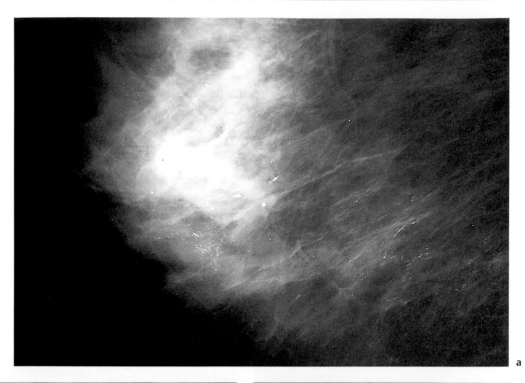

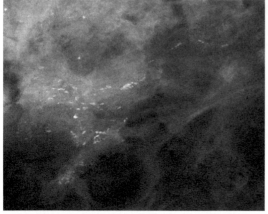

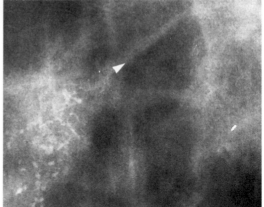

Fig. 14.**2 a–c**
a Typical segmental arrangement of microcalcifications, extending from the prepectoral region to the nipple: DCIS, comedo type
b The specimen radiograph (magnification) shows the elongated casts of individual calcifications and their branching pattern to better advantage
c Characteristic triangular group formation, with the apex of the triangle pointing toward the nipple. *Histology:* comedo DCIS

lar, club-shaped and butterfly-shaped formations, depending on the projection, may occur as well.
– Typical microcalcifications, so-called rod-like casting of the small lactiferous ducts with branching configurations (Y-shaped, V-shaped), linear and/or comma-shaped calcifications (Fig. 14.**3**).

– Typical, markedly pleomorphic, granular microcalcifications up to 2 mm in diameter (Fig. 14.**4**).

These calcifications frequently, but not invariably indicate the presence of DCIS, usually the comedo type, with a high degree of specificity (in about 80% of the cases). It should be pointed out that

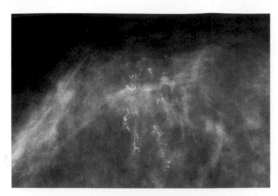

Fig. 14.**3** Magnification mammography with typical irregular, linear calcifications and branching pattern: comedo DCIS

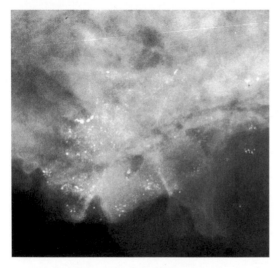

Fig. 14.**4** Predominantly larger granular, pleomorphic microcalcifications next to a few elongated casts. Specimen radiography: peripheral location of the calcifications

comedo-DCIS does not always calcify and that about 20–25% of the cases of calcified comedo-DCIS fail to exhibit this characteristic pattern.

2. *In the cribriform and micropapillary subtype of the non-comedo carcinoma* (Fig. 14.**5a–h**), the very tiny, often round cavities that are part of the typical histomorphologic architecture of these DCIS fill with secretion and calcify. Therefore, calcific manifestation of the non-comedo DCIS is:

– Frequently very delicate
– Occasionally fine granular, irregular to bizarre
– But sometimes also fine granular, relatively monomorphic

This means that the rod-like casts characteristic of comedo-DCIS are less common.

– As for comedo-DCIS, the *arrangement* of the calcifications may often be ductal or segmental

Such microcalcifications are considered less characteristic—in particular, if a ductal or segmental arrangement is not definitely recognizable—since they are very frequently encountered in benign changes as well and are indicative of a malignancy in only 5–20% of the lesions.

In addition to these uncharacteristic calcifications, less frequently non-comedo DCIS may develop comedo-type calcifications, facilitating early detection and differentiation from benign changes.

Altogether, exact mammographic assignment to a certain histologic subtype only succeeds in some cases. The list presented above should be seen as a basis for a better understanding of the microcalcific formations, but by no means as a substitute for histology. Moreover, a subtype rarely manifests itself, alone. More often, the various subtypes are mixed and occur together. Additionally, since the basement membrane cannot be seen mammographically, and because in some cases of pure ductal carcinoma in situ a mass can be present (corresponding to the ductal carcinoma in situ itself or to a reactive component adjacent to it), ductal carcinoma in situ cannot be differentiated from invasive cancer based on imaging. Therefore, the radiologist should not attempt to predict the histology of DCIS on the basis of the mammographic pattern of calcifications or predict invasion based on the presence of a mass or density.

In a prospective study, the comedo subtype was more likely accompanied by linear calcifications (78%)[5] than the non-comedo subtypes, which was more likely associated with fine-granular calcifications (53%).

Methodical Prerequisites for the Analysis of Microcalcifications

The comprehensive evaluation of microcalcifications requires mammography in at least two projections. High image quality concerning optimized contrast, correct exposure of the area in question, good contrast, and acceptable noise level are absolute prerequisites.

For demonstrating the teacup appearance of benign microcalcifications, one mediolateral view, perhaps as an added view, should be ob-

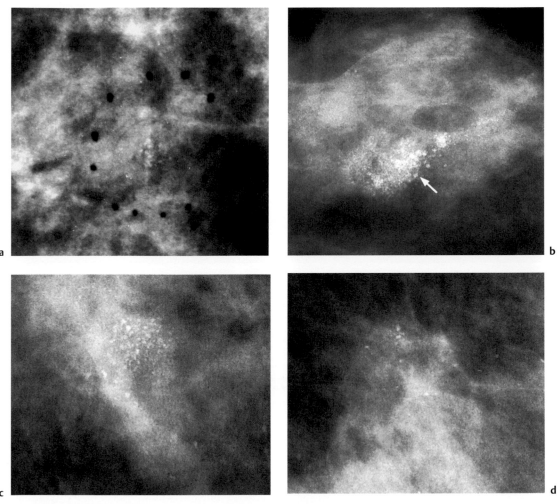

Fig. 14.**5 a–h** Magnification × 4

a Magnification mammography shows very fine granular calcifications arranged like a string of pearls.
Histology: low-grade ductal carcinoma in situ
b The specimen radiograph clearly depicts the individual fine granular configuration as well as the ductal distribution. *Histology:* micropapillary cribriform DCIS

c Fine granular pleomorphic microcalcifications, in clusters, which, however, contain casting shapes as well: cribriform DCIS
d Faint spiculated mass with several fine granular calcifications: cribriform–papillary DCIS

tained in a 90° lateral projection, usually with magnification.

Magnification mammography is of utmost importance for improving the analysis of the morphology of the individual calcifications and their extent.

■ **Other Mammographic Presentations**
(Figs. 14.6 a–d)

Other presentations of ductal carcinoma in situ include a spiculated lesion with or without a cen-tral density or a mass with smooth or irregular contours (usually without microcalcifications). Some ductal carcinomas in situ neither present as a mass nor as an architectural distortion nor with microcalcifications. These may be detected incidentally by histology (obtained for other reasons). In some cases a ductal carcinoma in situ may present by nipple discharge, and can be detected by galactography (unless otherwise apparent by mammography). Very rarely may a ductal carcinoma in situ be apparent on the mammogram as a thickened duct only (Fig. 14.6c).

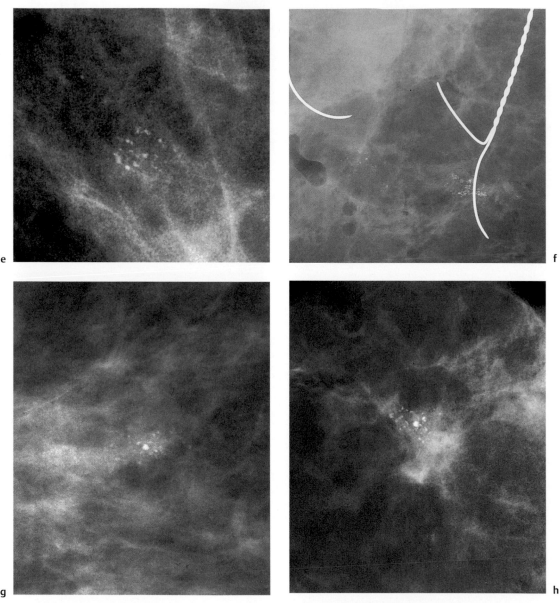

Fig. 14.**5 e** Small cluster of fine granular microcalcifications: DCIS, papillary type
f Magnification specimen radiograph (excision after vacuum biopsy) shows very small, partially punctated, partially elongated fine granular microcalcifications in 2 areas arranged in a branching, ductal distribution: DCIS with micropapillary and solid subtypes

g Small group of predominantly fine granular microcalcifications within a focal mass with delicate spiculation: small-cell DCIS, 5 mm in size, with desmoplastic reaction
h Magnification specimen radiography

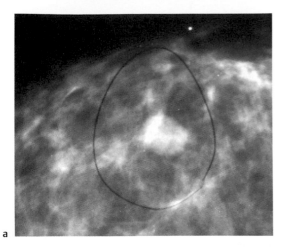

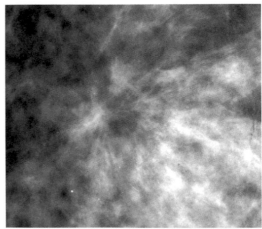

a

b

Fig. 14.**6** Other presentations of ductal carcinoma in situ

a Rarely a ductal carcinoma in situ may present as a mass, which more often is well-circumscribed as in this case. It was biopsied because it had newly developed.
Histology: highly differentiated papillary ductal carcinoma in situ

b Some ductal carcinoma in situ may arise in radial scars. This radial scar has a dense center („white scar") and contains some microcalcifications, two features which make it even more suspicious
Histology: low-grade ductal carcinoma in situ within a radial scar

c and **d** Some ductal carcinomas in situ become apparent by nipple discharge. Galactography is indicated

c In this patient there is a cutoff directly behind the nipple. However, a dilated duct is visible for another 2 cm behind the stop (arrows)

d In this patient the tissue behind the nipple exhibits slight architectural distortion. On the galactogram multiple filling defects and cutoffs are seen in the ductal system of this region

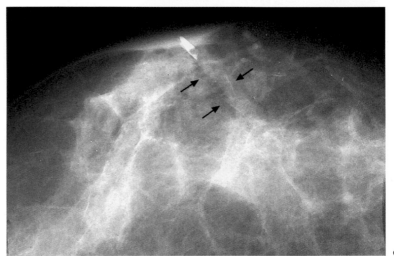

c

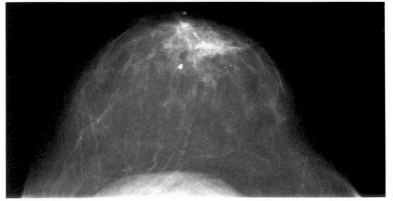

d

■ Accuracy of Mammography for the Detection and Differential Diagnosis

Mammography alone has made it possible to detect DCIS on a large scale. It is therefore the decisive method for detecting and diagnosing carcinomas in situ. Since carcinomas in situ not visible mammographically are generally clinically asymptomatic, the true sensitivity is unknown.

DCIS presenting as "characteristic calcifications" or spiculated density is mammographically detectable with a very high sensitivity and good specificity. DCIS with less characteristic calcifications that are aggregated in groups too small for analysis as well as DCIS presenting as an uncharacteristic or a smoothly outlined density may not always be diagnosable by imaging. Since these changes are uncharacteristic, they cannot all be pursued by immediate biopsy in order to maintain an acceptable specificity.

It is well known that some DCIS may not be visible mammographically and may only be discovered as an incidental histologic finding. Prevalence as well as significance of mammographically invisible DCIS cannot be assessed at the present time.

■ Additional Roles of Mammography for DCIS

In addition to detecting DCIS (usually on the basis of microcalcifications), mammography is given the important role of providing information concerning its extent (as feasible through microcalcifications) as accurately as possible. This is necessary since a complete removal of DCIS is of great therapeutic significance and since DCIS generally is neither palpable nor macroscopically demarcated.

The mammographic assessment of size, however, is only a crude estimate, since noncalcified components of the DCIS are usually mammographically not apparent. This means that *the extent of intraductal carcinomas is often mammographically underestimated.* To assess the extent as best as possible:

- *Preoperative mammography* must be performed using optimal technique (magnification).
- *Specimen radiography* should be used routinely and with optimal technique, i.e., as standard and magnification views.
- All *microcalcific foci* (especially those close to the cut surface) are *to be marked* on the specimen for the pathologist.

- Postoperative mammography of the surgical site should be performed if breast-preserving surgery is planned, including standard and magnification views. This is important in order to detect any remaining calcifications that might necessitate a second resection or mastectomy, and to document residual benign calcifications for future mammograms obtained as part of the follow-up care.[22]

■ Sonography (Fig. 14.7)

■ Image Presentation

Most carcinomas in situ have no characteristic sonographic presentation, i.e., they cannot be distinguished sonographically from normal parenchyma. Only in a few carcinomas in situ—in particular, if a high resolution transducer is used—larger microcalcifications may be visualized or suspected by relatively strong echoes, or dilated hypoechoic ductal structures be interpreted as evidence of DCIS. However, numerous other causes exist for dilated ducts.

Ductal carcinoma in situ, which presents as a mass, may be detected by ultrasound within dense tissue.[33, 34]

■ Accuracy

All evidence considered, sonography does not afford a reliable diagnosis of DCIS.

■ Importance

Consequently, sonography does *not* contribute to the detection, exclusion, or differential diagnosis of DCIS.

■ Magnetic Resonance Imaging

The experiences of several investigators concerning the presentation of ductal carcinoma in situ on contrast-enhanced MRI is summarized:[35–39]

■ Image Presentation

In contrary to initial expectations most ductal carcinomas in situ (80–90%) enhance with contrast agent. However, the enhancement pattern of part of the ductal carcinoma in situ overlaps with enhancement patterns seen in benign changes.

The following features, which occur in ductal carcinoma in situ, have to be considered suspicious of malignancy and can thus lead to the correct diagnosis of ductal carcinoma in situ based on MRI:

- Early enhancing lesion with irregular contours
- Early enhancement and early washout (associated with any type of morphology)
- Peripheral enhancement, which is more frequently present in invasive carcinoma
- Ductal or branching enhancement (irrespective of enhancement dynamics)
- Segmental enhancement (irrespective of enhancement dynamics)

If one of the above signs is present, biopsy should be considered even in the absence of abnormal findings on conventional imaging. A distinction between invasive carcinoma and ductal carcinoma in situ or between the different types of ductal carcinoma in situ is not possible by MRI. About 50–80% of the ductal carcinoma in situ will fulfil at least one of the above criteria and can be correctly recognized by MRI. In addition a correct biopsy recommendation may be made in ductal carcinoma in situ with nonspecific enhancement (focal lesion with delayed enhancement), if the area in question is considered abnormal by other imaging modalities as well, or if the patient is at high risk (e.g., preoperative MRI before breast-conserving therapy). The latter recommendations depend on the chosen interpretation guidelines.

■ Accuracy

Depending on patient preselection and interpretation rules, sensitivities ranging from 50% to over 90% have been reported by different authors.

In general, guidelines that yield a higher sensitivity are usually associated with lower specificity, and vice versa. It should, however, be understood that some ductal carcinomas in situ (10–20%) do not enhance.

■ Significance

In order to avoid false negative diagnoses on otherwise suspicious lesions, MRI is not recommended for differentiation of mammographically suspected DCIS. If suspicious microcalcifications or other signs compatible with the potential presence of ductal carcinoma in situ (radial scar)

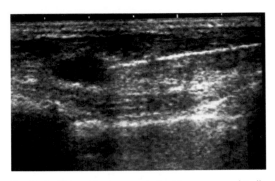

Fig. 14.**7**   This patient presented with a sonographically visible 7-mm hypoechoic mass, which corresponded to a discrete palpable abnormality detected by the patient herself. No abnormality was seen on the mammogram, which showed very dense breast tissue.

exist on conventional imaging, biopsy is necessary irrespective of the MRI findings.

However, MRI is capable of detecting ductal carcinoma in situ not visualized by other methods. Whether MRI should be recommended for preoperative local staging to assess the extent or multicentricity of ductal carcinoma in situ is controversial.

■ Percutaneous Biopsy

The accuracy of conventional percutaneous biopsy is lower for ductal carcinoma in situ than for invasive carcinoma.[40–42] The reason may be that many ductal carcinomas in situ exhibit discontinuous growth and that microcalcifications indicative of ductal carcinoma in situ may be remote from the malignant cells. Thus sampling error may occur. Entities for which an increased risk of sampling error exists, include lesions that present with microcalcifications only and radial scars. Since vacuum biopsy allows aquisition of a much higher volume of tissue, an improved accuracy may be expected, provided a sufficient volume of tissue is acquired (see Chapter 7, p. 134).

Advantages of vacuum biopsy over conventional biopsy have been confirmed for microcalcifications[43–45]; the role of vacuum biopsy in radial scars, however, which may be associated with ductal carcinoma in situ in their periphery, is under investigation. Ductal carcinoma in situ, which presents as a mass, may be worked-up by conventional percutaneous biopsy or vacuum biopsy under stereotactic or sonographic guidance.

Whenever ductal carcinoma in situ is a differential diagnosis and biopsy does not confirm the suspicion, correlation of imaging and histopathology is required to check representative removal. A percutaneous biopsy diagnosis (conventional or vacuum biopsy) should lead to appropriate surgical treatment (re-excision with or without irradiation or—in case of extended involvement—mastectomy). If the ductal carcinoma in situ is associated with an invasive component, axillary dissection or sampling is required. Whereas fine needle aspiration cannot distinguish between invasive and in situ carcinoma, vacuum biopsy is able to correctly diagnose associated invasion in a much higher percentage than core needle biopsy.[46, 47] This is advantageous for treatment planning.

■ Summary

LCIS cannot be diagnosed clinically or mammographically. It is often discovered incidentally through excisional biopsies performed because of questionable abnormal palpation or indeterminate mammographic findings. The therapeutic consequence consists of categorizing a patient with histologically proven LCIS as a patient at risk, i.e., to subject her to annual clinical and mammographic examinations for the early detection of a developing invasive carcinoma.

The term DCIS encompasses a group of histologically and prognostically heterogeneous noninvasive carcinomas. Its discovery has risen with the increasing use of mammography. Microcalcifications are the cardinal finding in DCIS. Therefore mammography is the primary imaging method since it alone permits the detection and analysis of microcalcifications.

While the comedo subtype produces a mammographically characteristic (ductal) pattern of individual forms and distribution, the noncomedo subtypes are more difficult to differentiate from the numerous microcalcifications that are associated with benign breast conditions. The rigorous use of magnification mammography adds significantly to increasing the accuracy.

Sonography plays no role in the detection, exclusion, or differential diagnosis of DCIS.

The experience with contrast-enhanced MRI is limited at the present time and MRI does not contribute to the differential diagnosis of microcalcifications.

At present, further investigations and data are necessary to determine whether and under which conditions percutaneous biopsy methods (aspiration cytology, core needle biopsy) might eventually be able to replace excisional biopsy for evaluating microcalcifications. Presently, the limitations of percutaneous biopsy must be critically taken into account, particularly when suspected microcalcifications are to be evaluated.

■ References

1   Stegner HE. Histopathologie der Mammatumoren. Licht- und elektronenmikroskopischer Atlas. Stuttgart: Enke; 1986
2   Beute BJ, Kalisher L, Hutter RV. Lobular carcinoma in situ of the breast: clinical, pathologic, and mammographic features. AJR. 1991;157:257–65
3   Ringberg A, Andersson J, Aspegren K, Linell F. Breast carcinoma in situ in 167 women: incidence, mode of presentation, therapy and follow-up. Eur J Surg Oncol. 1991; 17:466–76
4   Goldschmidt RA, Victor TA. Lobular carcinoma in situ of the breast. Semin Surg Oncol. 1996;12:314–20
5   Schnitt SJ, Silen W, Sadowsky NL, Connolly JL, Harris JR. Ductal carcinoma in situ (intraductal carcinoma of the breast). N Engl J Med. 1988;318:898–903
6   v. Dongen JA, Harris JR, Petersen JL, Fentiman IS, Holland R, Salvadori E, Stewart HJ. In situ breast cancer: The EORTC consensus meeting. Lancet. 1989;25–7
7   Holland R, Hendriks JHCL, Verbeek ALM, Schuurmans Stekhoven JH. Extent, distribution and mammographic/histological correlations of the breast ductal carcinoma in situ. Lancet. 1990;335:519–22
8   Stomper PC, Conolly JL. Ductal carcinoma in situ of the breast: correlation between mammographic calcification and tumor subtype. AJR. 1992;159:483–5
9   Dershaw DD, Abramson A, Kinne DW. Ductal carcinoma in situ: mammographic findings and clinical implications. Radiology. 1989;170:411–15
10 Lagios MD, Margolin FR, Westdahl PR, Rose MR. Mammographically detected duct carcinoma in situ: frequency of local recurrence following tylectomy and prognostic effect of nuclear grade on local recurrence. Cancer. 1989;63:618–24
11 Silverstein MJ. Intraductal breast carcinoma (DCIS). Clinical factors influencing treatment choice. Abstract: 7th International Congress on Senology, Island of Rhodes. 1992
12 Lagios MD, Westdahl PR, Margolin FR, Rose MR. Duct carcinoma in situ: relationship of extent of noninvasive disease to the frequency of occult invasion, multicentricity, lymph node metastases and short-term treatment failures. Cancer. 1982;50:1309–14
13 Ashikari R, Huvos AG, Snyder RE. Prospective study of noninfiltrating carcinoma of the breast. Cancer. 1977;39:435–9

14 Millis RR, Thynne GSJ. In situ intraduct carcinoma of the breast: a long term follow-up study. Br J Surg. 1975;62:975–62

15 Eusebi V, Foschini MP, Cook MG, Berrino F, Azzopardi JG. Long-term follow-up of in situ carcinoma of the breast with special emphasis on clinging carcinoma. Semin Diagn Pathol. 1989;6:165–73

16 Solin LJ, Yeh IT, Kurtz J et al. Ductal carcinoma in situ (intraductal carcinoma) of the breast treated with breast-conserving surgery and definitive irradiation. Correlation of pathologic surgery and definitive irradiation. Correlation of pathologic parameters with outcome of treatment. Cancer. 1993;71:2532–42

17 Bellamy COC, McDonald C, Salter DM, Chetty U, Anderson J. Noninvasive ductal carcinoma of the breast: the relevance of histologic categorization. Hum Pathol. 1993;24:16–23

18 Holland R, Petersen JL, Millis RR et al. Ductal carcinoma in situ: a proposal for a new classification. Semin Diagn Pathol. 1994;11:167

19 Holland R, Hendriks JHCL. Microcalcifications associated with ductual carcinoma in situ: mammographic-pathologic correlation. Semin Diagn Pathol. 1994;11:181–92

20 Silverstein MJ, Lagios MD, Craig PH et al. A prognostic index for ductal carcinoma in situ of the breast. Cancer. 1996;77:2267–74

21 Schwartz GF, Finkel G, Garcia JC, Patchefsky AS. Subclinical ductal carcinoma in situ of the breast. Treatment by local excision and surveillance alone. Cancer. 1992;70:2468–74

22 Fisher F, Constantino J, Fisher B, Palekar A, Redmond C, Mamounas E. Pathologic findings from the National Surgical Adjuvant Breast Project (NSABP) Protokol B –17. Intraductal carcinoma (ductal carcinoma in situ). Cancer. 1995;75:1310–19

23 Page DL, Dupont WD, Rogers LW, Landenberger M. Intraductal carcinoma of the breast: Follow-up after biopsy only. Cancer. 1982;49:751–8

24 Solin LJ, Recht A, Fourquet A et al. Ten-year results of breast-conserving surgery and definitive irradiation for intraductal carcinoma (ductal carcinoma in situ) of the breast. Cancer. 1991;68:2337–44

25 Silverstein MJ, Poller DN, Waisman JR et al. Prognostic classification of the breast ductal carcinoma in situ. Lancet. 1995;345:1154–7

26 Poller DN, Silverstein MJ, Galea M et al. Ductal carcinoma in situ of the breast: a proposal for a new simplified histological classification association between cellular proliferation and c-erb B 2 protein expression. Mod Pathol. 1994;7:257–62

27 Holland R, Hendriks JH. Microcalcifications associated with ductal carcinoma in situ: mammographic-pathologic correlation. Semin Diagn Pathol. 1994;11:181–92

28 Hermann G, Keller RJ, Drossman S et al. Mammographic pattern of microcalcifications in the preoperative diagnosis of comedo ductal carcinoma in situ: histopathologic correlation. Can Assoc Radiol J. 1999;50:235–40

29 Evans AJ, Wilson AR, Burrell HC et al. Mammographic features of ductal carcinoma in situ (DCIS) present on previous mammography. Clin Radiol. 1999;54:644–6

30 Di Piro PJ, Meyer JE, Denison CM et al. Image-guided core breast biopsy of ductal carcinoma in situ presenting as a non-calcified abnormality. Eur J Radiol. 1999,30.231–6

31 Dessole S, Meloni GB, Capobianco G et al. Radial scar of the breast: mammographic enigma in pre- and post-menopausal women. Maturitas. 2000,34:227–31

32 Alleva DQ, Smetherman DH, Farr GH, Cederbom GJ. Radial scar of the breast: radiologic-pathologic correlation in 22 cases. Radiographics. 1999;19:S27–35

33 Skaane P. The additional value of US to mammography in the diagnosis of breast cancer. A prospective study. Acta Radiol. 1999,40:486–90

34 Berg WA, Gilbreath PL. Multicentric and multifocal cancer: whole-breast US in preoperative evaluation. Radiology. 2000;214;59–66

35 Gilles R, Zafrani B, Guinebretiere JM et al. Ductal carcinoma in situ. MR imaging: histopathologic correlation. Radiology. 1995;196:415–9

36 Soderstom CE, Harms SE, Copit DS et al. Three-dimensional RODEO breast MR imaging of lesions containing ductal carcinoma in situ. Radiology. 1996;201:427–32

37 Westerhof JP, Fischer U, Moritz JD, Oestmann JW. MR Imaging of mammographically detected clustered microcalcifications; is there any value? Radiology. 1998;207:675–81

38 Orel SG, Medonca MH, Reynolds C et al. MR imaging of ductal carcinoma in situ. Radiology. 1997;202:413–20

39 Viehweg P, Lampe D, Buchmann J, Heywang-Köbrunner SH. In situ and microinvasive breast cancer: Morphologic and kinetic features on contrast-enhanced MR imaging. MAGMA 2000, in press

40 Liberman L, Dershaw DD, Glassman JR et al. Analysis of cancers not diagnosed at stereotactic core breast biopsy. Radiology. 1997;203:151–7

41 Mainiero MB, Philpotts LE, Lee CH et al. Stereotaxic core needle biopsy of breast microcalcifications correlation of target accuracy and diagnosis with lesion size. Radiology. 1996,198:665–9

42 Brenner RJ, Fajardo L, Fisher PR et al. Percutaneous core biopsy of the breast: effect of operator experience and number of samples on diagnostic accuracy. AJR. 1996;166:341–6

43 Meyer JE, Smith DN, Dipiro PJ et al. Stereotactic breast biopsy of clustered microcalcifications with a directional, vacuum-assisted device. Radiology. 1997;204:575–6

44 Jackman RJ, Marzoni FA, Nowels KW. Percutaneous removal of benign mammographic lesions: comparison of automated large-core and directional vacuum-assisted biopsy techniques. AJR. 1998;171:1325–30

45 Heywang-Köbrunner SH, Schaumlöffel U, Viehweg P et al. Minimally invasive stereotactic vacuum core breast biopsy. Eur Radiol. 1998;8:377–85

46 Burbank F. Stereotactic breast biopsy of atypical ductal hyperplasia and ductal carcinoma in situ: improved accuracy with a directional, vacuum-assisted biopsy instrument. Radiology. 1997;202:843–8

47 Brem RF, Behrndt VS, Sanow L, Gatewood OMB. Atypical ductal hyperplasia: histologic underestimation of carcinoma in tissue harvested from impalpable breast lesions using 11-gauge stereotactically guided directional vacuum-assisted biopsy. AJR. 1999;172:1405–7

15. Invasive Carcinoma

Invasive carcinoma is by far the most frequent carcinoma of the female breast, and is, in fact, the most frequent malignancy in women. For unknown reasons, the incidence of breast carcinoma continues to increase. Currently, it can be expected that about every 8th American woman will develop a breast carcinoma in her lifetime. In populations not yet subjected to screening, mortality due to breast carcinoma remains high in spite of improved therapy. All things considered, breast carcinoma is the most frequent cause of death for women between the age of 39 and 58 years.[1, 2]

■ Definition and Problems Posed

With the development of invasion—recognizable by the extension of tumor cells through the basement membrane—*the possibility of metastases, and therefore death, exists. It is therefore desirable to detect the invasive carcinoma when it is as small as possible.* This is confirmed by studies[3] that suggest worsening of the prognosis of tumors exceeding 15 mm in size. Of course, breast carcinomas smaller than 15 mm can metastasize, but early detection will prevent metastases in most of these carcinomas. Delay in diagnosis with increasing tumor size suggests a worsening prognosis.

■ Spectrum and Detectability

While detecting the carcinoma that is already large and exhibits characteristic findings usually does not represent a problem, the timely detection of tumors in their early stage or with atypical manifestations remains a diagnostic challenge. Both breast carcinomas and various benign breast conditions exhibit a considerable range of variability, and the signs of an early carcinoma frequently overlap with those of benign conditions, making detection and diagnosis more difficult. With all modalities, the detectability of the breast carcinoma depends on size, histology (e.g.,

difficult recognition of lobular carcinoma), growth pattern (difficult recognition of diffusely growing carcinoma), and surrounding tissue (difficult recognition of carcinomas within dense tissue).

It should be kept in mind that so far no available clinical diagnostic method can detect all invasive carcinomas. False negative findings can be encountered in diffusely growing carcinomas, rarely even in large focal carcinomas, but above all in small carcinomas surrounded by dense tissue.

The positive predictive value, which indicates the percentage of carcinomas found among recommended biopsies, is variable.

The positive predictive value primarily depends on

- Age distribution of the screened population
- Examination intervals (with long screening intervals, the number of large and consequently unequivocal findings increases in comparison with shorter, e.g., annual intervals)
- The extent of utilizing additional methods, e.g., sonography, percutaneous biopsy, MRI, and
- The individual threshold of the examiner[4-9]

All things considered, there is an inversely proportional relationship between sensitivity and positive predictive value (number of carcinomas per number of recommended biopsies). Selecting a very low threshold for a positive diagnosis (recommending a biopsy even for findings with a low likehood of being malignant) increases the number of found malignancies by a few percent. The positive predictive value, however, decreases markedly because more benign changes have to be removed. Selecting a very high threshold for a positive diagnosis increases the positive predictive value, but several carcinomas that would have been detected with a lower threshold remain undetected.

Considering the possibilities and limitations of imaging methods, it remains important to combine imaging with palpation, inspection, and patient history for symptomatic patients.

For the interpretation of imaging methods in asymptomatic patients, a compromise has to be made between a detection rate that is as high as possible and the number of additional examinations and biopsies that can be justified medically and economically.

The evaluation of symptomatic patients with an uncertain finding requires the utilization of supplemental methods to avoid unnecessary biopsies combined with the highest safety for the patient.

■ Diagnostic Strategy and Goals

The diagnostic methods for detecting and evaluating breast carcinomas have the following goals:

● In asymptomatic patients, diagnostic methods are used as *screening* for early detection of breast carcinoma. The only method currently appropriate for screening is mammography. The effectiveness of mammographic screening to reduce mortality by 30–50% through improved early detection has been established in numerous studies (see Chapter 21).

● In clinically symptomatic patients and in patients with abnormal screening examinations, further *evaluation* is indicated to avoid unnecessary biopsies and to reveal or exclude possible additional findings. For this diagnostic evaluation, special supplemental mammographic techniques (magnification views, additional projections, galactography) and other imaging modalities, such as sonography and MRI, are available, as well as percutaneous biopsy techniques.

● In the presence of a suspicious finding, the available imaging methods are used for preoperative *staging*. This involves assessing the extent of the known tumor, detecting or excluding multifocality or multicentricity, and assessment for possible tumor in the other breast (possible detection of involved lymph nodes, see p. 270). Findings with significant therapeutic consequences (e.g., detection of a second lesion) must be confirmed histologically.

■ Screening

Screening refers to examinations performed on asymptomatic patients at regular intervals with the goal of early detection with increased likelihood of cure. Because of its high sensitivity and acceptable specificity and because of its fast and well-reproducible performance and interpretation as well as its reasonable costs, mammography is currently the only imaging method suitable for screening for breast cancer.

Due to the high false positive rate and increased expense of the clinical examination, most screening programs do not combine mammography with a clinical examination.

When mammographic screening is performed without palpation, it should be remembered

- That about 10% of detectable cancers will be palpable, but not visible mammographically.
- That a mammographically negative screening finding is not sufficient for the exclusion of malignancy in the presence of clinical symptoms.

The task of mammography is to detect suspicious findings with the highest possible sensitivity. Comparison of the current mammogram with prior mammograms is desirable. Not infrequently, such comparison can markedly improve accuracy.

For some indeterminate mammographic findings, a positive predictive value of only 10–30% can be expected. Further workup serves to avoid excisional biopsies for benign findings as much as possible, thus increasing the positive predictive value.

Too many diagnostic biopsies performed on asymptomatic patients for safety's sake is neither medically nor economically justified for a screening program. Consequently, the desired positive predictive value for biopsies recommended after complete evaluation should exceed 20% (US) or 30% (most European screening programs). At the same time, the rate of interval carcinomas (carcinomas that become clinically apparent in the "interval" between screening examinations) should be monitored and kept as low as possible.

Because of the utmost importance of technical quality for reducing mortality,[10, 11] all institutions that perform screening examinations need to have a quality-assurance program in place for monitoring their own accuracy.

■ Imaging Methods for Further Workup

Preceding any additional evaluation of a potentially malignant finding, a technically adequate mammogram consisting of two views should be available.

Regardless of whether an indeterminate or even a suspicious finding has been found clinically or mammographically, the role of the additional evaluation consists of separating benign from potentially malignant findings with the highest achievable certainty.

The goal of the additional diagnostic workup is
- To avoid unnecessary biopsies (e.g., simple cysts)
- To refer a potentially malignant finding to biopsy.

This difficult task can be approached with additional mammographic views, sonography, MRI, galactography. Percutaneous biopsy methods can be used to reduce the number of patients sent for surgery.

- *Mammographically,* additional views should be obtained for palpable findings that are not included on the standard views because of atypical location, for mammographically suspicious densities possibly caused by superimposition, and for microcalcifications. For the evaluation of microcalcifications, mammography (lateral view and magnification view) is the crucial imaging method.
- *Sonography* is the supplemental modality for palpable changes in mammographically dense tissue and for all changes that might be attributable to simple cysts. Sonography is also valuable for assessing the margins of a mass, especially when it lies in dense tissue. It should always be remembered that a negative sonographic finding does not exclude a suspected malignancy, since carcinomas that are small and preinvasive can be inapparent sonographically.
- *Percutaneous biopsy* is appropriate for further evaluation of findings that are indeterminate by palpation, mammography, sonography, or MRI. Its use is contingent on high-quality technique, procurement of adequate tissue, and review of the accuracy of one's own patient material. A positive finding can confirm malignancy. A negative finding must be critically checked as to the accuracy of the localization procedure and the possibility of sampling error. If the histologic result and the imaging findings are nonconcordant, a repeat percutaneous or open biopsy is necessary.
- *Contrast-enhanced MRI* may presently be the most sensitive method for detecting breast cancer. It has proven capable of detecting invasive and sometimes even non-invasive foci not visible by the other methods. Because of the relatively high false positive rate encountered in proliferative benign changes, contrast-enhanced MRI is currently not recommended for work-up of indeterminate lesions, which is possible by percutaneous biopsy. Furthermore, it is not suitable for offering a differential diagnosis of indeterminate microcalcifications. Used in conjunction with conventional imaging, MRI has, however, proven useful in patients at increased risk, in whom the breast tissue is difficult to assess. These indications include: diagnostic problems due to multiple (surgical) scars, radiation fibrosis, or silicone implants; exclusion of multicentricity in difficult-to-assess breast tissue before breast-conserving therapy; search for primary tumor in cases with positive axillary lymph nodes—if the other imaging modalities were unsuccessful. Furthermore, MRI may be helpful in selected cases where exact localization of a suspected lesion is not possible by other methods (progressive nipple retraction, pathologic discharge, and unsuccessful galactogram, suspected density visible on one view only, not visible by ultrasound). The value of contrast-enhanced MRI in patients at high genetic risk is presently being evaluated in several large studies. Even though absent enhancement is associated with a high probability of benignity (approximately 95%) neither MRI nor percutaneous biopsy alone can dismiss a highly suspicious lesion whose assessment is negative with these techniques.
- *Galactography* should follow mammography as the method of choice for further evaluation of the breast with pathologic discharge.

Legal aspects. Because of the increasing number of lawsuits claiming that carcinomas have been discovered too late, it is important to document one's own accuracy. This applies not only to screening but also to diagnostic examinations performed for further evaluation.[11] This is particularly important considering that a high percentage of interval carcinomas and up to 50% of all carcinomas detected by screening can, in retrospect, be seen as discrete abnormality in the preceding examination.[12-17] The dividing line is blurred between findings that unquestionably need further evaluation and findings that cannot be differentiated, even by an experienced mammographer, from benign lesions. Having one's own accuracy well documented is particularly advantageous for cases subject to litigation.

■ **Staging**

Therapeutic planning must consider the

- Extent of the cancer in the breast
- Exclusion/detection of additional foci in the ipsilateral or contralateral breast
- Nodal involvement

If imaging methods suggest extension of findings over a wide area or the presence of a second focus, this has to be verified (e.g., through percutaneous biopsy or excision after localization).

Therapy should only be changed after adequate confirmation.

Extent of Tumor

The following findings have to be observed since their presence precludes a breast-preserving therapy:

- Tumor size too large to permit resection with good cosmetic results, or evidence of widely separated multifocal or multicentric carcinoma.
- Invasion of the nipple or subareolar ducts, or a narrow space between the tumor and these structures, precluding an excision with an adequate margin while preserving the nipple. This does not preclude conservation but requires sacrificing the nipple.
- Invasion of the skin.
  - To *assess the extension* in fatty or normal breasts, the examination with standard methods is generally sufficient. In mammographically dense, small, and normal-sized breasts, supplemental sonography has been used. High-resolution ultrasound is capable of detecting additional foci or demonstrating larger extension than shown on mammography.[18,19] If multicentricity has been detected by ultrasound and confirmed by percutaneous biopsy, treatment planning will be influenced. If this is not the case, and the breast tissue is difficult to evaluate, further workup for staging may be considered. Contrast-enhanced MRI proves to be the most sensitive method for invasive foci or for demonstration of the complete extension of a carcinoma. Even though only 80–90% of carcinomas in situ enhance (half of which enhance slowly or diffusely), MRI has proven to be able to complement conventional imaging by also showing additional in situ extent or foci, which may be undetected mammographically.[20–24] Since both MRI and ultrasound have a high rate of false positive calls, however, any finding suggestive of in situ or invasive carcinoma that would change treatment needs verification (e.g., by US- or MR-guided biopsy).
  - To assess the extension into the *subareolar region*, MRI is advantageous as well. Ultrasound may be limited in this area due to the posterior nipple shadow.
  - To detect *ductal carcinoma in situ* found by *microcalcifications,* mammography is the definitive method. Assessing the full extent of microcalcifications often requires additional magnification views.

Care should be taken to *excise all suspicious microcalcifications* and to *mark them in the specimen* so that they can be found and evaluated by the pathologist to determine the extent of the tumor. *Otherwise, small foci of microcalcifications can—being nonpalpable—remain undetected by the surgeon as well as by the pathologist.*[25] On the other hand, the pathologist might find mammographically occult carcinomas in situ.

If specimen radiography reveals marginal or possibly incompletely excised areas of microcalcifications, a wider resection at the time of the lumpectomy should be considered by the surgeon. If microcalcifications are detected remote from the primary area of concern, preoperative vacuum biopsy is recommended. It usually allows a reliable histopathologic diagnosis of the second area of concern and may thus provide the information that is decisive for treatment planning.

- In suspected incomplete excision or unsuccessful excision following a wider resection, a postoperative mammogram should be obtained if the original tumor contained calcifications. Residual uncalcified tumor, which often cannot be adequately assessed by postoperative mammography, can be evaluated by MRI up to the 10th postoperative day (before granulation tissue will develop). While neither method can exclude residual microscopic foci, they can disclose most remaining foci $\geq$ 3 to 5 mm.

Exclusion and Detection of Additional Foci

Preoperative evaluation to find or exclude additional foci is important for three reasons:

- Any additional suspicious focus as well as a contralateral suspicious finding should, if possible, be removed during the same surgical procedure or be worked up by percutaneous conventional or vacuum biopsy preoperatively.
- If multicentric growth* is confirmed, breast-preserving therapy is no longer appropriate because of the expected high recurrence rate and the deformity of the breast resulting from removal of tumor at multiple sites
- If the primary finding proves to be benign, the suspected secondary finding might become the relevant primary finding

For these reasons, *a thorough diagnostic evaluation of both breasts* is indicated before any scheduled breast surgery.

Surgery on the basis of palpable findings alone without further diagnostic evaluation is no longer considered standard care.

The preoperative exclusion or detection of additional foci begins with the standard diagnostic evaluation.

Microcalcifications as suggestive evidence for additional foci can be detected by additional magnification views. Ultrasound may complement mammography in dense breasts and may detect additional foci not seen by mammography.

Contrast-enhanced MRI is the most sensitive method for detecting any possible secondary foci (without microcalcifications) before breast-conserving therapy, whenever the breast tissue is difficult to assess by conventional imaging. Based on the present literature, additional unexpected foci may be detected in 10–35% (average 15%) of the patients with breast cancer. A suspected secondary focus should be confirmed, as described above, before altering the therapy.

Diagnostic Evaluation of the Lymph Nodes

Axillary lymph nodes. Targeted imaging of the regional lymph nodes is generally not done because no imaging method can detect or exclude prognostically relevant microscopic nodal metastases. Instead, it is customary to perform an axillary dissection or sampling, the extent of which varies with different surgeons, or a sentinel node biopsy. Imaging evaluation of the axillary lymph nodes is so far not considered necessary prior to surgery. If imaging is performed in an individual case, typical features should be known (Chapter 16).

Detecting microscopic metastases in the internal mammary lymph nodes (medial or central location of the tumor) is also difficult for imaging methods. Whether diagnostic tests can detect macroscopic metastases with adequate certainty and whether this has any prognostic significance is controversial.

Metastases are rarely found in intramammary lymph nodes. Macroscopic metastases appear as focal findings, while micoscopic metastases escape detection by imaging methods.

In general, the regional lymph nodes are evaluated clinically. A microscopic metastasis, which is of considerable importance for the therapeutic approach, cannot be visualized by any imaging method.

Consequently, there is no substitute for histopathologic assessment of the lymph-nodes.

Sonography is the method of choice for clinically suspected involvement of the axillary lymph nodes requiring preoperative confirmation.[26–28]

Mammography (axillary view) may show evidence of involvement when suspicious microcalcifications are visualized within a lymph node, its margins assume an irregular shape, or a lymph node increases in density and loses its central fat.[29–31]

The confirmation of a suspicion is possible by means of a fine-needle aspiration, which is usually performed under sonographic guidance, but a negative outcome of the FNA cannot exclude nodal involvement.

Recurrent disease (above all, axillary, supraclavicular, or infraclavicular recurrence) can be best evaluated by sonography. Contrast-enhanced CT and contrast-enhanced MRI (using a different technique than for breast imaging) may be helpful as well.

■ Histology

A major reason for the difficulty encountered in recognizing and differentiating breast carcinomas is the multitude of patterns and types observed. Therefore, knowledge of the histologic growth

---

* The definition of multicentricity is variable. Some define multicentricity as presence of foci in other quadrants than the primary carcinomas, others as presence of foci that are 4 or 5 cm distant from the primary carcinoma. Overall, multicentricity suggests foci in more than one duct system, whereas multifocality suggests foci just in one duct system

patterns and tumor types is of particular importance for diagnosing breast carcinoma.

The growth patterns are generally characterized as:

- Spiculated as well as lobulated growing carcinomas with irregular margins
- Nodular and lobulated carcinomas
- Round as well as smoothly demarcated carcinomas
- Diffusely growing carcinomas

The intracystic carcinoma is by definition a carcinoma in situ as long as it does not penetrate the cyst wall. If it has penetrated the cyst wall, it becomes an invasive carcinoma.

■ **Types of Carcinomas**

The most frequent type of carcinoma is the invasive ductal carcinoma not otherwise specified (NOS) (60–80% of carcinomas), followed by the invasive lobular carcinoma (about 15%) as well as special types of invasive ductal carcinoma, including medullary carcinoma (3–4%), mucinous (about 3%), papillary (about 2%), and tubular (about 2–3%) carcinoma. There are other rather rare types of carcinoma. Paget carcinoma of the nipple and inflammatory carcinoma are breast carcinomas with unique clinical presentation.

Ductal carcinoma is the most frequent type. It arises in the region of the terminal ductolobular segment. Many of these carcinomas have no distinctive histologic findings and are, therefore, classified as NOS.

Wide variations in the morphology of the tumor cells can be found, ranging from relatively uniform, small cells to pleomorphic, large cells.

The cells can grow in parenchymal formations, in nests or cords, or, similar to intraductal carcinoma, along the existing ductal structures where they penetrate the basement membrane at one or several sites. A marked fibrotic component can often be found. Infrequently, extensive areas of carcinoma in situ are present within and in the tissue surrounding the invasive ductal carcinoma. When present, an extensive intraductal component that cannot be completely removed can often lead to tumor recurrence after breast-conserving therapy. Histopathologic grading has a significant influence on the prognosis.

Growth patterns that determine the image presentation vary considerably.

- Most frequently, ductal carcinoma shows a *spiculated and nodular growth* with an irregular outline. Histologically, these tumors often contain marked fibrosis that can be very pronounced in the center of the tumor.
- Medullary, mucinous, and papillary carcinomas characteristically show a round, nodular growth. They are less frequent in number. Similar growth patterns can also be seen in ductal carcinomas NOS.
- The *diffusely growing* types are particularly difficult to recognize with imaging methods since the carcinomatous cells extend through the parenchyma or adipose tissue without forming a localized mass. Consequently, they may be invisible mammographically or sonographically. Unless these diffusely growing carcinomas contain microcalcifications, they often become visible only after accompanying fibrosis has caused an increase in the density of the parenchyma. Fibrosis can also lead to retraction and even reduce the size of the entire breast.
- About 30–40% of invasive ductal carcinomas contain microcalcifications. These calcifications can—as in DCIS—characteristically appear as rod-like casts along the ductal system, but calcifications exhibiting less characteristic manifestations can occur. Central necrotic areas in large tumors can harbor coarse calcifications.

Lobular carcinoma is the second-most frequent type. Characteristically, it exhibits a *diffuse* growth pattern or architectural distortion. It may also produce lobulated or spiculated masses or, rarely, even a fairly well-circumscribed mass. The cells of invasive lobular carcinoma are small, round, and uniform. They often contain mucinous vacuoles. If these mucinous vacuoles are large and dominate the entire cellular pattern, it is a sign of the prognostically unfavorable signet ring carcinoma. The cells of lobular carcinoma often grow diffusely, individually, or in a string-like arrangement into the stroma.

Frequently, invasive lobular carcinoma also contains areas of lobular carcinoma in situ (LCIS).

Invasive lobular carcinoma forms no microcalcifications. Some LCIS may be rarely associated with areas of microcalficiations, but usually the calcifications are adjacent to the tissue containing LCIS.

The prognosis of lobular carcinoma depends on its stage and is similar to that of invasive ductal carcinoma. Because of its frequently diffuse growth, it is often discovered late. Lobular carcinoma is often multicentric or bilateral.

Medullary carcinoma belongs to the special types of invasive ductal carcinoma and is a highly cellular tumor. It occurs in all age groups. The *typical medullary carcinoma* consists of large tumor cells with prominent nuclei, frequent mitoses, and atypical nuclei (a presentation that appears to contradict the relatively good prognosis). These cells lie close to each other—without forming glandular structures—and are characteristically surrounded by extensive infiltrates of inflammatory cells (lymphocytes and plasmocytes).

Characteristically, the tumor is smoothly outlined, but it can be lobulated. Indistinct image presentation of a characteristic medullary carcinoma can occur because of superimposed surrounding tissue or through inflammatory infiltrates. Not infrequently, large medullary carcinomas develop central necroses that can calcify.

If a carcinoma fulfills some but not all of the mentioned criteria of a medullary carcinoma, it is categorized as *atypical medullary carcinoma*. Its prognosis corresponds to that of a ductal carcinoma NOS.

Mucinous (colloid) carcinoma also has a favorable prognosis in its pure form. *Atypical mucinous carcinoma* can be considered a ductal carcinoma with a mucinous component, and its growth pattern and prognosis correspond to that of the ductal carcinoma NOS. The *typical mucinous (gelatinous or colloid) carcinoma* appears primarily in older age. It consists of cell groups or cords, or individual cells that float in large lakes of extracellular mucin. The individual cells are small and uniform and show only minimal atypia. The characteristic mucinous carcinoma growth is smoothly marginated, sometimes also lobulated. Calcifications can occasionally develop in mucinous carcinomas.

Papillary carcinoma is the third, also relatively rare, subtype of invasive ductal carcinoma. It exhibits a predominantly nodular growth. Histologically, epithelial papillae with a fibrovascular core are characteristic. Papillary carcinomas can contain microcalcifications. The microcalcifications encountered here are—corresponding to their formation in small cavities within the tumor—characteristically fine and granular, similar to those found in papillary DCIS.

If the papillary carcinoma is intracystic, the surrounding cyst wall can give it an entirely smooth outline. Only after penetration of the cyst wall does it become an invasive papillary carcinoma. Penetration beyond the cyst wall can be seen mammographically as irregularity of the margin if visualized tangentially. The cyst itself frequently contains blood.

Cribriform carcinoma is a rare, well-differentiated carcinoma. Similar to the cribriform DCIS, solid cell-aggregates are formed with characteristic cribriform interspaces.

Tubular carcinoma is a highly differentiated carcinoma with a favorable prognosis. It frequently arises in the region of radial scars (see pp. 182, 184, and 188). Histologically, it is characterized by highly differentiated, parenchyma-like tubules. It frequently induces very intense fibrotic reaction with spicules, producing the mammographic features that suggest this subtype of carcinoma. Microcalcifications can be present. They are often found in intraductal components that accompany some tubular carcinomas (usually noncomedo DCIS).

Other very rare carcinomas include the adenoid cystic carcinoma, squamous cell carcinoma, and mucoepidermoid carcinoma as well as the metaplastic carcinomas, such as the carcinosarcoma, spindle cell carcinoma, etc. These carcinomas are not distinguishable from other types of carcinoma by imaging methods and consequently are diagnosed exclusively histologically. They will not be discussed further here.

Special types of breast carcinoma that may be characterized by their clinical findings are Paget carcinoma and inflammatory carcinoma.

Paget carcinoma is characterized by the presence of tumor cells in the nipple and areola. Clinically, this induces an inflammatory reaction with erythema, moisture, and ulceration. Paget carcinoma may be caused by an invasive carcinoma or a true carcinoma in situ. The tumor arises from a subareolar duct and extends to the nipple and areola, to produce its characteristic findings. Cancer can also be found elsewhere within the breast. Paget involvement of the nipple is then caused by seeding of this tumor.

Paget carcinoma of the nipple is diagnosed by cytologic smear of the weeping nipple-eczema or by excisional biopsy of the suspicious lesion. This diagnosis must lead to a thorough search for a carcinoma in the parenchyma away from the nipple.

Inflammatory carcinoma has an extremely poor prognosis. It can arise from any type of breast carcinoma. The diagnosis is made by excisional biopsy with a punch biopsy of the skin showing emboli of tumor cells in the lymphatic vessels of the skin, which are responsible for the clinical presentation of edema, erythema, and hyperthermia. Inflammatory carcinoma is not treated surgically unless it can be shrunk with radiation or chemotherapy.

■ Clinical Presentation

Corresponding to the multifarious histologic presentation, the clinical presentation also varies considerably.

Since mammography, the only screening method, and other imaging methods are not able to detect all breast carcinomas, clinical examination continues to play an important role in the detection of breast carcinoma. It is relevant that some carcinomas smaller than one centimeter and even some carcinomas in situ present clinically, usually as palpable finding (about 10%). This means *that the clinical examination is important in the early detection of the carcinoma.*

■ History

In addition to assessing risk factors, attention should be paid to all changes reported by the patient (palpable abnormality, newly developed pain, discharge, nipple changes).

While pain related to the menstrual cycle is common in benign changes, unilaterally localized pain, which generally is not related to the menstrual cycle, should be taken seriously. Such pain should always prompt a thorough evaluation.

■ Clinical Findings

While inspecting the patient, *skin retraction* should be looked for. It can be caused by reactive fibrosis that can even be induced by a small carcinoma.

It is noteworthy that retraction can precede a definite palpatory finding.

During the clinical examination, retraction can be elicited by asking the patient to raise her arms and thereafter to lean on them. (By contracting the pectoral muscle, discrete retraction can be accentuated). Finally, the breast must be systematically evaluated for the Jackson phenomenon (see p. 10). Any skin retraction must be considered suggestive until proven otherwise and should lead to a thorough evaluation.

Any possible *deviation, decreased erectility of the nipple*, or a definite *retraction of the nipple* should be thoroughly looked for. In particular,

unilateral nipple changes must be considered suspicious unless unequivocally explained by scar formation or mastitis. (Bilateral nipple retraction can be associated with the so-called plasma cell mastitis).

In the presense of eczematous changes of the *nipple or areola*, Paget disease of the nipple must be excluded by cytologic smear as well as by mammography, including a magnification view of the retroareolar region.

Localized skin changes (edema, erythema, induration, peau d'orange) overlying a palpatory finding can be evidence of tumor infiltration.

Diffuse skin changes, such as thickening, edema, and erythema, as well as peau d'orange and induration of the breast, warrant the exclusion of an inflammatory carcinoma unless it can be definitely explained by an underlying benign condition (mastitis).

Palpation (technique see p. 10) must pay attention to any area different from its surroundings or from the corresponding area of the contralateral breast. It should be remembered that breast carcinomas do not always present as discrete nodules. Often only a diffuse, viscous (rubber-like) consistency and impaired moveability of the soft tissue is found. Some medullary and mucinous carcinomas, as well as the phyllodes tumor when it is still small, can be relatively soft to palpation. Some of these malignancies are also moveable.

Each palpatory abnormality must be correlated with the image presentation. Vice versa, it may be helpful to review mammographically and sonographically abnormal areas in context with the palpatory finding.

A palpatory finding larger than the corresponding mammographic finding increases the suspicion of a carcinoma since many scirrhous carcinomas elicit a palpable reaction in the surrounding area. However, a mammographically large, irregularly outlined density immediately under the skin without a corresponding palpatory finding reduces the likelihood of a malignancy.

Any spontaneous abnormal discharge that is hemorrhagic or clear, cytologically suspicious, or unilateral and, above all, attributable to a single duct needs further evaluation.

It is often worthwhile obtaining a *cytologic smear in the evaluation of every discharge* despite the unreliability of a negative cytologic finding and the cytologic evaluation of nipple discharge in general. The smear cytology can be repeated at

Table 15.**1** Mammographic signs of breast carcinoma

Direct signs of a focally growing invasive carcinoma
1. Focal lesion of increased density in comparison with the parenchyma
2. Focal lesion equal in density in comparison with the parenchyma

To 1 and 2:
The outline of the density can be:
 – Spiculated or irregular,
 – Similar to parenchyma, lobulated, geographically ill-definded (= indeterminate mass),
 – Round or rarely entirely smooth
3. Microcalcifications (with or without surrounding soft-tissue density)
4. Distorted architecture
5. Asymmetry in comparison with the contralateral side
(6. Single dilated duct)

Indirect signs of a focally growing invasive carcinoma (secondary signs of malignancy)
1. Nipple retraction (sometimes only mammographically apparent)
2. Local retraction of the skin or the parenchyma overlying the lesion
3. Thickening of Cooper's ligaments in the vicinity of the lesion (subcutaneous or prepectoral)
4. Local thickening of skin overlying the lesion
5. Trabecular thickening in the subcutaneous space or in the prepectoral adipose tissue
6. Retraction or fixation on the pectoral muscle
7. Enlarged, multiple, homogeneously dense, smoothly or unsharply outlined lymph nodes in the axillary extension

Signs of a diffusely growing carcinoma
1. Diffuse microcalcifications
2. Diffuse density, hyperdense in comparison with the contralateral parenchyma
3. Diffuse density, isodense in comparison with the parenchyma, but asymmetric in location compared to the contralateral side
4. Contour deformity
5. Thickened Cooper's ligaments
6. Distorted architecture
7. Indistinctness of the structures of the mammary tissue
8. Trabecular–reticular marking in the subcutaneous and prepectoral fatty tissue
9. Skin thickening (generally in inflammatory carcinoma)

any time and occasionally discover nonmalignant causes underlying a persistent galactorrhea.

Regardless of the cytologic findings, the source of the pathologic discharge must be further assessed by galactography.

■ Mammography

Mammographically, invasive carcinoma—corresponding to its various histologic patterns—has many features.

Since mammography as the only screening method is the primary imaging modality, it is particularly important to know the various presentations of breast carcinomas.

While spiculated and nodular breast carcinomas are diagnosed without difficulty in fatty breasts, it is a challenge even for the experienced mammographer to detect carcinoma in its early stage when its features are often still indeterminate, to find carcinoma without microcalcifications within dense tissue, and, in particular, to diagnose the diffusely spreading carcinoma.

Table 15.1 summarizes the direct and indirect findings for detecting focally growing invasive breast carcinomas.

The listed findings can be present alone or in combination (Figs. 15.1 a–e).

Before explaining and illustrating these findings further, the principles that govern the radiographic density of breast carcinomas will be briefly discussed.

Radiographic density of breast carcinomas. All breast carcinomas visible as density have a higher mass attenuation coefficient than fat. The mass attenuation coefficient can also be higher than that of parenchyma, though this only applies, unfortunately, to some carcinomas. Indeed, only about half of carcinomas have a higher attenuation than parenchyma, while the parenchyma may well show considerable variations in its attenuation. The remaining carcinomas have equal or even less mass attenuation in comparison with parenchyma or dense tissue (Figs. 15.2 b, c, f–m).[32]

In particular, early carcinomas frequently have the same density as parenchyma.[33] In those cases, other morphologic criteria are important (configuration, architectural distortion, asymmetry, secondary signs of malignancy, etc.).

Furthermore, mammographically increased density can be technical in nature. In the majority of cases, areas with increased density found in the normal mammogram are caused by the summation of several parenchymal lobules or lobules of dense tissue.

Foci with truly increased radiodensity must be identifiable in several planes. Otherwise, the increased radiodensity only represents superimposition.

a Spiculated mass or architectural distortion

Spiculated mass with center (frequent)

Indistinctly outlined mass (frequent)

Spiculated mass without central mass   or   architectural distortion

b Lobulated mass

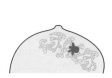 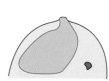 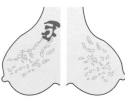

Visualized in two views

Visualized because of atypical location

Visualized as asymmetry

Visualized through changes on serial examinations

As neodensity

By increase in size

By decrease in size and retraction

c Nodular mass

Not entirely smoothly outlined, sometimes with microlobulation

Smoothly outlined with indistinct areas

Smoothly outlined (<2% of all malignancies)

d Malignant microcalcifications

Pleomorphism of the individual calcification (linear or granular)

Casting rod-like, v-, or y-shaped individual calcifications (multiple or in one group) with irregular shape.

Pleomorphic, granular microcalcifications (new finding, typical distribution)

Fig. 15.**1 a–e**   Most frequent mammographic appearance of focally growing breast carcinomas
a Spiculated and/or indistinctly outlined mass
b Lobulated mass
c Nodular mass
d Malignant microcalcifications

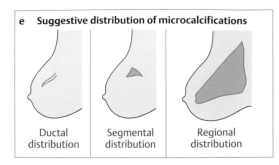

e   **Suggestive distribution of microcalcifications**

| Ductal distribution | Segmental distribution | Regional distribution |

Fig. 15.**1 e**   Suggestive distribution of microcalcifications

■ **Direct Signs of Focally Invasive Breast Carcinoma**

(Figs. 15.**2 a–t**)

A schematic summary of the most frequent features of the focal breast carcinoma is presented in Figure 15.**1**.

The *focal, irregularly outlined, and spiculated mass* is a very important and frequent sign of breast carcinoma. If surrounded by adipose tissue or tissue of less density, such a change can be perceived very early (Fig. 15.**2 a**).

In mammographically dense tissue, these carcinomas are often detected by their spiculated extensions, i.e., their characteristic morphology (Figs. 15.**2 b** and **d**). Some of them may present with increased density in comparison with the surrounding parenchyma. As already stated, this increased density is neither necessary nor confirmatory.

Some carcinomas show a *lobulated parenchyma-like growth pattern.* Some of these carcinomas are recognized by increased density, while others are only recognized by a disturbance of the normal distribution pattern of the parenchyma, by architectural distortion, by asymmetry, or by atypical location (Figs. 15.**2 f–k**).

Depending on the severity of the changes, size of the lesion, and density of the surrounding tissue, these indistinct masses may or may not be readily identifiable. Magnification mammography, palpatory findings, sonography, MRI, and percutaneous biopsy help in their detection and differentiation.

Again, depending on the density of surrounding tissues, *nodular and round carcinomas may or may not be readily visible.*

Medullary, mucinous, papillary, and intracystic papillary carcinomas are characteristically nodular or smoothly outlined carcinomas. Because of its high prevalence, however, ductal carcinoma NOS is the most frequent round carcinoma. (Other noncarcinomatous malignancies that can present as round masses include malignant lymphomas, phyllodes tumors, malignant lymph nodes, and rare sarcomas of the breast, as well as metastases.)

Because of the frequent benign round lesions (mastopathic nodules, fibroadenomas, etc., see also p. 212), the differentiation of these round carcinomas from the many benign findings with similar presentation can be difficult, compromising their detection (Figs. 15.**2 l–p** and 15.**8 d**).

In the approximately 5–10% of the carcinomas that show a round growth pattern, indistinctness of the contour is frequently observed and, until proven otherwise, should be considered a sign of malignancy. It is rare that carcinomas exhibit an entirely smooth outline or are surrounded by a halo (Fig. 15.**2 p**, see also Fig. 15.**9 b**).

Actually, less than 2% of the lesions entirely smooth in outline are malignant.[33]

This implies that all nodular or round lesions with a contour that is not entirely distinct need further evaluation. If considered suspicious (e.g., increase in size), even lesions with entirely smooth outlines need further workup.

As a general rule, follow-up examinations at intervals of 6, 12, 24, and 36 months are sufficient for those focal lesions that are smoothly outlined.

Depending on the radiodensity and composition of the surrounding tissue and of the carcinoma itself, not all focal carcinomas are visible as focal densities. They can be obscured by or be equal to—and indistinguishable from—dense surrounding tissue.

Therefore, it is important to look for other signs, such as distorted architecture, asymmetry, as well as for any possible secondary signs of malignancy (see Table 15.**1**). Very rarely a single dilated duct may be the only hint of a carcinoma.

Finding architectural distortion and asymmetry means looking for distortion of normal structures:

– Looking for masses (which can resemble parenchyma) outside the normal parenchymal distribution. Most parenchymal tissue is in the upper outer quadrant and extends toward the nipple. Any parenchyma-like density in atypical location (asymmetry in comparison with the contralateral side, increased density anterior, medial, and, especially, deep to the

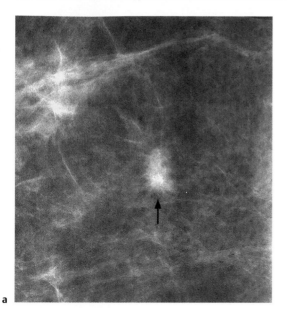

a

Fig. 15.**2a–p** Focally growing carcinomas with irregular contour.

a Two spiculated masses in different patients. The large mass (top) shows typical long spiculations extending across the breast. A few fine microcalcifications are also present in the mass. The density of the mass is much higher than the density of the surrounding fatty tissue.

The other, very small mass (bottom) is also well-recognized within the surrounding prepectoral fat. It exhibits an irregular contour but no long spiculations. Its density equals the density of the glandular tissue (in the retroareolar region). Nevertheless, this lesion, too, is highly suspicious and proved to be a ductal carcinoma with tubular differentiation

b and **c** Oblique view and craniocaudad view of a spiculated *ductal scirrhous carcinoma* (arrow) at the posterolateral margin of the breast parenchyma. The carcinoma is easily descernible by its spiculation and its location (atypical site for normal tissue) at the periphery of the parenchyma on the MLO view. On the craniocaudal view the carcinoma is difficult to recognize within the overlying dense tissue. It does, however, produce a slight retraction of the parenchyma (arrow)

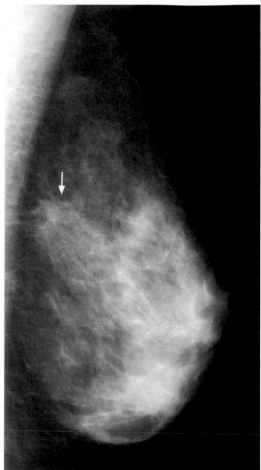

b

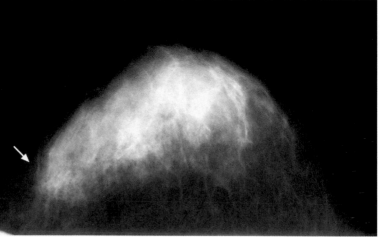

c

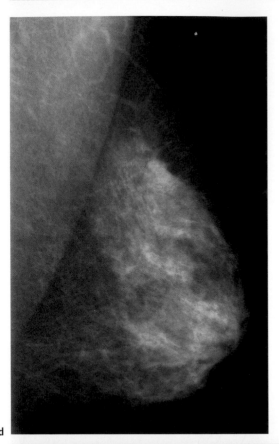

Figs. 15.**2d** and **e**   Oblique and craniocaudal views of a *ductal carcinoma* that mimics the lobular architecture. On the MLO view the mass is apparent by its increased density. Very faint spiculations may be perceived. Note the slight retraction of the glandular tissue over the carcinoma. On the craniocaudal view, the ducts appear to converge toward the mass, disturbing their usual orientation toward the nipple

d

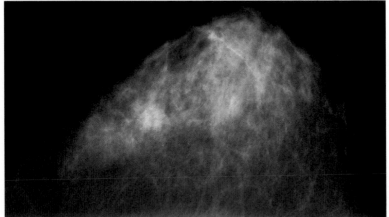

e

parenchyma) needs thorough evaluation, for example, by means of magnification mammography, additional projections, or other imaging modalities (Figs. 15.2 b, h, l, m).

– Looking for any distortion in the usual course of the parenchyma toward the nipple. Such distortions are suspicious, regardless of whether a real center can be recognized or not (Figs. 15.2 f, g, h, i, k).

– Looking for any retractive changes in the parenchyma (Figs. 15.2 c, d, f, g and 15.6 a).

– Looking for secondary signs of malignancy in the skin and subcutaneous tissue (Table 15.1 and Fig. 15.4).

f and **g** This patient presented with a palpable thickening medial to the nipple. Even though the tissue in the upper outer quadrant is denser than in the area of the palpable abnormality, the latter is suspicious: while the tissue density is not increased on the craniocaudal view the ducts appear to converge toward at least 2 centers (located about 3 cm behind the nipple). The ducts are thus disturbed during their course toward the nipple. On the mediolateral view this area appears dense, partly due to superimposition of the 2 centers shown in the craniocaudal view. Except for the architectural distortion, this lobular carcinoma imitates breast tissue very well

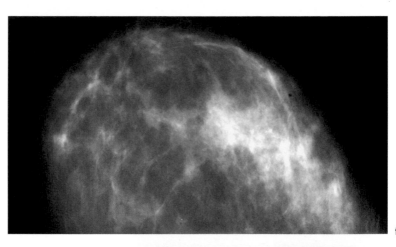

f

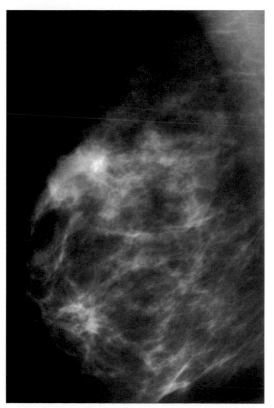

g

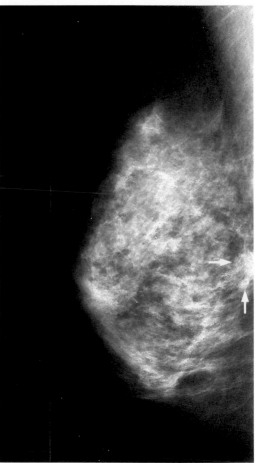

h

h Another *ductal carcinoma* imitating the growth pattern of the parenchyma. The carcinoma, which is isodense with the parenchyma, can be suspected because of the increased density of the ductolobular structures in the posterior aspect of the parenchyma (arrows).

The oblique view is not correctly positioned since it does not delineate the pectoral muscle at the level of the nipple. Consequently, the carcinoma, which extends into the retromammary space, is only partially visualized. The predominantly medially distributed tissue in the caudal portion of the breast ist not completely included. (Presumably, the patient was not rotated far enough toward the film holder). A small group of intraductal calcifications is discernible at the periphery of the carcinoma

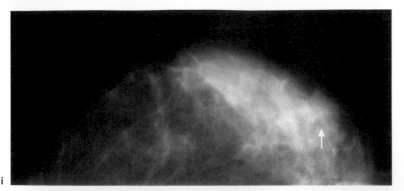

i

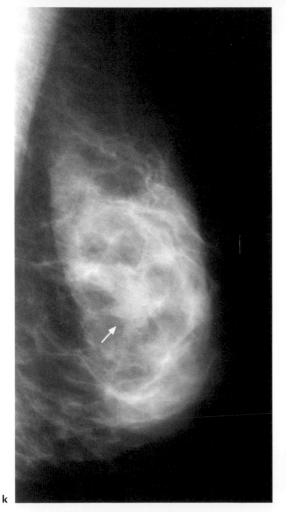

k

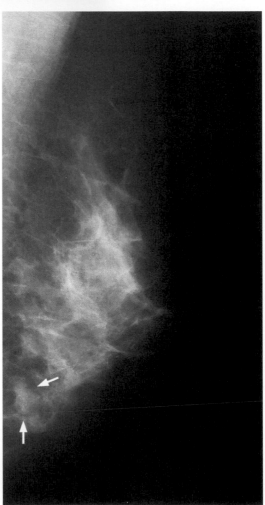

l

Fig. 15.**2i** and **k** In dense breast tissue carcinomas may be completely obscured. In this case the carcinoma is visible (arrows) in both views as an irregular mass. It is only diffi-cult to perceive since it has identical density as the breast tissue. It does not show retraction, but the usual architec-ture of ducts converging toward the nipple is disturbed *Histology*: ductal breast cancer (NOS)

l Nodular *invasive ductal carcinoma*, isodense with the glandular tissue. The nodular carcinoma (arrows) is not re-liably distinguishable from other nodules in breast tissue

Fig. 15.**2m** Same carcinoma as shown in 15.**2l**. In the craniocaudal view (medially exaggerated), it is conspicuously delineated by its location deep to the parenchyma. Asymmetric densities in the retromammary fat are to be considered suspect until proven otherwise

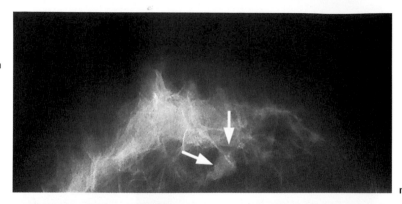

m

Fig. 15.**2n** A round fairly well-circumscribed mass is seen. Biopsy is warranted since it had newly developed. *Histology*: ductal carcinoma NOS. Ductal carcinomas are the most frequent histology encountered among well-circumscribed carcinomas

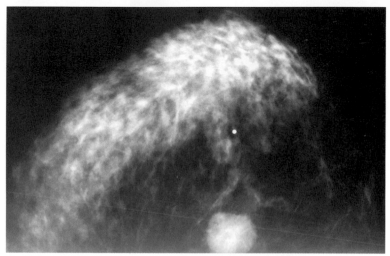

n

The likelihood of malignancy based on these signs depends primarily on their severity. If any of these signs are present, they must be further evaluated in all cases (mammographic compression or magnification views, additional projections, repeat and targeted palpation, sonography, MRI, or core biopsy).

A very rare sign of malignancy is the appearance of a single dilated *duct*. Multiple dilated ducts, in contrast, are usually caused by benign changes (such as duct ectasia or papillomas). The likelihood of malignancy increases with additional suggestive findings (microcalcifications, ductal discharge, progressing nodularity, or retraction (Fig. 15.**3g** and Fig. 14.**6c**).

As with the detection and diagnosis of intraductal carcinomas, finding *microcalcifications* is also of great importance for invasive carcinomas. The percentage of invasive carcinomas with microcalcifications is, however, less than that of intraductal carcinomas. Depending on the patient

selection, microcalcifications can be found in only 30–40% of invasive carcinomas.

This means that microcalcifications are important evidence for diagnosing a carcinoma, but they are by no means mandatory for such a diagnosis.

The malignant criteria for microcalcifications found in invasive carcinomas correspond to those found in carcinomas in situ and are, therefore, only briefly repeated here (Table 15.**1** and Fig. 15.**3a–g**).

Linear, V-shaped, and Y-shaped calcifications as intraductal casts are very suggestive of malignancy.

Clustered, larger granular, pleomorphic calcifications, usually ranging between 0.3 and 2 mm, are strongly suspicious for malignancy. Furthermore, fine granular calcifications ≤ 0.3 mm that follow a segmental distribution may be indicative of malignancy, in particular, if they are new. Any distribution pattern (segmental or ductal) that suggests a ductal origin of the microcalcifications must be considered suspicious for malignancy.

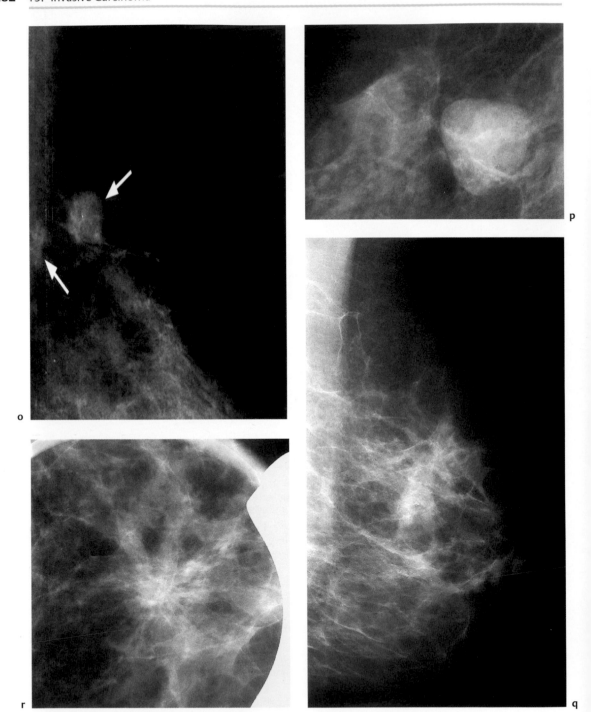

Fig. 15.2**o** and **p** Further well-circumscribed breast carcinomas are shown. Papillary carcinomas may appear as round, fairly well-circumscribed mass

p Here, an entirely smoothly outlined carcinoma with halo is shown. Despite the smooth outline and a relatively soft moveable lesion on palpation, it is not a benign lesion but a *mucinous carcinoma*. The lesion was newly discovered in this 63-year-old patient

q and **r** Ductal carcinoma with distorted architecture. The oblique view shows an increased density. The course of the ductal structures toward the nipple is altered, and these structures appear to converge toward this area. This impression is confirmed by the magnification view **(r)**, which better demonstrates this spiculated mass

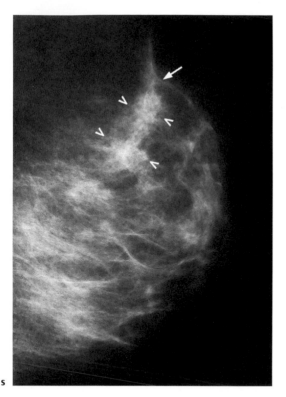

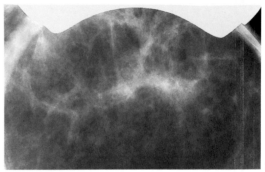

Fig. 15.**2 s** and **t**   Only the mediolateral view disclosed a suspicious dense area (arrowheads). In addition to the density, the subcutaneous fascia is displaced by a focal retraction. The magnification craniocaudal view confirms the presence of an area of slightly increased density, which persists despite spot compression. The excisional biopsy revealed an intraductal carcinoma with early invasion

Indeterminate microcalcifications may be more worrisome if they are clearly localized and asymmetric to the contralateral side, or if they have increased in comparison with the previous examination (Figs. 15.**3 d–g**). Calcifications that are clearly benign (e.g., coarse calcifications), however, do not need to undergo biopsy.

An associated soft-tissue density (if it is distinguishable from dense tissue) may be an additional sign of malignancy, in particular, if it is irregularly outlined or if it follows the ductal structures (Fig. 15.**3 e**).

Whenever the mass or the microcalcifications or both appear suspicious, further evaluation is indicated.

Surrounding soft-tissue density does not indicate that a carcinoma is invasive. Though such a soft-tissue density may be caused by invasion, it can also represent reactive fibrosis induced by DCIS without invasion. Absent soft-tissue density does not exclude an invasive growth.

■ **Indirect Signs (Secondary Criteria of Malignancy) of Focally Growing Invasive Carcinomas**

● Secondary signs of malignancy (Table 15.1) often *accompany advanced breast carcinomas.* Together with a focal finding, they increase the likelihood of malignancy (Fig. 15.**4**) and *often suggest a widespread extension:*
  – Nipple retraction → extension into the subareolar space or even nipple
  – Reticular subcutaneous thickening, thickening of Cooper ligaments → extension into the subcutaneous space or into the prepectoral adipose tissue
  – Skin thickening or retraction → extension into the skin
  – Retraction or fixation on the musculature → extension into the musculature
  – Axillary adenopathy

These signs, however, do not prove a direct infiltration.

● They can be caused by *reactive changes* (retraction or edema) *in the vicinity of a carcinoma*, e.g.:

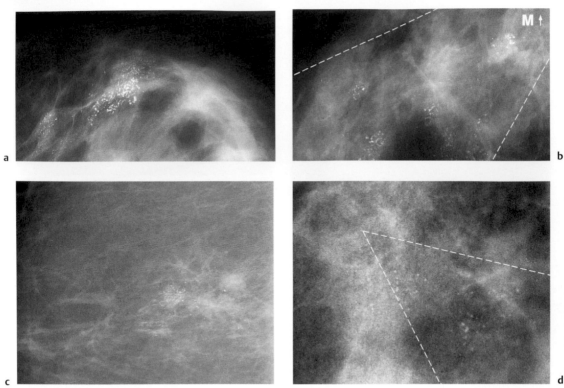

Fig. 15.**3 a–g** Malignant microcalcifications as evidence of a carcinoma

a Extensive pleomorphic granular microcalcifications measuring up to 2 mm in diameter. These microcalcifications are characteristic of a carcinoma. Rarely do early calcifying fibroadenomas exhibit similar individual forms. The typical distribution along the ducts (segmental) is consistent with malignancy: histologically, invasive ductal carcinoma with large in situ comedo component. Concomitant soft-tissue changes—if present—are indistinguishable from the dense surrounding tissue

b Very pleomorphic microcalcifications. Despite the almost round configuration of individual clusters, the overall pattern is clearly suspicious for malignancy: extensive pleomorphism, several elongated, in part very fine calcifi-

cations (casts), and a segmental arrangement (triangular configuration) with the apex pointing toward the nipple (M). Extensive carcinoma in situ with microcalcifications

c Fine microcalcifications with typical elongated casts. Also in this case, the calcifications are oriented along the ductal system toward the nipple (not visualized). There may be some minimal associated architectural distortion and soft-tissue density. *Histology:* comedo DCIS

d Extremely fine, granular microcalcifications, barely discernible (twice the magnification of that shown in Fig. 15.**3 a, c**), with minimal pleomorphism. They are less typical of a carcinoma than those shown in **a–c** and similar calcifications are also found in the various benign changes. *Histology:* ductal carcinoma with extensive intraductal component

Fig. 15.**4 a** Secondary signs of malignancy. A large oval ▷ mass is shown in the lower aspect of this breast. The lesion has spiculations. Furthermore, there is increased interstitial density around the lesion compatible with lymphangiosis. The lower aspect of the breast is flattened; the overlying skin and partly also the Cooper ligaments are thickened. Note the dense axillary lymph nodes. The faint density and the bizarre dystrophic calcifications in the upper breast are due to previous trauma

b A large, spiculated carcinoma has retracted adjacent breast tissue and the overlying skin (arrows)

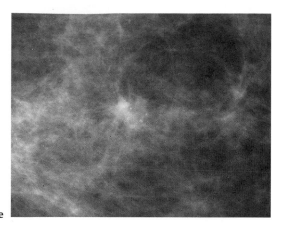

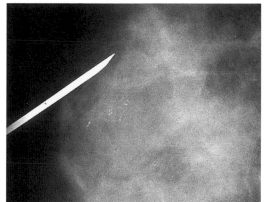

e

f

Fig. 15.**3 e** An irregularly outlined mass with microcalcifications is suggestive of a carcinoma, even if it contains only a few or uncharacteristic calcifications. *Histology:* ductal carcinoma, 6 mm

f–g Less characteristic groups of microcalcifications as evidence of malignancy. In particular, the analysis is limited with only very few tiny microcalcifications. Because of their pleomorphism and clustering, they were biopsied

f Intraductal noncomedo carcinoma with microinvasion (the trace of a segmental distribution as well as individual casting elongated forms should be noted)

g Subtle ductal thickening and typical arrangement of very few pleomorphic calcifications with a ductal distribution. Small ductal breast carcinoma

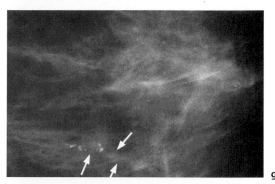

g

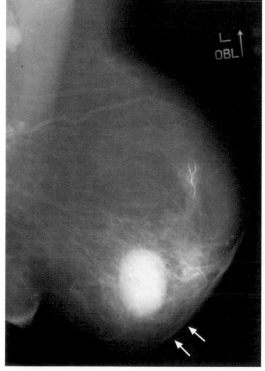

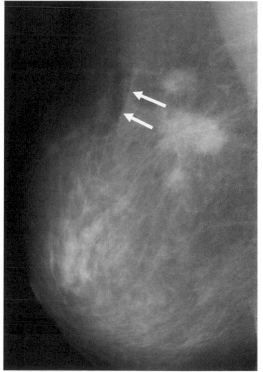

a

Fig. 15.**4**

b

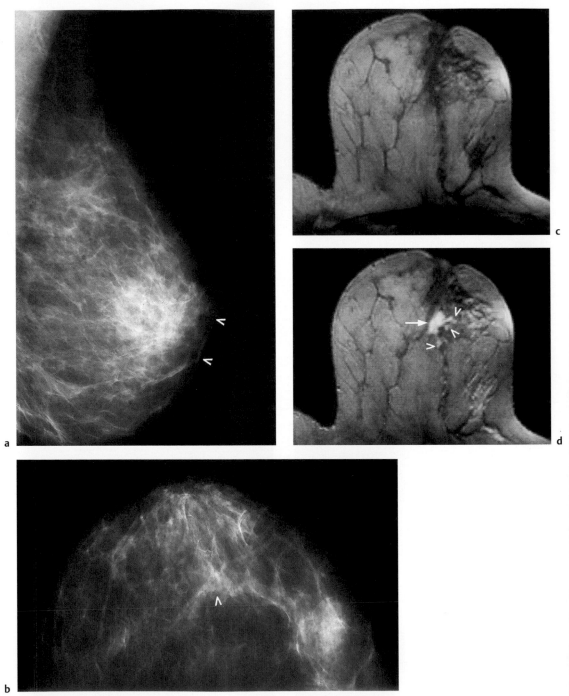

Fig. 15.**5**

◁ Fig. 15.**5** Secondary signs may rarely also be the first hint of a small carcinoma. Forty-year-old patient who noticed impaired erectility of the nipple
a Only the mediolateral view—provoked by good compression—reveals flattening of the areola (arrowheads). The central parenchyma appears slightly thickened but without definite evidence of malignancy
b This craniocaudal view, as well as the corresponding oblique view, was interpreted as negative by an experienced radiologist. Retrospectively, focal mass and architectural distortion (arrowhead) can be discerned deep in the breast but without corresponding finding in the mediolateral view
c Transverse MRI image at the level fo the nipple before administration of contrast medium
d The same image shown in (**c**) but after injection of contrast medium. There is strong, rapid focal enhancement in the breast tissue, strongly suggestive for malignancy (arrow). The small satellite foci should be noted (arrowheads). The laterally situated parenchyma shows moderate enhancement in this patient. Without mammographic–clinical suspicion, this speaks for an enhancing mastopathy (e.g., proliferative mastopathy)

- Dimpling and retraction of the skin caused by reactive fibrosis affecting the extended surrounding of the tumor
- Parenchymal retraction along the subcutaneous or retromammary fascia caused by reactive fibrotic strands
- Nipple retraction caused by reactive fibrotic strands (Fig. 15.5)
- Thickening confined to Cooper ligaments caused by reactive fibrosis and peritumoral edema.
- Reticular linear thickening in the subcutaneous or prepectoral fatty tissue caused by lymphedema

Finally, such changes can also be observed in nonmalignant findings, such as scars, inflammatory changes, or fat necrosis.

In the presence of a carcinoma, it can only be determined histologically whether these signs represent reactive changes or direct tumor invasion.

● If the reactive changes are induced by small tumors, they may be the only evidence of a *small malignancy within dense mammary tissue.* Accentuated by good mammographic compression, they can become visible on the mammogram before they are clinically apparent (Figs. 15.5, compare also with Figs. 15.2 t and s). Therefore, searching for secondary malignant criteria, such as *retraction*

affecting skin, subcutaneous tissue, prepectoral space, or nipple, is also important for *early diagnosis.* Even in the absence of a focal finding, the cause of these changes has to be investigated (magnification mammography or further modalities).

■ Signs of Diffusely Growing Carcinomas

The detection of diffusely growing carcinomas may be quite difficult, especially if these carcinomas do not contain microcalcifications.

If *microcalcifications* are present, the same differentiating criteria are valid as applied to the evaluation of microcalcifications in general. Especially V-shaped and Y-shaped casts and larger granular or pleomorphic microcalcifications are suggestive for malignancy, as is the ductal distribution pattern. Fine granular monomorphic calcifications may, on occasion, require further evaluation as well,

- if they follow a ductal distribution pattern,
- if they are new,
- if additional soft tissue changes are present, or,
- if associated with a clinically suspicious finding.

The problem of early mammographic detection of diffusely growing, *noncalcifying carcinoma* is the divergent spread of these carcinomas without inducing any mammographically visible increase in density. Increased density or retractive changes or both often become visible only after a clinically apparent finding has developed. Therefore, *clinical correlation* is very important for the detection of diffusely growing carcinomas.

To detect *diffusely growing carcinomas* without microcalcifications, the following has to be looked for (Figs. 15.**6** and 15.**7**):

- *assymmetry* in comparison to the contralateral side (close correlation with palpation, and possibly with sonography and MRI),
- already present or newly developed *increased density,*
- increased *blurring* of the ligamentous structures in the parenchyma (caused by cellular infiltrates or edema),
- *densities in the subcutaneous region* and in the *retromammary fatty tissue* (usually caused by accompanying inflammation or direct infiltration),
- any *retractive changes,*

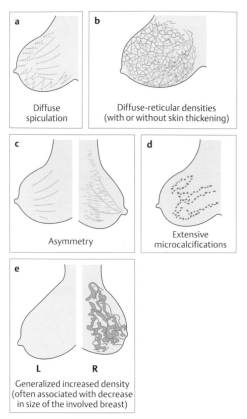

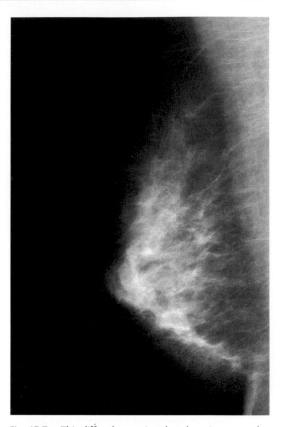

Fig. 15.**6 a–e**   Diffusely growing carcinoma (diagram)—mammographic appearance

Fig. 15.**7 a**   This diffusely growing *ductal carcinoma* can be recognized by subtle spicules and thickening of the Cooper ligaments along the border of the parenchyma, as well as early retraction and thickening of breast parenchyma

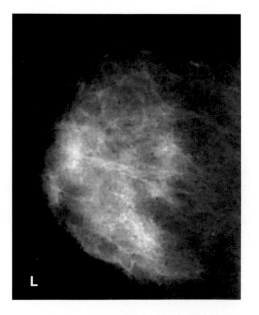

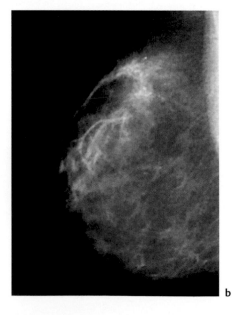

Fig. 15.**7 b–c**
b This diffusely growing *lobular carcinoma* asymmetrically shows more radiodense tissue on the left in comparison to the right. The density of this tissue within the innate fat density equals, in contrast to the right breast, that of normal parenchyma. In addition to a palpable asymmetry, the mammographic asymmetry was the only evidence of this diffusely growing lobular carcinoma that masqueraded as normal parenchyma
c Inflammatory carcinoma. There is diffuse thickening of the entire parenchyma as well as definite skin thickening that is most pronounced in the central periareolar region. The reticular densities in the subcutaneous and retromammary fat can be explained as edematous thickening. In the axilla, a large and a small, very dense lymph node are partially visualized

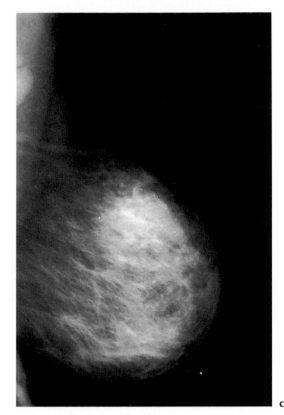

c

– as well as *thickening of Cooper ligaments*, whereby this thickening usually begins deep in the ligament near the parenchyma rather than more superficially (Fig. 15.**7 a**).

The signs of an *inflammatory carcinoma*, which is generally clinically apparent, are:

– skin thickening,
– *trabecular thickening* in the subcutaneous space and prepectoral space, and
– *blurring* of structures caused by edema (Fig. 15.**7 c**).

All of these signs are typically present in an inflammatory carcinoma. While these signs can also be found in inflammation, the presence of additional malignant-type calcifications strongly suggests the diagnosis of an inflammatory carcinoma.

■ **Value of Follow-up and Previous Studies**

For the detection of discrete changes, a comparison with previous mammograms is important. If available, *previous mammograms should be compared with the current mammogram*.[34]

A mammographic finding that has increased in size or is new suggests a malignancy (Fig. 15.**8 a–d**).

But even a *decrease in size* can be *evidence of malignant retraction* caused by invasion with accompanying fibrosis. It is unfortunate that this finding, which can be observed in focally as well as diffusely growing carcinomas, is often misinterpreted (Fig. 15.**8 e** and **f**).

Therefore, a *change in a finding*, be it an increase, a new appearance, or a decrease, raises the possibility of a *carcinoma*.

The *value of serial mammograms* for excluding malignancy is, however, somewhat restricted by the observation that carcinomas, particularly carcinomas in situ as well as low-grade malignancy, can remain unchanged for years.[35] This implies that a stable appearance makes malignancy less likely but can exclude it only after follow-up examinations over an extended period of time (Fig. 15.**8 g–h**). In particular, this must be considered in the evaluation of microcalcifications and smoothly outlined lesions.

Suspicious changes—even if unchanged in comparison with the previous examination—have to be further evaluated by biopsy.

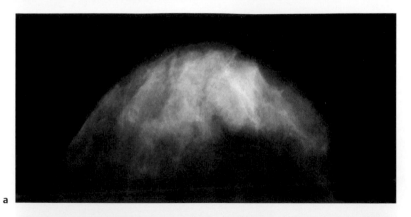

a

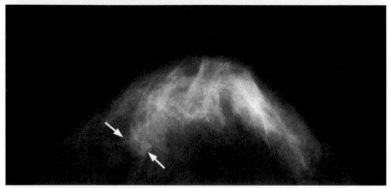

b

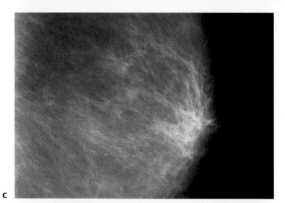

c

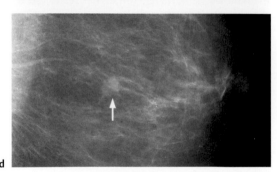

d

Fig. 15.**8 a–h**   Follow-up mammography
a and **b** Current craniocaudal view (**b**) and previous craniocaudal view (**a**) obtained 3 years earlier. In comparison with the previous view, the current a new density equal to the density in the remaining parenchyma (arrows). Since it is new or has increased in size, it must be considered suspect despite its radiodensity equal to that of the parenchyma. Retrospectively, a subtle structural alteration can already be appreciated in the same area 3 years ago, i.e., the parenchyma in this area is not oriented toward the nipple. *Histology:* ductal carcinoma, multifocal

Fig. 15.**8 c** and **d**   A round structure measuring a few millimeters is shown here. It could represent a small cyst, a very small fibroadenoma, or a papilloma in the parenchyma. The next follow-up examination revealed an increase in size, rendering this structure (arrow)—in particular, since it does not correspond to a cyst sonographically—very suspicious for malignancy (close-up of an oblique view). *Histology:* intraductal carcinoma with minimal invasion (pT1a)

Fig. 15.**8e** This mammogram of a 46-year-old patient reveals asymmetric densities with distorted architecture and slightly increased density medially, which were not mentioned as suspicious by the interpreting radiologist

f Three years later, the density of the mass has increased, and its margins are now spiculated. (The density of the entire parenchyma appears increased since a high-contrast film was used.) Decrease in size is certainly not a sign of benignity and can be explained by retraction due to fibrosis. Another small mass has appeared adjacent to the thoracic wall. *Histology:* well-differentiated, slowly growing tubular carcinoma

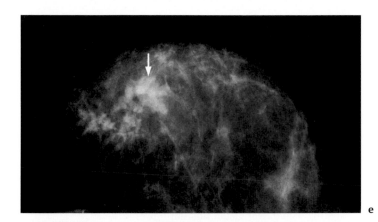

e

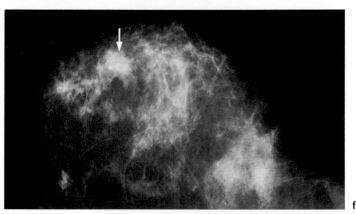

f

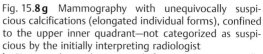

g

h

Fig. 15.**8g** Mammography with unequivocally suspicious calcifications (elongated individual forms), confined to the upper inner quadrant—not categorized as suspicious by the initially interpreting radiologist

h Six years later, the microcalcifications are essentially unchanged. The surrounding soft tissues have even decreased in density due to postmenopausal involution. Because of the suspicious appearance of the individual calcifications and despite the lack of any interval change, excisional biopsy was recommended. *Histology:* extensive DCIS with microinvasion. This finding confirms that any progression seen on follow-up examination mandates prompt definitive evaluation, but that stability—as illustrated in this case—cannot be taken as assurance of benignity of an otherwise suspicious finding

To follow changes judged to be benign, the generally accepted approach is:

- The *invervals* should—because of the usual slow doubling time of breast carcinomas—generally not be shorter than *six months.*
- Follow-up examinations must be continued for a sufficient time span (in general, at least three years).
- If possible, the current mammogram should be compared with *previous mammograms older than two years.* If the intervals are too short, discrete and slowly developing changes are not sufficiently appreciated or cannot be distinguished from usual fluctuations of technique (different projection, compression, distance to the film).

■ **The Influence of Histology on Mammographic Presentation**

As already mentioned, histologic type and growth pattern of the carcinoma affect the mammographic presentation. Knowing the histologic features and the different manifestations of the various types of carcinomas is important for detecting breast carcinomas. Though the histopathologic classification cannot be deduced, it can sometimes be suspected from the particular presentation of the carcinoma.

In this context, the relationships between histology and mammographic features are recapitulated.

Invasive ductal carcinoma can have diverse manifestations, and any of the signs of malignancy listed in Table 15.1 can be present, alone or with others (e.g., irregularly outlined mass, circumscribed mass, diffuse growth pattern, focal microcalcifications, diffusely distributed microcalcifications, or no microcalcifications).

Invasive lobular carcinoma frequently grows along established tissue planes without forming a mass and without inciting fibrosis. Therefore, it is often difficult to recognize. Occasionally a spiculated mass or other focal lesion (not infrequently similar to the density of the normal parenchyma) is observed. Very rarely even a round mass can be present. Because of its diffuse growth, lobular carcinomas have the highest percentage of mammographically overlooked carcinomas. Lobular carcinoma does not form microcalcifications.

Tubular carcinoma frequently presents as a spiculated mass with long, reactive, fibrotic strands. It can contain microcalcifications. Re-gardless of the individual shapes of these microcalcifications, the spiculated mass is an indication for biopsy. Microcalcifications often are the manifestation of DCIS accompanying a tubular carcinoma and can assume characteristic configuration or arrangement.

Medullary, mucinous and papillary carcinomas belong to the types of carcinoma that present as round lesions. However, the most frequent round, well-defined carcinoma histologically is the invasive ductal carcinoma, not otherwise specified (Figs. 15.2 n–p). Round carcinomas frequently show areas of indistinctness or subtle undulation (microlobulation) that speak against benignity (Fig. 15.9 a). Some of these carcinomas, however, can be smoothly outlined throughout and might even be surrounded by a halo. *Intracystic papillary carcinoma can be completely round if the papillary cancer is in situ.* Any macroscopic infiltration is detected only if the affected portion of the cyst wall is seen tangentially (Fig. 15.9 b), showing irregularity with extension into adjacent tissue. Carcinomas with a completely smooth outline (some with a halo sign) constitute less than 2% of the smoothly outlined solid lesions. While medullary and mucinous carcinoma only rarely show microcalcifications (usually single and atypical), some papillary carcinomas, such as papillary carcinoma in situ, can have microcalcifications.

Paget disease of the nipple becomes clinically apparent through eczema of the nipple or areola. The eczema is induced by seeding of malignant cells into the nipple or areola or both. It can arise from any carcinoma within the breast that extends to the areola through the ductal system. A direct retroareolar site of origin in the major ducts is also possible. Eczema suggestive of Paget disease of the nipple always demands a thorough evaluation of the breast to the level of the thoracic wall (mammography, magnification mammography, supplemental methods). In most cases, Paget disease of the nipple has no mammographic findings. Occasionally focal changes in the nipple–areolar complex are seen. Mammography should be obtained, however, to try to detect an underlying carcinoma within the breast.

Inflammatory carcinoma (Fig. 15.7 c) is characterized by diffuse thickening of the skin as well as by increased trabecular markings in the subcutaneous tissue and parenchyma, caused by carcinomatous lymphangiosis. Focal thickening as well as malignant-type microcalcifications can be present.

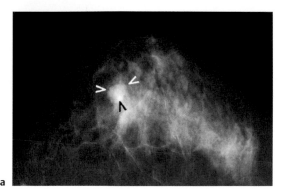

a

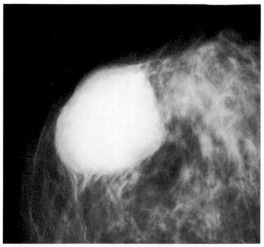

b

Fig. 15.**9a–c** Additional specific manifestations
a Medullary carcinoma, 1 cm in size. In this case, the outline of the round carcinoma is relatively sharp, but microlobulation (arrowheads) raises the possibility of a malignancy (sonography, see Fig. 15.**12b**)
b and **c** Mammographically smoothly outlined lesion
b Some areas of indistinctness might be explained by superimposed tissue, but the pattern should raise concern about possible spiculation
c Sonography shows that the smoothly outlined lesion with good sound transmission consists of a solid and a liquid component. *Histology:* papillary carcinoma. Remark: A small focus of invasion outside the wall of the cyst is only detectable if this segment of the wall (not illustrated here) is tangentially projected on the mammographic view. Sonographically, macroscopic invasion can be noted as irregular interface with the adjacent tissue

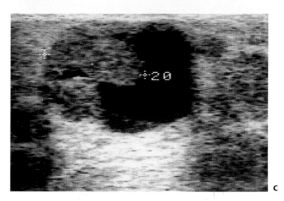

c

Breast carcinoma associated with nipple discharge. Pathologic discharge is always an indication for mammography; supplemental cytologic examination may be helpful. Positive cytology confirms an underlying malignancy, but negative cytology does not exclude it. The majority of discharge-inducing breast carcinomas are mammographically detectable. Rarely can such breast carcinomas be hidden in mammographically dense tissue. To localize these carcinomas, *galactography* is indicated.

Filling defects in the ductal system and truncated ducts speak for a carcinoma (Fig. 15.**10**). A definite differentiation between papillomatosis, benign papilloma, or papillary carcinoma can not be achieved by galactography. This means that galactographically suggestive changes must be clarified histologically. The rare cases of negative galactography despite a definite positive cytology should be considered for MRI.

■ **Sensitivity and Specificity of Mammography**

Qualitatively excellent mammography approaches a sensitivity of 90%. The sensitivity of detecting lesions in fatty tissue is close to 100%. With increasing density of tissue, the accuracy of mammography decreases because small carcinomas without microcalcifications or diffusely growing malignancies can be hidden in isodense tissue.[36, 37] In a screening situation, when mammography is performed in asymptomatic women only, sensitivity ranges around 80%.[16,17,37]. Depending on their histology and growth pattern, large carcinomas are in most cases obvious. However, diffusely growing carcinomas may sometimes be difficult to detect. Since mammography may also miss palpable carcinomas, it is recommended to complement mammography by clinical evaluation. Both in symptomatic patients and in patients with any indeterminate mammographic abnormality, which might be palpable or

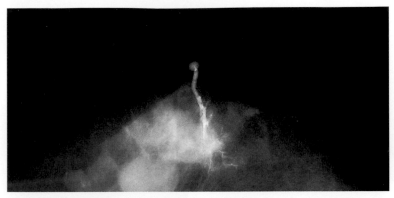

Fig. 15.**10**   Galactography of a patient with pathologic nipple discharge and suspicious cytologic smear. Mammography, sonography, and palpation were unremarkable. Galactography, craniocaudad view: There are small persistent filling defects, best explained as remnants of debris. There is an appreciable change in caliber and ductal cut-off 2–3 cm behind the nipple. This region must be considered suspicous. *Histology:* extensive, partially intraductal, partially invasive, poorly differentiated ductal carcinoma

otherwise symptomatic, correlation between mammography and clinical findings is indispensable for decisions on future workup.

The specificity of mammography depends on the finding itself. In general, the appearance of an early carcinoma may be less characteristic than that of an advanced palpable carcinoma. To detect as many early carcinomas as possible, biopsies for benign changes cannot be avoided. Adequate evaluation, regular review of one's own accuracy, and selecting an acceptable threshold for detecting carcinomas are required to keep both sensitivity and specificity in an acceptable range.

■ Differential Diagnostic Considerations

Any mammographic pattern, even if most suspicious for carcinoma, can be caused by benign entities.

Spiculated masses have a high likelihood of malignancy, unless they correspond to a surgical scar. The appearance can be mimicked by the superimposition of breast tissue, which can be excluded further by a compression view or views in additional projections. Other causes of a spiculated mass include radial scar, fat necrosis, hematoma, abscess, and extra-abdominal desmoid.

A lobulated mass has a moderate probability of malignancy. The differential diagnosis should include asymmetrically developed parenchyma, mastopathic changes, superimpositions, hormone-induced changes, fat necrosis, and scar formation.

Round and smoothly outlined changes can be a manifestation of malignancy. The probability of malignancy, however, is low. It is less than 2% for lesions exhibiting an outline that is entirely smooth. After sonographic exclusion of a cyst, the differential diagnosis of benign entities with this presentation includes fibroadenomas, papillomas, or masses caused by fibrocystic alteration (see also Chapter 22, pp. 223 and 397).

Microcalcifications are found in about 30% of invasive carcinomas and can be a sign of malignancy, with or without surrounding soft-tissue density. Depending on their features, various benign conditions are to be considered as well, primarily microcalcifications in benign changes with or without atypia, in fibroadenomas, "plasma cell mastitis", or scarring (see also Chapter 22, pp. 436–452).

Diffuse changes, such as *asymmetry, increased density, thickening, and indistinctness of structures,* are particularly suspicious if associated with an abnormal palpatory finding. If the palpation is normal, the likelihood of malignancy is low, but further evaluation (supplemental image studies, percutaneous biopsy) may still be indicated, depending on the severity of the abnormality. The differential diagnosis should include developmental asymmetries, benign fibrocystic changes, hormone-induced changes, and postsurgical or postradiation changes (see also Chapter 22, pp. 411–415).

Architectural distortion and diffuse retraction are suggestive, particularly if found unilaterally. They are often—if caused by a malignancy—associated with diffusely increased consistency to palpation. The differential diagnosis should primarily consider chronic mastitis, in addition to postsurgical scarring and radial scar. Thorough evaluation (MRI, core biopsy, and surgical biopsy) is necessary.

Diffuse skin thickening, if associated with peau d'orange, hyperthermia, and erythema, should first raise the possibility of an inflammatory carcinoma rather than a nonpuerperal mastitis, in particular, in patients who are not pregnant, nursing, or postpartum. Furthermore, other rare causes of skin thickening should be mentioned, such as lymphoma, metastatic involvement, and venous, or lymphatic stasis. A biopsy of the representative skin should be the next diagnostic procedure unless further imaging studies have already revealed a suspicious focus. In case of such a finding, these methods will also be applied to guide biopsy.

■ Sonography

■ Diagnostic Role

Sonography is the most important method supplementing mammography and is primarily used for *further diagnostic evaluation*. It can provide the following important information complementing mammography.

Since many palpable carcinomas are sonographically hypoechoic compared to normal breast tissue, sonography can frequently directly visualize a carcinoma, that, on mammography, is hidden in dense tissue. Therefore, sonography can contribute to immediate further evaluation of an abnormal palpatory finding in mammographically dense breasts.

Furthermore, sonography is indicated for all localized findings that might represent a cyst. The sonographic documentation of a cyst as cause of the local finding can avoid unnecessary biopsies.

Neither *absence of a sonographic finding* nor the *presence of a sonographically benign-appearing solid (noncystic) finding* can exclude a mammographically or clinically suspicious carcinoma.[38–44]

The reason for this conclusion is that:
1. Benign and malignant changes show overlapping sonographic features
2. Sensitivity of sonography is limited, primarily for small nonpalpable or preinvasive carci-

nomas that can be overlooked for the following reasons:

a) If surrounded by hypoechoic fatty tissue, hypoechoic carcinomas exhibit minimal contrast, particularly if no characteristic echogenic rim or acoustic shadowing is present. Furthermore, when surrounded by mixed fatty and glandular tissue, small hypoechoic carcinomas can be mistaken for hypoechoic fat lobules imbedded in the parenchyma.

The differentiation between fat lobules and small tumors (compressibility, examination in several planes) is operator-dependent and time-consuming as well as unreliable for small lesions.

b) Especially small carcinomas and carcinomas in situ can also be isoechoic compared with glandular tissue and cannot be distinguished from parenchyma. Only differences in elasticity or acoustic shadowing might suggest the presence of such a carcinoma.

Furthermore, sonography cannot be used to exclude malignancy in mammographically detected suspicious lesions that do not prove to be cysts. Because of its limited sensitivity for detecting carcinomas in situ and small invasive carcinomas, sonography is not recognized as a screening method—*not even* for the mammographically dense breast.[38–43]

■ Indications

For the diagnostic evaluation of breast carcinoma, sonography has the following *indications:*

– Exclusion of a simple cyst as cause of a mammographically or clinically indeterminate focal finding (avoidance of unnecessary biopsies!).
– Detection of malignancy in the presence of uncharacteristic and questionable palpatory findings in mammographically dense tissue. Sonographic exclusion of a malignancy, however, apart from the diagnosis of a simple cyst, is unreliable.
– Sonographically guided puncture (for percutaneous biopsy or preoperative localization of focal findings), often done faster than mammographically guided stereotactic puncture. In addition, it allows direct documentation of the correct position of the needle (in contrast to the stereotactic localization that only

shows the correct *projection* of the needle during the procedure) (see also Chapter 7).

■ **Image Presentation of the Breast Carcinoma**

Sonographically, breast carcinoma is characteristically seen as a mass with the following findings:

- Hypoechoic, often with varying echogenicity throughout the mass
- Poorly to moderately compressible or moveable
- Irregularly outlined with or without hyperechoic rim
- With or without acoustic shadow

This presentation is highly suggestive of malignancy, but cannot prove malignancy since a similar appearance is found in a few benign lesions. Moreover, only some breast carcinomas show these characteristic features. In general, the breast carcinoma expresses a wide sonographic spectrum (Figs. 15.11–15.13).

1. Echogenicity

- Characteristically, a *hypoechoic mass* is found. In general, it is easily recognized if surrounded by more hyperechoic parenchyma (Figs. 15.12 a–c and d). The differentiation from interposed hypoechoic fat lobules as well as its demarcation within fat can be difficult, primarily in the absence of an echogenic rim or acoustic shadow (Fig. 15.12 d, g).
- About 10% of carcinomas (Fig. 15.12 h, i) (primarily early carcinomas and carcinomas in situ) are isoechoic with the parenchyma. In general, they are indistinguishable from breast tissue and therefore sonographically undetectable.

2. Demarcation (Margins)

- *Irregular* margins are a characteristic feature of most carcinomas (Fig. 15.12 c). Evaluating the lateral margin of a mass may be more difficult sonographically than mammographically, but the superficial margins can be more accurately assessed with sonography than with mammography.
- A smooth outline (compare Figs. 17.5 b, 15.12 e, g, and 15.13 d) can be found in nodular malignancies, and its incidence is comparable to that found in mammography. If a thick hyperechoic rim is encountered, a malignancy

should be considered first, even if the mass is relatively smooth in outline.

- A *hyperechoic* thick rim (as opposed to the thin hyperechoic capsule seen in fibroadenoma) (Figs. 15.12 a and b) is a strong indication for malignancy but is by no means found in all carcinomas (Figs. 15.12 d and g). It could correspond to the zone of carcinomatous infiltration into the surrounding tissue, representing the numerous lamellated interfaces induced by this infiltration.

3. Orientation

A lesion with a sonographic *height exceeding its width* is strongly suspicious for a malignancy. This finding is only seen in some malignancies (Fig. 15.12 b). An oval lesion oriented parallel to the transducer (its width exceeding its height) favors a fibroadenoma if it is smoothly outlined, but this does not exclude a malignancy (Fig. 15.13 d).

4. Internal structure

Many carcinomas show heterogeneous internal echoes (Fig. 15.13 b), (exceptions see Figs. 15.12 f and 15.13 d).

5. Attenuation

- A *central or eccentric acoustic shadow* seen behind one or more areas within the lesion and not characteristic of a delicate edge shadow is strongly *suspicious for malignancy* if a (partly) calcified fibroadenoma is excluded mammographically. Extensively fibrosed noncalcified fibroadenomas can have this feature as well. They can often be distinguished from malignancy by MRI. The acoustic shadow can be explained by sound absorption in fibrotic tissue. The posterior border of the lesion is not always distinguishable from the acoustic shadow (Figs. 15.11 e and 15.12 a).
- Presence of a *thickened edge shadow* also speaks against a benign lesion (compare also Fig. 11.3 e).
- Some carcinomas show *no significant attenuation difference* in comparison with the surrounding structures (Figs. 15.12 c–f).
- Some ductal, medullary and mucinous carcinomas can even exhibit a more or less intense posterior *acoustic enhancement* (Fig. 15.13 d).
- *Acoustic shadows without focal findings* in the tissue itself—but not originating from Cooper ligaments (compare also p. 93)—can be evidence of a diffusely growing carcinoma, but

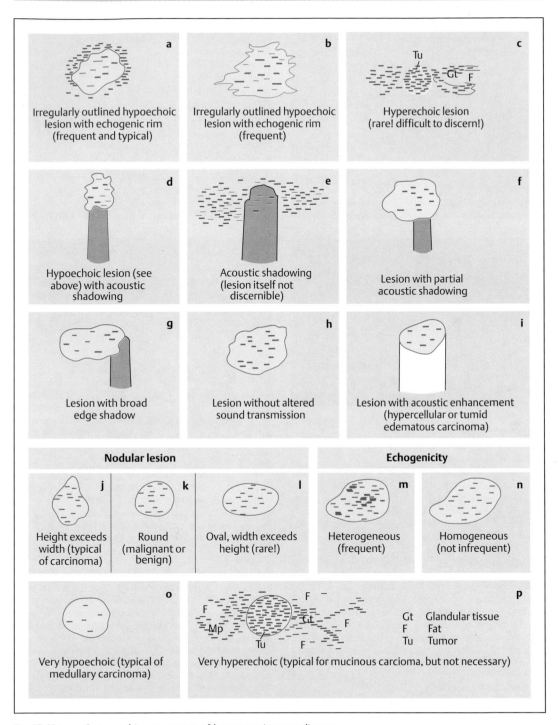

a — Irregularly outlined hypoechoic lesion with echogenic rim (frequent and typical)

b — Irregularly outlined hypoechoic lesion with echogenic rim (frequent)

c — Hyperechoic lesion (rare! difficult to discern!)

d — Hypoechoic lesion (see above) with acoustic shadowing

e — Acoustic shadowing (lesion itself not discernible)

f — Lesion with partial acoustic shadowing

g — Lesion with broad edge shadow

h — Lesion without altered sound transmission

i — Lesion with acoustic enhancement (hypercellular or tumid edematous carcinoma)

Nodular lesion

j — Height exceeds width (typical of carcinoma)

k — Round (malignant or benign)

l — Oval, width exceeds height (rare!)

Echogenicity

m — Heterogeneous (frequent)

n — Homogeneous (not infrequent)

o — Very hypoechoic (typical of medullary carcinoma)

p — Very hyperechoic (typical for mucinous carcioma, but not necessary)

Gt Glandular tissue
F Fat
Tu Tumor

Fig. 15.**11 a–p** Sonographic appearance of breast carcinomas: diagram

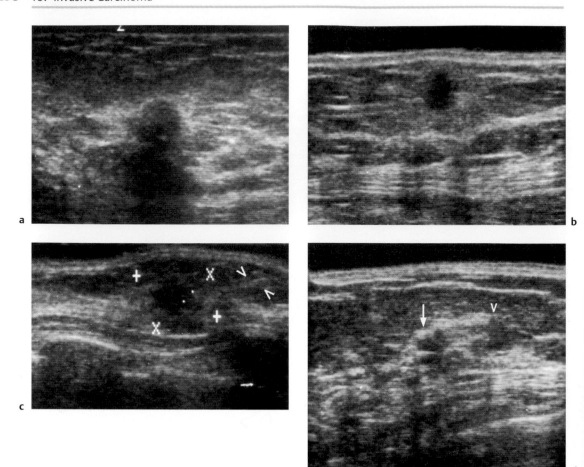

Fig. 15.**12 a–i**
a Typical hypoechoic breast carcinoma with acoustic shadowing. The carcinoma, situated within moderately hyperechoic tissue, is not entirely smoothly outlined and exhibits a delicate hyperechoic rim. *Histology:* ductal carcinoma
b Hypoechoic carcinoma, appearing relatively smoothly outlined with very homogeneous internal echoes.
(Mammographically seen microlobulation is not visualized sonographically because of inherent resolution limits.) The broad, isoechoic rim suggests a malignancy. It corresponds to the histologically identifiable inflammatory zone. Another sign of malignancy is the observation that the lesion's height exceeds its width. This rim of the carcinoma interrupts the hypoechoic fat, i.e., it distorts the architecture of the subcutaneous fat. *Histology:* Medullary carcinoma (mammography see Fig. 15.**9**).
c Typical hypoechoic carcinoma. The carcinoma causes neither appreciable sound attenuation nor appreciable

acoustic enhancement. This carcinoma also is surrounded by a barely hyperechoic rim.
Histologically, both the rim, corresponding to the infiltrative zone, and the hypoechoic central region are part of the carcinoma. A thickened Cooper ligament is incidentally visualized (arrowheads). *Histology:* invasive ductal carcinoma
d Small hypoechoic invasive ductal carcinoma (mammographically detectable through microcalcifications), without causing any appreciable sound attenuation or enhancement. It cannot be determined with certainty whether the surrounding hyperechoic tissue corresponds to breast tissue or whether a hypoechoic rim is present surrounding the tumor. Overall, the carcinoma (arrow) is not easily discernible from a parenchymal nodule surrounded by fatty tissue. Applied compression appears to deform the carcinoma less than the surrounding tissue and an adjacent fat lobule (arrowhead)

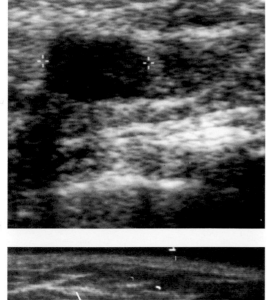

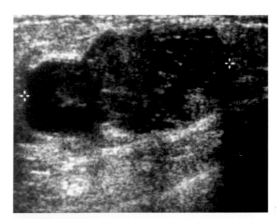

e

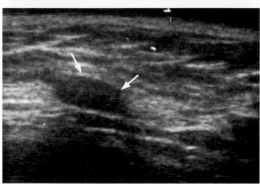

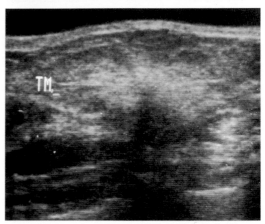

g

f

h

Fig. 15.**12 e** This patient presented with a rapidly enlarging breast mass. Sonography shows that it is solid and largely well-defined. Its lengthened diameter is more than 1.5 x its transverse diameter and its long axis is parallel to the transducer. However, some smaller lobulations are seen and no capsule is shown. Histologically it proved to be infiltrating ductal carcinoma
f This oval, wider than tall, inhomogenous but largely hypoechoic mass shows some lobulation of its margins and distal enhancement of the sound beam. Histologic analysis showed this to be a mucinous carcinoma

g Hypoechoic lesion (arrow) within prepectoral fat, without rim or appreciable sound alteration and with very homogeneous echo structure. The carcinoma was sonographically diagnosed in conjunction with the known mammographic findings (Fig. 15.2 l and **m**). *Histology:* hypercellular ductal carcinoma
h Predominantly hyperechoic carcinoma with distal acoustic shadowing. *Histology:* invasive ductal carcinoma

such acoustic shadows are nonspecific since they can frequently be seen in fibrotic benign changes (fibrocystic alterations) (Figs. 15.**12 k, l, m**).

6. Distorted architecture

Sonographically, *architectural distortion* (Fig. 15.**12 b** and **c**) can be identified and suggests a malignancy. It corresponds to an interruption

– Of the parenchyma that is oriented parallel to the transducer, caused by hypoechoic structures not corresponding to fat lobules (Fig. 15.**12 c**);
– Of the subcutaneous adipose layer caused by structures isoechoic with the parenchyma (Fig. 15.**12 b**). This corresponds to fibrotic reactions or accompanying edematous reaction in the vicinity of a mass. Architectural distortion is difficult to recognize sonographically because of the variable echo pattern of the normal breast.

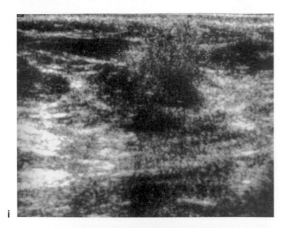

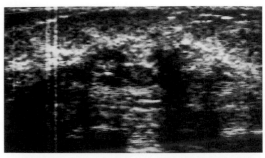

i

k

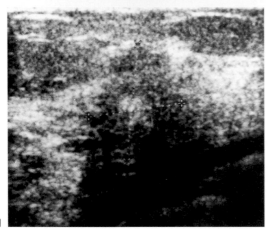

l

m

Fig. 15.**12 i** Another hyperechoic carcinoma is shown. It is located subcutaneously (arrow)
k Diffusely growing lobular carcinoma.
The carcinoma is not directly visualized. Increased echogenicity and diffuse acoustic shadowing in the parenchyma as well as a trace of hypoechoic structures behind hyperechoic tissue. *Histology:* extensive, diffusely growing lobular carcinoma.
l This G3 carcinoma is only visible as architectural distortion on sonography

m Hypoechoic tubular structures with discrete acoustic shadows are suspected within the hyperechoic parenchyma.
In this extensive, diffusely growing *invasive carcinoma*, the tubular structures probably correlate with ducts filled with malignant cells.
This finding could be missed without knowledge of the mammographic findings. It might also be caused by ducts with periductal fibrosis, extensive mastopathy, or debris-filled ducts

7. Elasticity

Corresponding to their palpable findings, many carcinomas also exhibit sonographically detectable diminished elasticity (for evaluation of the elasticity see p. 94) (see also Fig. 15.**13 b**). This can assist in the differentiation of less elastic carcinomas from fat lobules and in the very difficult detection of isoechoic carcinomas. However, good compressibility may be found with some carcinomas. Since such differences in elasticity are only in the millimeter range, compressibility is only applicable to larger and superficial lesions.

8. Mobility

Restricted mobility, i.e., less displacement by the palpating finger, is also a property of most carcinomas.

Exceptions include the papillary intracystic carcinoma and metastases.

Moreover, the following *secondary signs* of a malignancy can be sonographically observed:

1. Thickening and possibly shortening of Cooper ligaments (which may be responsible for the vertical orientation of malignant lesions)

2. Skin infiltration recognizable as interruption of the interface between the hyperechoic skin and hypoechoic subcutaneous tissues and as thickening of the skin
3. Skin thickening which can occur locally or, in case of the inflammatory carcinoma, diffusely

■ Correlation Between Sonographic Image Presentation and Histology

The sonographic detectability of carcinomas, like their mammographic detectability, is affected by their size, type, growth pattern, and surrounding tissue.

Understanding the different manifestations of breast carcinomas in relation to their histology is—as in mammography—an important prerequisite for the correct interpretation of sonography and sensitive detection of carcinomas. As in mammography, however, it is only rarely possible to deduce the exact histology from the sonographic presentation.

- Corresponding to its diverse composition and growth pattern, *ductal carcinoma* also has a variable sonographic presentation.
  The usual ductal carcinoma with definite scirrhous component has a discrete acoustic shadow, a hyperechoic rim, and decreased elasticity. Hypercellular types can also be round, occasionally even oval, and be smoothly outlined with delicate lateral acoustic shadows. Because of its homogeneous structure, the hypercellular carcinoma often shows distal acoustic enhancement, similar to that seen with the hypercellular fibroadenoma. The diffusely growing ductal carcinoma is often difficult to recognize. Occasional hypoechoic foci are found in areas with nodular growth. Dilated hypoechoic ductal structures are sometimes noticed. Diffuse shadowing and diminished elasticity can also be occasionally detected. Finally, small carcinomas are often sonographically isoechoic and consequently difficult to identify.
- *Lobular carcinoma* can grow focally or diffusely (Figs. 15.**12 k** and 15.**13 b**). In the latter case, it presents like a ductal carcinoma whereby diffuse malignant growth is difficult to recognize.
- In addition to the nodular manifestation of some ductal carcinomas (Fig. 15.**13 d**), *medullary* (Fig. 15.**12 b**), *mucinous*, and *papillary* (Fig. 15.**9 c**) carcinomas are carcinomas with a

characteristically nodular or round appearance. These types of carcinomas are not always easily differentiated from fibroadenomas because they can also exhibit regular internal echoes and deep acoustic enhancement. If a sharply outlined focus shows only moderate compressibility, moderate mobility, or even is oriented vertically (e.g., its height exceeds its width), a carcinoma must be seriously considered. If these findings are not present, a carcinoma cannot be excluded with certainty. An increase in size always requires further evaluation.

- It should be mentioned as a peculiarity that the *mucinous carcinoma* can be hypoechoic, but usually is isoechoic and consequently shows little difference relative to surrounding tissue. If an oval lesion shows an isoechoic pattern, a mucinous carcinoma should be considered first, not a fibroadenoma.
- *Papillary carcinoma* can, in addition to showing a nodular growth or a growth along the ducts, also be intracystic and is then sonographically easily recognizable as a hypoechoic intracystic structure. A differentiation between intracystic papilloma and papillary carcinoma is generally not possible, unless definite infiltrative signs (fixation to the surrounding, etc.) are seen.
- *Inflammatory carcinoma* presents sonographically with marked skin thickening, thickened Cooper ligaments, and edematous changes in the subcutaneous space. Additional foci of tumor nodules might be detectable within the parenchyma. Detecting such foci can be helpful in mammographically dense tissue to select areas for biopsy.

■ Accuracy and Differential Diagnosis

It is generally felt [38–44] that the accuracy of sonography is not adequate without mammography in the patient above 35 years of age.

Because of limited accuracy, time commitment (physician time), and strong operator-dependence, sonography is not suitable for screening.

If sonography is used selectively as a supplemental method to solve problems, it can increase accuracy.

- If palpation reveals an questionable finding, sonography can contribute to the correct diagnosis in mammographically dense tissue

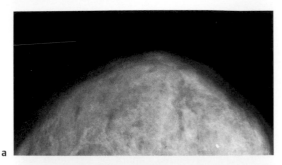

a

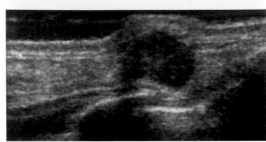

b

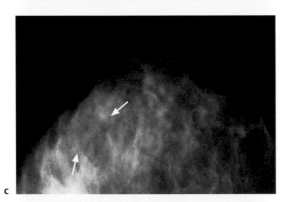

c

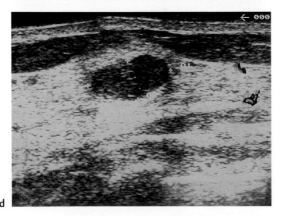

d

Fig. 15.13 a–d Advantages and limitations of sonography

a Dense mammogram, compromised evaluation, without evidence of malignancy. Because of the dense tissue and the consequently impaired evaluation, a suspicious palpable finding of about 2 cm in diameter directly medial and caudal to the nipple requires further evaluation

b In the region of the palpable finding, a hypoechoic lesion with heterogenous internal echoes is easily recognized sonographically. It is not entirely smoothly outlined and exhibits variable sound absorption (in comparison to the surrounding structures, subtle acoustic shadowing, and, on the right, subtle acoustic enhancement). In conjunction with the clinical findings, the lesion has to be considered suspicious.

Sonography complements mammography. *Histology:* focally growing *lobular carcinoma*

c nd **d** Young patient with smoothly outlined, relatively soft palpable finding in the upper outer quadrant

c In the mammographically dense breast, only a discrete oval density is suspected in the region of the palpable finding (arrows). Further evaluation of the palpable finding is mandatory

d Sonographically, smoothly outlined oval lesion oriented parallel to the transducer with a moderate degree of compressibility. These properties were the reasons why an experienced examiner diagnosed the lesion incorrectly as fibroadenoma. *Remark:* this case illustrates that sonographic exclusion of malignancy is unreliable even when (almost) all benign criteria are fulfilled. (Retrospectively, the bulging parenchyma in the region of the lesion might be regarded as sign of moderate compressibility. Moreover, the slightly increased echogenicity of the subcutaneous space over the lesion could be a discrete sign of edema that surrounds the lesion, speaking against benignity). *Histology:* hypercellular, poorly differentiated carcinoma

and in this way contributes in the timely detection of carcinomas (= avoidance of false negative findings).

- In clinical and mammographic findings that can be sonographically explained as one or several simple cysts, sonography can markedly eliminate unnecessary biopsies (= avoidance of false positive diagnoses).
- The sensitivity of sonography is markedly limited for the detection of small and preinvasive carcinomas. Therefore, negative sonography with a noncystic finding does not refute a mammographic or clinical suspicion.
- Because of the wide range of variations found with benign as well as malignant tumors (smooth or irregular outline, acoustic shadowing to acoustic enhancement, different compressibility of benign and malignant findings), sonography has no advantage over

mammography in differentiating solid findings that are visualized mammographically. Applying it for the differentiation of such lesions is not indicated.

- In all sonographically detected findings:
  - Fat lobules and tumors must be carefully distinguished (accuracy depends on the examiner, his/her experience, size and depth of the lesion).
  - The differential diagnosis of hypoechoic findings includes (in addition to malignant tumors) complex cysts, fibroadenomas, and papillomas, as well as hypoechoic areas that can be multiple in the presence of pronounced fibrocystic changes or adenosis. Depending on the degree of suspicion, follow-up examinations in 6 months, sonographically guided percutaneous needle biopsy or excisional biopsy is indicated.
- All things considered, the sonographic accurary of detecting tumors in sonographically homogeneous, echogenic tissue (mastopathy, dense parenchyma) is better than in heterogenous tissue (fibrocystic changes with hypoechoic areas and acoustic shadowing, or glandular tissue with multiple interspersed fat lobules). In adipose tissue, mammography is the method of choice.

Magnetic Resonance Imaging

Contrast-enhanced MRI currently is the most sensitive method for the detection of invasive carcinomas or additional foci. At least 95% of the invasive carcinomas show moderate to marked enhancement following injection of Gd-DTPA, so that contrast-enhanced MRI, as a method complementary to mammography, can provide valuable additional information. As a screening method, contrast-enhanced MRI is not feasible, particularly in view of the detection of numerous benign changes (fibroadenomas or papillomas) that require further evaluation.

Imaging Presentation of Carcinomas

Invasive carcinomas can be visualized as follows[45-51] (Figs. 15.**14a–i**, see also Chapter 5).

- Focal, moderate to marked enhancement is the cardinal finding for detecting 85–90% of the carcinomas. The focal enhancement is:
  - Mostly irregularly outlined (Figs. 15.**14a–b**)
  - Occasionally linear or segmental by follow-

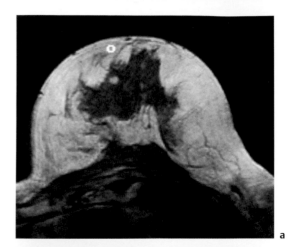

a

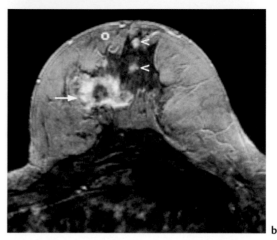

b

Fig. 15.**14a–i** MRI appearance of carcinomas
a and **b** Preoperative MRI of the same patient shown in Fig. 15.**8a** and **b**, before (**a**) and after (**b**) i.v. injection of the paramagnetic contrast agent Gd-DTPA. In addition to the large, medially located focus (large arrow) corresponding to the mammographic finding, there are several additional foci (arrowheads) that are not visualized mammographically. The central zone without enhancement corresponds to central necrosis. *Histology:* multifocal ductal carcinoma

ing ductal structures (this corresponds histologically to a partial intraductal growth [Figs. 15.**14c–e**])
- Occasionally nodular (Fig. 15.**14f–g**)
- Rarely smoothly outlined (see also Figs. 15.**14a–b**, second focus and 15.**14f**)
- More intense or earlier enhancement along the periphery is characteristic of a carcinoma. The peripheral areas of early and intense enhancement generally correspond to the hypercellular growth zone of the carcinoma (Fig. 15.**14g**).

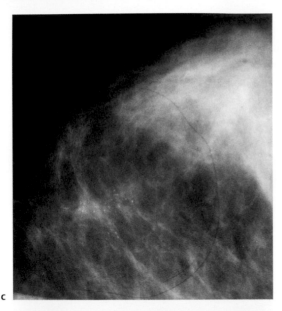

c

Figs. 15.**14 c–e** Preoperative MRI in a patient with suspicious microcalcifications, performed as part of a clinical trial (from Heywang-Köbrunner SH.[28])
c Mammographically pleomorphic microcalcifications with a suggested ductal arrangement
d Transverse image at the level of the suspicious microcalcifications.
e Intense rapid enhancement of the involved ductal system (arrows) after administration of the contrast agent. In contrast to the enhancing ductal segments, the transected vessels (arrowheads) appear punctate or linear and follow a curved course in the subcutaneous space but do not converge toward the nipple. *Histology:* intraductal carcinoma with microinvasion

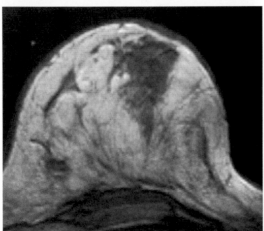

d

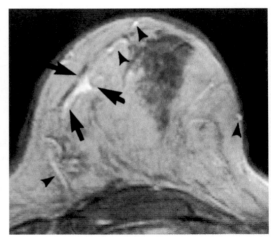

e

- Diffuse enhancement (= milky or patchy-confluent enhancement, without distinct border, covering large areas of the parenchyma) is seen in about 10–15% of carcinomas. About half of these cases with diffuse enhancement correspond to diffusely growing carcinomas (Figs. 15.**14 h** and **i**). In the remaining cases, a histologically focal tumor is surrounded by diffusely enhancing, mostly proliferative fibrocystic changes, rarely by inflammatory tissue. In these cases of enhancing surrounding tissue, the tumor cannot reliably be delineated and can usually not be detected by MR alone.

- Most carcinomas show rapid enhancement, i.e., the maximum enhancement is achieved 1–3 minutes after injection of the contrast medium.[45] About 50% of these carcinomas show a decrease in signal intensity, beginning 3–5 minutes after the injection and corresponding to a washout effect. Washout is associated with a high probability of malignancy. However, as mentioned above, only about half of the cancers exhibit washout.
- Slow enhancement, i.e., enhancement without reaching its maximum within the initial 3 minutes after the injection, was observed in our patients in 12% of the carci-

Fig. 15.**14f** Contrast-enhanced MRI (from left upper corner to right lower corner), unenhanced and 1, 3, and 5 minutes after i.v. injection of Gd-DTPA, shows a slowly enhancing nodule corresponding to an uncertain palpable finding. Even delayed enhancement (maximum at 3 minutes or later after injection) is an indication for biopsy of a lesion found to be suspicious by other imaging modalities or clinically. *Histology:* papillary carcinoma with microinvasion (5 mm) (from Heywang-Köbrunner SH.[28])

g Ring-like enhancement in a focal finding. The contrast-enhanced MRI (from left upper corner to right lower corner), unenhanced and 1, 3, and 5 minutes after i.v. application of Gd-DTPA, shows a ring-like enhancement. This pattern of enhancement must be considered as highly suggestive of a malignancy. *Histology:* ductal carcinoma

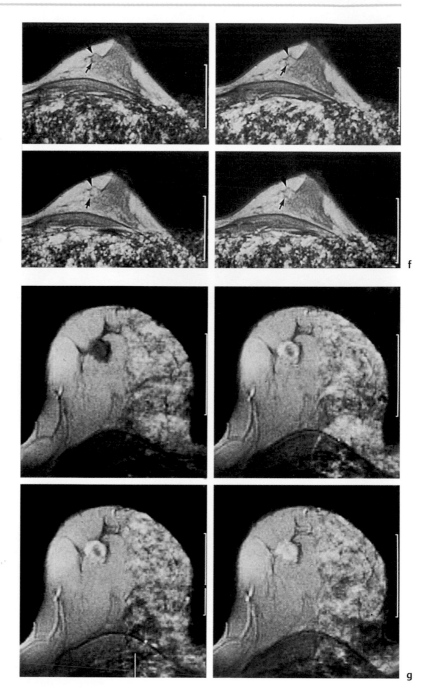

f

g

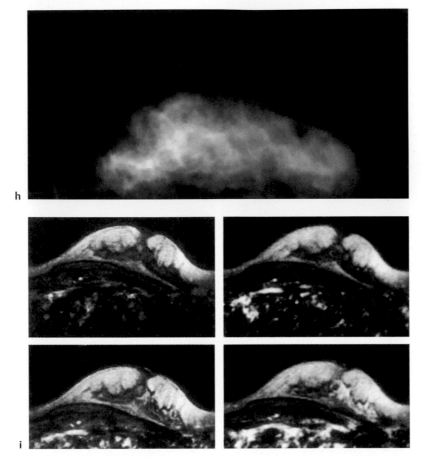

h

i

Fig. 15.**14h** and **i** Diffuse
and delayed enhancement in
a carcinoma permeating the
upper outer quadrant
h Mammographically, the
carcinoma, noticed as palpable finding, was unde-
tectable in the dense
parenchyma
i MRI before scheduled biopsy (from left upper corner
to right lower corner), unenhanced and 1, 3, and 5
minutes after i.v. application
of Gd-DTPA, shows a
delayed enhancement in the
entire upper outer quadrant
(arrows).
As explained in conjunction
with the case illustrated in
Fig. 15.**14f**, the excision of
an area found to be suspicious by other imaging modalities is always indicated—
even if the enhancement is
diffuse or slow. *Histology:*
lobular scirrhous carcinoma
(from Heywang-Köbrunner
SH and Beck R.[29])

nomas. In *view of these slowly enhancing carcinomas, slow enhancement that is otherwise
characteristic of benign changes cannot be used
to exclude malignancy in cases with mammographic, clinical, or sonographic suspicion.*

■ Correlation between MRI and Tumor Extension

Based on the present experience the following
may be stated:[20–24]

- In focally growing invasive carcinomas, the
area enhancing on MRI corresponds very well
to the histologically determined size of the invasive carcinoma.
- If an area with a poorly differentiated carcinoma in situ (e.g., comedo carcinoma) is histologically found next to an invasive carcinoma, the contrast enhancement of the carci-

noma in situ is similar to that of the invasive
carcinoma and consequently cannot be distinguished from it. In these cases, the enhancing
area seen on MRI often correspond to the site
of the invasive carcinoma plus the site of the
carcinoma in situ.

- Some ductal carcinomas in situ enhance less
and more slowly than the invasive carcinoma.
These may be demarcated from the invasive
carcinoma, with the focally strong enhancement corresponding to the invasive carcinoma itself. In some cases the in situ component may enhance as strongly as the invasive carcinoma. In other cases, the in situ component may be indistinguishable from benign
proliferative changes. In few cases it may not
enhance and may thus only be detectable by
mammography (by presence of microcalcifications) or by histopathology.

- Diffuse enhancement can (see above) correspond to diffuse carcinomatous growth but does not prove it. This appearance may also be caused by a focal carcinoma that is surrounded by benign tissue with a marked enhancement.
- According to most authors' experiences, however, MRI proved to be the method that depicted tumor extent most accurately.[20-24]

■ Variations and Pitfalls

The following situations should be dealt with cautiously:

- Carcinomas with pronounced scirrhous component, mainly the lobular scirrhous carcinoma, can have moderate, diffuse or delayed enhancement (Figs. 15.**14h** and i). Such enhancement should not lead to the exclusion of a carcinoma, even if it is most often associated with benign changes.
- While most invasive carcinomas demonstrate strong enhancement, individual cases with very low or even absent enhancement have been observed. Histologically, they were of the mucinous or lobular scirrhous subtype.
- For the differential diagnosis of microcalcifications, mammography rather than MRI is still the method of choice.

■ Indications

Current indications for MRI include questions for which MRI can provide relevant information in addition to conventional methods, and cases for which evaluation by conventional methods is impaired.[51]

These include:
- Detection or exclusion of malignancy in a breast that is severely scarred after multiple surgeries, after conservative therapy for breast carcinoma with or without radiation, and after silicone implants (see also Figs. 18.**14**, 18.**15** and 18.**20**, as well as Fig. 22.**9**).[51-59]
- Detection or exclusion of multicentricity or bilateral involvement before planning conservative therapy of a suspected small breast-carcinoma, mainly in patients with dense parenchyma[20-24]
- Search for primary tumor in cases with positive axillary lymph nodes and no findings on conventional imaging[60-62]

- Monitoring of neoadjuvant chemotherapy. While MRI (like any other imaging modality) cannot exclude microscopic residual tissue, it may allow recognition of poor response and depiction of macroscopic residual tissue preoperatively[63,64]
- Complementary use for questions that could not be adequately answered with conventional methods and are not suitable for percutaneous biopsy (nipple retraction of unclear origin, nipple discharge and unsuccessful galactogram, evaluation of multiple unclear findings, findings that are problematic to puncture, such as densities only visible on one mammographic view)
- The value of contrast-enhanced MRI in patients at high risk (genetic breast cancer) is presently under study.[65-67]

It is mandatory that all nonpalpable findings seen only by MRI and considered suggestive are further evaluated by MR-guided percutaneous biopsy or by excision after MR-guided localization, which is necessary for the surgeon and pathologist.

All things considered, MRI can *add important and decisive information to the diagnostic evaluation of carcinomas*. As a general rule, it should be exclusively reserved as a *complementary method* for specific indications.

■ Percutaneous Biopsy Methods

For further evaluation of clinically, mammographically, and sonographically abnormal findings or even abnormal findings by MRI, percutaneous needle biopsy is currently the most cost-effective method.

Cognizance of the achievable *accuracy* of the particular percutaneous biopsy method is crucial for the *appropriate application* and *correct assessment* of the cytologic or histologic results in the diagnostic work-up. The accuracy can be estimated from data in the literature but should also be continuously validated for the respective diagnostic team and the given technical conditions (correlation of percutaneous biopsy with the results of surgery or subsequent follow-up).

The accuracy achieved for diagnosing or excluding breast carcinoma indeed depends on several factors (see Chapter 7):

- Experience of the diagnostic team
- Methodical factors
- Biologic factors

Sensitivity of core needle biopsy ranges around 92–98% and specificity approximates 100%. The accuracy in the diagnosis of masses exceeds that of microcalcifications or architectural distortion.[71–74] Further improvement, particularly concerning the diagnosis of microcalcifications, has been reported for vacuum biopsy.[75–77] For image-guided cytology, sensitivities of 53–98% and specificities of 89–100% have been reported.[68–71]

■ Methodical Factors Affecting the Accuracy

The following factors can affect the accuracy.

- Cytology is able to cover a larger area by obtaining several passes in a fan-like fashion. The evaluation of the procured material, however, is more difficult for the cytologist. Furthermore, due to the much smaller overall volume of tissue acquired, sampling error may occur more easily, particularly in diffusely spreading or discontinuously growing cancers.

  The quality of the aspirated material is determined by the speed of the needle insertion but also by the skill of the examiner, who can, if experienced, often predict the correct location of the malignant finding by the consistency encountered when penetrating the tissue.

- In core biopsies, the number of the procured cores has great influence on the archievable accuracy (see Chapter 7). Also of great importance is the diameter of the needle as well as how far it is advanced. Most data in literature refer to 3–10 passes per lesion with 14 gauge (2.1 mm) needles and a needle advancement of at least 15 mm. Improved accuracy using vacuum biopsy can be explained by its capability to acquire much more tissue, by suction (allowing pulling of displaced tissue into the cutting window and avoidance of hematoma during the procedure, which might displace the lesion), and by the fact that in most cases visualization of the defect allows direct countercheck of representative tissue acquisition.

- With mammographically guided stereotactic biopsy, the following errors can occur:
  - Error due to patient motion during or after the localizing film was obtained. This, however, should be apparent on the documenting films, which always must be re-

viewed very critically. Even deviation of only a few mm on the localizing films can result in a misrepresentation of more than 1 cm, primarily when localizing deep structures.
  - Errors in assessing the depth through problems with the selected target point. These errors can occur primarily with indistinctly outlined findings or with multiple microcalcifications, since this might make it difficult to identify the same target point in both stereotactic views. Errors in determining the target point annihilate the precision of the depth assessment (see above).
  - Displacement through needle deviation. Even with good guidance of the needle outside the breast, the needle can be deflected in one direction—particularly when passing through thick tissue—caused by the bevel of the needle tip. This deviation can be considerable with thin needles, but it can still amount to several mm with thick needles.

- For sonographically guided puncture, the correct identification of the lesion as well as its correct puncture depends on the examiner's experience. Difficulties can be expected with small lesions (less than 10 mm).

■ Biologic Factors Affecting the Accuracy

Both size and growth pattern of the carcinoma may affect the accuracy.

- If the finding is small (less than 10 mm), accuracy, particularly for those less experienced with these techniques, may diminish (greater influence of patient motion, instrument-related imprecision, examiner's experience in recognizing and identifying the findings and guiding the needle to the lesion with all methods).
- The following applies to the growth pattern:
  - Irregularly outlined densities are suitable for sonographically guided percutaneous biopsies if they are unequivocally identifiable by sonography. With stereotactically guided punctures, problems can arise if the lesion is not clearly identifiable in both stereotactic views.
  - The accuracy of percutaneous biopsy may be less for microcalcifications than for masses.

– Diffusely growing carcinomas, such as the small cell (lobular) carcinoma, can escape detection through aspiration because of their dispersed growth.

■ Indications

Based on the experience so far, percutaneous biopsies have gained increasing importance for the diagnostic evaluation of carcinomas. Assuming proficiency of the diagnostic team, the following approach is recommended:

● Questionable or uncharateristic findings: If— as in the American experience—the cases for biopsy are already selected with a low threshold (positive predictive value [PPV] 20–25%), the availability of percutaneous biopsy should not increase the number of biopsies performed in a practice. If—as in many European centers—the PPV ranges around 50%, additional core biopsy may be considered in some more cases with moderate suspicion, which would otherwise only have been followed.
● With a suspicious finding, a percutaneous biopsy can confirm the diagnosis before surgery and chemotherapy or radiation, or both.
● A suspicious clinical or imaging finding is to be dismissed judiciously on the basis of the results of percutaneous biopsy. Both accuracy of the localization and possibility of sampling error must be critically considered in view of both imaging and histologic findings.

■ Disposition after Percutaneous Biopsy

After percutaneous biopsy, it is the task of the examining physician *to correlate* the *histologic or cytologic findings with the available information* obtained through imaging and clinical examination. Only then should the recommendation of the further approach be issued.

Together with the pathologist or cytologist, it has to be decided whether the obtained result is or could be representative. Depending on the certainty of the result, a decision has to be made between follow-up examinations, repeat core biopsy, or surgical excision of the finding in question. Discordant or uncertain findings should be further evaluated by excision or at least by repeat percutaneous biopsy.

■ Summary

Because of their histologic variability and their multiple patterns of growth, invasive breast carcinoma can have diverse presentations. Knowing these variations is important for early detection.

Mammography with or without clinical correlation is the only recognized screening method. Mammography and clinical examination are complementary. The accuracy of mammography depends on the type of tumor, growth pattern, and surrounding tissue. While the sensitivity of mammography in adipose tissue approaches 100%, it markedly decreases in mammographically dense tissue. In this situation, a negative mammogram cannot be taken to dismiss a clinical suspicion of malignancy. Since most nonpalpable carcinomas are first diagnosed or suspected on the basis of the mammographic finding, optimal technique, continued education, and review of one's own accuracy are important prerequisites for good results.

While mammography and clinical examination as screening methods aim to detect suggestive findings as early as possible, supplemental methods serve to evaluate these findings further.

By delineating cysts, sonography can prevent unnecessary biopsies of uncertain palpatory findings or mammographic masses caused by cysts. In mammographically dense tissue, sonography used as a complementary method can improve the detection of carcinomas (particularly in the presence of palpable changes). Sonographic exclusion of a malignancy in sonographically visualized solid or nonvisualized findings is not possible.

MRI is the most sensitive method for detecting secondary foci in mammographically dense tissue and is particularly suitable for detecting or excluding malignancy in scarred tissue. Apart from these indications, use of MRI should be limited to findings that could not be resolved otherwise or where a lesion cannot be exactly located with conventional methods for percutaneous biopsy (e.g., search for primary tumor, strong suspicion in a mammographically very dense or scarred tissue).

Percutaneous biopsy represents a fast and cost-effective method for evaluating suspicious lesions. The small core of retrieved tissue can render a complete histologic diagnosis. The quality of the core determines the accuracy of the method. It depends on size, location, and morphology of the lesion, accuracy of hitting the lesion, needle diameter, needle advance, and number of passes.

Histologic results of percutaneous biopsy must be critically assessed to determine whether the procured material is representative and, consequently, the result definitive. A negative finding in the face of a highly suspicious lesion cannot exclude a malignancy. If uncertainty remains, repeat percutaneous or surgical biopsy must be considered.

■ References

1   Fentiman IS. Detection and treatment of early breast cancer. London: Dunitz; 1990:58
2   Seltzer V. Cancer in women: prevention and early detection. J Womens Health Gend Based Med. 2000;9:483–8
3   Tabar L, Fagerberg G, Day NE et al. Breast cancer treatment and natural history: new insights from results of screening. Lancet. 1992;339 (8790):412
4   Kopans DB. Mammography screening for breast cancer. Cancer. 1993;72:1809
5   Meyer J, Timothy J, Stomper P, Sonnenfield M. Biopsy of occult breast lesions: analysis of 1261 abnormalities. JAMA. 1990;263:2341–3
6   Moskowitz M. The predictive value of certain mammographic signs in screening for breast cancer. Cancer. 1983;51:1007
7   Sickles EA, Ominski SH, Sollitto RA et al. Medical audit of a rapid throughput mammography screening practice: methodology and results of 27 114 examinations. Radiology. 1990;175:323
8   Elmore JG, Wells CK, Lee CH et al. Variability in radiologists' interpretations of mammograms. N Eng J Med. 1994;331:1493–9
9   Taplin SH, Rutter CM, Elmore JG et al. Accuracy of screening mammography using single versus independent double interpretation. AJR. 2000;174:1257–62
10 Baines CJ, Miller AB, Kopans DB et al. Canadian National Breast Screening Study: assessment of technical quality by external review. AJR. 1990;155:743
11 Sickles EA. Quality assurance: how to audit your own mammography practice? Radiol Clin North Am. 1992;30:265
12 Bird RE, Wallace TW, Yankaskas BC. Analysis of cancers missed at screening mammography. Radiology. 1992;184:613
13 Van Dijck JAAM, Verbeek ALM, Hendricks JHCL, Holland R. The current detectability of breast cancer in a mammographic screening program. Cancer. 1993;72:1933
14 Harvey JA, Fajardo LL, Innis CA. Previous mammograms in patients with impalpable breast carcinoma: retrospective versus blinded interpretation. AJR. 1993;161:1167
15 Ikeda DM, Andersson I, Wattsgard C et al. Interval carcinomas in the Malmö mammographic screening trial:

16 Saarenmaa J, Salminen T, Geiger U et al. The visibility of cancer on earlier mammograms in a population-based screening programme. Eur J Cancer. 1999;35:1118–22
17 Duncan KA, Needham G, Gilbert FJ, Deans HE. Incident round cancers: what lessons can we learn? Clin Radiol. 1998;53:29–32
18 Skaane P. The additional value of US to mammography in the diagnosis of breast cancer. A prospective study. Acta Radiol. 1999;40:486–90
19 Berg WA, Gilbreath PL. Multicentric and multifocal cancer: whole-breast US in preoperative evaluation. Radiology. 2000;214;59–66
20 Fischer U, Kopka L, Grabbe E. Breast carcinoma: effect of preoperative contrast-enhanced MR imaging on the therapeutic approach. Radiology. 1999;213:881–8
21 Krämer S, Schulz-Wendtland R, Hagedorn K et al. Magnetic resonance imaging and its role in the diagnosis of multicentric breast cancer. Anticancer Res. 1998;18:2163–4
22 Oellinger H, Heins S, Sander B et al. Gd-DTPA-enhanced MR breast imaging: the most sensitive method for multicentric carcinomas of the female breast. Eur Radiol. 1993;3:223–8
23 Mumtaz H, Hall-Craigs MA, Davidson T et al. Staging of symptomatic primary breast cancer with MR imaging. AJR. 1997;169:417–24
24 Drew PJ, Chatterjee S, Thurnbull LW et al. Dynamic contrast-enhanced magnetic resonance imaging of the breast is superior to triple assessment for the pre-operative detection of multifocal breast cancer. Ann Surg Oncol. 1999;6:599–603
25 Kollias J, Gill PG, Beamond B et al. Clinical and radiological predictors of complete excision in breast-conserving surgery for primary breast cancer. Aust N Z J Surg. 1998;68:702–6
26 Bruneton JN, Maestro C, Marcy PY, Padovani B. Echography of the superficial lymph nodes. J Radiol. 1994;75:373
27 Moriggl B, Steinlechner M. Ultrasono-anatomy for evaluation of the local lymphatic groups of the mamma. Surg Radiol Anat. 1994;16:77
28 Turoglu HT, Janan NA, Thorsen MK et al. Imaging of regional spread of breast cancer by internal mammary lymphoscintigraphy, CT and MRI. Clin Nucl Med. 1992;17:482
29 Dershaw DD, Selland DG, Tan LK, Morris EA, Abramson AF, Liberman L. Spiculated axillary adenopathy. Radiology. 1996;201:439–42
30 Walsh R, Kornguth PJ, Soo MS, Bentley R, Delong DM. Axillary lymph nodes: mammographic, pathologic, and clinical correlation. AJR. 1997;168:33–36
31 Leibman AJ, Wong R. Findings on mammography in the axilla. AJR. 1997;169:1385–90
32 Jackson VP, Dines KA, Bassett LW et al. Diagnostic importance of the radiographic density of noncalcified breast masses: analysis of 91 lesions. AJR. 1991;157:25
33 Sickles EA. Nonpalpable, circumscribed, noncalcified solid breast masses: likelihood of malignancy based on lesion size and age of patient. Radiology. 1994;192:439
34 Thurfjell MG, Vitak B, Azavedo E et al. Effect on sensitivity and specificity of mammography screening with or without comparison of old mammograms. Acta Radiol. 2000;41:52–6
35 Lev-Toaff AS, Feig SA, Saitas VL et al. Stability of malignant breast microcalcifications. Radiology. 1994;192:153
36 Rosenberg RD, Hunt WC, Williamson MR et al. Effects of age, breast density, ethnicity, and estrogen replacement therapy on screening mammographic sensitivity and

radiographic appearance and prognostic considerations. AJR. 1992;159:187

cancer stage at diagnosis: review of 183, 134 screening mammograms in Albuquerque, New Mexico. Radiology. 1998;209:511–8

37 van Gils CH, Otten JD, Verbeek AL et al. Effect of mammographic breast density on breast cancer screening performance: a study in Nijmegen, the Netherlands. J Epidemiol Community Health. 1998;52:267–71

38 Balu-Maestro C, Bruneton JN, Melia P et al. High frequency ultrasound detection of breast calcifications. Eur J Ultrasound. 1994;3:247

39 Bassett LW, Kimme-Smith C. Breast sonography. AJR. 1991;156:449–55

40 Ciatto S, Roselli-del-Turco M, Catarzis M et al. The diagnostic role of breast echography. Radiol Med (Torino). 1994;88:221

41 Heywang SH, Dunner PS, Lipsit ER, Glassman LM. Advantages and pitfalls of ultrasound in the diagnosis of breast cancer. J Clin Ultrasound. 1985;13:525–532

42 Pamilo M, Soiva M, Anttinen I et al. Ultrasonography of breast lesions detected in mammography screening. Acta Radiol. 1991;32:220–5

43 Potterton AJ, Peakman DJ, Young IR. Ultrasound demonstration of small breast cancers detected by mammographic screening. Clin Radiol. 1994;49:808

44 Skaane P, Sauer T. Ultrasonography of malignant breast neoplasms. Analysis of carcinomas missed as tumor. Acta Radiol. 1999;40:376–82

45 Heywang-Köbrunner SH, Beck R. Contrast-enhanced MRI of the Breast. Berlin, Heidelberg, New York: Springer; 1996

46 Fischer U, Vosshenrich R, Probst A et al. Preoperative MR mammography and patients with breast cancer—useful information or useless extravagance. Fortschr Rontgenstr. 1994;161:300

47 Kuhl CK, Mielcarek P, Klaschik S et al. Dynamic breast MR imaging: are signal intensity time course data useful for differential diagnosis of enhancing lesions? Radiology. 1999;211:101–10

48 Ikeda O, Yamashita Y, Morishita S et al. Characterization of breast masses by dynamic enhanced MR imaging. A logistic regression analysis. Acta Radiol. 1999;40:585–92

49 Nunes LW, Schnall MD, Orel SG. Breast MR imaging interpretation model. Radiology. 1997;202:833–41

50 Heywang-Köbrunner SH, Bick U, Bradley WG et al. International Investigation of breast MRI: results of a multicenter study (11 sites) concerning diagnostic parameters of contrast-enhanced MRI based on 519 histopathologically correlated lesions. Eur Radiol. In press.

51 Heywang-Köbrunner SH, Viehweg P, Heinig A, Küchler Ch. Contrast-enhanced MRI of the breast: accuracy, value, controversies, solutions. Eur J Radiol. 1997;24:94–108

52 Heywang-Köbrunner SH, Schlegel A, Beck R et al. Contrast-enhanced MRI of the breast after limited surgery and radiation therapy. J Comput Assist Tomogr. 1993;7:891–900

53 Gilles R, Guinebretiere JM, Shapeero LG et al. Assessment of breast cancer recurrence with contrast-enhanced subtraction MR imaging: preliminary results in 26 patients. Radiology. 1993;188:473–8

54 Mussurakis S, Buckley DL, Bowsley SJ et al. Dynamic contrast-enhanced magnetic resonance imaging of the breast combined with pharmacokinetic analysis of gadolinium-DTPA uptake in the diagnosis of local recurrence of early stage breast cancer. Invest Radiol. 1995;30:650–62

55 Drew, PJ, Kerin MJ, Turnbull LW et al. Routine screening for local recurrence following breast-conserving therapy for cancer with dynamic contrast-enhanced magnetic resonance imaging of the breast. Ann Surg Oncol. 1998;5:265–70

56 Krämer S, Schulz-Wendtland R, Hagedorn K et al. Magnetic resonance imaging in the diagnosis of local recurrences in the breast cancer. Anticancer Res. 1998;18:2159–62

57 Viehweg P, Heinig A, Lampe D et al. Retrospective analysis for evaluation of the value of contrast-enhanced MRI in patients with breast conservative therapy. MAGMA (Magnetic Resonance Materials in Physics, Biology and Medicine). 1998;7:141–52

58 Heinig A, Heywang-Köbrunner SH, Viehweg P et al. Wertigkeit der Kontrastmittel-Magnetresonanztomographie der Mamma bei Wiederaufbau mittels Implantat. Radiologe. 1997;37:710–7

59 Boné B, Aspelin P, Isberg B et al. Contrast-enhanced MR imaging of the breast in patients with silicon implants after cancer surgery. Acta Radiol. 1995;36:111–6

60 Morris EA, Schwartz LH, Dershaw DD et al. MR imaging of the breast in patients with occult primary breast carcinoma. Radiology. 1997;205:437–40

61 Schorn C, Fischer U, Luftner-Nagel S et al. MRI of the breast in patients with metastatic disease of unknown primary. Eur Radiol. 1999;9:470–3

62 Orel SG, Weinstein SP, Schnall MD. Breast MR imaging in patients with axillary node metastases and unknown primary malignancy. Radiology. 1999;212:543–9

63 Mumtaz H, Davidson T, Spittle M et al. Breast surgery after neoadjuvant treatment. Is it neccessary? Eur J Surg Oncol. 1996;22:335–41

64 Rieber A, Zeitler H, Rosenthal H et al. MRI of breast cancer: influence of chemotherapy on sensitivity. Br J Radiol. 1997;70:452–8

65 Kuhl CK, Schmutzler R, Leutner CC et al. Breast MR imaging screening in 192 women proved or suspected to be carriers of a breast cancer susceptibility gene: preliminary results. Radiology. 2000;215:267–76

66 Tilanus-Linthorst MM, Bartels CC, Obdejin AI, Oudkerk M. Earlier detection of breast cancer by surveillance of women at familial risk. Eur J Cancer. 2000;36:514–9

67 Stoutjesdijk MJ, Boetes C, Van Die LE et al. Magnetic resonance mammography for breast cancer screening of patients from high risk populations: results of a prospective pilot study. Radiology. 1999;213:454

68 Azavedo E, Svane G, Auer G. Stereotactic fine-needle biopsy in 2594 mammographically detected non-palpable lesions. Lancet. 1989;1:1033

69 Pisano ED, Fajardo LL, Tsimikas J et al. Rate of insufficient samples for fine-needle aspiration for nonpalpable breast lesions in a multicenter clinical trial: The Radiologic Diagnostic Oncology Group 5 study. Cancer. 1998;82:678–88

70 NHS Breast Screening Programme. Guidelines for Cytology Procedures and Reporting in Breast Cancer Screening: Report by Cytology Sub-Group of the National Coordinating Committee for Breast Screening Pathology; NHSBSP Publication N. 22; Sept. 1993

71 PD Britton. Fine needle aspiration or core biopsy. The Breast. 1999;8:1–4

72 Liberman L, Dershaw DD, Glassman JR et al. Analysis of cancers not diagnosed at stereotactic core breast biopsy. Radiology. 1997;203:151–7

73 Mainiero MB, Philpotts LE, Lee CH et al. Stereotaxic core needle biopsy of breast microcalcifications correlation of target accuracy and diagnosis with lesion size. Radiology. 1996;198:665–9

74 Brenner RJ, Fajardo L, Fisher PR et al. Percutaneous core biopsy of the breast: effect of operator experience and number of samples on diagnostic accuracy. AJR. 1996;166:341–6

75 Meyer JE, Smith DN, Dipiro PJ et al. Stereotactic breast biopsy of clusterd microcalcifications with a directional, vacuum-assisted device. Radiology. 1997;204:575–6

76 Jackman RJ, Marzoni FA, Nowels KW. Percutaneous removal of benign mammographic lesions: comparison of automated large-core and directional vacuum-assisted biopsy techniques. AJR. 1998;171:1325–30

77 Heywang-Köbrunner SH, Schaumlöffel U, Viehweg P et al. Minimally invasive stereotactic vacuum core breast biopsy. Eur Radiol. 1998;8377–85

16. Lymph Nodes

Of all the prognostic factors in breast cancer, nodal involvement is the most important. Based on 30-year follow-up, Adair reported that those with negative nodes had a 75% survival. Women with level I involvement had only a 40% survival,[1] and this deteriorated with higher levels involved. The number of lymph nodes involved is also important. Vernonesi[2] reported on 60-month follow-up of women with breast cancer with 1–3, 4–10, and >10 nodes involved was 80%, 62%, and 35% respectively. He found that survival for nodal involvement is usually progressive, with nodes closest to the breast (level I) involved before those at higher levels. However, in about 9% of cases, skipped metastases occur with higher levels involved without evidence of level I nodal disease. This means that in about 95% of women, the status of level I nodes truly indicates the presence or absence of nodal disease.

Some breast cancers drain into internal mammary nodes. As is also the case for axillary lymph nodes, dissection or irradiation of internal mammary nodes does not improve survival.[3] However, involvement of these nodes appears to be an independent additional indicator for a worse prognosis. Thus, sampling of internal mammary lymph nodes, especially when they are identified on sentinel node imaging, may be performed in some patients.[4–5]

Overall, it is generally known and accepted that involvement of regional nodes is an important prognostic parameter.[1–7]

■ The Role of imaging

Traditionally, lymph-node imaging has not played a significant role in staging of patients with breast cancer. The reasons for this have included the inability of imaging to detect microscopic nodal metastases. Because it is the most accurate technique to determine the status of axillary nodes, axillary dissection has long been considered an indispensable part of cancer staging. To decrease

morbidity associated with axillary dissection, sentinel node sampling is increasingly used as an alternative procedure for histopathologic staging. Sentinel node mapping using radionuclides and/or blue dye helps to detect the lymph nodes that constitute the first node draining at the site of the tumor. After surgical removal of the sentinel node, histopathologic analysis of this node (or nodes) allows highly accurate determination of the presence or absence of nodal metastases.

At present imaging can be used for the workup of indeterminate findings in the axilla. Furthermore, lymph nodes of the lower axilla are often imaged during assessment of the breast. Because these nodes are frequently visualized, it is important to know the typical imaging features of normal and diseased axillary lymph nodes. Unfortunately, imaging techniques are often not able to differentiate inflammatory and neoplastic nodal disease.

■ Anatomy

The lymph nodes in the axilla are divided into three levels, defined by their relation to the pectoralis minor muscle (see also Appendix 2). Those nodes which are inferior and lateral to this muscle are level I, those that are deep to the muscle are level II, and those that are superior and medial to the pectoralis minor are level III. Nodes that are found between the pectoralis major and minor are called Rotter's nodes.

As noted above, a small percentage of breast cancers drain medially into the internal mammary chain. These nodes are parasternal, deep to the intercostal muscles and extrapleural. They follow the internal mammary vessels and are usually present in the first three intercostal spaces.

■ Normal Lymph Nodes

The normal mammographic pattern of lymph nodes is reniform or coffee-bean shaped with a

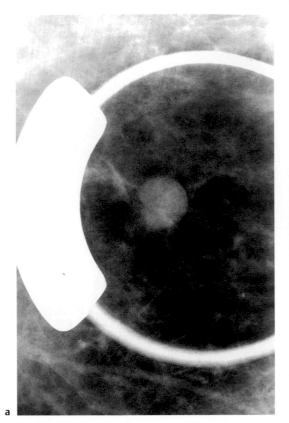

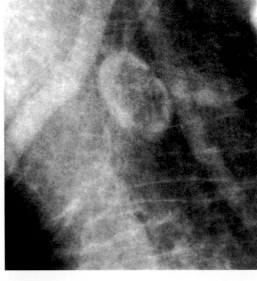

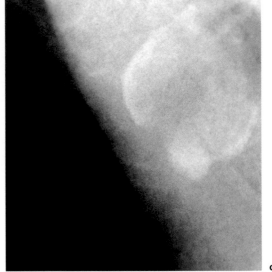

Fig. 16.**1 a–c** Mammography of normal lymph nodes
a This coned view of an intramammary lymph node shows the classic coffee-bean shaped pattern with the fatty notch of the nodal hilum. The node is well-defined, and its density is equal to that of breast tissue
b The fatty hilum of this node is more prominent, but the node is well-defined, and its density is not greater than surrounding normal tissues
c As fatty replacement of a node increases, it will progressively enlarge. This large, palpable axillary node is almost all fat with a thin rim of nodal tissue. Another, smaller node overlies the inferior portion of this large lymph node, suggesting a lobulated contour to the node

fatty hilum. It may take multiple views of a node to demonstrate this classic configuration. If smooth margins, a coffee-bean shape, and fatty hilum can be demonstrated, the mass can be definitely identified as lymph node. The size of normal nodes is variable, and the overall size of a lymph node is not of any clinical significance. Nodes with very large fatty hila and a small crescent of nodal tissue can measure up to 5 cm. If only the parenchyma (excluding the fatty hilum) of the small axis is determined, this measure-

ment allows some correlation with presence of malignant involvement (accuracy: 70–80%). However, an exact diagnosis is not possible because microscopic involvement does not lead to an increase in the lymph-node size, and benign lymph nodes may have an increased parenchymal diameter due to postinflammatory changes. Nodes are seen in about one-third of axillae on mammography. The mammographic density of the node is usually equal to or less than that of normal breast tissue. Furthermore, some lymph

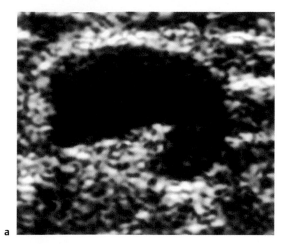

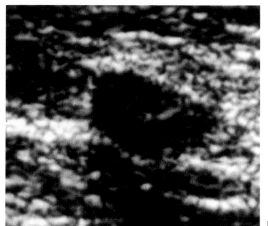

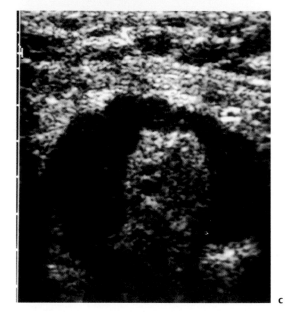

Fig. 16.**2a–c** Sonography of normal lymph nodes
a This hypoechoic mass has a pattern similar to that seen in Fig. 16.**1a**. The coffee-bean-shaped mass is well-defined, and the echo pattern throughout the mass is uniform. The fatty hilum appears sonographically as an echogenic area indenting the mass
b If the node is imaged in an orthogonal projection, the fatty, echogenic hilum can appear as an echogenic focus centrally positioned in the lymph node. Note that the mass is otherwise uniformly hypoechoic and well-defined
c As there is increasing fatty replacement of the node, the central echogenic fat becomes more prominent and the hypoechoic nodal tissue is draped over the large, echogenic hilum

nodes may occur within the breast. These are „intramammary lymph nodes." Although they may occur in any location within the breast, they are usually situated on the posterior half of the upper outer quadrant. Mammographically these nodes become apparent if they are not obscured by dense breast tissue. They are recognized as such if they exhibit the typical morphology of a lymph node.

When mammographic imaging of the axilla is desired, this can be optimized using the axillary view.[8] This view is performed using a small, rectangular compression paddle over the axilla and angling the view at 40°. Even with this optimized view, only about the lower half of level I can be imaged mammographically.

Sonographically, lymph nodes are also coffee-bean shaped, smoothly marginated, with an echo-poor cortex and a central, echogenic fatty hilum (Fig. 16.**2**). When a mass in the axilla or the breast cannot be definitively imaged mammo-

graphically as a lymph node, sonography can be helpful in imaging the classic nodal shape and pattern, due to the ease in obtaining images in multiple planes. The pattern of the cortex should be uniform. Unlike mammography, sonography is capable of imaging the entire axilla.

■ Metastatic Adenopathy

Women with metastatic disease in the axilla from breast cancer usually have a known primary in the breast. Rarely, enlarged lymph nodes are the first manifestation of a breast cancer, which is not

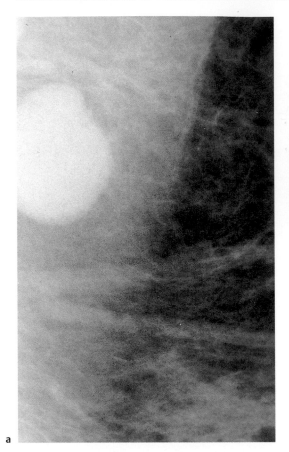

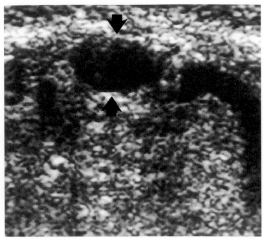

Fig. 16.**3a** and **b** Breast cancer metastases
a This axillary node contains metastatic disease from breast carcinoma. It is dense, and the fatty hilum has been replaced. In the context of known breast carcinoma, the pattern is suggestive of a metastasis
b Sonographically, nodes containing metastases can develop a lobulated configuration. The focal bulging in the contour of this node (arrows) was due to metastatic breast carcinoma

apparent clinically, mammographically, or sonographically. In most of these cases, axillary lymph-node involvement is detected clinically by palpation of suspicious nodes in the axilla. It is extremely rare to discover axillary or intramammary lymph-node involvement in such patients by imaging alone.

It should be remembered that nodes with metastatic involvement are often comingled with normal lymph nodes. It should also be remembered that, using any imaging modality, a lymph node with a normal appearance does not exclude the possibility of metastatic disease within the node.

If (by any imaging modality) enlargement of lymph-node parenchyma or replacement of the fatty hilum is noted, it is usually impossible to differentiate metastatic disease in axillary nodes from reactive hyperplasia without biopsy. Mammographically[9-12] metastatic nodes can have a density greater than that of normal breast tissue.

In addition to change in nodal density, lymph nodes containing metastases can also show loss of the normal fatty hilum (Fig. 16.**3a**).

Lymph nodes containing metastatic disease are usually smoothly marginated. Irregularity and gross spiculation of the node can occasionally occur. (Figs.16.**4a** and **b**) This pattern is due to extranodal extension of tumor into perinodal fat and indicates a biologically aggressive cancer, especially when three or fewer nodes are involved.

Although calcifications are common in primary breast cancers, they are rarely present within sites of metastatic disease, including axillary nodes. If a node contains microcalcifications, metastatic involvement should be suspected (Fig. 16.**5**).

Sonographically[13-14] the following changes should raise the suspicion of lymph-node involvement in women with known breast cancer or other malignancies. Partial or complete replace-

Fig. 16.**4a–d** Spiculated axillary adenopathy. In the context of known breast carcinoma, spiculated axillary nodes are due to extranodal extension of metastatic disease into perinodal fat
a This axillary node has a spiculated contour due to perinodal extension of metastatic disease from a primary carcinoma within this breast
b The sonographic pattern of the lymph node in **a** shows a very poorly defined hypoechoic mass (arrows)
c Sonography of another spiculated lymph node shows an irregular contour, particularly the upper portion of the node. Again, this was caused by perinodal extension of metastatic breast carcinoma

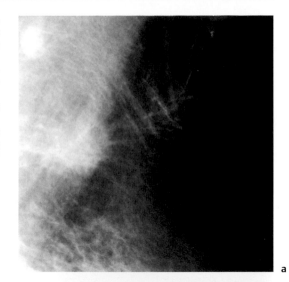

a

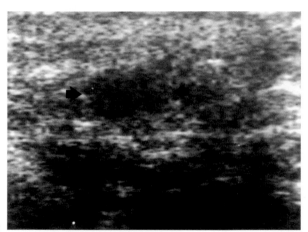

b

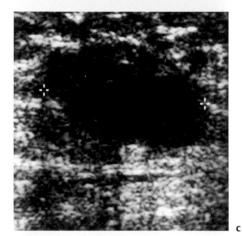

c

ment of the echogenic fatty hilum (Fig. 16.3b), focal or diffuse decrease of echogenicity within the nodal cortex (Figs. 16.3b and c; Figs. 16.4c and d), and focal bulges or marginal irregularity (Figs. 16.4c and d) in some cases or increased transverse diameter of the lymph-node parenchyma can occur. Overall size, however, does not have clinical significance.

In a recent publication[15] a statistically significant difference between benign and malignant lymph nodes was shown for the following features: longitudinal-transverse axis ratio and presence of peripheral versus central flow pattern. Even though the difference is statistically significant, overlap existed. Future evaluations will have to show whether or how these observations may

be prospectively helpful in decisions concerning individual cases.

Malignancies other than breast cancer can be responsible for metastatic axillary adenopathy. The most common of these are lymphoproliferative malignancies such as lymphomas and leukemias, especially chronic lymphocytic leukemia. Nodes in lymphoproliferative malignancies are usually grossly enlarged and dense. These nodes are usually well-defined and often massive (Fig. 16.6). Other common sites of metastatic disease to the axilla include contralateral breast, lung, melanoma, gastrointestinal, thyroid, and ovarian cancers. There are no characteristic patterns to these metastases.

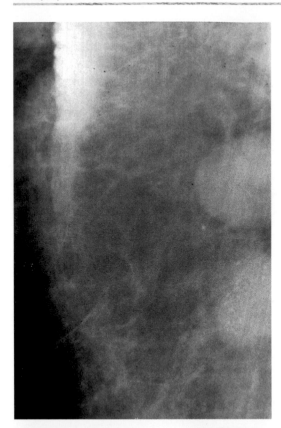

Fig. 16.**5**   Faint calcifications are present in the lower of these two enlarged, dense axillary nodes containing metastatic breast carcinoma

Fig. 16.**6 a–c**   Malignant axillary adenopathy not due to breast carcinoma
a Multiple, enlarged, dense axillary nodes are present in this patient with metastatic thyroid carcinoma. A similar pattern was present in both of her axillae
b This bulky, dense mass of large nodes was readily palpable and is due to chronic lymphocytic leukemia
c Another woman with multiple, bulky lymph nodes. These are due to lymphoma. Lymphoproliferative diseases can produce some of the most impressive adenopathy seen in the axillae
▽

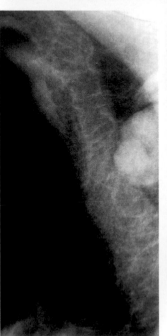

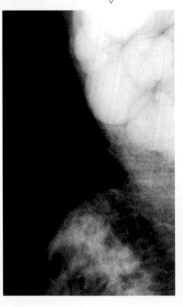

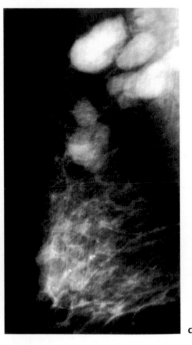

a   b   c

■ Other Causes of Adenopathy

The most common cause of axillary nodal involvement is nonspecific benign adenopathy. A series by Walsh[11] reported this as the cause in 29% of cases, although this percentage will depend upon the population under study. Causes of this change can include skin and nail infections or inflammatory processes in the arm, breast infections, or inflammation and breast surgery. A large number of non-malignant diseases have been reported as causing axillary lymphadenopathy. These include tuberculosis, HIV and AIDS, sarcoidosis, rhematoid arthritis, psoriasis, and other collagen vascular diseases (Fig. 16.7). When the significance of adenopathy is uncertain, questioning the patient about systemic diseases may make it possible to ascertain the etiology of nodal enlargement.

Interval enlargement of lymph nodes on serial mammography can be a source of worry, but without a history of cancer, this is only unfrequently the first indication of malignant disease. In 24 women with lymph nodes enlarging by 20% to over 300% on serial mammograms, Lee[16] found that metastatic disease was only found in two, both of whom had a known history of cancer. Reactive nodal enlargement has been reported to be associated with medullary carcinoma without metastatic disease.[17] Interval nodal enlargement also commonly occurs in the axilla after breast surgery. In women who have recently had surgery for breast carcinoma, enlargement of axillary nodes is invariably benign and should not be a source of concern.

In order to avoid unnecessary interventions patient history and short-term follow-up may be considered first.[18]

■ Nodal Calcifications

Occasionally, calcifications will be present in axillary nodes.[19-21] These can be due to benign and malignant causes (Fig. 16.8). Coarse calcifications due to old granulomatous disease or fat necrosis can be found. Punctate calcifications from gold given for treatment of rheumatoid arthritis can also be seen. Dense nodes, simulating those con-

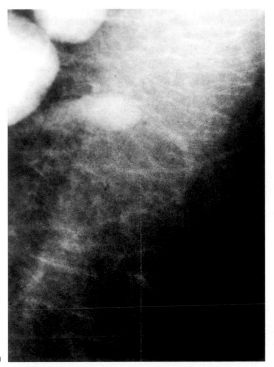

a

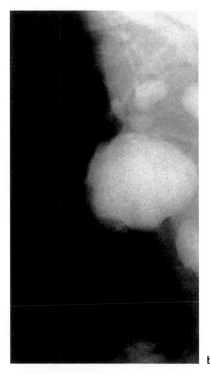

b

Fig. 16.7 a and b Benign etiologies of axillary adenopathy. Axillary nodal enlargement due to benign causes can appear identical to malignant axillary nodal enlargement

a Multiple, dense nodes without central fatty hila are seen in this woman with adenopathy due to HIV disease b Marked axillary adenopathy in this patient is caused by histiocytosis X

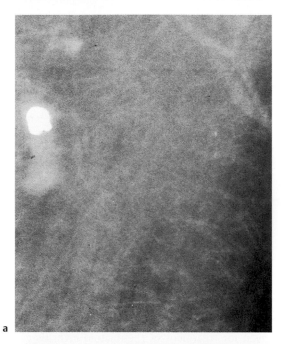

a

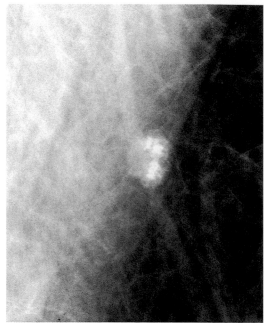

b

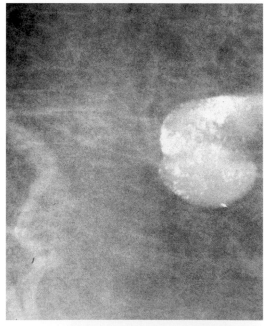

c

Fig. 16.**8 a–c** Benign axillary nodal calcifications
a As can be seen in nodes elsewhere in the body, coarse, benign dystrophic calcifications, probably due to old inflammatory disease, can be seen in axillary lymph nodes. The calcification in this node was unchanged over many years and is presumably due to old inflammation
b Dytrophic calcification is also seen in this axillary node
c Fine calcifications and increased nodal density in this patient were caused by gold treatment given for rheumatoid arthritis

taining calcifications, can also be found in women with silicone injected into the breast or silicone leaks from breast augmentation prostheses. Silicone drains into the axilla and can be taken up by axillary nodes, causing them to appear extremely dense.

Although calcification is present in about 50% of invasive breast cancers on mammography, calcifications are rarely present at sites of metastatic disease, including the axilla. When metastatic adenopathy due to breast carcinoma contains calcifications, these calcifications are usually pleomorphic and often faint (Fig. 16.**5**). Similar calcifications within nodes can also be seen with metastatic ovarian and thyroid carcinoma. A case of papillary carcinoma of the breast has been reported as presenting as axillary nodal calcifications.

■ Sentinel Node Imaging

To decrease the morbidity associated with axillary lymph-node dissection, sentinel lymph-node mapping has been developed to identify the node or nodes that are the first site of drainage of a carcinoma.[22] If these are negative, there is a likelihood of over 90% that no metastatic disease is present within the axilla. This technique may help to decrease the extent of axillary surgery and may thus help to reduce postoperative sequelae of axillary dissection, including lymphedema.

The technique involves injecting a blue dye or isotope in the breast and locating the first node or nodes to which it travels, this node being the "sentinel node" (Fig. 16.**9**). This node is then removed. If it does not contain metastatic disease, no further axillary dissection is performed. If it is positive for metastatic disease, a full axillary dissection is done. Controversy exists over which agent should be injected to identify the sentinel node, but many studies suggest that the greatest accuracy of the technique is obtained when both dye and isotope are injected. There is also controversy over whether agents should be injected into the breast around the tumor or in the overlying skin.

Imaging may only be used when isotope is injected. Injection is done several hours before surgery and images are obtained to identify the location of the first draining nodes of the tumor. Mostly these will be located in the axilla. Occasionally, sentinel nodes are located in the internal mammary chain or in the breast (intramammary nodes). Intraoperatively, after isotope injection, the surgeon locates the sentinel nodes using a hand-held detector. When these first draining lymph nodes are removed, the detector indicates a high concentration of activity within the excised node and reduction of activity in the biopsy site to a level approaching that of background.

Sentinel node mapping is particularly useful in patients with small primary carcinomas, which are most likely node negative or which only exhibit microscopic lymph-node involvement. It is less reliable in advanced cancers because lymph nodes, which are largely replaced by metastatic involvement, may not take up isotope dye. These macroscopically involved lymph nodes may go undetected, and the dye or isotope will accumulate in different lymph nodes due to changed routes of drainage. Also because of altered drainage routes sentinel node mapping is not reliable in women who have had prior axillary surgery or have palpable, suspicious adenopathy. When sentinel node mapping is being done as part of definitive surgery after a prior lumpectomy, care should be taken not to inject tracer into the lumpectomy cavity.

■ Percutaneous Biopsy

If further diagnostic workup in addition to imaging is required, needle biopsy can be performed, and fine needle aspiration is very useful in this setting.[23-25] Although a negative diagnosis cannot

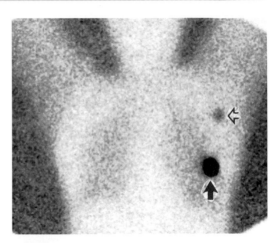

Fig. 16.**9**   Sentinel node imaging. The intense concentration of tracer is at the site of injection of Tc-99 m over the site tumor site (closed arrow). The fainter concentration of istope (open arrow) is within the sentinel node, the initial site of drainage of the tumor

definitely exclude malignant involvement, a positive diagnosis is quite reliable and can be used to influence treatment decisions.

■ New Techniques in Nodal Imaging: MRI and PET

Some studies have suggested that MRI using Gd-chelate as contrast agent has a high positive predictive value for axillary nodal metastates[26,27] (Fig. 16.**10**). In a study including 75 axillae in women with breast carcinoma, Mumtaz found sensitivity of 90 % and specificity of 82 % in detecting nodal metastases using criteria including a nodal size greater than 5 mm, higher than soft-tissue intensity on short inversion time inversion recovery images, and enhancement after the injection of Gd-dimeglumine. Mussurakis demonstrated that of 51 women studied with MR after the adminstration of gadopentetate dimeglumine, uptake patterns in lymph nodes in about one quarter of women made it possible to define groups with <5 % or >95 % likelihood of nodal metastases.

The use of ultra small particles of iron-oxide (USPIO) as so-called specific contrast agent is presently being investigated.[28,29] USPIO accumulates in the reticuloendothelial system of normal lymph-node tissue and causes a decrease of signal intensity on T2-weighted images by its ferromagnetic properties. However, in metastatic tissue

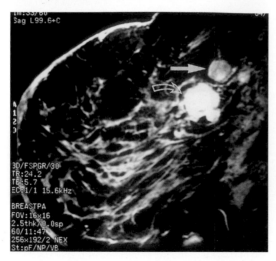

Fig. 16.**10** MRI of axillary adenopathy. Postcontrast T1-weighted image shows an irregular, enhancing mass (open, curved arrow) that is an infiltrating ductal carcinoma. An adjacent mass with patchy enhancement (closed, straight arrow) is an adjacent lymph node containing metastatic tumor. A second lymph node, also containing metastatic disease, is present just posterior to this larger node

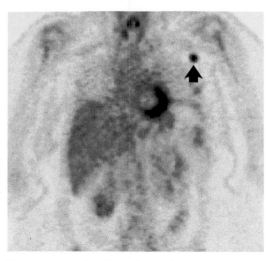

Fig. 16.**11** PET of axillary adenopathy. FDG-PET imaging of a woman with known metastatic breast carcinoma shows an axillary node containing metastatic disease (arrow)

USPIO does not accumulate, and therefore signal intensity does not change. Initial experiences show improved accuracy compared to T2-weighted non-enhanced MRI. Overlap has also been observed. Whether with the appropriate optimizations this technique might become useful for regional lymph-node imaging in breast cancer has to be evaluated.

In another set of women with nodal disease, MRI may be especially helpful: In those women who present with axillary metastases and no known primary, MRI may be able to detect the primary tumors in a high percentage of cases.[30–32]

Positive emission tomography (PET) using [fluorine-18]2-deoxy-2-fluoro-D-glucose (FDG) may also be useful in assessing axillary lymph nodes[33,34] (Fig. 16.11). Adler[34] demonstrated a sensitivity and negative predictive value of 95%, specificity of 66%, and accuracy of 77% in 50 women undergoing 52 axillary dissections. Similar results had also been reported by Scheidhauer[33]. Whereas detection of small or microscopic malignant foci in lymph nodes is not possible by PET, and reliability may decrease in obese patients, the major advantage of PET appears to be its capability to image distant metastases simultaneously. Thus, in selected patients its use may be cost-effective despite the expense of this technique. This is especially true for follow-up of women with multiple sites of metastatic disease.

■ Internal Mammary Nodes

In some instances internal mammary lymph nodes may become apparent on imaging. They may prove to be the first draining nodes of a medially located breast cancer on sentinel node radionuclide mapping. If obviously enlarged, they may be seen on CT. Occasionally enhancing internal mammary lymph nodes can be imaged between the ribs on contrast-enhanced breast MRI or on a PET study.

If imaging of internal mammary nodes is desired, ultrasound can be very useful.[35,36] Biopsy of internal mammary lymph nodes is associated with some risk due to the proximity of both internal mammary vessels and the lung. It should therefore only be considered if biopsy results will change treatment.

In general, imaging of internal mammary nodes has so far not been considered necessary for staging of breast cancer.

■ Summary

Targeted imaging of regional lymph nodes is not usually done, since only tissue sampling can reliably determine the status of these nodes. However, imaging can be useful for the workup of clinical findings.

Furthermore, lymph nodes located within the breast or lower axilla may be visualized on imaging studies of the breast. For this reason the imager should be familiar with the usual pattern of these nodes.

Mammographically, a benign lymph node typically has a fatty hilum and smooth contour. Its parenchyma has a density comparable to breast parenchyma. Overall size is of no importance. Replacement of the hilum by dense tissue, irregular contours, and the rare presence of microcalcifications may be indicators of malignant involvement.

Sonographically smooth contours, homogeneous texture of the lymph node parenchyma, and presence of a hyperechoic hilum are usually seen in benign lymph nodes. Irregular contours, bulging of the parenchyma, and visualization of hypoechoic parenchymal foci suggest malignant involvement.

If biopsy of indeterminate or suspicious imaging findings is required, this can be done by imaging-guided percutaneous biopsy, usually fine-needle aspiration cytology.

New imaging modalities such as MRI with different contrast agents or PET have proven capable of assessing macroscopic lymph-node involvement.

Further investigations will be needed to assess their added value and to check the overall value of imaging evaluation as a supplement to new surgical methods.

It must, however, be recognized that so far no imaging modality is capable of reliably detecting or excluding microscopic lymph-node involvement.

■ References

1 Adair F, Berg J, Joubert J et al. Long-term follow-up of breast cancer patients: the 30-year report. Cancer. 1974;33:1145–50
2 Veronesi U, Galimberti V, Zurrida S, Merson M, Greco M, Lini A. Prognostic significance of number and level of axillary node mestases in breast cancer. Breast. 1993;2:224–8
3 Veronesi U, Marubini E, Mariani L et al. The dissection of internal mammary nodes does not improve the survival of breast cancer patients. 30-year results of a randomized trial. Eur J Cancer. 1999;35:1320–5
4 Freedman GM, Fowble BL, Nicolaou N et al. Should internal mammary lymph nodes in breast cancer be a target for the radiation oncologist? Int J Radiat Oncol Biol Phys. 2000;1;46:805–14
5 Sugg SL, Ferguson DJ, Posner MC, Heimann R. Should internal mammary nodes be sampled in the sentinel node era? Ann Surg Oncol. 2000;7:188–92
6 Boora RS, Bonanni R, Rosato PE. Patterns of axillary nodal involvement in breast cancer. Predictability of level I dissection. Ann Surg. 1982;196:642–4
7 Hartveit F. Axillary metastases in breast cancer: when, how and why? Semin Surg Oncol. 1989;5:126–36
8 Dershaw DD, Panicek DM, Osborne MP. Significance of lymph nodes visualized by the mammographic axillary view. Breast Dis. 1991;4:271–80
9 Meyer JE, Ferraro FA, Frenna TH, DiPiro PJ, Denison CM. Mammographic appearance of normal intramammary lymph nodes in an atypical location. AJR. 1993;161:779–80
10 Dershaw DD, Selland DG, Tan LK, Morris EA, Abramson AF, Liberman L. Spiculated axillary adenopathy. Radiology. 1996;201:439–42
11 Walsh R, Kornguth PJ, Soo MS, Bentley R, Delong DM. Axillary lymph nodes: mammographic, pathologic, and clinical correlation. AJR. 1997;168:33–6
12 Leibman AJ, Wong R. Findings on mammography in the axilla. AJR. 1997;169:1385–90
13 Vaidya JS, Vyas JJ, Thakur MH et al. Role of ultrasonography to detect axillary node involvement in operable breast cancer. Eur J Surg Oncol. 1996;22:140–3
14 Strauss HG, Lampe D, Methfessel G, Buchmann J. Preoperative axilla sonography in breast tumor suspected of malignancyûa diagnostic advantage? Ultraschall Med. 1998;19:70–7
15 Yang WT, Chang J, Metreweli C. Patients with breast cancer: differences in color Doppler flow and gray scale US features of benign and malignant axillary lymph nodes. Radiology. 2000;215:568–73
16 Lee CH, Giurescu ME, Philpotts LE, Horwath LJ, Tocino I. Clinical importance of unilaterally enlarging lymph nodes on otherwise normal mammograms. Radiology. 1997;203:329–34
17 Neuman mediolateral, Homer MJ. Association of medullary carcinoma with reactive axillary adenopathy. AJR. 1996;167:185–6
18 Dershaw DD. Question and answers. AJR. 1996;166:1491
19 Hooley R, Lee C, Tocino I, Horowitz N, Carter D. Calcifications in axillary lymph nodes caused by fat necrosis. AJR. 1996;167:627–8
20 Bruwer A, Nelson GW, Spark RP. Punctate intranodal gold deposits simulating microcalcifications on mammograms. Radiology. 1987;163:87–8
21 Dunnington GL, Pearce J, Sherrod A, Cote R. Breast carcinoma presenting as mammographic microcalcifications in axillary lymph nodes. Breast Dis. 1995;8:193–8
22 Giulano AE, Kirgan DM, Guenther JM, Morton DL. Lymphatic mapping and sentinel lymphadenectomy for breast cancer. Ann Surg. 1994;220:391–401
23 Bonnema J, van Geel AN, van Ooijen B et al. Ultrasound-guided aspiration biopsy for detection of nonpalpable axillary node metastases in breast cancer patients: new diagnostic method. World J Surg. 1997;21:270–4
24 Verbanck J, Vandewiele I, De Winter H et al. Value of axillary ultrasonography and sonographically guided punc-

ture of axillary nodes: a prospective study in 144 consecutive patients. J Clin Ultrasound. 1997;25:53–6

25 De Kanter AY, van Eijck CH, van Geel AN et al. Multicentre study of ultrasonographically guided axillary node biopsy in patients with breast cancer. Br J Surg. 1999;86:1459–62

26 Mumtaz H, Hall-Craggs MA, Davidson T et al. Staging of symptomatic primary breast cancer with MR imaging. AJR. 1997;169:417–24

27 Mussurakis S, Buckley DL, Horsman A. Prediction of axillary lymph node status in invasive breast cancer with dynamic contrast-enhanced MR imaging. Radiology. 1997;203:317–21

28 Heywang-Köbrunner SH, Taupitz M, Hamm B et al. Iron oxide enhanced intravenous MR-lymphography in patients with suspected breast cancer: Results of a clinical phase III trial. Eur Radiol. 2000;10(suppl. 1):250

29 Stets C, Gilbert FJ, Buchmann J, Wallis F, Lautenschläger C, Heywang-Köbrunner SH. Statistical analysis of various qualitative and quantitative parameters in the evaluation of axillary lymph nodes in breast cancer patients. Submitted to Clinical Radiology

30 Morris EA, Schwartz LH, Dershaw DD, Van Zee KJ, Abramson AF, Liberman L. MR imaging of the breast in patients with occult primary breast carcinoma. Radiology. 1997;205;437–40

31 Schorn C, Fischer U, Luftner-Nagel S et al. MRI of the breast in patients with metastatic disease of unknown primary. Eur Radiol. 1999;9:470–3

32 Orel SG, Weinstein SP, Schnall MD. Breast MR imaging in patients with axillary node metastases and unknown primary malignancy. Radiology. 1999;212:543–9

33 Scheidhauer K, Scharl A, Pietrzyk U et al. Qualitative 18F-FDG-positron emission tomography in primary breast cancer: clinical relevance and practicability. Eur J Nucl Med. 1996;23:618–23

34 Adler LP, Faulhaber PF, Schnur KC, Al-Kasi NL, Shenk RR. Axillary lymph node metastases: screening with /F-18}2-deoxy-2-fluoro-D-glucose (FDG) PET. Radiology. 1997; 203:323–7

35 Konishi Y, Hashimoto T, Okuno T et al. Preoperative diagnosis of internal mammary node metastases in patients with breast cancer by using ultrasonography. Nippon Geka Gakkai Zasshi. 1992;93:1330–6

36 Bruneton JN, Maestro C, Marcy PY, Padovani B. Echography of superficial lymph nodes. J Radiol. 1994;75:373–81

17. Other Semi-malignant and Malignant Tumors

Phyllodes Tumor (Cystosarcoma Phyllodes)

The phyllodes tumor is a rare tumor (about 0.5% of all breast tumors). Its histologic spectrum includes benign tumors, of which up to 30% *recur*, and malignant tumors, which can metastasize. In toto, only about 5% of phyllodes tumors may metastasize. In view of its biologic property, timely detection and complete excision with an adequate safety margin is critical. Larger tumors require a mastectomy (axillary dissection should not be performed because these tumors metastasize hematogenously, not lymphogenously). Clinically and by imaging methods, the phyllodes tumor usually presents as a smoothly outlined nodule. It can develop in all age groups and generally shows a rapid growth.

■ Histology

The phyllodes tumor is a rare fibroepithelial neoplasm exhibiting the pattern of a fibroadenoma.

It is characterized by a hyperplastic, i.e., hypercellular, stroma, by wide leaf-like (phyllodes) interspaces covered with epithelium, and by epithelial metaplasias.[1]

Its hallmark is a fibromyxoid hypercellular stroma that contains fibroblasts, myofibroblasts, or even giant cells in a uniform or nonuniform distribution. The classification is determined by the degree of proliferation and differentiation of the quantitatively dominating stroma.[1-4]

Benign phyllodes tumor (prevalence 60–70%): Sharp demarcation, no atypical cells, no pleomorphic cells, low mitotic rate.

Malignant phyllodes tumor (prevalence: 25–30%): infiltrative growth, atypical cells, pleomorphic cells, obliteration of the fibroepithelial configuration, high mitotic rate: >5/10 HPF.

Borderline phyllodes tumor: usually sharply demarcated, minimal atypia of the pleomorphic cells, mitotic rate ~5/10 HPF.

Following incomplete excision, the phyllodes tumor has a high recurrence rate of 20–30%, whereby the proportion of multiple recurrences is relatively high if a wide margin of normal breast tissue is not included at the time of surgical excision.

■ Clinical Findings

The phyllodes tumor is generally palpable as:

- Smoothly marginated, round or lobulated mass, which is more or less elastic.
- Small tumors are generally moveable, but this characteristic is often lost with larger tumors.
- *Rapid growth* is suggestive of a phyllodes tumor. It can arise from a known fibroadenoma that was stable over a long period of time and is then noted by its increasing growth. It can also be found as a mass that increases in size.

At the time of the diagnosis, the majority of these neoplasms have reached a size of 3–5 cm, but occasionally small phyllodes tumors are also discovered (see also Fig. 22.**17**).

Due to the tension of the overlying skin, very large phyllodes tumors can cause erythematous or bluish discoloration of the skin, or even ulcerations.

■ Diagnostic Strategy and Goals

It is the major diagnostic goal *to differentiate* the phyllodes tumor from other nodular masses and mainly from the far more common solid nodular lesions that are *benign*. Only some phyllodes tumors have criteria that distinguish them from smoothly outlined benign lesions.

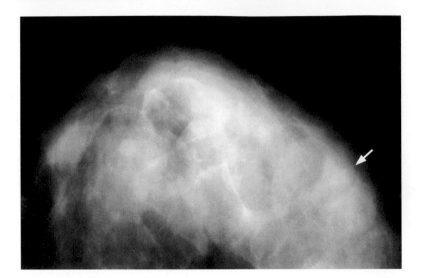

Fig. 17.**1 a–e**   Phyllodes tumor
a The phyllodes tumor, as an oval, smoothly outlined lesion, can only be suspected in the very dense parenchyma amid numerous sonographically documented cysts

It is therefore important that a phyllodes tumor should be considered whenever a smoothly outlined mass increases in size. If suspected, excision is indicated.

The definitive therapy for large tumors may require simple mastectomy, and for small tumors generous excision to obtain a tumor-free margin.

■ Mammography

(Fig. 17.**1 a** and **f**)

Mammographically[5-7], the phyllodes tumor often resembles a fibroadenoma. This means, it often presents as:

–   Oval, round, or lobulated mass.
–   Some of the phyllodes tumors are sharply outlined with or without a halo.
–   Depending on the surrounding tissue, the margin can be partially or completely obscured. In this situation, the phyllodes tumor is seen as a semicircular density or can be undetectable in dense parenchyma (Fig. 22.**17**).
–   Some irregularities in the contour are frequently, but not always, present. This can be caused by superimposition, vascular invasion, or infiltrating growth, and if present, indicates etiologies other than a fibroadenoma.
–   Rarely, bizarre or coarse calcifications (as seen in fibroadenomas) can be found in portions of phyllodes tumors.

The indistinct outline of some phyllodes tumors can serve as evidence against the presence of a fibroadenoma.

If an indistinct outline is absent or only minimal, there are, aside from a rapid increase in size and the often large extension, *no reliable mammographic differentiating criteria* between the phyllodes tumors and other smoothly or relatively smoothly outlined (usually benign) lesions.

■ Sonography

(Fig. 17.**1 b** and **g**)

Even sonographically,[5-8] the phyllodes tumor can resemble other smoothly or relatively smoothly outlined tumors. This means it often presents as:

–   Oval, round, or lobulated mass
–   With good acoustic enhancement, and
–   With usually good compressibility and moveability,
–   Its contour is generally smooth

Though occasionally also exhibited by fibroadenomas, the *following findings* suggest the correct diagnosis:

–   Indistinct outline (found in some phyllodes tumors) (Fig. 22.**17**), heterogeneity of the internal echo structure (in some phyllodes tumors, but often also in fibroadenomas, hamartomas, and malignancies)
–   Cystic spaces within the solid tumor (corresponding to the gelatinous, cystic, or necrotic areas) are sonographically characteristic of the phyllodes tumor and should suggest its diagnosis.

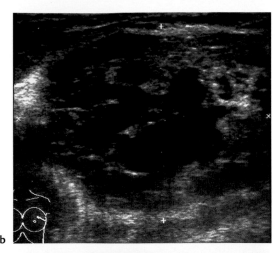

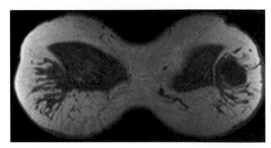

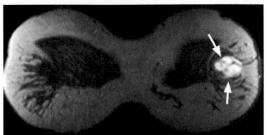

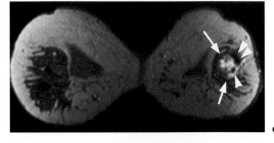

Fig. 17.**1 b**   Sonographically, the lesion is heterogeneous with intervening cystic spaces
c MRI (coronal plane) delineates a lesion of homogeneously low signal intensity and smooth outline before administration of contrast medium

d and **e** After i.v. administration of contrast medium, the lesion (arrows) shows a lobulated internal structure (intense enhancement within the lobules, slight enhancement in the septa), with some nonenhancing clefts (arrowheads) seen in adjacent sections (**e**). *Histology:* benign phyllodes tumor

■ Magnetic Resonance Imaging

(Fig. 17.**1 c–e**)

Experience with contrast-enhanced MRI is limited at present.[9, 10] As known so far, phyllodes tumors enhance rapidly and intensely. The enhancement pattern does not permit a reliable differentiation from hypercellular fibroadenomas or from smoothly outlined malignancies. Heterogeneities or cystic spaces may be disclosed by MRI, as also seen on sonography. If present, they strongly suggest the diagnosis of a phyllodes tumor.

All things considered, contrast-enhanced MRI offers no significant advantage over mammography or sonography in the differential diagnosis. The excellent visualization of the entire extent, in particular the relation of very large tumors to the thoracic wall, can be of interest to the surgeon.

■ Percutaneous Biopsy

Because of the multifarious changes of the stroma, which are decisive for establishing the diagnosis of phyllodes tumor, percutaneous biopsy may not allow an unequivocal diagnosis of the tumor in all cases.

If a phyllodes tumor is suspected owing to the rapid growth of a smoothly outlined mass, excisional biopsy should be considered to establish the diagnosis.

■ Summary

Microscopically, clinically, and by imaging, the phyllodes tumor presents as smooth or relatively smoothly outlined mass. *Reliable differentiation from other relatively smoothly outlined masses* and, in particular, from benign lesions is *often impossible.*

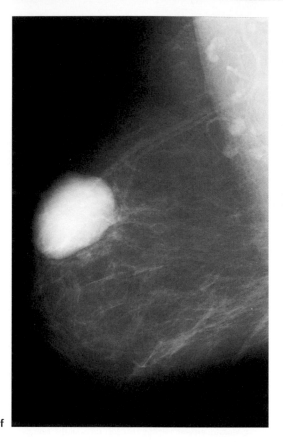

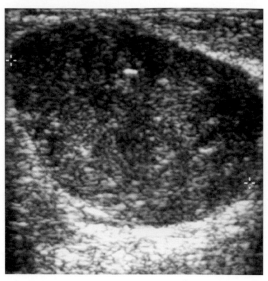

g

Fig. 17.**1 f, g** Fifty-seven-year-old woman who felt a lump in her breast
f Mammogram shows a dense, well-defined mass
g On sonography, a well-defined, solid mass with variable internal echogenicity, not cystic. *Histology:* malignant phyllodes tumor

f

In addition to the clinically noticed, usually rapid, increase in size, mammographic or sonographic irregularities of the outline as well as sonographically revealed heterogeneous internal echo structure suggest the presence of a fibroadenoma. Cystic spaces within the solid, smoothly outlined tumor disclosed by sonography or MRI are considered characteristic and should raise the suspicion of a phyllodes tumor.

Because of the unreliable differentiation of smoothly outlined solid masses that increase in size, a phyllodes tumor must always be considered. The diagnosis of such a tumor should be established by excisional biopsy.

Sarcomas

Sarcomas are rare tumors of the breast, comprising about 1% of all malignant neoplasms of this organ. Considering all sarcomas, they are found in the breast in 3% of women and in 0.5% of men. Sarcomas can occur in any age group. The average age of the wide age distribution is somewhat below that of breast carcinoma.

Since the manifestation of most sarcomas—except for their rapid growth—is uncharacteristic, the *diagnosis must be made histologically*.

■ Histology

The sarcomas of the breast are classified as follows:

– Malignant fibrous histiocytoma (44–64%)
– Fibrosarcoma (17%)
– Stromal sarcoma (27%)
– Liposarcoma (24%)
– Angiosarcoma (10–28%)

- Leiomyosarcoma
- Rhabdomyosarcoma
- Osteochondrosarcoma, chondrosarcoma
- Radiation-induced sarcoma following radiotherapy; postmastectomy angiosarcoma

The stated prevalence (relative to the prevalence of all breast sarcomas) depends on the selected histologic classification.[11] Sarcomas listed here without relative frequency are very rare. The prognosis of breast sarcoma depends on the tumor size and, partly, on grading.

Angiosarcomas are vessel-forming sarcomas with a poor prognosis, which can be further defined by the degree of malignancy.[12-14]

While the growth pattern of most soft tissue sarcomas is generally nodular (round, oval, with or without formation of a pseudocapsule, with a well-defined or irregular outline), angiosarcomas can be nodular or multinodular, but can also spread diffusely and infiltrate into the connective tissue. From the differential diagnostic and radiologic standpoint, it is relevant that the very rare liposarcoma is the only malignant mesenchymal tumor containing neoplastically transformed fatty tissue.

■ Clinical Findings

Corresponding to their growth pattern, most sarcomas present as round, oval or lobulated lesions that are—depending on the degree of infiltration— smoothly or indistinctly outlined, moveable or fixed. While fibrous sarcomas and malignant fibrous histiocytomas present as palpable firm lesions, leiomyosarcomas as well as all liposarcomas are palpated as elastic to soft lesions. Some of the sarcomas might present clinically with pain. Angiosarcomas are palpated as soft and sponge-like lesions, based on their vascular composition, and in 15–20% of the cases present with a bluish skin discoloration.

The *cardinal finding* of all sarcomas is their rapid growth.

■ Diagnostic Strategy and Goals

Because of rapid growth, sarcomas are generally discovered clinically rather than by screening examinations. They lack any characteristic presentation. A rapidly growing lesion must, in addition to other considerations, raise the possibility of a sarcoma. Since rapidly growing lesions need surgical intervention, the diagnosis is generally made histologically.

■ Mammography

(Figs. 17.**2**a, **d** and **e**)

Mammographically,[14-21] soft tissue sarcomas generally present as nodular (round, oval, or lobulated) lesions. If seen without superimposition, their outline can be smooth, but also indistinct, or even show signs of infiltrating growth (compare Fig. 17.**2**c).

Coarse calcifications may develop in necrotic or vascular areas, and typical calcifications of osteoblastic or chondroblastic transformation have rarely been described in sarcomas of the breast.

Liposarcoma is the only malignant tumor containing fatty areas. Because of its very rare occurence, liposarcoma does not play a role in the differential diagnosis of fatty lesions but has to be considered if a fatty tumor shows rapid growth.

Angiosarcomas and lymphangiosarcomas usually cause indeterminate densities. If the growth is diffusely infiltrating—found in about one-third of cases—they cannot be disclosed mammographically within dense tissue. Less frequently, they present as solitary, smooth, or indistinctly outlined nodular lesions or even as multiple nodules. Very rarely (less than 10%), bizarre calcifications have been described within angiosarcomas.

■ Sonography

(Fig. 17.**2**b)

Sonographically, soft tissue sarcomas[17, 19-21] present as hypoechoic nodular lesions, with smooth or indistinct contour. Depending on the consistency of the underlying sarcomatous type (liposarcomas and angiosarcomas have a soft consistency, while fibrous histiocytomas and fibrosarcomas are very firm), very good to minimal compressibility can be encountered sonographically.

Because of frequently occuring central necrosis, the internal structure is often irregular, with central and sometimes very hypoechoic necrotic areas.

A rather variable echo pattern has been described for angiosarcomas: A nodular lesion or several smoothly or indistinctly outlined hypoechoic nodules may be found. Angiosarcoma can be hyperechoic, hypoechoic, or heterogeneously hypoechoic and hyperechoic, with the hyperechoic areas probably representing hemorrhagic foci.

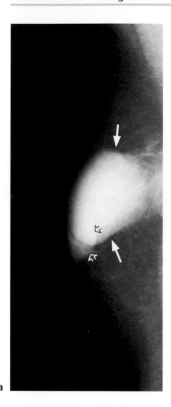

a

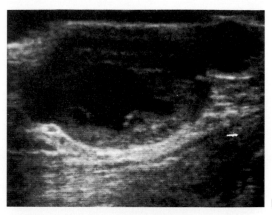

b

Fig. 17.**2** Various types of sarcomas
a, b Malignant fibrous histiocytoma in an 18-year-old man
a The mediolateral view, which was technically difficult because of infiltration of the thoracic wall, shows a large tumor (arrows), in part smooth (ventral), in part indistinct (dorsal) in outline. In addition (open arrow), directly behind the nipple a second nodule
b Sonographically, the tumor appears smoothly outlined on the section shown. It is apparent that the small nodule and the large nodule are connected. Like many sarcomas, this malignant fibrous histiocytoma shows extensive necrosis, which is anechoic

■ Magnetic Resonance Imaging

The current knowledge of the MRI property of soft tissue sarcomas is based on a few case reports so far[18, 10].

The recurrent fibrous histiocytomas among our patients showed homogeneous and pronounced enhancement in a smoothly outlined, oval tumor nodule. The enhancement was slightly delayed.

An angiosarcoma described by Liberman[18] showed a decreased signal in the T1-weighted image and an increased signal in the T2-weighted image, as seen with many malignancies. As a conspicuous finding, tubular structures of intense signal were found and attributed to vessels containing slowly flowing blood.

■ Percutaneous Biopsy

From an oncologic standpoint, percutaneous biopsy of a suspected sarcoma should be avoided.

■ Summary

Sarcomas are very rare tumors of the breasts. They usually present as a mass with well-circumscribed to ill-defined contour, rarely with diffuse extension. Almost exclusively, they are detected as an abnormal palpatory finding. Mammographically and sonographically, there are no characteristic findings differentiating them from other nodular or diffusely growing processes.

Mammography can reveal dystrophic calcifications. Very rarely, characteristic calcifications of chondrogenic or osteogenic transformation or fatty areas are found in liposarcomas. Sonographically, central necrotic areas are characteristic but not pathognomonic. Relatively characteristic for hypervascular tumors, such as the angiosarcoma, but not diagnostic and only seen in some of the cases, is the pattern of alternating hyperechoic and pronounced hypoechoic areas.

If a nodular lesion shows rapid growth, a rapidly growing carcinoma, a phyllodes tumor, or lymphoma must be considered, in addition to a sarcoma. The diagnosis must be made histologically.

Abb. 17.**2c** This large mass containing fat underwent biopsy. *Histology:* fibroadenoma
d A similar-appearing mass in another patient was also readily palpable. *Histology:* leiomyosarcoma. Even though both sarcomas shown here (**c, d,**) contain areas of fat, the general policy of considering fat-containing masses as benign should not be changed unless rapid growth is noted. The reason is that sarcomas and in particular fat-containing sarcomas are very rare
e A soft ill-defined mass developed in the posterior aspect of this breast. *Histology:* angiosarcoma

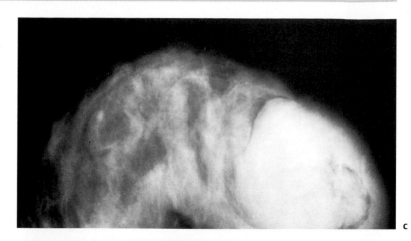

c

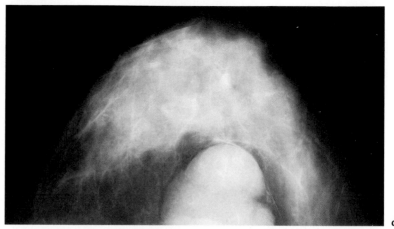

d

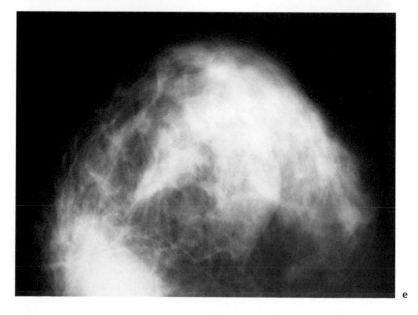

e

Malignancies of the Breast of Hematologic Origin

Listed in the order of frequency, malignancies of the breast of hematologic origin include non-Hodgkin lymphoma, leukemia, and the very rare Hodgkin lymphoma, as well as the extremely rare plasmocytoma, chloroma, and pseudolymphoma, which can precede a lymphoma for several years.[1, 22–24]

Involvement of the breast is secondary (1–5% of the malignancies), but in rare instances (less than 0.1–0.5%) the breast is the primary site of the disease, with or without involvement of the axillary lymph nodes.

The age distribution is—comparable to the hematologic malignancies involving other sites—wide and cannot be incorporated in the differential diagnosis. In the presence of an extramammary malignancy of hematologic origin, suspicious changes in the breast must raise the possibility of a concomitant mammary involvement. The histologically established diagnosis is the basis for the therapy, which differs considerably from the therapy of the breast carcinoma.

■ Morphology

Hematologic malignancies of the breasts do not vary from corresponding malignancies at other sites within the body. Macroscopically, most hematologic malignancies present as a localized finding. These foci (singular or multiple) generally grow in a nodular fashion. They are oval to round or lobulated. They can be sharply demarcated (with a complete or partial halo). In general, they show some irregularities and indistinctness of the contour. A spiculated configuration as seen with scirrhous carcinoma is not found. Diffuse infiltration of the breast has been observed with hematologic malignancies.

Characteristic differences in the macroscopic growth pattern between the individual hematologic malignancies (non-Hodgkin lymphoma, Hodgkin lymphoma, leukemia and so forth) have not been established.

The non-Hodgkin lymphomas of the breast are exclusively B-cell lymphomas, with a high proportion of germinal center lymphomas. The highly malignant lymphoblastic Burkitt lymphomas are primarily found in young women during pregnancy and lactation, and present as bilateral bluish macromastia.

Hodgkin lymphomas, plasmocytomas, chloromas, and leukemic involvement are very rare. They, too, manifest themselves as lesions of nodular or diffuse growth.

To establish the primary diagnosis (in particular the differentiation between small cell lymphoma and a lobular carcinoma), and to determine the exact type, retrieving an adequate tissue sample by excisional biopsy is important. Special stains and immunohistology are mandatory today.

It should be mentioned that hematologic malignancies can occasionally be receptor positive and that estrogen receptor positivity by no means proves the presence of a breast carcinoma.

■ Clinical Findings

Corresponding to their growth pattern, hematologic malignancies can present as:

● Diffuse skin thickening, increased consistency of the breast, enlargement of the breast, rarely erythema, or
● As a palpable nodule that is:
– More or less moveable
– Mostly elastic, relatively soft, and (therefore difficult to distinguish from a fibroadenoma)
– Rarely associated with pain or erythema
– Palpable axillary adenopathy may be present

Rapid growth is characteristic.

■ Diagnostic Strategy and Goals

In a patient with known systemic lymphoma, new changes in the breasts must raise the possibility of a lymphomatous involvement. If a malignancy of hematologic origin elsewhere in the body is not known, lymphomatous involvement of the breast is usually only suggested as one possibility in the differential diagnosis of nodular or diffusely growing lesions.

Excisional biopsy is essential for the primary diagnosis and exact classification.

■ Mammography

(Figs. 17.3 a–d, 17.4).

Hematologic malignancies[22-28] generally occur as:

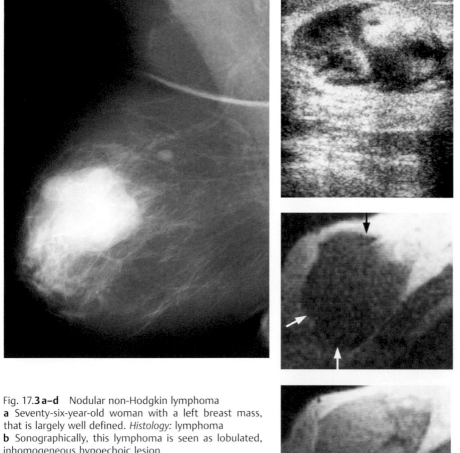

Fig. 17.**3 a–d**   Nodular non-Hodgkin lymphoma
a Seventy-six-year-old woman with a left breast mass, that is largely well defined. *Histology:* lymphoma
b Sonographically, this lymphoma is seen as lobulated, inhomogeneous hypoechoic lesion
c It is low signal on the T1-weighted images (arrows)
d Lobulation is apparent on the T2-weighted images (contrast medium was not available at the time of this examination), whereby the areas of high signal-intensity corresponded histologically to lymphomatous tissue. The linear signals of low intensity turned out to be fibrous structures

- Nodular mass (round, oval, or lobulated, frequently with irregularities of its contour rather than a completely smooth contour)
- Irregularly outlined lesion (less frequently) or
- Asymmetrically increased density

Extensive spiculations or microcalcifications are not part of the appearance found with a malignancy of hematologic origin. Furthermore, hematologic malignancies may sometimes present as:

- Diffuse pattern with skin thickening, trabecular coarsening, and generalized increased density
- Axillary adenopathy may be present

Hematologic malignancies have no pathognomonic changes.

Diffuse involvement can only be distinguished histologically from diffuse lymphedema secondary to axillary nodal metastases, with therapeutic implications. A reliable differentiation is mammographically impossible.

■ Sonography

(Fig. 17.**3 b**)

Nodular involvement is charaterized by more or less hypoechoic foci.[26, 29] They are:

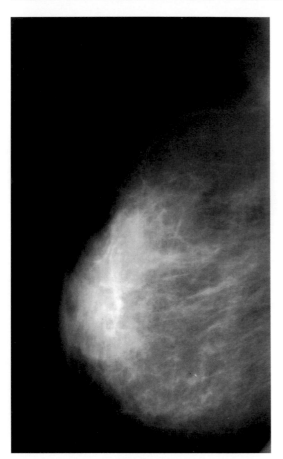

Fig. 17.**4**   Diffuse non-Hodgkin lymphoma
In addition to predominantly periareolar skin thickening, this older mediolateral mammogram shows diffuse interstitial thickening throughout the mammary tissue

- Generally round, oval, lobulated
- Partially sharply outlined, rarely with irregularities
- Generally with homogeneous internal structure, sometimes very hypoechoic (and can be mistaken for a cyst!), and

- Often with very good distal acoustic enhancement, less frequently with heterogeneous or absent enhancement

Because of the generally good elasticity and partly because of the encountered moveability, the lesions may be mistaken for fibroadenomas or, if very hypoechoic, for cysts.
Diffuse involvement is characterized[26, 29] by:

- Skin thickening
- Diffusely decreased echogenicity (uncharacteristic)

■ Magnetic Resonance Imaging

(Figs. 17.3 c and **d**)
The lymphomas may show focal (partly smoothly outlined) or diffuse contrast enhancement. The enhancement may be delayed or rapid.[10, 28]

■ Percutaneous Biopsy

The diagnosis of a lymphoma can generally be made by fine needle or core biopsy of tumorous infiltrates. Malignant lymphomas are often diagnosed by excisional biopsies. The immunohistochemical subclassification is generally based on the adequate material obtained from an excisional biopsy.

■ Summary

Hematologic malignancies can present as a focal lesion or as an indistinct diffuse process. There are no morphologic criteria to distinguish the individual hemotologic malignancies, nor are there reliable differentiating criteria toward benign tumors (for well-circumscribed masses), carcinomas (for irregularly outlined lesions) or inflammatory carcinoma, lymphedema, or inflammation (for diffuse involvement). The final diagnosis and exact classification rest on the excisional biopsy.

Metastases

Metastases in the breasts are rare (about 1–5% of the malignancies). They can arise from:

1. An extramammary tumor of any origin
2. A contralateral breast carcinoma
3. A malignancy of hematologic origin

Metastases should be considered in findings with multiple masses or diffuse increased breast density in cases with a history of known primary carcinoma or metastases, but a specific manifestation is not known.[30–34]

The therapeutic approach depends on the overall prognosis.

■ Histology

The most frequently observed metastases arise from the opposite breast, followed by malignant melanomas, bronchial carcinomas, ovarian carcinomas, and sarcomas. Moreover, metastases can arise from gastrointestinal carcinomas, cholangiocarcinomas, thyroid carcinomas, head and neck carcinomas, and urogenital carcinomas, including cervix carcinoma in women and prostate carcinoma in men. The metastases of most extramammary *malignancies* exhibit a *nodular* growth: rather round than oval, and sometimes lobulated.

Metastatic spread can produce *single or multiple* lesions. Metastases are usually distinct in outline and rarely somewhat indistinct. Spiculations do not occur. They are usually located in subcutaneous fat rather than in the core of the breast tissue.

Some extramammary malignancies also have metastases that show a *diffuse growth pattern.* This is most frequently observed in ovarian carcinomas, but has been occasionally described with other malignancies.

Metastases from a carcinoma of the contralateral breast can be hematogenous or lymphogenous via the lymphatics crossing the sternum.

■ Clinical Findings

If adequate in size and situated superficially, *focal metastases* may be palpated as:

- Smoothly outlined, round
- Usually moveable, rarely fixed
- More often firm than soft lesions (depending on the property of the primary tumor)
- The size of the palpable finding approximates the mammographic size (since reactive changes of the surrounding tissue—as found, for instance, in scirrhous carcinoma—are absent)[29]
- Frequently located in subcutaneous fat.

Reliable criteria differentiating these from fibroadenomas and cysts do not exist. History of rapid growth often suggests the diagnosis.

If the *involvement is diffuse*, skin thickening and diffuse swelling are observed. Pain is infrequent.

Metastases from a carcinoma of the contralateral breast usually occur via direct extension. They are detectable through skin thickening, palpable thickening, peau d'orange, nodules, or swelling.

■ Diagnostic Strategy and Goals

With the appropriate history, metastases should be considered if single or multiple, new or growing lesions are found clinically or mammographically, or if diffuse changes of undetermined etiology are encountered.

If the excisional biopsy of a breast lesion—without appropriate history—suggests a metastasis, the search for a primary tumor is warranted.

Appropriate special stains and immunohistology of the excised tissue may assist in determining the origin of the metastasis.

■ Mammography

(Figs. 17.**5** a and 17.**6**)

Focal metastases are generally visualized mammographically:[30, 33, 34]

- As round, sharply outlined lesions, frequently without any significant marginal indistinctness. Particularly suggestive is the perfectly round shape.
- Single or multiple.
- They can also be partially or totally hidden in dense tissue.
- Aside from coarse calcifications involving necrotic areas, calcifications are extremely rare and, as far as we know, only described as amorphic calcifications in ovarian carcinoma.
- Multiple round lesions containing subgroups of lesions that are about equal in size—reflecting intermittent dissemination—are characteristic and considered important evidence of the presence of metastases.

Reliable criteria that distinguish individual metastases from smoothly outlined benign lesions (fibroadenomas) *do not exist.*

Elongated, polymorphic or ductally oriented microcalcifications, or spicules preclude, for all practical purposes, a metastasis.

Diffuse metastases can become manifest as:

- Skin thickening
- Thickened trabecular markings
- Diffuse, asymmetrically increased density of the parenchyma

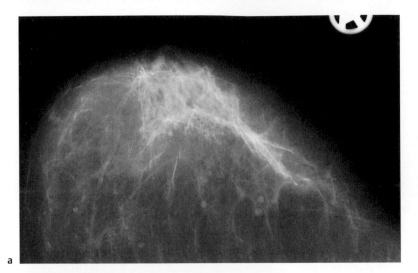

a

Fig. 17.**5a** and **b**   Multiple small nodular metastases in a patient with known metastatic malignant melanoma
a Craniocaudal mammogram. The multitude of nodules with several nodules equal in size suggests (even without the clinical history) a metastatic process. Despite the smooth outline, the perfectly round configuration favors metastases over benign lesions
b Sonography of a small metastasis—also exhibiting a perfectly round configuration.

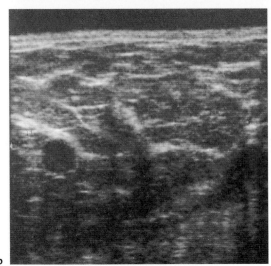

b

– Usually present as sharply outlined, round, hypoechoic lesions, with homogeneous internal structure, and with no or only minimal reactive changes in the surrounding tissue
– Usually have distal acoustic enhancement, sometimes no enhancement or acoustic shadowing (in the presence of intense fibrosis) is seen
– A certain indistinctness of the outline might be appreciated
– Heterogeneity of the internal structure can develop with central necrosis
– Metastases often are easily moveable, rarely fixed
– The consistency varies from firm to soft elastic

Consequently, *sonography does not allow a reliable differentiation* from benign lesions that are sharply outlined, such as adenomas.
Diffuse metastatic spread is sonographically:

– Recognized by diffuse skin thickening and obliteration of the echogenic interface with the subcutaneous layer
– Cooper's ligaments may be thickened and appear hypoechoic, secondary to lymphatic stasis caused by tumor cells
– The changes of the parenchyma are often uncharacteristic; overall, the parenchyma appears somewhat hypoechoic

Metastases from a carcinoma of the contralateral breast can involve the entire breast diffusely, or appear as cutaneous and subcutaneous thickening extending from the parasternal region laterally (Fig. 17.**6**).

■ Sonography

(Fig. 17.**5 b**)

Sonography is used to exclude a simple cyst and to verify the presence of palpable findings in mammographically dense tissue.
    Sonographically localized metastases:[32, 34]

■ Magnetic Resonance Imaging

The experience is based on only a few individual cases, which showed the metastases as smoothly outlined, nodular, enhancing lesions.

Fig. 17.**6** The medially rotated craniocaudal mammogram shows subtle skin thickening medially, and slightly accentuated interstitial markings in a locally metastasizing contralateral breast carcinoma. (Slightly rotated view for better visualization of the medial skin and subcutis)

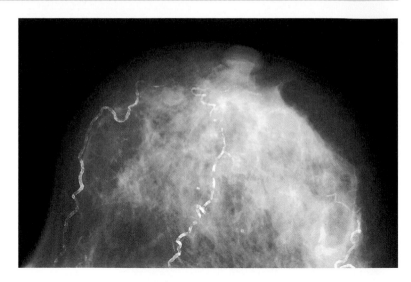

■ Percutaneous Biopsy

Percutaneous biopsy is very well suited to confirm the presence of malignancy. The diagnosis of a "metastasis" is usually made by excisional biopsy. The larger tissue sample obtained with excisional biopsy may permit better histologic evaluation and immunohistologic examination, but even then the site of origin of the primary tumor cannot be determined in all cases.

■ Summary

Metastatic spread can become manifest as diffuse, ill-defined changes (skin thickening, increased consistency) or by forming single or several nodular lesions.

Reliable criteria distinguishing metastases from other nodular, usually sharply outlined lesions or from other diffuse changes (mastitits, inflammatory carcinoma) do not exist. Several round lesions, including subgroups of equal size, suggest a metastasizing process.

With the history of a known carcinoma, metastases should be considered if nodular or diffuse changes are found. Confirmation and analysis as to their site of origin rest on the histologic examination.

Other Very Rare Tumors

The following very rare tumors, classified as semimalignant tumors, are listed here:

- fibromatosis
- hemangiopericytoma
- hemangioendothelioma

■ Fibromatosis (= Extra-abdominal Desmoid)

The fibromatosis of the breast grows locally invasive. Local recurrence occurs frequently following incomplete excision. It arises from the fascia and consequently is frequently fixed to the pectoral muscle. *Histologically,* it consists of proliferative fibroblasts and extensive fibrosis.[35]

Mammographically [34, 36], it is seen as irregular thickening with fibrous strands and retractions, and cannot be distinguished from the geographic growth of a scirrhous carcinoma.

Sonographically, extensive acoustic shadowing can be expected, as found in scirrhous carcinoma.

There is no experience with MRI. Excision is recommended for diagnosis and therapy.

■ Hemangiopericytoma and Hemangioendothelioma

Both tumors are rare. The diagnosis is made histologically.

■ References

1 Bässler R, Zahner J. Über Rezidive und Metastasen des Cystosarcoma phylloides (Phylloide Tumor, WHO). Geburtshilfe Frauenheilkd. 1989;49:1

2 Cohn-Cedermark G, Rutquist LE, Rosendahl I et al. Prognostic factors in cystosarcoma phylloides: clinicopathologic study of 77 patients. Cancer. 1991;68:2017

3 de Roos WK, Kaye P, Dent DM. Factors leading to local recurrence of death after surgical resection of phyllodes tumors or the breast. Br J Surg. 1999;86:396–9

4 Barth RJ Jr. Histologic features predict local recurrence after breast conserving therapy of phyllodes tumors. Breast Cancer Res Treat.1999;57:291–5

5 Buchberger W, Strasser K, Heim K et al. Phylloides tumor, findings on mammography, sonography and aspiration in 10 cases. AJR. 1991;157:715

6 Blanco JA, Serrano VB, Romero RR, Candejas ME. Phyllodes tumor of the breast. Eur Radiol. 1999;9:356–60

7 Liberman L, Bonaccio E, Hamele-Bena D, Cohen MA, Abramson AF, Dershaw DD. Imaging characteristics of benign and malignant phyllodes tumors. Radiology. 1996;198:121–4

8 Geisler DB, Boyle MJ, Malnar KF et al. Phyllodes tumor of the breast: a review of 32 cases. Am Surg. 2000;66:360–6

9 Grebe P, Wilhelm K, Brunier A, Mitze M. MR-Tomographie des Cystosarcoma phylloides. Ein Fallbeispiel. Akt Radiol. 1992;2:376

10 Heywang-Köbrunner SH, Beck R. Contrast-enhanced MRI of the breast. Heidelberg, New York: Springer; 1996

11 Gutman H, Pallock PE, Ross MJ et al. Sarcoma of the breast: implications for extent of therapy. Surgery. 1994;116:505

12 Chen KTK, Kickegaard DD, Bocean BB. Angiosarcoma of the breast. Cancer. 1980;46:368

13 Rosen PP, Kimmel M, Ernsberger D. Mammary angiosarcoma, the prognostic significance of tumor differentiation. Cancer. 1988;62:2145

14 Ciatto S, Bonardi R, Cataliotti L, Cardona G. Sarcomas of the breast: a multicenter series of 70 cases. Neoplasia. 1992;39:375–9

15 Tunon de Lara C, Roussillon E, Rivel J et al. Liposarcoma of the breast. A case report. J Gynecol Obstet Biol Reprod. 1998;27:201–4

16 Elson BC, Ikeda DM, Anderson I et al. Fibrosarcoma of the breast: mammographic findings in 5 cases. AJR. 1992;158:993

17 Ng CS, Taylor CB, O'Donnell PJ et al. Case report: mammographic and ultrasound appearances of Kaposi's Sarcoma of the breast. Clin Radiol. 1996;51:735–6

18 Liberman L, Dershaw DD, Kaufmann R, Rosen PP. Angiosarcoma of the breast. Radiology. 1992;183:649–54

19 Zincone GE, Perego P, Rossi GM, Bovo G. A case of breast angiosarcoma: diagnostic imaging and review of the literature. Tumori 1995;81:387–96

20 Brown AL, Holwill SD, Thomas VA et al. Case report: primary osteosarcoma of the breast: imaging and histological features. Clin Radiol. 1998;53:920–2

21 Son HJ, Oh KK. Multicentric granulocytic sarcoma of the breast: mammographic and sonographic findings. AJR. 1998;171:274–5

22 Giardini R, Piccolo C, Rilke F. Primary non-Hodgkin's lymphomas of the female breast. Cancer. 1992;69:725

23 Hugh JC, Jackson FJ, Hanson J et al. Primary breast lymphoma: an immunohistologic study of 20 new cases. Cancer. 1990;66:2602

24 Kennedy BJ, Bornstein R, Brunning RD et al. Breast involvement in acute leukemia. Cancer. 1970;25:693

25 Liberman L, Giess CS, Dershaw DD, Deutch BM, Louise DC. Non-Hodgkin's lymphoma of the breast: imaging characteristics and correlation with histopathology. Radiology. 1994;192:157–60

26 Paulus DD. Lymphoma of the breast. Radiol Clin North Am. 1990;28:833

27 Pameijer FA, Beijerinck D, Hoogenboom HH et al. Non-Hodgkin's lymphoma of the breast causing miliary densities on mammography. AJR. 1995;164:609–10

28 Mussarakis S, Carleton PJ, Turnbull LW. MR imaging of primary non-Hodgkin's breast lymphoma. Acta Radiol. 1997;38:104–7

29 Tohno E, Cosgrove DO, Sloane JP. Ultrasound Diagosis of Breast Diseases. Edinburgh: Churchill Livingstone; 1994

30 Bohmann LG, Bassett LW, Gold RH et al. Breast metastases from extramammary malignancies. Radiology. 1982;144:30

31 Paulus DD, Libshitz HJ. Metastases to the breast. Radiol Clin North Am. 1982;20:561

32 Derchi LF, Rizzato G, Guiseppetti GM et al. Metastatic tumors in the breast; sonographic findings. J Ultrasound Med. 1985;4:69

33 McCrea ES, Johnston C, Haney PJ. Metastases of the breast. AJR. 1983;141:685

34 Feder JM, de Paredes ES, Hogge JP, Wilken JJ. Unusual breast lesions: radiologic-pathologic correlation. Radiographics. 1999;19 Spec No:11–26

35 Wargotz ES, Norris HJ, Austin KM et al. Fibromatosis of the breast: a clinical and pathological study of 28 cases. Am J Surg Pathol. 1987;11:38

36 Ormandi K, Lazar G, Toszegi A, Palko A. Extraabdominal desmoid mimicking malignant male breast tumor. Eur Radiol. 1999;9:1120–2

18. Post-traumatic, Post-surgical, and Post-therapeutic Changes

Post-traumatic and Post-surgical Changes

Following surgery or trauma, characteristic tissue changes can develop.

Acute changes can be separated from late changes:

1. **Acute changes:** hematoma, seroma, edema, fat necrosis (acute)
2. **Late changes:** scar formation, retraction, dystrophic calcifications, fat necrosis (chronic): oil cyst, lipophagic granuloma

■ Histology

Hematomas and seromas occupy either a surgical cavity or a traumatic tear, or spread into the surrounding parenchyma, connective tissue, and adipose tissue.

After the formation of these fluid collections, resorption takes place. Tissue necrosis is generally called "fat necrosis," even though it only in part concerns fat cells. It is caused by traumatic injury of the cell membrane. The subsequent healing process is marked by the appearance of foam cells as well as of leukocytic, round cell and histiocytic infiltrates, permeating the affected area or causing resorption and repair along the border of the cavity. Beginning along the border, granulation tissue, rich in fibroblasts, grows centripetally. Initially, this tissue is hypervascular and is later transformed into a poorly vascularized, densely packed scar fibrosis. Confluent foci of necrotic fat can liquefy centrally, producing oil cysts, which have a tendency to calcify.

■ Clinical History and Findings

Following surgery or major injury, location and time of the trauma are well known. Both hematoma and fat necrosis can, however, also occur "spontaneously." The eliciting trauma is often not remembered. Instead, the patient notices a nodule, which may or may not be painful and is caused by a hematoma or fat necrosis. Sometimes an associated subcutaneous hematoma suggests the site of the trauma or hemorrhage.

Hematomas are generally completely resolved and transformed into scar tissue, while fat necroses present as tumor-like lipophagic granulomas or oil cysts. The lipophagic granuloma presents as a clinically suggestive palpable nodule, usually of medium to firm consistency and of poor demarcation. Despite their smooth mammographic demarcation, oil cysts are also generally palpated as indistinctly demarcated fixed nodules.

■ Diagnostic Strategy and Goals

Fresh hematomas and seromas are easily diagnosed by sonography in the context of preceding surgery and corresponding clinical findings.[1] This is, however, rarely necessary. An oval, sometimes even ill-defined mass at the surgical site may normally be present up to a year after surgery. For objective exclusion of a malignancy, mammographic evaluation of the lesion is necessary in all cases where doubts exist whether the suspected hematoma, seroma, or fat necrosis may explain all of the changes. The patient's statement of a preceding trauma may not prove a traumatic etiology, and it should be verified that findings are consistent with trauma rather than malignancy.

Old hematomas also can usually be diagnosed correctly by mammography in context with the clinical history, but a centrally necrosing malignancy must be excluded in the differential diagnosis.

Fat necroses are readily diagnosed by mammography if they present as calcifying liponecrosis or oil cysts but not as lipophagic granuloma, which requires histopathologic verification unless it can be diagnosed by its characteristic clinical course.[2–4]

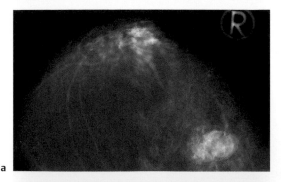

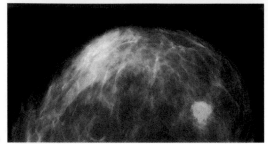

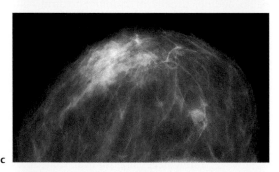

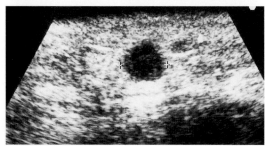

Fig. 18.**1 a–d**

a Patient after trauma. A soft, circumscribed resistance is palpated beneath a cutaneous hematoma, corresponding mammographically to a lobulated, indistinctly outlined soft-tissue density: hematoma

b and **c** Trauma while working in the garden. Irregularly outlined focal lesion in the medial half of the breast (**b**), 9 days later (**c**) markedly resolved

d Sonography (13 MHz). Round hypoechoic area, measuring 6.5 mm in diameter, with distal acoustic enhancement

Most scars have characteristic mammographic features and generally are positively diagnosed by correlation with the clinical findings, possibly aided by marking of the skin. On occasion it may be difficult, however, to exclude a malignant lesion without further workup.

Selected cases with palpable nodules or increased consistency on clinical examination can pose a problem as to the exclusion of residual or newly evolving malignancy, with mammographically increased density and architectural distortion, atypical dense center of the scar, or suspicious calcifications. MRI might supplement mammography, in particular in the presence of extensive scar formation, and biopsy of suspicious findings my be necessary.[5-6]

Dystrophic calcifications are usually clearly identified by mammography on the basis of their form, size, and location within or along scars. When these calcifications are first forming, differential diagnostic problems can be encountered.

■ Mammography

■ Acute Changes

Fresh hematomas/seromas are seen as an ill-defined mass (Figs. 18.**1 a–c**), sometimes only appreciated as a difference between both sides. Hematomas, which occupy a surgical cavity, usually present as round to oval masses with some contour irregularity. Air–fluid levels can be found in the acute postoperative period (Fig. 18.**2 a–c**). Fresh fat necrosis initially produces an ill-defined mass that can be more or less radiolucent. It may then progress to an oil cyst or to a lipophagic granuloma. Often skin thickening is visualized along the scar.

■ Late Changes

Scars in the skin are visualized as focal skin thickening seen if seen tangentially (Figs. 18-**2 b** and **c**), or as more or less round to elongated streaky densities if seen en face. Fibrous stranding into the subcutaneous fat may be present.

Scars within the breast usually are seen as elongated or spiculated and are usually associated with architectural distortion. In the majority of cases they can be correctly diagnosed as scars. In some cases (Fig. 18.**3 a** and **b**), differential diagnostic problems occur when differentiating scars from carcinomas or other spiculated masses. Whereas scars usually do not have a central mass and present differently on different pro-

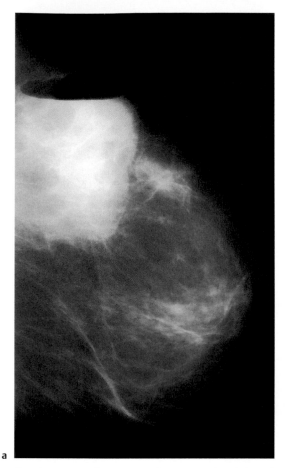

a

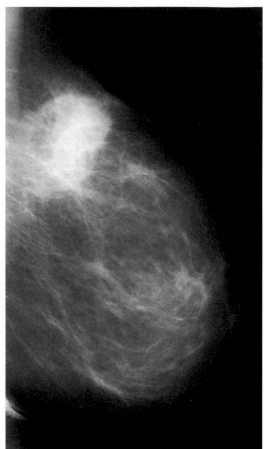

b

Fig. 18.**2 a–c** Evolving scar formation (mediolateral views)
a–c Follow-up of large fluid retention with air–fluid level 5 days after surgery (**a**)

Five weeks later, decrease in size of the mass, decreased radiodensity, and increasing spiculation as well as thickening and retraction of the skin (**b**). Three months later, scar formation with progressing retraction and demarcation of two oil cysts (arrows) (**c**)

jections compatible with a flat extension, carcinomas tend to grow more concentrically. The following options exist to define a radial structural change as a scar-related change as accurately as possible:

1. Marking the location on the skin by placing a thin metal wire over the scar on the skin. In general, the surgeon will select the most direct approach so that the parenchymal scar can be expected underneath the cutaneous scar.
2. An additional projection can help to clarify the findings. Scars can often be seen better on one orthogonal view than on the other and change their appearance in different projections (Figs. 18.**3 a** and **b**). Cancers, however,

mostly but not always have a similar pattern in different projections.
3. Spot compression views can often better prove the absence of a focal central mass. Fat can frequently be present in the center of the scar. Neither absence of a focal density nor presence of fat, however, can exclude a carcinoma with absolute certainty—a few carcinomas can only elicit spiculation without forming a hyperdense center—but detecting a newly developed central mass strongly suggests a neoplasm arising in a scar.
4. The interpretation of scar-related parenchymal structural changes is most definitive if serial postoperative mammographic studies can be reviewed. Changes caused by a scar are a

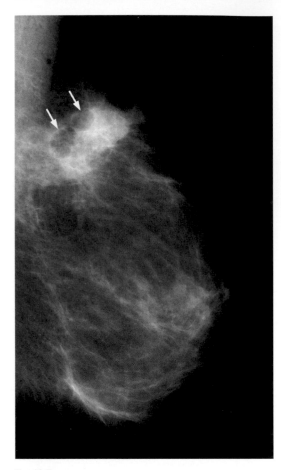

Fig. 18.**2c**

definite possibility if the findings remain unchanged or decrease in density.

Length of thickness of the spicules are not criteria for the *differential diagnosis:* markedly fibrosed ductal carcinomas and tubular carcinomas can have very long thick or delicate radial extensions mammographically.

5. The lipophagic granuloma is a special manifestation of granulomatous fat necrosis. It is visualized as an ill-defined mass (Fig. 18.**3c**). It cannot be distinguished from malignancy by imaging and consequently necessitates biopsy.[2]

Dystrophic calcifications within a scar are caused by deposition of calcium salts in necrotic tissue.
    The following calcifications occur:

– Calicifications of the stroma
– Calcifications within fat necroses
– Calcifications around suture material

Calcifications in the stroma have a characteristic coarse oblong form and are located within the scar (Fig. 18.**4a** and **e**). Furthermore, they can appear amorphous and plaque-like (Fig. 18.**4b**).
    Calcifications in fat necrosis can present as:

– Calcifying liponecrosis: small fat droplets are formed and become calcified, producing coarse, round, or ring-like calcifications (Fig. 18.**4a** and **c**).
– Oil cysts: a large cystic mass containing oily necrotic material may evolve. It produces a round or oval radiolucency surrounded by a capsule. Furthermore, typical eggshell-like calcifications can develop in the capsule (Fig. 18.**4d**, **g–i**).
– Small, circumscribed, calcified cellular necrosis: in this case, pleomorphic, clustered microcalcifications can evolve that are not always distinguishable from ductal calcifications (Fig. 18.**4f**).

Calcifying liponecrosis and oil cysts are definitively diagnosed by mammography and do not require further evaluation. Evolving microcalcifications in fat necrosis, however, can appear rather pleomorphic as well as clustered (Fig. 18.**4f**). Magnification mammography can improve the morphologic evaluation by better visualizing any evolving round and ring-like configurations as signs of benignity. Furthermore, demonstrating the relationship to a typically round or oval radiolucent area (Fig. 18.**4f**) can be helpful. If uncertainty remains, biopsy is indicated.
    Calcified suture material is identified as elongated string-like structures, sometimes with knots. Their double contour resembles periductal calcifications and chronic galactophoritis ("plasma cell mastitis").

■ Sonography

■ Acute Changes

Diffuse hemorrhage into the tissue can appear sonographically as an area:

– of increased echogenicity (usually indistinctly outlined) (Fig. 18.**5b**),
– of decreased echogenicity (Figs. 18.**5a**, 18.**1d**), or
– of suspicious architectural distortion.

In the acute stage, *hematomas* are visualized as an irregularly outlined hypoechoic area on sonography.

Fig. 18.**3 a–c**
a and **b** Scar formation in the upper outer quadrant with skin retraction and thickening, architectural distortion as well as retraction of the pectoral muscle (arrows). The craniocaudal view reveals a localized mass with a central density, which is not visible in the mediolateral view (scar). Different appearance on different views is typical for scarring
c Granuloma: in the upper half of the breast, a 7 mm focal finding with relatively thick spicules (mediolateral view)

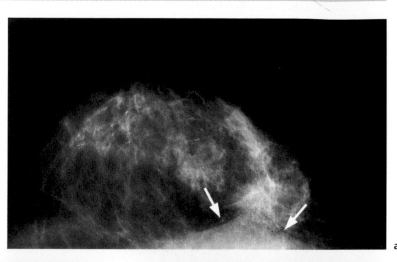

a

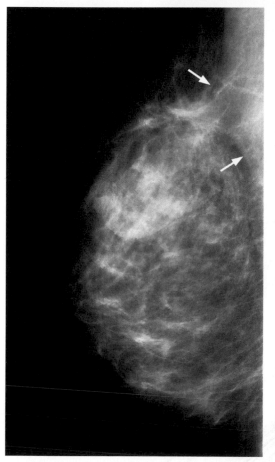

b

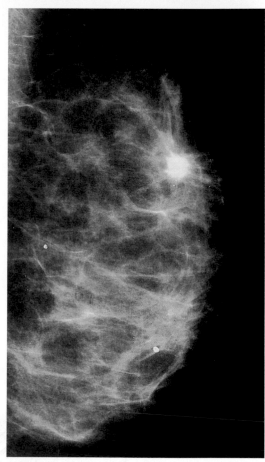

c

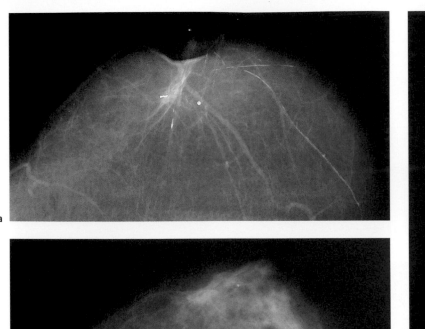

a

c

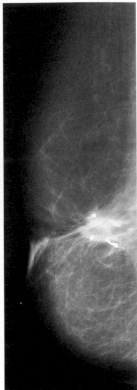

b

Fig. 18.**4a–i**   Calcifications after breast-conserving therapy

a–f Calcifications seen in scarring

a Cicatricial periareolar skin thickening and retraction, linear scarring causing thickened parenchymal structures and elongated coarse stromal calcification with adjacent calcifying liponecrosis. Extensive vascular calcifications (craniocaudal view)

b At the periphery of the architectural distortion, coarse amorphous stromal calcifications. Areolar retraction (mediolateral view)

c Coarse calcifications adjacent to a spiculated mass are due to fat necrosis following lumpectomy and breast conservation

With increasing age of the hematoma, it becomes more sharply demarcated from surrounding tissues. The hematoma can contain hypoechoic fluid but also echogenic components (e.g., clots), which are distinguished from solid lesions by showing fluctuating echoes on palpation.

Seromas present like hematomas. Echogenic internal structures are generally absent. Oil cysts may exhibit very variable appearance on ultrasound. Usually they present as solid or complex masses with variable sound transmission. They are usually not movable. Even though they mostly have smooth external contours, they usually have to be classified as indeterminate or suspicious based on usual ultrasound criteria.[7–9] Sometimes their appearance may mimic an intracystic mass. Irrespective of the sonographic appearance, oil cysts do not require further workup if mammography is characteristic (Fig. 11.**5**).

The diagnosis is unequivocal if reviewed together with the mammogram.

Fig. 18.**4d** Magnification mammography. Oval radiolucency with delicate capsule and typical eggshell-like calcifications: oil cyst

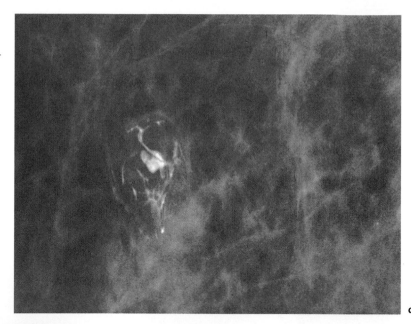

d

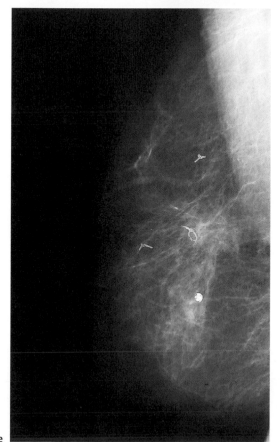

e

Fig. 18.**4e** Calcified suture material and calcifying liponecrosis

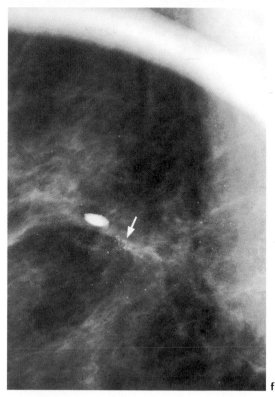

f

Fig. 18.**4f** This small group of pleomorphic microcalcifications newly appeared on one of the post-therapeutic follow-up studies. Based on the individual shapes, the arrangement, and the new development of the microcalcifications, biopsy was indicated. Histology revealed fat necrosis with microcalcifications and a foreign body granuloma

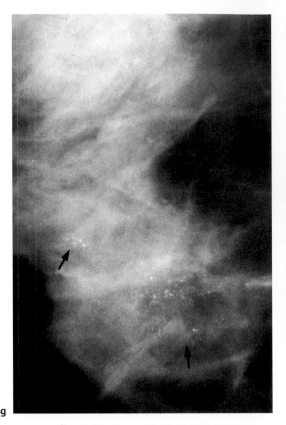

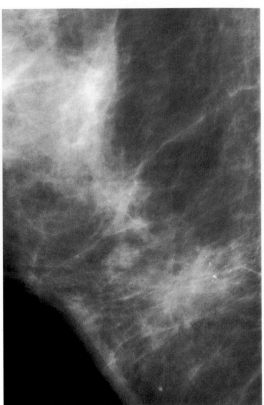

Fig. 18.**4g**   Preoperative mammography of the primary tumor in the upper half of the breast: two groups of granular microcalcifications: invasive ductal carcinoma, measuring 21 mm in diameter, as well as DCIS
h Four years after therapy of the primary tumor, new pleomorphic microcalcifications are seen. On magnification mammography (**i**), they can be unequivocally assigned to two small oil cysts

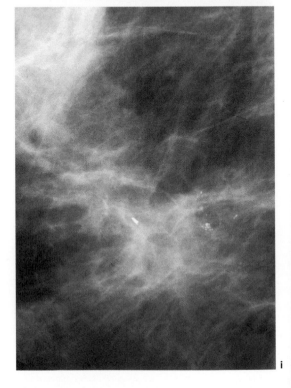

Fresh *fat necroses* containing necrotic and granulation tissue generally are seen as ill-defined masses with or without distal acoustic shadowing. A differentiation between fat necrosis and malignancy is, therefore, not possible on the basis of sonographic criteria or by any other method.

Hypoechoic areas in a scar that increase in size require further workup to exclude tumor. Such changes can also be caused by impaired wound healing. A differentiation between fat necrosis and tumor is sonographically impossible.

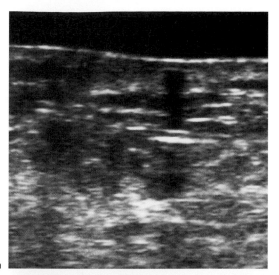

a

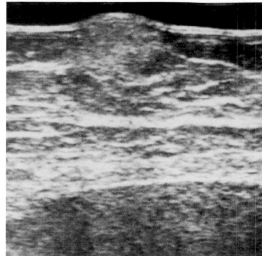

b

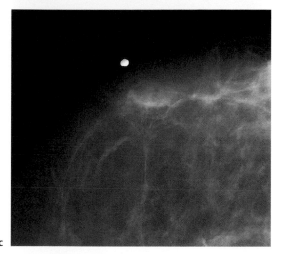

c

Fig. 18.**5a–c** Sonographic (**a** and **b**) and mammographic (**c**) visualization of hematomas
a Several hypoechoic areas as well as sound attenuation: bleeding
b Oval, hyperechoic lesion in the subcutaneous space with bulging of the overlying skin: hematoma following trauma
c The same patient as in Fig. 18.**5b**: magnification mammography with lead marker over the palpable finding shows an ill-defined subcutaneous soft-tissue density corresponding to a hematoma

■ **Late Changes**

Scar formation. With progressive scar formation, the hypoechoic areas caused by fresh fat necrosis and granulation tissue decrease in size.

In the final stage, the following findings remain (Fig. 18.**6a–e**):

– A more or less pronounced skin thickening along the scar in the skin
– Discrete to marked architectural distortion with occasional hypoechoic structures in the subcutaneous space, acoustic shadowing, interruptions, or distortion of the parenchyma
– Occasionally one or more hypoechoic, indistinctly outlined areas with or without distal acoustic shadowing
– Areas with marked acoustic attenuation

Above all, the sonographic exclusion or detection of a malignancy can be considerably impaired or even impossible in the presence of hypoechoic areas and marked acoustic shadowing. Well-documented serial sonographic studies, if available, can be helpful.

■ **Magnetic Resonance Imaging**

■ **Acute Changes**

Hemorrhage can—depending on its age—have a variable signal intensity on precontrast T1-

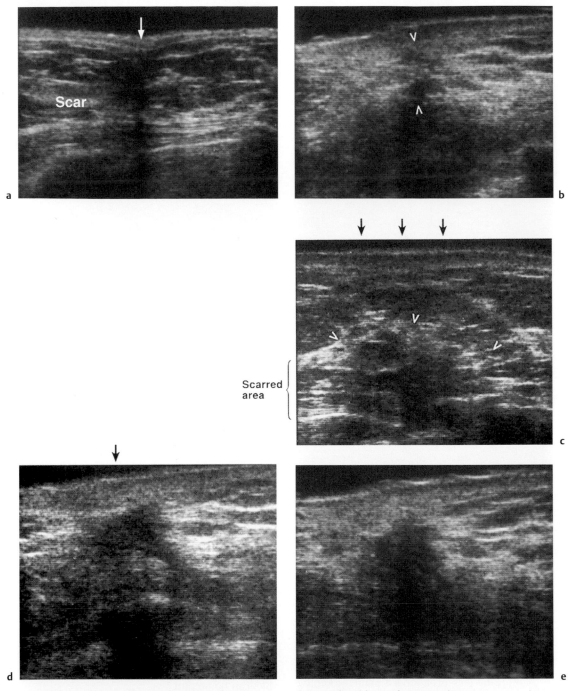

Fig. 18.**6 a–e**   Sonographic manifestations of scars
a Typical scar with acoustic shadowing (arrow) starting at the skin level and interrupting all tissue layers
b Scar-related architectural distortion (arrowheads)
c Extensive distortion of the architecture with hypo-echoic areas (arrowheads)

d Scar-related hypoechoic area that appears as a hypo-echoic mass
e Hypoechoic, irregularly outlined scar with acoustic shadowing

weighted images. Following injection of Gd-DTPA, minimal to moderate, usually somewhat delayed enhancement can be observed. Early or intense enhancement or both may occur infrequently.

Hematomas and seromas are visualized as a cavity of low to high signal-intensity, depending on their age and fluid composition. Following injection of contrast medium, the signal intensity of the nonenhancing content of the seroma or hematoma remains unchanged. The capsule—as far as it is developed—and the traumatized surrounding tissue usually show minimal to moderate enhancement, which generally is delayed.

Fresh granulation tissue within scarring usually enhances moderately and delayed. However, in some cases fast enhancement may occur, which may cause false positive calls.[5,6]

Utility. MRI is usually not necessary to image hemorrhage, seromas, or hematomas. Due to the usual pattern of moderate and mostly delayed enhancement, assessment is slightly impaired. (Delayed enhancing in situ carcinoma would not be recognized. Furthermore, it is important to understand that microscopic residual tumors can never be excluded.) If granulation tissue causes fast enhancement, which may also be focal, false positive calls may result. Therefore, it is recommended to perform a contrast-enhanced MRI later than 3–6 months after surgery or major interventions (vacuum biopsy) whenever possible. If, however, residual or missed tumor (without microcalcifications) is suspected within mammographically dense tissue, contrast-enhanced MRI might provide valuable additional information. In spite of the above mentioned limitations, MRI is often capable of diagnosing residual or missed tumor if present, because most tumors enhance faster, exhibiting a typical washout or a typical morphology that allows distinction even from

fresh scarring. Since presence of residual or missed non-calcified tumor may be even more difficult to assess by mammography or sonography early after therapy, MRI should be considered if residual or missed tumor has to be excluded in equivocal cases[10,11] (see chapter 5).

■ Late Changes

While fresh scar tissue generally shows minimal to moderate enhancement, old scar tissue after complete fibrosis no longer exhibits relevant enhancement.

This usually is the case after the 3rd to 6th postoperative month, and thereafter MRI allows a reliable differentiation between scar tissue and malignancy.

Utility. As a supplemental method, contrast-enhanced MRI offers new information relevant for the detection or exclusion of malignancy whenever evaluation is difficult or diagnostic uncertainty persists.

Mammography remains the method of choice to detect and to assess microcalcifications.

■ Percutaneous Biopsy

Scar tissue can compromise percutaneous biopsy because of needle deviation and the difficulty of retrieving an adequate specimen from fibrotic tissue. This is most important for aspiration cytology. Whenever a definite mass exists clinically, mammographically, sonographically, or on MRI, evaluation by core biopsy may be useful.[2, 12]

■ Summary

See p. 364

Changes Following Breast-conserving Therapy without Irradiation

■ Definition

Breast-conserving treatment involves surgical removal of the breast cancer, often with axillary node dissection, and is usually followed by breast irradiation. In numerous studies, survival rates have been comparable to those achieved with mastectomy. In selected controlled studies, ir-

radiation has been replaced by chemotherapy or antihormonal therapy; however, many consider this experimental treatment.

■ Clinical and Imaging Findings

Both clinical and imaging findings are identical to the findings after surgery described above. The amount of scarring and deformity of the breast is usually related to the volume of tissue excised. In addition, edematous changes due to lymphedema after axillary resection can be superimposed.

■ Differential Diagnosis and Diagnostic Strategy

Differential diagnosis and diagnostic strategy are the same as explained for postoperative scarring in general.

Changes Following Breast-conserving Therapy and Irradiation

■ Definition

Breast-conserving therapy combined with irradiation consists of surgical removal of the tumor, which should be performed with a tumor-free margin,* followed by radiotherapy of the breast.

It has become the standard therapy of breast carcinomas up to a size of 3–5 cm, with an increasing number of patients benefiting from this therapeutic approach today. Optimal interdisciplinary cooperation between surgeon, radiologist, radiotherapist, and pathologist is decisive for the success of this approach.

The role of radiology is:

– Accurate preoperative staging possible
– Preoperative localization of nonpalpable lesions
– Intraoperative specimen radiography to detect obvious areas of incomplete resection
– Postsurgical documentation of complete removal of calcifications
– Regular follow-up mammography, possibly supported by additional imaging methods
– Assessment of any clinically evident changes that may develop

In addition to postsurgical changes (see above) of the breast, changes following axillary node dissection and radiotherapy also can occur.

In contrast to the pattern discussed above for postsurgical scars, the changes induced by breast-conserving therapy with irradiation affect the entire breast and are superimposed on the changes at the surgical site. Furthermore, changes following breast-conserving therapy can be more severe than after excisional biopsy alone. Post-therapy changes can both mimic and obscure malignancy. To avoid diagnostic errors, knowledge of and ex-

perience with the expected changes are a prerequisite for the radiologist caring for these women. The interpretation of systematically performed follow-up examinations and the selection of supplemental methods is an important part of their treatment.

■ Clinical Findings

Depending on the extent of postoperative edema, the breast is regionally or diffusely dense and swollen in the early postoperative phase. This limits the value of palpation.

Axillary dissection and radiotherapy can lead to acute lymphedema of the breast with swelling and peau d'orange. Furthermore, a postoperative seroma in the axilla can cause lymphedema of the breast.

Radiotherapy induces hyperemia caused by vascular dilatation and capillary damage as well as by disturbed microcirculation, increased transudation, inflammation, and development of microscopic, and, less frequently, also of macroscopic areas of fat necrosis and granulation tissue. This leads to erythema, skin thickening, and swelling of the entire breast. A dry epitheliosis of the skin and an edema-induced induration may develop, as well as hyperpigmentation to a variable degree, and, in large breasts, a wet epitheliosis along the inferior mammary fold.

The entire radiated tissue and particularly the surgical bed show delayed resorption of exudates, and fluid might remain detectable for many months after completion of therapy.

In general, erythema, edema, and skin thickening largely resolve during the first 2 years, but considerable variations can be observed.

The resolution of edema is particularly slow around the areola and in the dependent regions of the breast, i.e., in the lower half of the breast, especially in the lower inner quadrant.

During the first few years after radiotherapy, the acute radiation changes can diminish. Simul-

---

* The tumor free margin should be larger if in situ carcinoma is present versus mere invasive carcinoma. The exact required margin is still disputed.

taneously, scars are formed and dystrophic calcifications can appear. In some patients mammary fibrosis can develop.

While the scar region is palpable as a flat plateau-like consistency, new nodular, rather firm areas can develop. They can be induced by the evolution of large dystrophic calcifications and oil cysts, as well as by emerging lipophagic granulomas. Clinically, these changes can usually not be distinguished from recurrence.

Mammary fibrosis is palpable as diffusely increased consistency of the parenchyma in comparison with the contralateral breast. This fibrosis is often particularly pronounced in the lower half of the breast and around the scar. It may also be the cause of skin dimpling. Both pronounced fibrosis or skin dimpling can be the cause of diagnostic problems clinically or by conventional imaging.

A pronounced tissue defect can usually be palpated in the dissected axilla, in addition to various manifestations of cicatricial induration. In the case of supraclavicular radiation, a diffusely increased firmness can develop in this region as well.

■ Diagnostic Strategy and Goals

Important *goals* are:

- Early detection of recurrent disease.
- The lowest possible rate of diagnostic excisional biopsies on benign lesions, i.e., a high positive predictive value. Avoiding diagnostic biopsies of benign post-therapeutic changes is of particular importance because radiation changes can lead to impaired wound healing that can compromise the cosmetic result of breast conservation.

Approach:

- Mammography, combined with clinical examination, is the most important diagnostic modality.[13-17] The highest accuracy can be achieved if both the preoperative mammogram and the postoperative studies are regularly available at the time a new mammogram is obtained. Ultrasound may be useful as an adjunct in mammographically dense tissue. It allows good assessment of early changes if needed. Sonographic assessment may, however, also be impaired by scarring. This causes shadowing and hypoechoic areas, which may lead to false negative or false positive results. Therefore, the value of ultrasound in the irradiated breast is assessed differently by various investigators.[1, 18]

- If evaluation by conventional methods is impaired by dense tissue or scarring or if the findings are equivocal, supplemental contrast-enhanced MRI—which should not be obtained earlier than 1 year following termination of radiation therapy—can provide important information, allowing not only early detection of recurrences but also correct identification of scar-induced changes.

■ Mammography

■ Technical Difficulties

The following different conditions must be considered following breast conserving therapy.
Complete mammographic evaluation of the parenchyma, particularly of the scar region, is often more difficult because of retraction of skin and muscle towards the tumor bed.

The post-therapeutic scar-related structural changes may require

- The *exhaustive use of extra mammographic views* (compression cone, magnification view)
- *Serial examinations* with the exposure as constant as possible

Therefore, the mammographic technique should aim for:

- The same exposure conditions for serial examinations (documentation of kVp, type of anode, position of the photocell, degree of compression). Otherwise, discrete increases in size or density as early evidence of a recurrence can be overlooked amidst the cicatricial changes.
- Complete visualization of the entire scar and inclusion of all breast tissue and pectoral muscle, despite the known retractive changes, by using all technical resources (coned-down views, tilting of the X-ray tube, oblique projections tailored to the individual situation).[19]
- Generous use of magnification technique.

If breast density limits adequate penetration after radiation, the choice of target or filter, or both, by which the energy of the X-ray beam can be optimized, can influence image quality.

■ **Post-therapeutic Changes**

The following changes are usually seen:[20-29]

1. Diffuse changes including trabecular coarsening, skin thickening, and diffusely increased breast-density secondary to irradiation and axillary dissection
2. Localized parenchymal changes of the skin and breast tissue due to the surgical scar
3. Localized parenchymal changes secondary to fat necrosis manifested as liponecrosis, oil cysts, or a lipophagic granuloma
4. Calcifications caused by any of the above mentioned reasons

These various changes are only partially separable, and together they determine the mammographic pattern. For didactic reasons, these changes are treated separately.

Diffuse Changes of the Parenchymal Structure

(Figs. 18.**7**a–c)

Hyperemia with increased transudation as well as edema secondary to axillary dissection and radiotherapy cause mammographically:

– Diffusely increased parenchymal density
– Diffusely increased trabecular markings
– Thickening of the skin and areola

These acute changes can resolve slowly during the first 2 years after therapy. Chronic edema can resolve or undergo fibrotic transformation, which produces a similar mammographic pattern to that seen with edema.
     The slow transformation of a chronic persistent edema into fibrosis (Figs. 18.**8**a–c) can be recognized mammographically by

– Slight resolution of the diffusely increased parenchymal density corresponding to the replacement of fluids with connective tissue and partial resorption of the edema
– Thinner and sharper demarcation of the increased trabecular markings
– Some resolution of the initial thickening of the skin and areola
– Calcifications that can develop owing to cell necrosis

If the described resolution and transformation is reversed by a renewed increase in the diffuse changes, or if the diffuse changes remain unchanged without recognizable resolution, the following conditions have to be considered in the differential diagnosis:

– Secondary mastitis
– Venous stasis (heart failure, mediastinal or axillary space-occupying lesion)
– Carcinomatous lymphangiosis

Localized Changes of the Cutaneous and Parenchymal Structures

They may occur with:

– Scar formation following surgery
– Fat necrosis that can transform into *oil cysts*, calcifications, or a *lipophagic granuloma* secondary to radiation-compromised microcirculation and subsequent development of necrosis, (partial) resorption, or formation of granulation tissue.

Scar formation is characterized by:

– Parenchymal asymmetry
– Associated architectural distortion and spiculations that can have extensions to the skin, the pectoral muscle or chest wall (Fig. 18.**9**)
– Masses caused by delayed resorption of large hematomas or seromas (Fig. 18.**10**a–d), by dense fibrosis, or by lipophagic granulomas (Fig. 18.**11**)
– Calcifications (see p. 342)
– Localized thickening or retraction of the skin along the scar

Evaluating the course of these changes is of great importance for their correct interpretation.
     The postoperative mammogram is obtained before the initiation of radiation therapy. It is only needed in women whose cancer contained microcalcifications and is done to check for if residual calcifications that may signify residual tumor, requiring reexcision. These studies may show hematomas or seromas. Large hematomas may not resolve completely, resulting in a persistent mass of variable extent. Characteristically, follow-up examinations will document decrease in size and increase in scar formation with spiculation.
     A parenchymal scar seen as a spiculated structure without central density can be recognized by its variable morphologic presentation on different projections, in contrast to a spicular cancer that mostly extends in all spatial directions. The radial structure of a mature scar remains constant in configuration and density.
     After the completion of radiation, a new base-

Fig. 18.**7 a–c** Diffuse acute structural changes of the parenchyma

a Status post segmentectomy (tylectomy): 5 days after surgery, diffusely increased density in the lateral half of the breast with air pocket (arrow) and skin thickening

b Three weeks after completion of radiation therapy: thickening of the skin and areola, diffusely increased reticular markings, and delicate cicatricial radial structural transformation at the site of the excision

c Four years after completion of radiation therapy, almost complete resolution, with skin thickening confined to the region of the scar and underlying radial structural transformation

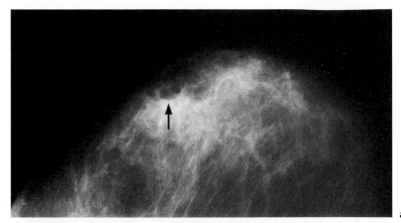

a

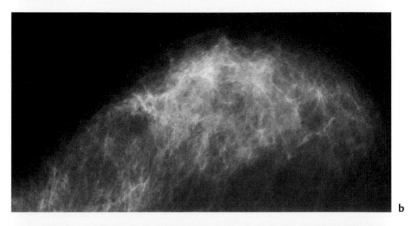

b

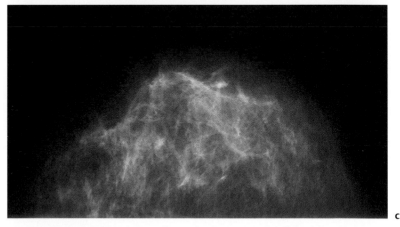

c

line mammogram of the treated breast should be done in 3 to 6 months, followed by another bilateral mammogram after 12 months. Policy varies for the following 2 years. In the United States, yearly mammograms are usually performed if no suspicion exists; in Germany, mammograms every 6 months are recommended for at least 3 years after irradiation. The contralateral breast is usually checked yearly.

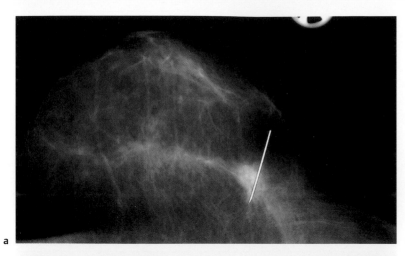

a

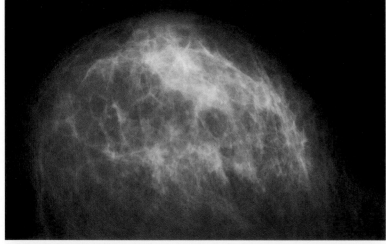

b

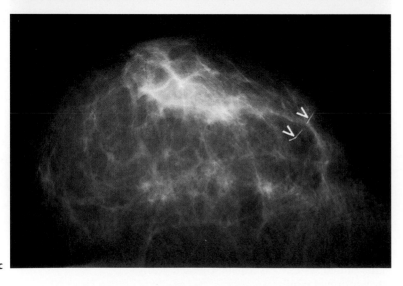

c

Fig. 18.**8a–c** Diffuse chronic structural changes of the parenchyma
a Localization mammogram of the primary tumor (1982)
b Mammography 3 weeks after completion of radiation therapy: swelling of the entire breast, tickening of the skin and areola, diffusely increased reticular markings
c Six years after therapy of the primary tumor, a thickening of the skin and areola persisted. The diffusely increased reticular markings are more distinct now, compatible with fibrosis. Calcified suture material at the site of the excision (arrowheads)

Oil Cysts

Oil cysts can arise from areas of fat necrosis. They are characterized by

- Round or oval radiolucencies of fat density (Fig. 18.**5a**).
- A smooth capsule.
- Eggshell-like calcifications within the capsule (Figs. 11.**5a, b**). They are very characteristic but are not always present. During their evolution, less characteristic thin calcifications may be observed.

Oil cysts often are clinically palpated as moderately moveable, suspicious nodules or induration, but they do not require further evaluation if they exhibit a mammographically typical appearance.

Lipophagic Granuloma

(Fig. 18.**11**)

It can be the manifestation of a post-therapeutic fat necrosis within scar tissue but may also develop at any other site within the irradiated breast outside the scar. It generally presents as newly developing mass with an irregular outline and can generally not be distinguished from a recurrence.[2, 20, 29] Therefore, biopsy is usually necessary.

Calcifications

Dystrophic calcifications frequently occur in conjunction with therapy-induced cell and tissue necrosis.

Concerning the individual configuration and arrangement, the following calcifications can be classified as typically benign (therapy-induced):

- Large, elongated, and coarse, as well as round, amorphous calcifications of the stroma (Figs. 18.**4a** and **b**)
- Typical ring-like calcifications occasionally beginning as semicircles as manifestation of a calcifying liponecrosis
- Eggshell-like calcifications around the radiolucency of an oil cyst (Fig. 18.**4c** and **d**)
- Scattered dystrophic microcalcifications
- Fine, punctate calcifications at the site of tumorectomy.

Calcifications evolving in the capsule of an oil cyst, a local aggregation of dystrophic calcifica-

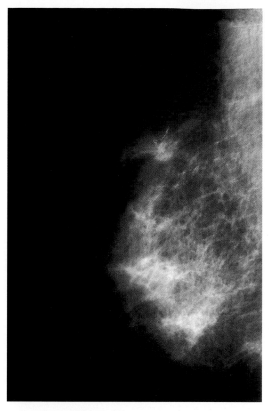

Fig. 18.**9** Localized cutaneous and parenchymal changes after breast-conserving therapy. Indistinctly outlined focal density in the upper outer quadrant of the breast with spiculation and retraction of the skin and pectoral muscle as well as dystrophic calcifications. Additional cutaneous and areolar thickening as well as diffusely increased reticular markings following axillary dissection and radiation therapy

tions, or calcifying liponecrosis can produce small pleomorphic clusters of microcalcifications. These are difficult to distinguish from malignant microcalcifications. Magnification mammography and short-term follow-up examinations may provide additional information.

Magnification mammography is necessary for an exact analysis of the contour and for finding all worrisome calcifications.

■ Detection of Recurrence and Differential Diagnosis

Recurrences can become mammographically visible as:

- Nodular or ill-defined mass
- Enlarging scar

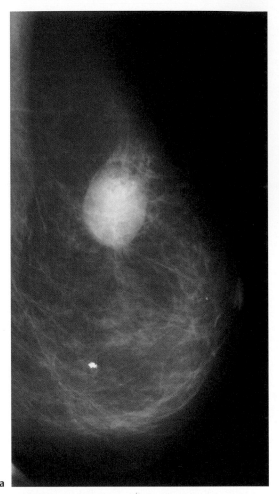

a

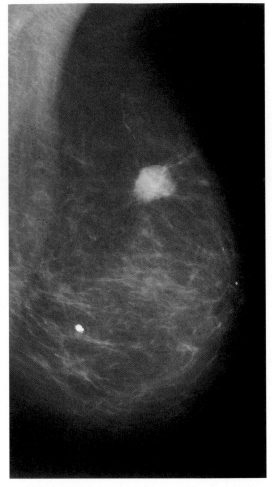

b

Fig. 18.**10**   Changes after breast conserving therapy may be focal and/or diffuse
a and **b** mediolateral and MLO views of a postlumpectomy breast at 6 and 18 months after breast conserva- tion. The rounded mass with adjacent surgical clips is a postoperative seroma. Note that it slowly involutes with time

– Microcalcifications
– Diffusely increased density (diffusely growing recurrence)

Focally Growing Recurrence

(Figs. 18.**12 a** and **b**)

About 70% of intramammary recurrences develop in the vicinity of the scar, and early treatment failures tend to be at the biopsy site. The most important feature of focal recurrences and also the best criterion for distinguishing them from post-therapeutic changes is the temporal evolution:

1. Newly occuring mass and/or tumor calcifications
2. Enlarging mass or scar
3. Increasing radiodensity
4. Increasing architectural distortion

These changes can be very discrete and can be underestimated or overlooked with variations in technique (different exposures) (see Technical Difficulties, p. 351).

A newly occurring mass and suspicious calcifications in quadrants other than the one harboring the primary tumor are generally easily recognized. Apart from recurrence, the differential diagnosis also includes benign changes, such as

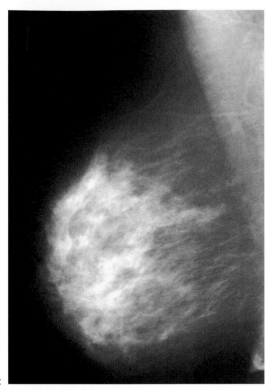

c

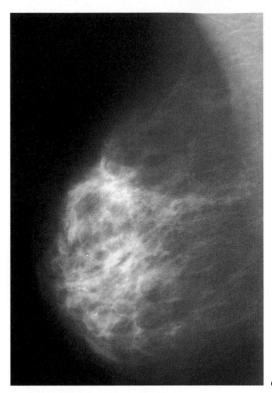

d

c and **d** In this patient a diffuse increased density is seen 6 months after breast-conserving therapy. Eighteen months after therapy the increased density has partly subsided. However, retraction is visible around the scar

cysts or fibroadenomas. Cysts should be excluded sonographically. A new lipophagic granuloma occurring after therapy cannot be distinguished from recurrent disease by any imaging method and therefore usually requires biopsy.

Microcalcifications as Evidence of Recurrence

Mammography is necessary to detect microcalcifications that can be an early sign of recurrence. Since microcalcifications can develop after radiation, thorough analysis of their individual configuration and their distribution is of great importance (Figs. 18.12c and d).

The criteria for the analysis of microcalcifications are also applicable to recognizing recurrent disease (see Chapter 20). Calcifications associated with recurrent breast cancer have a pattern identical to those found with de novo breast cancers.

It is important to consider the *time of the appearance* in the differential diagnostic consideration.

If the entire tumor was removed, documented by specimen radiography, histopathologic examination, and postoperative mammogram, a recurrence within 12–18 months after irradiation would be unusual. Instead, dystrophic calcifications tend to evolve during this time span.

Diffusely Increased Density as Evidence of Recurrence

Diffusely growing recurrences are most difficult to diagnose. They can be multicentric, present as carcinomatous lymphangiomatosis, or they can even be manifested by the growth of dispersed small-cell malignancies. They can be diagnosed as recurring or increasing diffuse density and structural coarsening, and as areas of increasing parenchymal density, together with a clinical increased consistency and possibly with a reduction in size and retraction of the breast (Figs. 18.12e and f). In our experience, more than half of diffusely growing recurrent tumors were early re-

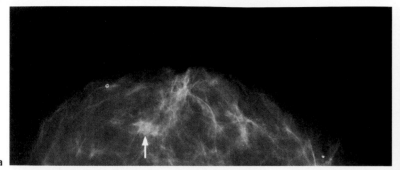

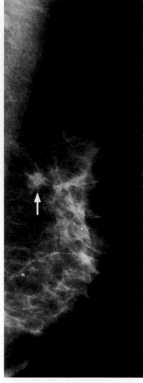

Fig. 18.**11 a–d** Lipophagic granuloma mimicking a malignancy. This patient had a mammogram 18 months after biopsy of a suspicious finding that turned out to be a proliferative mastopathy. A previous postoperative mammogram was not obtained.
This mammogram again shows a suspicious density in the region of the scar (arrow)
a Mammography, craniocaudal view
b Mammography, mediolateral view
c and **d** Because of the suspicious finding, an excisional biopsy was recommended. A supplemental contrast-enhanced MRI was obtained as part of a trial designed for preoperative patients. Representative section through the lesion before i.v. administration of contrast medium (**c**)
d shows the same section as in **c** after injection of the contrast medium Gd-DTPA. The lesion shows a rapid intense enhancement with irregular margins to be considered as suspect. *Histology:* Lipophagic granuloma (from Heywang-Köbrunner SH[5])

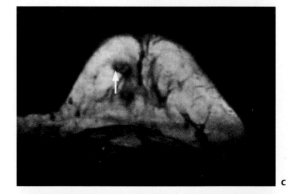

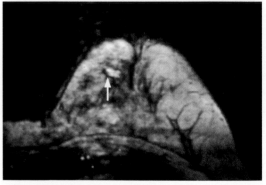

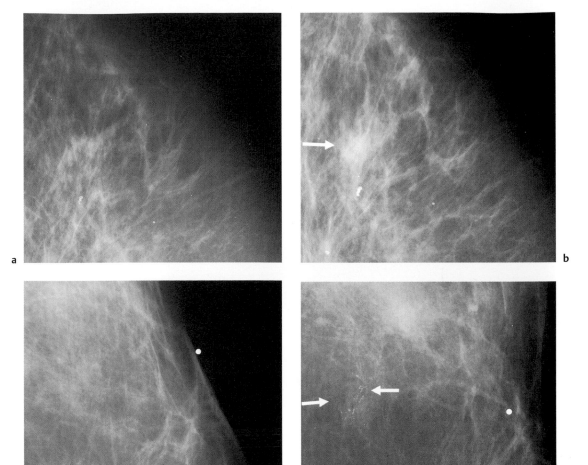

a

b

c

d

Fig. 18.**12 a–f** Mammographic presentations of recurrences
a Four years after breast conservation, a few coarse calcifications are present at the surgical site due to fat necrosis
b Three years later, a new mass (arrow) has developed at the scar due to a 1 cm recurrent infiltrating ductal carcinoma

c Two years after breast conservation, some deformity is noted in the lateral aspect of the breast. A skin marker localizes the scar
d A year later, new pleomorphic linear calcifications (arrows) have developed. These were due to new DCIS

currences with unusually rapid tumor growth, primarily affecting young women.[2]

■ Sonography

■ Diffuse Structural Changes

Early changes. Radiation induces varying degrees of skin thickening. In the acute stage, the edema-related echogenicity increases in the subcutaneous space and decreases in the parenchyma, leading to a loss of the normal echo pattern (Figs. 18.**13 a** and **c**).

Resolution. Over a period of 1–2 years, skin thickening and other early changes slowly regress. Some skin thickening may persist. Increased fibrosis found in the irradiated tissue frequently causes diffusely increased echogenicity.

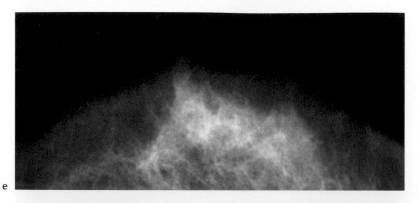

e

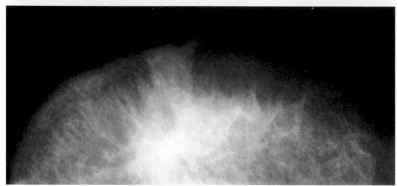

f

Fig. 18.**12 e** and **f**   Two years after breast-conserving therapy, scar-induced cutaneous thickening in the medial half of the breast, ill-defined reticular markings. Because of edematous changes and dense parenchyma, it is difficult to assess. Eleven months later (**f**): clinically decreased size and increased consistency of the right breast. Corresponding increase in the mammographic density throughout the entire remaining parenchyma and progressing spiculation: diffusely growing recurrence

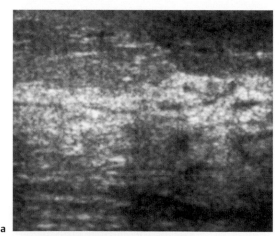

a

Fig. 18.**13 a–c**   Sonographic presentation of the breast after tumorectomy (lumpectomy) and radiation
a Extensive lymphedema 3 months after completion of radiation therapy. Increased echogenicity is seen in the subcutaneous tissue as well as in the prepectoral fat, with loss of the demarcation between the subcutaneous soft tissue and thickened dermis as well as poor separation of parenchyma from fatty tissue

■ **Focal Structural Changes**

They can occur as

– Scar formation
– Fat necroses in the form of *oil cysts* or *lipophagic granuloma*

In its early stage, *the scar region*, similar to nonirradiated scars (see pp. 342–6), often contains a seroma or hematoma; the resolution of either can be well-monitored sonographically. With increasing granulation tissue and fibrosis, small or large hypoechoic areas, and acoustic shadows—as also seen after surgery alone (see also Figs. 18.**6** and 18.**14 c**)—can develop in the region of the scar and compromise the evaluation. Well-documented serial examinations may be helpful.

Oil cysts (compare p. 207) are in general correctly diagnosed only when the ultrasound is interpreted together with mammography.

A *lipophagic granuloma* is visualized as hypoechoic lesion with or without acoustic shadowing and cannot be sonographically distinguished from a primary or recurrent carcinoma.

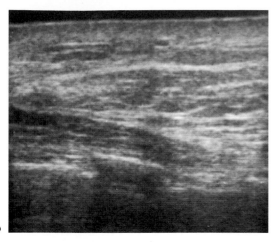

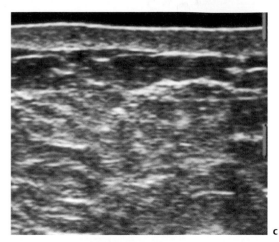

b

c

Fig. 18.**13 b** and **c** Slow resolution of increased echogenicity of the fatty tissue with increasingly improved demarcation of the ligamentous structures 9 months (**b**) and
18 months (**c**) after therapy

■ Utility

In the follow-up of these patients, sonography

– can be helpful to distinguish the mammographically visible or palpable hematoma
from a mass, if doubts exist.
– can be helpful to detect a recurrence (visible
as persistent mass that does not resolve) if the
breast tissue is very dense. However, the
policy regarding regular use of ultrasound
in the follow-up of dense breasts after irradiation varies. It may be able to detect additional
recurrence in dense breast tissue. However,
sensitivity and specificity are reduced due to
post-therapeutic hypoechoic areas and
shadowing. In order to avoid unnecessary
false positive calls, a high level of experience
is needed.
– is—as in other women—helpful in determining whether a new mass is due to a cyst.

More than 18 months after therapy, contrast-enhanced MRI is superior to sonography in the detection or exclusion of small recurrences and
should be preferred if the mammographic evaluation is difficult.[30–38]

■ Magnetic Resonance Imaging

■ Acute Stage

Immediately after radiation,[5, 32] as well as within
the subsequent 12 months, the irradiated tissue
and the scar may show enhancement. Often a

moderate and diffuse, but sometimes also patchy,
strong enhancement is seen. This enhancement
usually decreases within the initial 12 months
with considerable individual variation. Later than
12 months after radiotherapy, the irradiated
tissue can still exhibit some diffuse, usually
delayed enhancement.

Cutaneous thickening and enhancement usually regress more slowly than the parenchymal
enhancement. Some authors[39] have reported such
changes early after radiation therapy to a lesser
degree and thus also apply MRI earlier after irradiation (>6 months).

■ Late Stage

More than 12 months after therapy, diffuse and
delayed enhancement is only seen in individual
cases. In the vast majority of cases only minimal
("absent") enhancement exists. Residual skin
thickening and focal, scar-related architectural
distortion can be diagnosed by absent contrast
enhancement and do not interfere with the evaluation by MRI (Figs. 18.**14 d** and **e**).

■ Utility

Within the first 12 months after radiotherapy, the
information provided by MRI may be compromised by diffuse and enhancement. Patchy
and sometimes focal enhancement (probably due
to ongoing granulation) may cause false positive
calls.

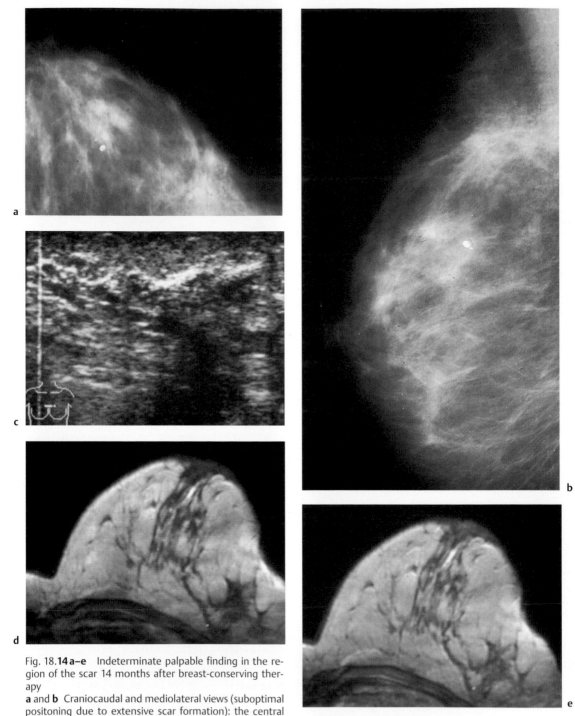

Fig. 18.**14 a–e** Indeterminate palpable finding in the region of the scar 14 months after breast-conserving therapy

a and **b** Craniocaudal and mediolateral views (suboptimal positoning due to extensive scar formation): the central radiolucency within the scar is consistent with a scar rather than a recurrent cancer

c Sonographically, the evaluation of the region of the scar is limited, showing acoustic shadowing. This finding is consistent with scar, but is identical to the pattern that can be seen with carcinoma

d Representative section through the scar region before administration of contrast medium

e The same section after i.v. administration of Gd-DTPA shows no appreciable enhancement: no evidence of a recurrence. Conclusion confirmed by clinical–mammographic follow-up for more than 3 years

With increasing fibrosis, the enhancement markedly decreases. Beginning 12 months after radiotherapy, detection and exclusion of recurrent disease in irradiated tissue is considerably improved.

Beginning about 12 months after radiotherapy, the evaluation by MRI is generally excellent[30-38] since the fibrosed parenchymal tissue enhances even less than normal mammary parenchyma. Supplemental MRI can detect very small recurrent tumors in dense or even irregularly structured tissue with great sensitivity (Fig. 18.15a–d) or excludes them with a high degree of certainty. Therefore, contrast MRI is the ideal method to complement mammography for otherwise difficult to evaluate tissue and for solving problems later than 12–18 months after breast-conserving therapy. However, mammography remains the modality of choice to detect suggestive microcalcifications, should they develop.

Possibly due to different radiation technique and individually differing response to radiation therapy, different observations have been reported during the first year after irradiation and the use of MRI during this period is discussed controversially.[38, 39] We would recommend using MRI later than 12 months after therapy, whenever possible. Only if severe diagnostic problems concerning the presence of residual tumor cannot be solved by conventional imaging MRI should be considered.

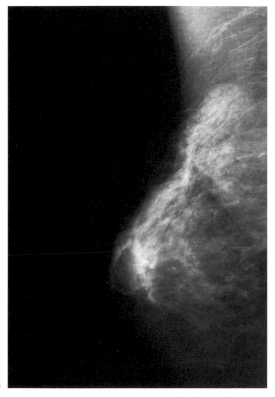

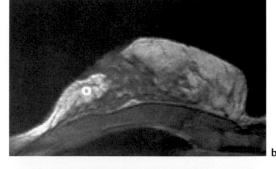

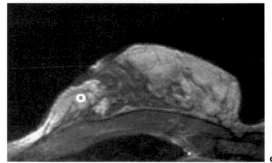

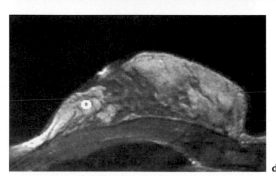

Fig. 18.**15a–d** Clinically, status post breast-conserving therapy 5 years ago, unchanged palpable finding
a The mammogram shows spiculation in the upper half of breast at the lumpectomy site, unchanged since the previous examination. Diffuse microcalcifications known for years, unchanged (the primary tumor had no microcalcifications). Supplementary MRI was offered as part of a clinical trial
b–d MRI: representative section through the scar before (**b**) as well as immediately after (0–5 minutes) (**c**), and delayed (6–11 minutes) (**d**) after Gd-DTPA. Suggestive focal enhancement (arrow) is apparent in the scar region. It characteristically enhances early and shows so-called washout (**d**). The focus discovered by MRI was excised after MR-guided localization. *Histology:* recurrence of an invasive ductal carcinoma

■ Percutaneous Biopsy

Percutaneous biopsy can be diagnostically helpful in the therapeutic decision, particularly since diagnostic excisional surgery on nonmalignant post-therapeutic changes should be avoided owing to the possibility of impaired healing.

The patient should be informed that the rate of infectious complications is possibly increased early after irradiation. With percutaneous biopsy, however, fewer complications may be expected than with surgical biopsy.

Note:

– Accuracy can decrease in markedly fibrosed tissue due to needle deviation and due to insufficient or nonrepresentative tissue,
– Histologic accuracy may be reduced due to procuring smaller specimens in the presence of marked fibrosis or due to early post-therapeutic cellular changes (inflammation, necrosis)

Nonetheless, reported data have shown that needle biopsy is able to accurately differentiate recurrent cancer from fibrosis.

■ Summary

Depending on whether a hematoma, seroma, or fat necrosis is present, acute post-traumatic and postsurgical changes can have a variable mammographic presentation.
If a malignancy (residual tumor) has to be excluded in freshly traumatized or surgical tissue, mammography should always be used.

Scar-related changes in their late stage after trauma or surgery (more than 3 months) or after radiation (more than 12 months) can cause characteristic mammographic features (architectural distortion or spiculated areas mostly without central density, coarse, or ring-like dystrophic calcifications) or sonographic phenomena (acoustic shadowing or hypoechoic areas). Because of architectural distortion following surgery and increased density following radiation, the overall evaluation can be compromised, and the differential diagnosis can pose problems. For the scarred breast following (multiple) surgeries as well as for the breast with radiation changes, mammography remains the primary diagnostic method, together with clinical examination.

Next to the selected use of additional projections, coned-down compression, and magnification views, an important diagnostic role is given to serial mammograms, whereby the accuracy can be improved by keeping exposure conditions constant.

In the breast that is difficult to evaluate, the selected use of contrast-enhanced MRI is important. In particular, if the evaluation is impaired owing to increased density and scars, contrast-enhanced MRI permits a markedly improved and earlier detection of recurrence and a correct identification of scar-related fibrotic changes beginning 1 year after radiotherapy.

Percutaneous biopsy can be considered as an additional diagnostic step in problem cases.

Changes Following Reconstruction, Augmentation, and Reduction

Reconstruction

■ Definition

Reconstruction refers to the surgical reconstitution after mastectomy.

■ Surgical procedures

Breast reconstruction can be achieved by means of implants or myocutaneous flaps.

Implants are placed underneath the pectoral muscle (subpectoral), generally preceded by implantation of an expander to create space for the prosthesis.

The submuscular implant is preferable to the subcutaneous implant because of its better cosmetic result and easier follow-up care. The silicone prostheses have frequently been used in this context. They come in different designs, the most important of which are (Fig. 18.**16**):

– *Single-lumen* silicone gel or saline-filled *prosthesis*

– The *inner lumen filled with silicone gel* forming a silicone cushion, surrounded by the outer lumen filled with a saline solution
– The *inner lumen filled with a saline solution* and the outer lumen filled with silicone gel is a less common configuration

Familiarity with these types is pertinent because each type is visualized differently, affecting the evaluation of the surrounding tissue.

Reconstruction with autogenous tissue transfer is most frequently done with the help of pedunculated or free myocutaneous flaps. The flaps are most frequently taken from the latissimus dorsi and transverse rectus abdominis muscle (TRAM-flap).

■ Diagnostic Strategy

Imaging is used to

– characterize clinically suspicious findings that may be due to malignancy, to benign changes within remaining breast tissue, or to postsurgical changes and
– detect a rupture of the prosthesis.

Symptomatic patients with myocutaneous flaps can be imaged and assessed by mammography,[40, 41] since muscle and fat can be penetrated by X-ray. Whether sonography might be useful is not yet established. In case of diagnostic problems, contrast-enhanced MRI may be useful for its excellent capability of distinguishing scarring from carcinoma. Indeterminate masses, which may, however, be caused by fat necrosis, require histopathologic workup; this can usually be obtained by percutaneous biopsy.

For asymptomatic patients with silicone implants, only the clinical examination is standard following mastectomy and reconstruction.

An abnormal palpatory finding can be further evaluated by mammography and sonography. MRI has proven very helpful in patients with scarring around implants that is difficult to assess and in patients with increased risk (after previous recurrence, multifocal disease).

■ Mammography

■ Implants

Breasts with silicone implants, which were placed after mastectomy for breast reconstruction, usually cannot be adequately imaged by mammography. This is because the tissue (which should just

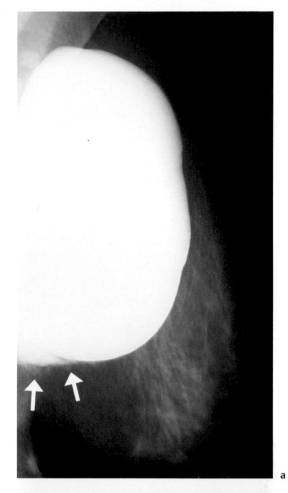

a

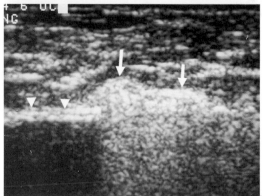

b

Fig. 18.**16 a–d**   Presentation of implant rupture
a and **b** Extracapsular rupture
a Routine mammogram 17 years after augmentation shows an extracapsular rupture with silicone outside the implant (arrows)
b Sonographic image of this rupture shows echogenic silicone (arrows) beyond the homogeneous echo of the implant (arrowheads)

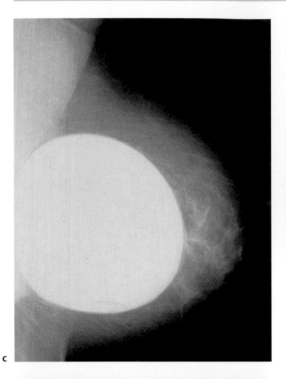

c

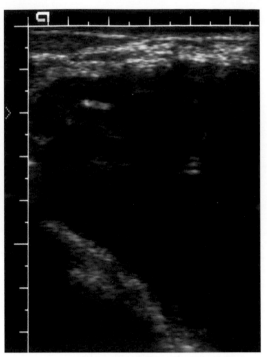

d

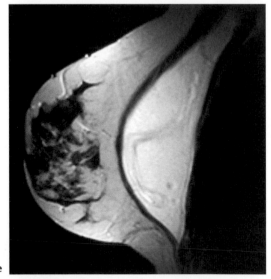

e

Fig. 18.**16 c–e** Intracapsular rupture
c, d Forty-nine-year-old woman 12 years after breast augmentation
c Mammographically, the silicone implant is intact
d Sonographically, multiple echoes, including several linear echoes, indicate an intracapsular rupture
e Intracapsular rupture on MRI (linguini sign). Low signal linear structures within the high signal silicone are due to the collapsed implant shell

be scar tissue and subcutaneous fat) cannot be displaced from the implant, as is performed in augmented breasts (see p. 56–9). Thus the implant would obscure most of the surrounding tissue. For this reason these patients are usually just followed clinically and sometimes by ultrasound or MRI. Mammographic tangential or coned views should be obtained if a palpable finding exists. Any palpable finding must be further evaluated by means of projection with appropriate tilting of the X-ray tube for tangential visualization of the tissue in question.[42–46] The rare saline-filled implants, however, are not as roentgendense as silicone implants. Patients with this type of implant may be examined using the usual mammographic technique. Assessment may be moderately impaired by overlying saline and by changes due to scarring. However, microcalcifications, which may be an important hint for a recurrence, can usually be imaged and assessed.

Normally, the prosthesis, which is surrounded by a thin rim of scar tissue, is covered by subcutaneous fat and skin. In submuscular implants, the muscle is visualized as a band-like density directly overlying the prosthesis. In patients with silicone implants, only those tissues, which are imaged tangentially beside the implant, can be evaluated, while the rest is obscured by the radiopaque implant (Fig. 18.**17**).

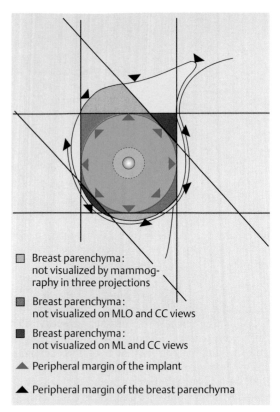

☐ Breast parenchyma:
not visualized by mammog-
raphy in three projections

▨ Breast parenchyma:
not visualized on MLO and CC views

▧ Breast parenchyma:
not visualized on ML and CC views

▲ Peripheral margin of the implant

▲ Peripheral margin of the breast parenchyma

Fig. 18.**17**   The different shading shows the parenchymal areas obscured by the implant on the standard projections (craniocaudad, mediolateral, and oblique views) (from Eklund and Cardenosa[19])

Fig. 18.**18**   Recurrence in a patient with a submuscular prosthesis for breast reconstruction. Oblique mammography: an irregularly outlined focal density with suggestive calcifications is mammographically seen in the axillary parenchymal extension, corresponding to a palpable finding marked with a lead BB: recurrent intraductal and papillary intracystic carcinoma

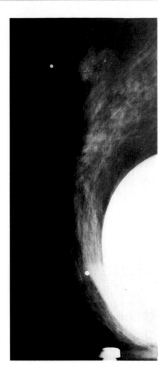

Utility

Because of the partial mammographic visualization of the tissue surrounding the prosthesis, mammography plays a limited role in the evaluation of any scar formation or detection of recurrent disease.

The mammographic exclusion of malignancy, particularly if clinically suspected, is often impossible (exception: oil cysts). The role of mammography—in contrast to MRI—is mainly restricted to the detection of suspicious microcalcifications (Fig. 18.**18**).

Rarely, an implant rupture may be detected by mammography if silicone can be recognized outside the implant or if the contour of the implant is irregular (Fig. 18.**16a**).

■ Myocutaneous Flap

(Fig. 18.**19a**)

Mammography is indicated for diagnostic evaluation of clinically suspicious abnormalities.[40, 41] When performed after breast reconstruction with autogenous tissue transfer, the mammographic evaluation of areas with dense scars or muscle tissue is limited. Regressive dystrophic changes of the adipose and connective tissue, such as oil cysts, are frequently found, producing clinically conspicuous palpatory findings. They can be correctly diagnosed as benign by mammography. Microcalcifications or ill-circumscribed masses may indicate recurrence. However, dystrophic microcalcifications, fat necroses, and scarring may mimic malignancy.

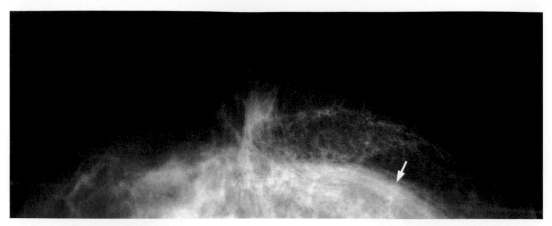

Fig. 18.**19**   Myocutaneous flap.
The craniocaudad view delineates the coarse fascicular structure of the implanted myocutaneous flap in the upper outer quadrant as well as the coarse subcutaneous reticular connective tissue structure, in comparison with the other side

■ Sonography

Sonography is suitable for the evaluation of the tissue surrounding the prosthesis. Its accuracy is limited too by the difficult differentiation of changes caused by scar formation. It is used for further evaluation of palpatory findings. Here, it may support the suspicion for a malignancy.

Even in the absence of mammographic and sonographic findings or in the presence of uncharacteristic findings, any clinical suspicion of malignancy cannot be dismissed. Aside from large silicone granulomas, which can produce a sonographically characteristic finding (see p. 248), small granulomas cannot be distinguished mammographically and sonographically from small malignant foci.

Sonography is able to diagnose pseudomasses, which are palpable and due to unusual folds. It may also be capable of demonstrating bleeding or siliconomas.[47, 48, 49, 50] In our experience sonographic assessment is often more difficult by ultrasound than by MRI, particularly in implants with multiple folds.

■ Magnetic Resonance Imaging

It is very well-suited for the evaluation of the breast with a silicone implant. It visualizes the entire tissue surrounding the prosthesis with excellent demarcation of small malignant foci from nonenhancing scar tissue (Fig. 18.**20**).

Because of its high sensitivity for detecting invasive foci, it can be employed as a supplemental examination for patients at risk, as well as for focal findings in need of further evaluation. Results from patients examined with conventional imaging and MRI have shown that recurrences around implants can be detected earlier with MRI than with any other imaging modality.[51, 52] Lack of enhancement cannot absolutely exclude malignancy, but allows a fairly high degree of certainty and may therefore be helpful in areas that are difficult to assess. Enhancing granulomas or diffuse inflammatory reactions can pose a problem, but small lesions (often representing granulomas solely detected by MRI) can be distinguished from malignancies by short-term follow-up examinations.

For the detection of even small prosthetic defects, MRI (without contrast enhancement) has now become the method of choice. Using a combination of pulse sequences,[53–60] even small defects can be detected with high sensitivity (approximately 90%) and specificity (approximately 90%).

Percutaneous biopsy should only be used when the needle can be inserted parallel to the prosthesis without risk of damaging it.

Augmentation

■ Definition

Augmentation refers to enlargement of the breast for the correction of congenital or acquired anisomastia or micromastia, or for cosmetic reasons.

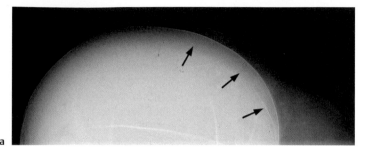

a

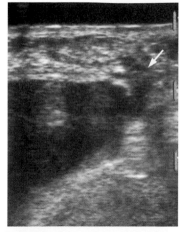

b

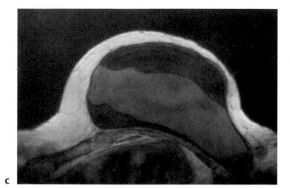

c

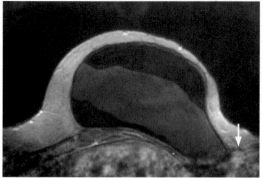

d

Fig. 18.**20 a–d** Detection of the carcinoma in the presence of a silicone prosthesis
a The mammographic evaluation is considerably compromised by the narrow mantle of tissue surrounding the prosthesis. The mobility is impaired because of scarring along the thoracic wall. No evidence of densities or calcifications suspicious for malignancy in several projections, with the craniocaudal view shown here (the arrows point at the outline of the inner compartment of the double-lumen prosthesis)

b Sonography: the small carcinomatous focus at the dorsolateral aspect of the outer margin of the prosthesis was not noted clinically or sonographically. It was apparently mistaken as part of the prosthesis itself. Only retrospectively could a corresponding area be identified (arrow)
c Representative MRI section before administration of contrast medium at the level of subsequent suspicious enhancement (**d**)
d After application of contrast medium, highly suspicious enhancement adjacent to the prosthesis (arrow): *Histology:* recurrence of a ductal carcinoma (from Heywang-Köbrunner et al.[5])

■ Surgical Procedures

Prostheses containing silicone gel or saline or both are used to enlarge the breast. Because of the risk of the development of fibrotic changes or contractures, submuscular prostheses are preferred to retroglandular prostheses. The prosthesis is implanted using a laterocaudal (along the inferior mammary fold) or perimamillary approach. Direct silicone injections are prohibited, as are injections of wax and autogenous adipose tissue.

■ Diagnostic Strategy

In the presence of submuscular prosthesis, the visualization of most of the parenchymal tissue can sometimes be achieved by two views using the technique described by Eklund. If this is not feasible, more views in additional projections are necessary. Retroglandular prostheses usually require a combined mammographic technique (Eklund views and supplemental views).

If the parenchymal tissue can be visualized free of any superimposition of the implant, the diagnostic approach for detecting or excluding malignancies is identical to that used for the non-augmented breast.

Portions of the parenchyma that cannot be evaluated despite combined mammographic techniques can be further evaluated by supplemental sonography or contrast-enhanced MRI. Large defects of the prosthesis are rarely mammographically visible but are generally seen sonographically. Large deposits of silicone have a typical sonographic presentation.

The most reliable method for detecting or excluding defects of the prosthesis is MRI, which is performed without contrast enhancement in this case.

Mammography

Technical Peculiarities

- After breast augmentation the breast tissue anterior to the implant is usually screened using so-called implant displacement views (see pp. 56–9). If relevant amounts of breast tissue are close to the chest wall or overlying the implant, they may not be adequately imaged by the above-described views. In such cases, additional coned or tangential views with the implant in place may be needed.
- Since portions of the augmentation prosthesis can be superimposed on the photocell (Fig. 18.**17**), manual exposure is necessary.
- If previous films are not available, a preliminary exposure in one projection should be obtained to find the best technique.
- Since the view described by Eklund does not compress the prosthesis, normal compression can be applied to the breast parenchyma when this view is obtained.
- If compression of the prosthesis cannot be avoided, the compression pressure should only be adequate to immobilize the breast. Otherwise, rupture of the capsule—though rare—can be induced.

Findings

Mammographically, only the contour of the prosthesis can be evaluated. Intracapsular rupture (rupture of the prosthesis with the surrounding fibrous capsule intact and keeping the silicone in place) cannot be diagnosed mammographically. Only an extracapsular rupture, in which silicone extends beyond the capsule into the breast, can be diagnosed by mammography. The fibrous capsule is seen as a band-like density of variable width, possibly containing calcific deposits, around the implant. This, however, does not imply a diagnosis of capsular fibrosis, which is predominantly a clinical diagnosis. With a submuscular location of the prosthesis, the pectoral muscle is seen as a broad band of increased density draping around the top and front of the prosthesis.

In the presence of a localized bulge or polylobulated contour of the prosthesis, mammography cannot distinguish between a rupture, herniation, or focal weakening of the prosthesis, unless silicone is seen outside the prosthesis, indicating an extracapsular rupture.

The detection of localized findings is impaired if portions of the parenchymal tissue are superimposed on the prosthesis and cannot be projected free of any superimposition, or if extensive scar formation is present.

Calcifications can occur as postsurgical dystrophic calcifications, capsular calcifications, and calcifications in extruded silicone. The calcifications can be extensive and plaque-like, but also eggshell-like or coarse.

As in patients without implants, magnification mammography can be used for the differential diagnosis of microcalcifications.

All symptomatic patients should have appropriate tangential projections if necessary, and magnification should be added as needed.

Sonography

Sonographic presentation and accuracy depend on

- the type of parenchymal tissue and
- the extent of scar formation

The position of the prosthesis in relation to the pectoralis muscle does not affect the sonographic evaluation.

Magnetic Resonance Imaging

It can be helpful to visualize changes deep to the prosthesis or to assess areas with extensive scar formation.

Percutaneous Biopsy

Whenever percutaneous biopsy is considered, care must be taken not to damage the implant. If percutaneous biopsy cannot be averted, the needle should be inserted parallel to the prosthesis to avoid any damage. It is wise to document on the informed consent form that the patient has been warned of the possibility of rupture during the biopsy.

Reduction

■ Definition

Reduction refers to making the breast smaller to achieve symmetry following mastectomy and reconstruction or because of anisomastia. Furthermore, macromastia is a frequent indication of reduction mammoplasty, which is also performed in conjunction with breast lifting.

■ Surgical Procedures

To reduce the volume of the breasts, portions of the parenchyma and skin are removed, and the areola and nipple are repositioned. This is achieved by means of a characteristic "key-hole" incision technique (Fig. 18.21 a–c), with a scar around the areola and along the inferior mammary fold, as well as a vertical scar in the 6-o'clock position connecting the periareolar scar with the inframammary scar.

■ Diagnostic Strategy

Palpable nodules that represent oil cysts or contain typical calcifications are easily diagnosed mammographically. It has proven helpful to have a baseline mammographic documentation, which is equally valuable for the correct evaluation of parenchymal asymmetries. The differential diagnosis of calcifications, which can be related to scar formation, rests on the meticulous analysis of microcalcifications.

In the presence of extensive scar formation and resultant impaired evaluation, contrast-enhanced MRI can provide useful supplemental information, beginning about 3 months after surgery.

■ Mammography, Sonography, Magnetic Resonance Imaging, Percutaneous Biopsy

The image evaluation of scars following reduction and of any focal findings within these scars (oil cysts, lipophagic granulomas, and calcifications) is the same as the evaluation of scars of other origin (see pp. 339–349).[3, 4]

Due to the architectural distortion that results from this special surgical procedure, it is recommended to obtain a baseline mammogram 3–6 months postoperatively.

■ Summary

Following breast reduction as well as reconstruction or augmentation with transplanted autogenous tissue, the resultant scar formation and architectural changes are determined by the surgical technique. For the diagnostic evaluation of these scars, the same principles apply as for scar tissue in general (see pp. 339–349).

Augmentation or reconstruction with silicone prostheses compromises the evaluation even further because the tissue behind the prosthe-

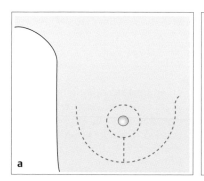
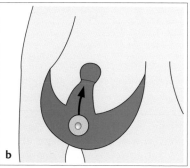

Fig. 18.**21 a–c**   Scars after reduction mammoplasty
a Incisions of the reduction mammoplastiy. Circumareolar incision connected by a vertical incision with the in-

framammary incision. At the end of the procedure, the nipple, which remains on a vascular pedicle, is pulled upward and reimplanted (**b**)

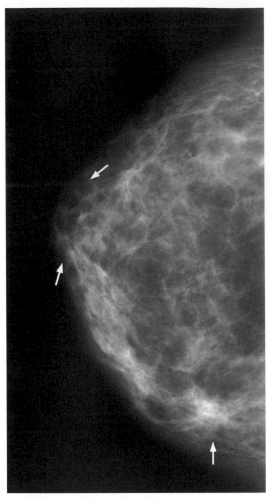
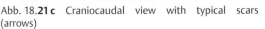
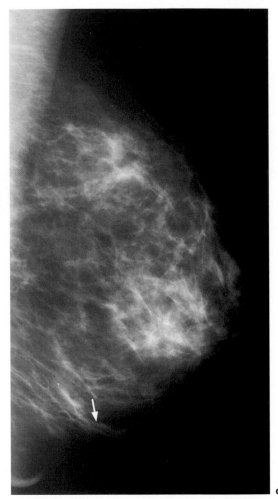

c

d

Abb. 18.**21c** Craniocaudal view with typical scars (arrows)
d Typical mammographic finding (mediolateral view) after bilateral reduction mammoplasty: cranial displace-
ment of the nipple, structural densities caused by linear scarring along the inframammary fold. Altogether, parenchymal arrangement different from the usual appearance

sis is clinically, mammographically, and sonographically inaccessible or superimposed. Mammography can only evaluate tissue visualized tangentially to the prosthesis. Additional projections as well as the implant displacement view can improve the evaluation, particularly of the augmented breast. For patients at risk as well as for diagnostic problems, contrast-enhanced MRI has proven to be an important supplemental method because of its excellent sensitivity.

Percutaneous biopsy should only be performed if the location of the finding in question permits an approach that avoids damage of the prosthesis.

To detect prosthetic defects, unenhanced MRI is the method of choice.

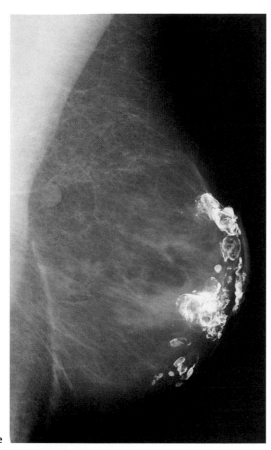

e

e Extensive calcification due to fat necrosis after reduction mammoplasty

■ References

1 Balu-Maestro C, Bruneton JN, Geoffray et al. Ultrasonographic posttreatment follow-up of breast cancer patients. J Ultrasound Med. 1991;10:1–7
2 Harrison RL, Britton P, Warren R, Bobrow L. Can we be sure about a radiological diagnosis of fat necrosis of the breast? Clin Radiol. 2000;55:119–23
3 Beer GM, Kompatscher P, Hergan K. Diagnosis of breast tumors after breast reduction. Aesthetic Plast Surg. 1996;20:391–7
4 Mandrekas AD, Assimakopoulos GJ, Mastorakos DP, Pantzalis K. Fat necrosis following breast reduction. Br J Plast Surg. 1999;47:560–2
5 Heywang-Köbrunner SH, Beck R. Contrast-enhanced MRI of the breast. Heidelberg, New York: Springer; 1996
6 Fischer U, Kopka L, Grabbe E. Magnetic Resonance guided localization and biopsy of suspicious breast lesions. Topics in Magnetic Resonance Imaging. 1998;9:44–59
7 Soo MS, Kornguth PJ, Hertzberg BS. Fat necrosis in the breast: sonographic features. Radiology. 1998;206:261–9
8 Harvey JA, Moran RE, Maurer EJ, De Angelis GA. Sonographic features of mammary oil cysts. J Ultrasound Med. 1997;16:719–24
9 Stavros AT, Thickman D, Rapp CL et al. Solid breast nodules: use of sonography to distinguish between benign and malignant lesions. Radiology. 1995;196:123
10 Soderstrom CE, Harms SE, Farell RS et al. Detection with MR imaging of residual tumor in the breast soon after surgery. AJR. 1997;168:485–88
11 Orel SG, Reynolds C, Schnall MD et al. Breast carcinoma; MR imaging before reexcisional biopsy. Radiology. 1997;205:429–36
12 Parker SH, Burbank F, Jackman RJ et al. Percutaneous large-core breast biopsy: a multiinstitutional study. Radiology, 1994;193:359–64
13 Schreer I. Radiodiagnostic aspects of the conservative treatment of malignant breast disease. Eur Radiol 1994;4:95–101
14 Berenberg AL, Levene MB, Tonnesen GL. Mammographic evaluation of the post-irradiated breast. In: Harris JR, Hellmann S, Silen W eds. Conservative Management of Breast Cancer: New Surgical and Radiotherapeutic Techniques. Philadelphia: Lippincott; 1983:265–72
15 Dershaw DD. Mammography in patients with breast cancer treated by breast conservation (lumpectomy with or without radiation). AJR. 1995;164:309–16
16 Orel SG, Troupin RH, Patterson EA, Fowble BL. Breast cancer recurrence after lumpectomy and irradiation: role of mammography in detection. Radiology. 1992;183:201–6
17 Voogd AC, von Tienhoven G, Peterse HL et al. Local recurrence after breast conservation therapy for early stage breast carcinoma: detection, treatment, and outcome in 266 patients. Dutch Study Group on Local Recurrence after Breast Conservation (BORST). Cancer. 1999;85:437–46
18 Bock E, Bock C, Belli P et al. Role of Diagnostic imaging of the breast in patients treated with postsurgical radiotherapy or presurgical radiotherapy or chemotherapy. Radiol Med (Torino). 1998;95:38–43
19 Eklund GW, Cardenosa G. The art of mammographic positioning. Radiol Clin North Am. 1992;30:21–53
20 Dershaw DD. Evaluation of the breast undergoing lumpectomy and radiation therapy. Radiol Clin North Am. 1995;33:1147–60
21 Dershaw DD, McCormick B, Cox L, Osborne MP. Differentiation of benign and malignant local tumor recurrence after lumpectomy. AJR. 1990;155:35–8
22 Gluck BS, Dershaw DD, Liberman L, Deutch BM. Microcalcifications on postoperative mammograms as an indicator of adequacy of tumor excision. Radiology. 1993;188:469–72
23 Harris KM, Costa-Greco MA, Baratz AB, Britton CA, Ilkhanipour ZS, Ganott MA. The mammographic features of the post-lumpectomy, post irradiated breast. Radiographics. 1989;9:253–68
24 Dershaw DD, McCormick B, Osborne MP. Detection of local recurrence after conservative therapy for breast carcinoma. Cancer. 1992;46:186–90
25 Solin LJ, Fowble BL, Troupin RH, Goodman RL. Biopsy results of new calcifications in the post-irradiated breast. Cancer. 1989;63:1956–61

26 Dershaw DD, Abramson A, Kinne DW. Ductal carcinomas in situ: mammographic findings and clinical implications. Radiology. 1989;170:411–5

27 Krishnamurty R, Whitman GJ, Stelling CB, Kushwaha AC. Mammographic findings after breast conservation therapy. Radiographics. 1999;19 Spec No.:S53–62

28 Giess CS, Keating DM, Osborne MP, Rosenblatt R. Local tumor recurrence following breast conservation therapy: correlation of histopathologic findings with detection method and mammographic findings. Radiology. 1999;212:829–35

29 Holli K, Saaristo R, Isola J et al. Effect of radiotherapy on the interpretation of routine follow-up mammography after conservative breast surgery: a randomized study. Br J Cancer. 1998;78:524–5

30 Lewis-Jones HG, Whitehouse GH, Leistner SJ. The role of magnetic resonance imaging in the assessment of local recurrent breast carcinoma. Clin Radiol. 1991;43:197–204

31 Dao, TH, Rahmouni A, Campana F et al. Tumor recurrence versus fibrosis in the irradiated breast: differentiation with dynamic gadolinium-enhanced MR imaging. Radiology. 1993;187:751–5

32 Heywang-Köbrunner SH, Schlegel A, Beck R et al. Contrast-enhanced MRI of the breast after limited surgery and radiation therapy. J. Comput Assist Tomogr. 1993;7:891–900

33 Gilles R, Guinebretiere JM, Shapeero LG et al. Assessment of breast cancer recurrence with contrast-enhanced subtraction MR imaging: preliminary results in 26 patients. Radiology. 1993;188:473–8

34 Mussurakis S, Buckley DL, Bowsley SJ et al. Dynamic contrast-enhanced magnetic resonance imaging of the breast combined with pharmacokinetic analysis of gadolinium-DTPA uptake in the diagnosis of local recurrence of early stage breast cancer. Investigative Radiology. 1995;30:650–62

35 Drew, PJ, Kerin MJ, Turnbull LW et al. Routine screening for local recurrence following breast-conserving therapy for cancer with dynamic contrast-enhanced magnetic resonance imaging of the breast. Ann Surg Oncol. 1998;5:265–70

36 Krämer S, Schulz-Wendtland R, Hagedorn K et al. Magnetic resonance imaging in the diagnosis of local recurrences in breast cancer. Anticancer Research. 1998;18:2159–62

37 Rieber A, Merkle E, Zeitler H et al. Value of MR mammography in the detection and exclusion of recurrent breast carcinoma. J Comput Assist Tomogr. 1997;21:780–4

38 Viehweg P, Heinig A, Lampe D et al. Retrospective analysis for evaluation of the value of contrast-enhanced MRI in patients with breast conservative therapy. MAGMA (Magnetic Resonance Materials in Physics, Biology and Medicine). 1998;7:141–52

39 Müller RD, Barkhausen J, Sauerwein W, Langer R. Assessment of local recurrence after breast conserving therapy with MRI. JCAT. 1998;22:408–12

40 Eidelman Y, Liebling RW, Buchbinder S et al. Mammography in the evaluation of masses in breasts reconstructed with TRAM flaps. Ann Plast Surg. 1998;41:229–33

41 Hogge JP, Zuurbier RA, de Paredes ES. Mammography of autologous myocutaneous flaps. Radiographics. 1999;19 Spec. No.: S63–72

42 Dershaw DD, Chaglassian TA. Mammography after prosthesis placement for augmentation or reconstructive mammoplasty. Radiology. 1989;170:69–74

43 Eklund GW, Busby RC, Miller SH et al. Improving imaging of the augmented breast. AJR. 1988;151:469–73

44 Handel N, Silverstein MJ, Gamagami P, Jensen JA, Collins A. Factors affecting mammographic visualization of the breast after augmentation mammoplasty. JAMA. 1992;268:1913–7

45 Leibman AJ, Styblo TM, Bostwick J 3rd. Mammography of the postreconstruction breast. Plast Reconstr Surg. 1997;99:698–704

46 Fajardo LL, Harvey JA, McAleese KA et al. Breast cancer diagnosis in women with subglandular silicone gel-filled augmentation implants. Radiology. 1995;194:859–65

47 Park AJ, Walsh J, Reddy PS et al. The detection of breast implant rupture using ultrasound. Br J Plast Surg. 1996;49:299–301

48 Lorenz R, Stark GB, Hedde JP. The value of sonography for the discovery of complications after the implantation of silicone gel prostheses for breast augmentation or reconstruction. RoeFo. 1997;166:233–7

49 Harris KM, Ganott MA, Shestak KC, Losken HW, Tobon H. Silicone implant rupture: detection with US. Radiology. 1993;187:761–8

50 Leibman AJ, Kruse B. Breast cancer: mammographic and sonographic findings after augmentation mammoplasty. Radiology. 1990;174:195–8

51 Heinig A, Heywang-Köbrunner SH, Viehweg P et al. Value of contrast enhanced magnetic resonance tomography of the breast after reconstruction with silicone implant. Radiologe. 1997;37:710–7

52 Boné B, Aspelin P, Isberg B et al. Contrast-enhanced MR imaging of the breast in patients with silicone implants after cancer surgery. Acta Radiol. 1995;36:111–6

53 Everson LI, Parantainen H, Detlie T et al. Diagnosis of breast implant rupture: imaging findings and relative efficacies of imaging techniques. AJR. 1994;163:57–60

54 Gorczyca DP, Sinha S, Ahn CY et al. Silicone breast implants in vivo: MR imaging. Radiology. 1992;185:407–10

55 Gorczyca DP, Schneider E, DeBruhl ND et al. Silicone breast implant rupture: comparison between three-point Dixon and fast spin-echo MR imaging. AJR. 1994;162:305–10

56 Monticciolo DL, Nelson RC, Dixon WT et al. MR detection of leakage from silicone breast implants: value of a silicone-selective pulse sequence. AJR. 1994;163:51–6

57 Mund DF, Fartia DM, Gorczyca DP et al. MR imaging of the breast in patients with silicone-gel implants: spectrum of findings. AJR. 1993; 161: 773–8

58 Ahn CY, DeBruhl ND, Gorczyca DP et al. Comparative silicone breast implant evaluation using mammography, sonography and magnetic resonance imaging: experience with 59 implants. Plast Reconstr Surg. 1994;94:620–7

59 Chilcote WA, Dowden RV, Paushter DM et al. Ultrasound detection of silicone gel breast implant failure: a prospective analysis. Breast Dis. 1994;7:307–16

60 Drake DB, Miller L, Janus CL. Magnetic resonance imaging of in situ mammary prosthesis. Ann Plast Surg. 1994;33:258–62

19. Skin Changes

Nodular Changes of the Skin and Subcutaneous Tissue

Nodular changes of the skin and subcutaneous tissue can be visualized on the mammogram and, if not seen in profile, can be mistaken for intramammary lesions. Therefore, mammographic interpretation should always include the results from inspection and palpation of the skin.

Most frequent are:

- Fibroepitheliomas (usually at the areola/ Mamilla)
- Moles
- Epithelial cysts (atheromas)
- Lipomas
- Keloids

Hemangiomas, lymphangiomas, neurofibromas, histiocytomas, and leiomyomas are rare nodular cutaneous or subcutaneous lesions.

■ Clinical Findings

While fibroepitheliomas most frequently account for small, sometimes pedunculated lesions at the nipple, moles and epithelial cysts can occur anywhere on the skin of the breast. Epithelial cysts (atheromas) form nodular tumors of variable size within the skin and occasionally become infected. Lipomas present as soft, subcutaneous nodules of variable size with more or less pronounced bulging of the overlying skin.

■ Diagnostic Strategy

All nodular changes of the skin and subcutaneous tissue are accessible to direct examination and therefore can be evaluated clinically, Since they can mimic intramammary lesions, imaging studies should always be interpreted in conjunction with the clinical findings.

■ Mammography

Moles and epithelial cysts can generally be assigned to a cutaneous location by their pattern of a mass surrounded by a radiolucent rim, which is caused by air between tumor, skin, and compression device (Figs. 19.1 a–d) and accounts for the characteristic mammographic appearance. Size and density of the focal findings are subject to wide individual variability. Moles also can contain calcific particles, potentially imitating an intramammary lesion with microcalcifications.

In general, the correct diagnosis is established by combining clinical and mammographic findings. If questions remain, a repeat view with a marker placed on the cutaneous finding is recommended for clarification.

Skin Thickening

■ Definition

The thickness of the skin can vary individually. Furthermore, small breasts presumably have a slightly thicker skin than larger breasts. According to Wilson et al., and Pope et al.,[1, 2] the lateral and cranial skin thickness as seen in the normal mammogram (craniocaudal projection and mediolateral projection, respectively) should not exceed 2.5 mm. Medially and caudally, the skin thickness can be up to 3 mm. However, in an individual patient skin thickness is best assessed by comparing both sides, since skin thickening is rarely bilateral and its presence is usually suspected based on clinical or other mammographic findings. Discrete pathologic skin thickening cannot always be distinguished from a normal variant. Suggestive of a pathologic process are: localized skin thickening, asymmetry in comparison to the contralateral side, a change with time (assuming

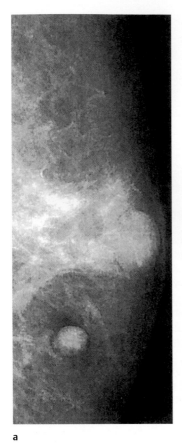
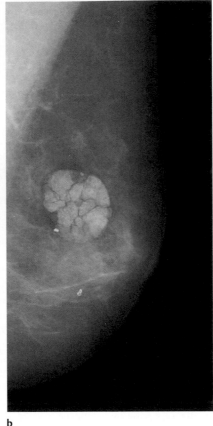
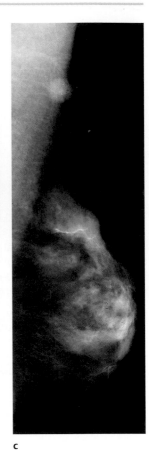

a   b   c

Fig. 19.**1 a–f**
a Oval, smoothly outlined mass measuring 10 mm in diameter, surrounded by a radiolucent halo, in projection of the lower half of the breast: verruca
b Seventy-seven-year-old woman with a large mole on her breast
c Smoothly outlined mass, measuring 14 mm in diameter, with central microcalcifications, in projection of the axillary extension of the breast, corresponding to a verruca senilis

comparable mammographic technique), as well as the association with increased trabecular markings in the subcutaneous tissue or elsewhere in the breast.

■ Incidence

Skin thickening can involve the breast locally (confined to one area) or diffusely.[3–7]

The most important causes of *localized skin thickening* include:

- Dermatologic conditions such as circumscribed scleroderma, psoriasis, etc
- band-like skin thickening as a manifestation of Mondor disease, which is a thrombophlebitis of a superficial vein. It presents as cord-like skin thickening along the course of the vein, associated with slight retraction if seen in the stage of scar formation
- Skin thickening in scarring
- Concomitant thickening of the skin overlying a localized process (representing localized reaction or direct infiltration), as seen, for instance, with an abscess, fat necrosis, carcinoma, metastasis, and hematologic malignancy (see also Fig. 15.4 a)

The most important causes of *diffuse skin thickening* are:

- Mastitis
- Inflammatory carcinoma, diffuse metastatic spread to the breast, diffuse infiltration of the breast as seen with hematologic malignancies
- Iatrogenic edema following surgery, radiotherapy (see p. 352), later evolving into a scar,

Fig. 19.**1 d**   Very dense, round, smoothly outlined mass, measuring 23 mm in diameter, in projection of the medial half of the breast, corresponding to an atheroma in the inner lower quadrant
e   To resolve diagnostic uncertainties, a lead BB placed as marker on the skin can confirm the suspected diagnosis
f   Convex mass with two central, partially visualized radiolucencies in projection of the medial half of the breast along the thoracic wall: Partially visualized tip of the nose

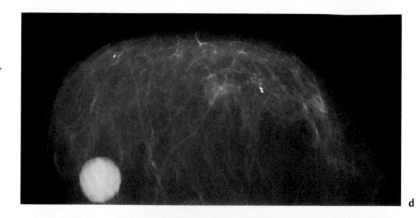

d

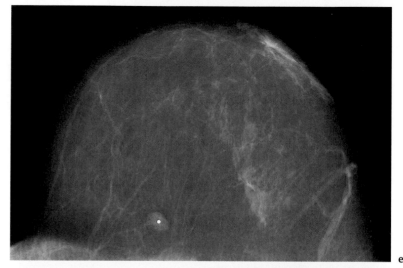

e

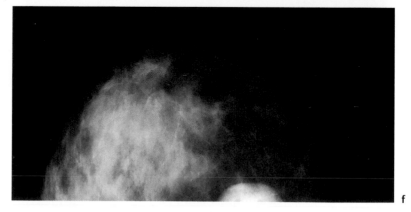

f

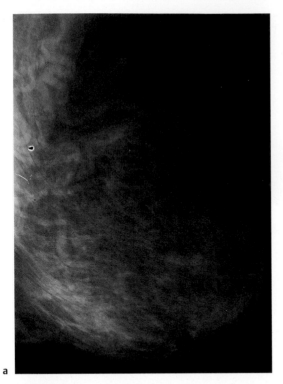

a

Fig. 19.2 a–e
a This patient has developed superior vena cava obstruction due to central venous catheters. Skin thickening, trabecular coarsening, and multiple dilated veins serving as collaterals are shown

and anticoagulation therapy (as manifestation of an acute mammary necrosis)
– Lymphatic stasis caused by interruption of the lymphatics (mainly axillary), secondary to axillary nodal metastases, inflammatory processes and status post axillary dissection, or radiation
– Generalized edema due to cardiac decompensation, obstructed venous drainage, fluid overload, renal insufficiency, severe hepatic disease, hypoalbuminemia

■ Diagnostic Strategy

The differential diagnosis for localized skin thickening can generally be narrowed down on the basis of the physical examination. The clinical findings must be incorporated in the interpretation of the imaging findings to establish the correct diagnosis of an imaged localized skin thickening. The nature of any underlying focal finding determines the differential diagnosis of the accompanying localized skin thickening.

Except for exclusively dermatologic conditions, diffuse skin thickening is invariably associated with edema of the connective tissue. It can be classified as follows:
- Symmetric appearance in both breasts can be evidence of generalized edema (cardiac decompensation, fluid overload, etc.), to be confirmed clinically. Important exceptions are asymmetric generalized edema following preferential lying on one side or bilateral edema, e.g., due to bilateral lymphatic stasis secondary to axillary metastases bilaterally or superior vena cava syndrome with obstructed venous drainage.
- The clinical history is of utmost importance (recent surgery or radiotherapy, exclusion of conditions associated with a generalized edema, etc.). The resolution of postradiation skin thickening and interstitial edema has to be monitored clinically and by imaging. An increase in skin thickening and interstitial edema should lead to a careful diagnostic evaluation to exclude or detect recurrent disease.
- For the difficult differential diagnosis between inflammatory carcinoma and mastitis (see p. 237–9, 287–9 and Figs. 13.1 and 15.7), imaging has to be used, as it should be used for newly suspected venous or lymphatic stasis (sonography, contrast-enhanced CT or MRI is available for evaluating the axillary findings).
- If imaging cannot establish a definitive diagnosis (as would be the case if microcalcifications suggestive for malignancy are present), imaging can be helpful to select the most appropriate site for the excisional biopsy with punch biopsy of the skin (see p. 241).
- If inflammatory skin thickening is suspected, a trial of anti-inflammatory therapy should be considered (to be monitored by serial imaging).

■ Clinical Findings

For the **differential diagnosis,** a carefully obtained clinical history (underlying malignancy, related to surgery or radiotherapy) is of great importance, as are inspection (in dermatologic conditions), general physical examination (in the presence of generalized edema), and clinical evaluation of the breast (erythema, hyperthermia, peau d'orange).

To **detect** skin thickening, imaging is superior to the clinical examination since inflammatory

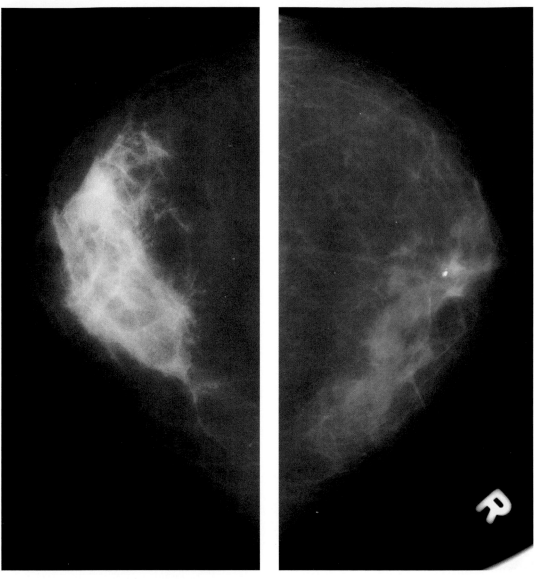

b

c

Fig. 19.**2b, c**   Skin thickening and diffuse increase in breast density are seen on the left due to bacterial mastitis, which resolved following antibiotic therapy

carcinoma, for instance, can cause skin thickening that is visible on imaging studies weeks prior to its clinical manifestation.[2]

■ Mammography

With correct exposure, skin thickening is reliably and readily seen mammographically.

In addition to detecting or documenting skin thickening (important, for instance, for monitoring changes following radiotherapy), mammography is mainly used to detect signs of malignancy (suggestive microcalcifications, suggestive lesion). Absence of a lesion or microcalcifications, however, does not exclude an otherwise suspected malignancy (see p. 241).

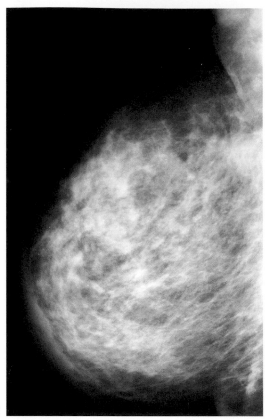

d

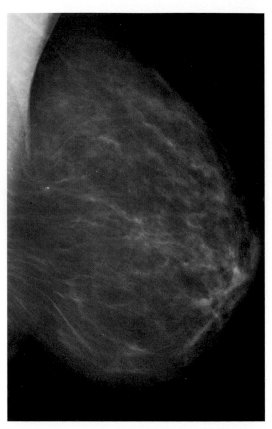

e

Fig. 19.**2d, e** Inflammatory carcinoma on the right (d) causes extensive skin thickening, diffusely increased breast density, and coarsened trabecular markings. Axil-lary adenopathy is also suggested. The pattern is identical to mastitis

■ Sonography

Sonography can also be employed to detect or document skin thickening. Detecting a hypoecho-ic focus in mammographically dense tissue can be relevant for the differential diagnosis.

■ Contrast-enhanced MRI

MRI can also reveal skin thickening. Worm-like enhancement in and around tumorous foci found in subcutaneous lymphatic vessels can be evidence of lymphangiomatosis but is not visible in all cases. Otherwise, skin thickening and enhancement in the thickened skin are nonspecific. Contrast-enhanced MRI can make an important contribution to the differential diagnosis by detecting or excluding otherwise occult focal lesions in mammographically dense tissue (e.g., after radiotherapy). But for the differentiation between mastitis and inflammatory carcinoma, contrast-enhanced MRI appears less suitable because enhancement is found in both conditions.

■ Biopsy Methods

Excisional biopsy including skin is the most suitable method for further evaluation of skin thickening. The histologic finding that is diagnostic for inflammatory carcinoma is the presence of tumor emboli in the dermal lymphatics. Imaging can be useful in selecting the site to be biopsied.

■ Summary

Skin thickening can be detected and documented with all imaging methods. For the differential diagnostic classification, clinical history, course of the skin thickening (status post radiotherapy), clinical findings (evidence of generalized edema), and inspection (dermatologic origin) are of particular importance. While skin thickening with or without edema is generally nonspecific, imaging is used to search for signs suggestive of malignancy, such as microcalcifications or additional highly suggestive focal findings, or to identify suspicious areas for biopsy.

■ References

1   Wilson SA, Adam EJ, Tucker AK. Patterns of breast skin thickness in normal mammograms. Clin Radiol. 1982;33:691–3
2   Pope TL Jr, Read ME, Medsker T et al. Breast skin thickness: normal range and causes of thickening shown on film screen mammography. J Can Assoc Radiol. 1984;35:365–8
3   Skaane P, Bautz W, Metzger H. Circumscribed and diffuse skin thickening (peau d'orange) of the female breast. ROFO 1985;14:212–9
4   Britton CA. Mammographic abnormalities of the skin and subcutaneous tissues. Crit Rev Diagn Imaging. 1994; 35:61–83. Review
5   Pluchinotta AM, De Min V, Presacco D et al. Unilateral edema of the breast secondary to congestive heart failure. Report of 2 cases. Minerva Chir. 1994;49:1171–4
6   Crowe DJ, Helvie MA, Wilson TE. Breast infection. Mammographic and sonographic findings with clinical correlation. Invest Radiol. 1995;30:582–7
7   Kushwaha AC, Whitman GJ, Stelling CB et al. Primary inflammatory carcinoma of the breast: retrospective review of mammographic findings. AJR. 2000;174:535–8

20. The Male Breast

In the male, the mammary gland consists of a small retroareolar nodule composed of a branched system of lactiferous ducts and collagenous connective tissue.

Since the male mammary gland is also subject to hormonal proliferative stimuli, temporary or permanent increases in the size can occur during the patient's life, such as in puberty or old age.

■ Clinical Findings

Depending on its individual form, the normally developed mammary gland is either not distinguishable from the areola itself, or it is palpable as a small circumscribed area of retroareolar resistance. Pain and enlargement of the glandular tissue occurs only in hyperplasia.

■ Mammography
(Fig. 20.1a)

At mammography, the glandular nodule appears as a funnel-shaped retroareolar density, with the base of the funnel pointing toward the chest wall. Substructures are not discernible. The glandular nodule is surrounded by fatty tissue, which can vary from patient to patient. In many men, no soft tissue density is seen behind the nipple, and the entire volume of the breast is fatty.

Gynecomastia

■ Definition

Gynecomastia is a unilateral or bilateral enlargement of the male breast under the influence of estrogens or substances having an estrogenic effect.

Physiologic forms of gynecomastia (gynecomastia in newborns, puberal hypertrophy, and senescent hypertrophy) can occur in the presence of endocrinopathy or liver disorders. Gynecomastia also frequently occurs as a result of medication (for example, in estrogen therapy of prostate therapy or diuretic therapy), or it may be a manifestation of a paraneoplastic syndrome.

■ Histology

Proliferation of the ductal system occurs with development and growth of alveoli, hyperplasia of the glandular epithelium, and an increase in stromal tissue.

■ Clinical Findings

Gynecomastia is often associated with pain or tenderness. The diagnosis is usually clinically suspected. Pseudogynecomastia is the result of deposition of fat in the subcutaneous tissue. It occurs bilaterally and is characterized by the soft consistency typical of fatty tissue. In genuine gynecomastia, the proliferative glandular tissue will be palpable unilaterally or bilaterally as a generalized or nodular localized area of increased soft, tender subareolar density. About 60% of patients with gynecomastia give a history of a medical condition that may be associated with gynecomastia or of medications known to cause gynecomastia.[1]

■ Diagnostic Strategy

The most important examination method aside from clinical examination is mammography. Sonography has only limited use since cysts rarely

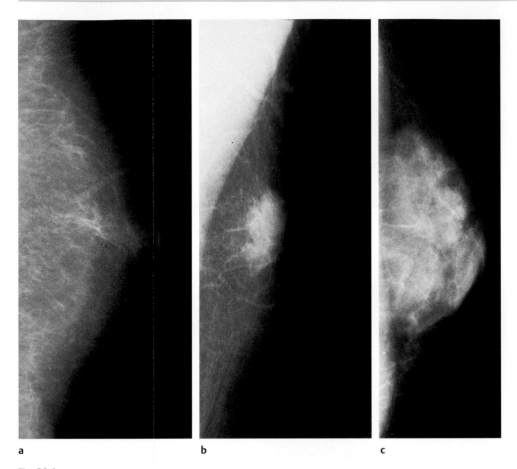

a   b   c

Fig. 20.**1 a–c**
a Normal male breast
b Gynecomastia, visible as focal area of increased density behind the nipple
c Pronounced gynecomastia showing diffuse nodular increased density throughout this enlarged breast, resembling fibrocystic changes

occur in the male breast, and this modality is not specific enough to identify solid findings as benign or malignant. No data are available on MRI in the male breast.

■ Mammography
(Figs. 20.**1 b** and 20.**2**)

Bilateral mammography should be performed. Although gynecomastia may only be clinically evident in one breast, it is frequently radiographically bilateral.

Depending on the severity of the gynecomastia, either a small circumscribed density posterior to the nipple will be visible, or, in the presence of more pronounced proliferation, nodular con-

fluent parenchymal densities will be discernible, which may even appear like a female mammary gland with fibrocystic changes (Fig. 20.**1 c**). The usual radiographic pattern is of glandular proliferation arising from the nipple with an irregular (flame-shaped) deep margin. Lateral margins may be smooth or irregular. Calcifications are not associated with gynecomastia.[2, 3]

■ Other Methods

Sonography can provide additional information in radiopaque areas. Probably due to the small size of male breasts, it has even been reported to have a higher sensitivity than mammography alone. Overall, the sensitivity of mammography and pal-

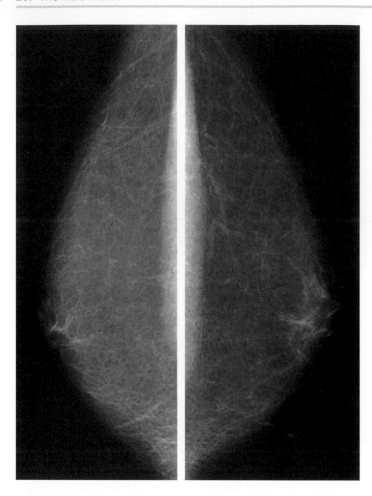

Fig. 20.**2** Pseudogynecomastia. The enlargement of the male breast is caused exclusively by fatty tissue

pation together, however, appears to be equal to ultrasound[4]. However, ultrasound does not allow differentiation between benign and malignant solid masses. For this reason, further workup is required in the presence of clinical or mammographic evidence of a suspected malignancy.

In our opinion, no other imaging modalities are indicated for gynecomastia.

Breast Cancer in Men

■ Definition

Breast cancer is a rare disease in men. In the United States about 1000 cases are reported annually. Stage for stage, prognosis is the same as for breast cancer in women. The disease in men is often related to increased levels of circulating estrogens, as is gynecomastia, and therefore the two may coexist, although gynecomastia is not premalignant. Breast cancer in men also can be caused by radiation and is increased in Klinefelter syndrome. Familial male breast cancer is reported and is often associated with the BRCA2 gene.

■ Histology

Men do not have lobules, so breast cancer in men is always ductal. Ductal carcinoma in situ can be diagnosed in men, and DCIS accounted for one-quarter of breast cancers reported in one series.[5]

Fig. 20.**3**   Palpable breast cancer in a 57-year-old male
a Sonogram
b Mammogram
c Mammogram of another patient. A hard, palpable, non-tender mass connected to the nipple in a male is characteristic for carcinoma

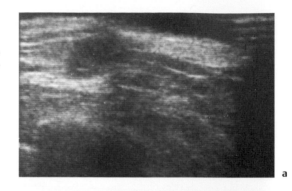

a

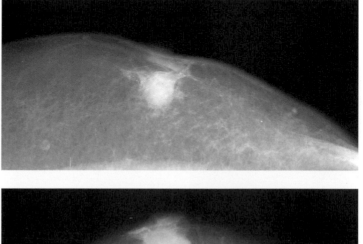

b

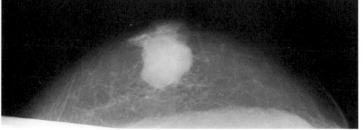

c

■ Clinical Findings

Breast cancer in men is usually subareolar, and changes in the nipple are commonly present. The palpable mass is hard and non-tender to the chest wall, not soft and tender as in gynecomastia. A bloody discharge from the nipple is always strongly suggestive of breast cancer in the man. Changes in the nipple can also occur.

■ Mammography

Unlike cancer in the woman, breast cancer in the man is usually attached to the nipple. The tumor mass is frequently smooth or lobulated; spiculation is rare. Microcalcifications are an unusual finding. Calcifications associated with breast cancer in the male may not be very pleomorphic. Secondary signs of nipple inversion and skin thickening are common.[6]

Coexistent gynecomastia may obscure a cancer. Despite mammographic findings of gynecomastia, a biopsy is indicated whenever the physical examination is worrisome. Detection of nonpalpable breast cancer in men followed with screening of the contralateral breast after mastectomy has been reported. However, the role of screening in this population and in BRCA positive men is unestablished.

■ Sonography

The sonographic pattern of breast cancer in men is usually that of a rounded, hypoechoic mass. The

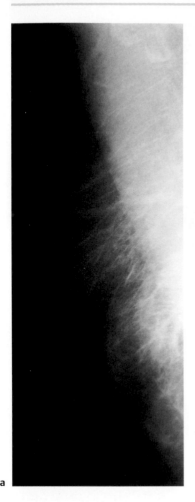

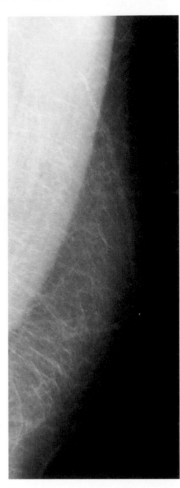

a

b

Fig. 20.**4 a, b** This man presented with a hard deformed breast fixed to the chest wall. The contour is distorted, the skin is thick, and breast density is diffusely increased at the involved side (**a**) compared to the normal breast (**b**). On biopsy, only chronic inflammatory changes without focal lesion were found

margins may be irregular and distal acoustic shadowing can occur (Fig. 20.**3 a**). On Doppler interrogation hypervascularity can be seen.

■ Summary

Gynecomastia is usually evident by clinical examination. Although often unilateral clinically, it is frequently bilateral mammographically. The pattern is usually asymmetric. Despite a pattern consistent with gynecomastia, if carcinoma is clinically suspected, biopsy should be performed. Mammographic and sonographic signs of malignancy are similar to those in the female breast.

■ References

1 Volpe CM, Rafferto JD, Collure DW et al. Unilateral male breast masses: cancer risk and their evaluation and management. Am Surg. 1999;65:250–3
2 Dershaw DD. Male mammography. AJR. 1986;146:127–31
3 Chantra PK, So GJ, Wollman JS, Bassett LW. Mammography of the male breast. AJR 1995;164:853–8
4 Ambrogetti D, Ciatto S, Catarzi S, Murala MG. The combined diagnosis of male breast lesions: a review of a series of 748 consecutive cases. Radiol Med (Torino). 1996;91:356–9
5 Dershaw DD, Borgen PI, Deutch BM, Liberman L. Mammographic findings in men with breast cancer. AJR. 1993;160:267–70
6 Cooper RA, Gunter BA, Ramamurthy L. Mammography in men. Radiology. 1994;191:66

III Application of Diagnostic Imaging of the Breast

21. Screening

Definition

Screening refers to examinations performed regularly on asymptomatic women. In Europe this term implies a program, in which women are systematically invited to participate according to a population registry with the goal to detect clinically occult breast cancer at an early stage. It includes quality control, exact documentation and systematic follow-up. Its task, however, is searching, not diagnosing.

Results of International Studies

■ Randomized Studies

The HIP (Health Insurance Plan of Greater New York)[1, 2] study is the oldest randomized study. Between 1963 and 1970, 31 000 women between the ages of 40 and 64 years were allocated to have a two-view mammogram together with a clinical examination, followed by three annual follow-up mammograms. This screening was not offered to the control group of 31 000 women. Five years after commencement of the study, a 50% reduction in mortality was found in the screened women aged 50 to 64 years. Reduced mortality was still found after 18 years but declined to 23% since women could only participate for 4 years. For women ages 40 to 49 years, a mortality reduction was only evident after a longer follow-up; it now is at 24.6%.

Three randomized trials were conducted in Sweden. The first (Two County Study) trial was undertaken in the counties of Kopparberg and Ostergotland starting in 1977. About 77 000 women were in the screening group and 56 000 women in the control group, i.e., passive study group. Single-view mammography without clinical examination was performed on women aged 40 to 49 years at 2-year intervals, for the older women at intervals of 33 months. The mortality reduction was 40% in women ages 50 to 74 years. Up to 12 years after the initiation of the study, no statistically significant reduction in mortality was observed in women aged 40 to 49 years.

The 2nd Swedish trial in Malmö[7, 8, 9] included 21 000 women older than 45 years who had a two-view mammogram for the first two screening examinations, followed by three single-view mammographic screenings, without clinical examination. The intervals were 18 to 24 months. In comparison with the control group, a reduction in breast cancer mortality of 19% could be achieved over a period of 12 years. For the correct interpretation of the rather disappointing data, it should be mentioned that 24% of the women in the control group had at least one mammogram, and this was obtained in 13% of the women aged 65 to 69 years and 34% of the women aged 45 to 49 years, and that 20% of the breast carcinomas were also mammographically diagnosed in the control group. Considering that 26% to 30% of the women in the study group had no mammography, the lack of any detectable benefit for the women aged 45 to 49 years should not be surprising. Adding to the first cohort (MMST I) the second cohort (MMST II) and pooling the data of the cohorts resulted in a statistically significant 36% reduction in breast cancer mortality in the intervention group of women under 50 years.

The 3rd Swedish randomized study in Stockholm began in 1981.[10, 11] Single-view mammography without clinical examination was performed on 43 000 women aged 40 to 64 years at 2½-year intervals. The reduction in mortality rate 7 years after initiation of the trial was 30% for all patients and 43% for patients older than 50 years. The reduction of the mortality rate 11.4 years after initiation of the trial was 20% for all patients.

Additional randomized studies were carried out in Scotland (Edinburgh)[13, 14] and Canada[15] (Table 21.1).

Table 21.**1**   Results of 7 randomized controlled trials

Study	Start	Age (yrs)	Modality	Interval (Mo)	Participation (%)	Follow-up (yrs)	Relative risk (95% Confidential interval) All	< 50 yrs
HIP	1963	40–64	2-view Mx + PE*	12	67	10	0.71 (0.55–0.93)	0.77 (0.50–1.16)
Two County	1977	40–74	1-view Mx	24 (< 50)	89	15.2	K⁺ 0.68 (0.52–0.98)	0.73 (0.37–1.4)
				33 (50+)		14.2	O⁺ 0.82 (0.64–1.05)	1.02 (0.52–1.99)
Malmö	1976	45–69	2-view Mx	28–24	74	12	0.81 (0.62–1.07)	0.64 (0.45–0.89)
Stockholm	1981	40–64	1-view Mx	24	81	11.4	0.80 (0.53–1.22)	1.08 (0.54–2.17)
Gothen-burg	1982	40–59	2-view Mx	18	84	12		0.56 (0.31–0.99)
All Swedish studies (Update 1997)		40–49		18–24		12.8 (median)		0.71 (0.57–1.89)
Edinburgh	1978	45–64	2-view Mx + PE (later 1-view Mx)	12 (PE) 24 (Mx)	61	14	0.79 (0.60–1.02)	0.75 (0.48–1.18)
Canada 1 (NBSS 1)	1980	40–49	2-view Mx + PE	12	100	10.5		1.14 (0.83–1.56)

* Mx: Mammography, PE: Physical examination, K⁺: Kopparberg, O⁺: Ostergotland

The Edinburgh study included 23 000 women ages 45 to 64 years who underwent annual physical examination alternating with annual mammography with physical examination. Fourteen years after initiation of the study, breast cancer mortality, which was calculated adjusting for socio-economic status, was reduced by 21 %. This reduction is of borderline significance (95 % [0.60–1.02]).

An important result of the Edinburgh trial was the observation that the detection rate of interval carcinomas was lower in the years with additional mammography than in the years with physical examination only.

In Canada, two randomized trials were undertaken, one of which concentrated exclusively on a younger age group (40 to 49 years). Commencing in 1980, a total of 25000 women underwent annual two-view mammography and physical examination for 5 years. No decrease in mortality could be detected in comparison with the control group that only had a single physical examination and usual care. This disappointing result can be attributed to several deficiencies of the trial design: only volunteers were examined, yielding a "pseudo-compliance" rate of 100%. Furthermore, symptomatic patients, some of whom had an advanced cancer, were included mainly in the mammography arm of the study*. Moreover, unbiased reviewers could document that within the first 5 years more than 50% of the mammographic studies were of a quality deemed poor to unacceptable, leading to the false assurance of normality and thus delaying the diagnosis. In addition, similar to the Malmö study, 20% of the women in the control group also had a mammogram. Finally, 25% of the recommended biopsies were not done.

Therefore, the negative outcome of the Canadian study, which was designed to provide data for the *cost-effectiveness* of breast cancer screening in women ages 40 to 49 years, should *not be considered proof of* ineffectiveness of screening younger women.

■ Case Control Studies

In addition to randomized studies, three case control studies were conducted in the Netherlands (Nijmegen, Utrecht)[16] and in Italy (Florence).[17] Only women who really participated in the study

---

* This is documented by the fact that 80% more carcinomas (including a high number of advanced stages) entered the study in the "mammography" arm than in the "palpation-only" arm.

were compared with nonparticipating women. This is in contrast to the randomized studies, where all women invited to undergo screening were compared to those who were not invited, regardless of whether the invited women participated or not. The results of the randomized studies are therefore distorted by the results of those women who were invited for mammography but did not undergo it, and by the inclusion of mammographically examined women in the control group. Because of this, randomized studies underestimate the impact of screening, while controlled studies may more accurately indicate the extent of its benefit. When well conducted, however, randomized studies are felt to be more biostatistically valid.

In *Nijmegen*, annual single-view (lateral) mammography was performed on women between the ages of 35 and 65 years, and a 50% reduction in the mortality rate was found. In *Utrecht*, the mortality rate could be reduced by 70% in women ages 50 to 64 years who underwent two-view mammography and clinical examination at short intervals of 12, then 18, and then 24 months.

In *Florence*, the reduction in the mortality rate was 68% for women ages 40 to 70 years who had a two-view mammogram every 2.5 years.

Since both the randomized and the case control studies do not include an adequate number of young women (40 to 49 years), the proof of a *statistically significant* reduction in mortality rate by some of these studies is still lacking. It can, however, be extrapolated based on the data of the BCDDP study.

These results correspond well with the outcome of both the Malmö and Gothenburg trials, for which a statistically significant mortality reduction of 36% and 44% was published for those women younger than 50 years.

Obviously, both excellent image quality and the use of two-view mammography allowed an increase in the detection rate of breast cancers, which appears to be of the utmost importance in young women with dense breast tissue.[21-25]

Further Screening Studies

■ Breast Cancer Demonstration Project

The Breast Cancer Detection Demonstration Project (BCDDP)[19, 20] is the largest nonrandomized multicenter study. It was conducted throughout the United States from 1973 to 1981 on a total of approximately 280000 women who were screened by annual two-view mammography combined with a physical examination. The pertinent results are compared with the data of the HIP study in Table 21.2.

The doubling of the detection rate of carcinomas (BCDDP vs. HIP), the markedly decreasing rate of interval carcinomas, and the increase in the number of small carcinomas clearly reflect the higher sensitivity due to improved mammographic quality of the BCDDP. This is especially apparent in young women, in whom 45% of the cancers were only detected by mammography in the BCDDP compared to 20% in the HIP study. Comparison of the tumor stages in the different age groups reveals a proportionately equal distribution of the tumor stages in women ages 40 to 49 years (Table 19.3) compared to those above age 50. From this, it can be deduced that a significant reduction in mortality can also be expected in young women.

The most recent summary of the results computed over a 15-year observation period revealed comparable mortality reduction for women ages 40 to 49 years in comparison to women ages 50 to 59 years.

Table 21.**2**   Comparison between the results of the more recent HIP trial and the old BCDDP trial

	BCDDP	HIP
Cancer detection rate*:		
First phase	5.54‰	2.73‰
Second phase	2.65‰	1.49‰
Interval cancer+	13%	34%
Cancers solely diagnosed mammographically+:		
40–49 years	45%	20%
50–59 years	47%	38%

* Relative to the screening population
+ Relative to the number of cancers

Table 21.**3** Results of the BCDDP multicenter study conducted: cancers of 280 000 women, tabulated according to patient age and tumor stage

Histology	Breast Cancer Detection Demonstration Project (BCDDP), Number of Cancers (%)			
	40–49 years	50–59 years	60–69 years	Total
In situ	166 (15)	232 (15)	130 (13)	528 (15)
Invasive	742 (75)	1180 (76)	761 (76)	2683 (75)
N–	544 (54)	866 (56)	599 (60)	2009 (56)
N+	198 (20)	314 (20)	162 (16)	674 (19)
Unknown	96 (10)	148 (9)	110 (11)	354 (10)
Total	1004 (100)	1560 (100)	1001 (100)	3565 (100)
Tumor size				
< 10 mm	78 (12)	117 (11)	106 (16)	301 (13)
10–19 mm	211 (32)	362 (35)	269 (40)	842 (35)
20–49 mm	181 (27)	286 (27)	144 (21)	611 (26)
> 50 mm	27 (4)	49 (5)	25 (4)	101 (4)
Total	663 (100)	1046 (100)	674 (100)	2382 (100)

United Kingdom Trial of Early Detection Breast Cancer (TEDBC)

In 1997 a non-randomised study[26] was set up to evaluate the effect of screening and education of breast self examination on breast cancer mortality. Eight centers were included: two screening centers (in Guilford and Edinburgh), two breast self-examination centers (in Huddersfield and Nottingham), and four comparison centers. Women aged 45–64 years were offered mammography and clinical examination every 2 years and clinical examination in the intervening year. Mortality rates were calculated comparing expected versus observed numbers of deaths. After a 16-year follow-up in cohort I (Guilford and Edinburgh), a 27 % mortality reduction (RR 0.73, CI 0.63–0.84) was reported. No reduction of mortality could be seen in the two breast self-examination centers. Combining all cohorts aged 45-64 years at entry a 34 % mortality reduction (RR 0.64, CI 0.50–0.86) was achieved. The authors concluded that „there was no evidence that the benefit might be less for those women who entered a screening trial at age 45–46, than for older women; the effect of screening in this age group begins to emerge already after 3–4 years."

Further community-based screening programs (University of California, San Fransisco, Mobile Mammography Screening Program; New Mexico Screening Program; British Columbia Program SMPBC; Uppsala Trial) were able to present age-independent results by use of so-called surrogate measures (tumor size, lymph-node status, ratio of ductal carcinoma in situ and higher staged tumors, sensitivity, specificity).

They thus confirmed the old BCDDP data.

Controversies and Answers

A recently published overview with a de novo analysis of all randomized screening studies tried to question the mortality reduction results.

A critical analysis of this overview article, however, shows that the main critique, which concerned small imbalances of the age distribution (a few months) between the study and control groups, cannot justify the conclusion that eight large randomized trials are invalid. Such differences cannot cause errors of the suspected order.

The fact that the criticism focused on such small imbalances while biases of much greater importance such as contamination of study and control group, patient compliance, screening interval, and image quality were neglected, shows that the real variables of the randomized breast-screening trials were not well understood. This impression is supported by the fact that the trials considered good by the authors were those seen to be flawed by experts in the field.

■ Summary

Ten of the 11 large international studies revealed a definite reduction in the mortality rate of 30% and approaching 70% in women older than 50 years. The only study that failed to show a mortality reduction is the Canadian study whose results, however, must be viewed critically (poor to very poor mammographic quality, insufficient physician training, corresponding delay in diagnosis, inadequate trial design as to randomization). The comparison of older studies with newer studies as well as the results of the Canadian study prove the great importance of excellent image quality and physician training. Furthermore, comparison of the data of the various studies allows the conclusion that screening by mammography combined with physical examination can reduce the mortality of women ages 40 to 49 years, though some believe that statistical confirmation is still lacking. The often considerable differences of the results of the individual studies can be attributed to differences in trial design (mammography alone vs. mammographic–clinical screening, single-view vs. two-view mammography, intervals of 1 to 3 years, randomization vs. case control study, etc.).

All things considered, these studies document excellent effectiveness. No other diagnostic or therapeutic measure so far can show a comparably high reduction in the mortality rates. By further optimizing the image quality and physician training, by employing regular two-view mammography, combined with physical examination whenever possible, and by selecting shorter examination intervals, further improvements can be expected.

Benefit–Risk/Benefit–Costs

■ Benefit–Risk

Our knowledge of the carcinogenic effect of radiation on the breast is based on populations that have been subjected to considerably higher dose levels (1–20 Gy) in comparison to the current mean absorbed parenchymal dose levels of about 2.5 mGy delivered by mammography in two projections. These populations include survivors of the atomic bomb explosions of Hiroshima and Nagasaki, women who had fluoroscopic exposure to one hemithorax exceeding that of the contralateral hemithorax to monitor the therapy of their tuberculosis (Massachusetts, Canada), and women who underwent anti-inflammatory radiation for therapy of mastitis (New York, Sweden).

Any mention of the radiation risk of mammography refers to the *estimated hypothetical and theoretical risk*. These estimates depend on the dose, fractionation, and age at the time of the exposure, as well as on the dose–effect model and latent period, i.e., it is a complex interaction of factors. The most recent report from the National Research Council Committee on the Biological Effects of Ionizing Radiation (BEIR) in 1990 is based on the results of atomic-bomb survivors, fluoroscopic studies performed in Canada and Massachusetts, and mastitis studies conducted in New York. The latent period is stated as 10 years after the exposure, and the assumption is based on age dependence and a linear dose effect relationship because this model encompasses the higher theoretical risk. This implies that repair mechanisms characteristically operative with solar and cosmic radiation remain excluded. Thus, the resultant estimates represent a worst-case scenario.

The estimates are as follows: If 100 000 women had a mammogram (2.5 mGy) at the age of 45 years, at the most one breast carcinoma (that is fatal in about 50%) could be induced throughout the entire life span of these women. This lifelong fatal risk corresponds to the risk of dying from smoking three cigarettes.

This has to be balanced against the fact that 1500 of each 1 million women ages 45 years will develop a breast carcinoma per year owing to the natural incidence of breast carcinomas and that 50% of them will succumb to it. In other words, 750 breast cancer deaths can be expected annually in 1 million women. If these women were subjected to a single screening examination and if a 20%, 40%, and 60% mortality reduction, respectively, is assumed, 150, 300, and 450 breast cancer deaths could be avoided with two-view mammography. A baseline mammogram at the age of 35 years and an annual screening mammogram beginning at the age of 40 years would increase the theoretical risk of a women developing a breast carcinoma in her lifetime from 9.3% (natural incidence) to at most 9.32 to 9.4%.[32, 33]

Therefore, the *theoretical radiation risk* as a disadvantage of regular screening mammography can be *ignored* by the individual woman if she considers the tremendous advantage of early detection, which, in addition to reducing her mortality, can offer her the possibility of breast-preserving therapy as well as possible avoidance of adjuvant therapy. As long as there is neither a primary prevention of breast cancer nor a 100% cure, screening for breast cancer by means of mammography and physical examination is the only and best method to exert a beneficial influence on the biologic course of this disease.

■ Benefit–Costs

Mammographic screening has made it possible to save lives. Even though the value of a woman's life saved from breast cancer cannot be expressed as a benefit–cost estimate, it is necessary to make benefit–cost calculations to obtain the financial support from the society necessary to implement screening programs.

A realistic estimate of the costs expressing the benefit in relation to the calculated numbers of years saved is extremely difficult since many of the determining factors are quite variable and are different to assess.[34]

The following factors are included in the calculation:

- The actual costs of the mammographic screening (costs for the material of single-view and two-view mammography, costs for equipment depreciation, wages for technologists and fees for physicians, frequency of screening examinations, e.g., annually, biannually, triennially).
- The costs of additional examinations (imaging, needle aspiration, surgical excision) performed because of suggestive or unclear findings on the screening examination. In all screening programs, the number of findings requiring further evaluation is considerably higher than that of the ultimately confirmed carcinomas. Thus the costs of workup strongly depend on the false positive rate of the initial screening.

- The effectiveness of the achievable early detection (number of carcinomas actually detected by screening, compiled from the distribution of the stages of the carcinomas and from the stage-dependent survival rates).
- Natural prevalence and mortality of breast carcinoma in the examined population.
- Compliance rate: Since most costs are caused by the examination itself as well as by the ensuing costs of workup mentioned above, the compliance rate has only limited influence on calculating the cost-effectiveness.
- Costs of primary therapy of the carcinoma (percentage of the performed breast-conserving therapies). Unfortunately, breast-conserving therapies, which have increased due to improved early detection, are more expensive than mastectomy and consequently are a cost-raising factor.
- The costs saved by reducing the number of cost-intensive therapies needed for advanced stages of the disease.
- Effect of years gained on the gross national product, on income, and on taxes (cost savings only for years gained before reaching retirement age).

Depending on the healthcare system, these factors vary from country to country.[35] From the above considerations, it is also apparent that the most cost-effective screening program unfortunately will not be the one with the highest detection rate of breast carcinoma. (For instance, more and earlier carcinomas are detected by annual screening in comparison to biannual screening. The number of detected carcinomas, however, increases less than the cost increments due to the additional screening examinations). The technical quality as well as the interpretive quality are of great importance. Both determine not only the number of prognostically favorable carcinomas detected at an early stage but also the false positive rate with its resultant cost-intensive additional examinations performed for confirmation.[36] There are studies that show high fluctuations of the false positive rate from country to country as well as markedly reduced false positive rates for centralized screening units.

Currently, the most cost-effective screening programs appear to be in the Netherlands and Great Britain.[4, 5] But even there, the costs (the screening itself, the ensuing examinations, and the expensive breast-preserving therapies) by far exceed the cost-savings (reduced expenses due to fewer palliative therapies). This means that approximately $3000 to $5000 is spent for each year of patient-life gained. Though these costs are considerable, they can compete with other health-related costs in our society, considering that screening for cervix carcinoma in the same countries is about three times as expensive.[6]

As already mentioned, these results of the Netherlands and Great Britain are not directly applicable to other countries with different populations and, above all, differently structured healthcare systems.

All things considered, the costs of screening and early diagnosis cannot be compensated by cost-savings in palliative therapy. This means that the screening programs, depending on their effectiveness, may induce costs for each year of a woman's life gained. However, in comparison to other healthcare costs, these costs are within an acceptable range. It can therefore be hoped that more countries implement lifesaving screening programs.

Recommendations on the Basis of the Trials

A consortium of American medical organizations including the American Cancer Society has issued the following recommendation: Beginning at age 40 women should undergo screening mammography every year. Physical examination should be part of breast cancer screening.

In Europe, the recommendations for the respective national screening programs differ from country to country. In Great Britain, women between the ages of 50 and 64 years are examined by single-view mammography every 3rd year. In the Netherlands, women between the ages of 50 and 70 years are examined every other year, with two-view mammography initially and single-view mammography thereafter. In Sweden, the screening interval is a year and a half for women ages 40 to 54 years and 2 years for women ages 55 to 74 years. The initial screening examination consists of two-view mammography, followed by single-view mammography. In Finland, women ages 50 to 62 years undergo a two-view mammography at 2-year intervals. In Iceland, the same scheme is used for women ages 40 to 69 years.

In general, screening should only be performed with the highest standard of quality. The intervals should be adapted to the individual risk, the expected tumor doubling time and the incidence. Since breast carcinomas with high growth potential can develop between the ages of *40 and 49 years,* women in this age group should have an annual physical examination and mammography for optimal early detection. *Beginning at the age of 50 years,* the incidence of breast carcinoma increases linearly. This is the reason for annual mammography and physical examination in these age groups. For older women (65 or older) as well as for women with partial or complete parenchymal involution, some have suggested

that the intervals be increased to 2 years. For diagnostic reasons (markedly improved accuaracy, fewer patient recalls because of diagnostic uncertainties), mammography should be performed in two views and combined with a physical examination. This can be concluded from the interval cancer rates reported by centers with single-view mammography.

Scientific studies have not established the upper age limit for screening.

■ References

1   Shapiro S, Venet W, Strax P et al. Periodic Screening for Breast Cancer. The Health Insurance Plan Project and Its Sequelae. 1963–1986; Baltimore: John Hopkins University Press, 1988
2   Shapiro S. Periodic Screening for Breast Cancer: The HIP randomized controlled trial. Monogr Natl Cancer Inst. 1997;22:27–30
3   Tabar L, Fagerberg G, Day NE et al. What is the optimal interval between mammographic screening examinations? An analysis based on the latest results of the Swedish two-county breast cancer screening trial. Br J Cancer. 1987;55:547–51
4   Tabar L, Fagerberg G, Suffy SW et al. Update of the Swedish two-county program of mammographic screening for breast cancer. Radiol Clin North Am. 1992;30:1987
5   Tabar L, Fagerberg G, Chen H-H et al. Efficacy of breast cancer screening by age. New results from the Swedish two-county trial. Cancer. 1995;75:2507–17
6   Tabar L, Fagerberg G, Chen H-H et al. Tumor development, histology and grade of breast cancers: Prognosis and progression. Int J Cancer. 1996;66:413–9
7   Andersson I, Aspregren K, Janzon L et al. Effect of mammographic screening in breast cancer mortality in an urban population in Sweden. Results from the Malmö mammographic screening trial (MMST). Boston Med J. 1988;297:943
8   Andersson I, Aspregren K, Janzon L et al. Mammographic screening and mortality from breast cancer: the Malmö mammographic screening trial. BMJ. 1991;297:943–8
9   Andersson I, Janzon L. Reduced breast cancer mortality in women under age 50: Updated results from the Malmö

mammographic screening program. Monogr Natl Cancer Inst. 1997;22:63–7

10 Frisell J, Eklund G, Hellstrom L et al. Randomised study of mammography screening: preliminary report on mortality in the Stockholm trial. Breast Cancer Res Treat. 1991;18:49–56

11 Frisell J, Lidbrink E. The Stockholm Mammographic Screening Trial: Risks and benefits in age group 40–49 years. Monogr Natl Cancer Inst. 1997;22:49–51

12 Bjurstam N, Björneld L, Duffy SW et al. The Gothenburg breast screening trial. First results on mortality, incidence, and mode of detection for women aged 39–49 years at randomisation. Cancer. 1997;80:2091–9

13 Alexander FE, Anderson TJ, Brown HK et al. The Edinburgh randomised trial of breast cancer screening: results after 10 years of follow-up. Br J Cancer. 1994;70:542

14 Alexander FE, Anderson TJ, Brown HK et al. 14 years follow-up from the Edinburgh randomised trial of breast-cancer screening. The Lancet. 1999;353:1903–8

15 Miller AB, To T, Baines CB et al. The Canadian National Breast Screening Study: update on breast cancer mortality. Monogr Natl Cancer Inst. 1997;22:37–41

16 Otten JDM, v. Deyck J, Peer PGM et al. Long-term breast cancer screening in Nijmegen, the Netherlands: The nine rounds from 1975–1992. Epidemiol Commun Health. 1996;50:353–8

17 Gøtzsche PC, Olsen O. Is screening for breast cancer with mammography justifiable? Lancet. 2000;355:129–34. Discussion and Editorial: Lancet. 2000;355:80–1, 747–58

18 Schreer I, Frischbier HJ. Breast Cancer Screening Projects: Results. In: Radiological Diagnosis of Breast Disease. M Friedrich, EA Sickles, eds. 1997:333–46

19 Smart CR, Hartmann WH, Beahrs OH, Garfinkel L. Insights into breast cancer screening of younger women: evidence from the 14-year follow-up of the Breast Cancer Detection Demonstration Project. Cancer. 1993;72:1449

20 Smart CR, Byrne C, Smith RA et al. Twenty-year follow-up of the breast cancers diagnosed during the Breast Cancer Detection Demonstration Project. CA Cancer J Clin. 1997;47:134–49

21 Blanks RG, Moss SM, Wallis MG. Use of two-view mammography compared with one-view in the detection of small invasive cancers: Further results from the National Health Service Breast Screening Programme. J Med Screening. 1997;4:98–101

22 Hunt KA, Rosen EL, Sickles EA. Outcome analysis for women undergoing annual versus biennial screening mammography: a review of 24, 211 examinations. Am J Roentgenol. 1999;173:285–9

23 Young KC, Wallis MG, Blanks RG, Moss SM. Influence of number of views and mammographic film density on the detection of invasive cancers: results from the NHS Breast Screening Programme. Br J Radiol. 1997;70:482–8

24 Anttinen I, Pamilo M, Soiva M et al. Double reading of mammography screening films: one radiologist or two? Clin Radiol. 1993;48:414–21

25 Wald NJ, Murphy P, Major P et al. UKCCCR multicentre randomized controlled trial of one and two view mammography in breast cancer screening. BMJ. 1995;311:1189–93

26 UK Trial of Early Detection of Breast Cancer Group: 16-year mortality from breast cancer in the UK Trial of early detection of breast cancer. Lancet. 1999;353:1909–14

27 Sickles EA. Breast cancer screening outcomes in women aged 40–49. Clinical experience with service screening using modern mammography. Monogr Natl Cancer Inst. 1997;22:99–104

28 Kerlikowski K, Barclay J. Outcomes of modern screening mammography. Monogr Natl Cancer Inst. 1997;22:105–11

29 Linver MN, Paster SB. Mammography outcomes in a practice setting by age: Prognostic factors, sensitivity, and positive biopsy rate. Monogr Natl Cancer Inst. 1997;22:113–7

30 Thurfjell EL, Lindgren JA. Breast cancer survival rates with mammographic screening: Similar favorable survival rates for women younger and those older 50 years. Radiology. 1996;201:421–6

31 Feig SA, Hendrick RE. Radiation risk from screening mammography of women aged 40–49 years. Monogr Natl Cancer Inst. 1997;22:119–24

32 Jung H. Mammographie und Strahlenrisiko. RöFo. 1998;169:336–43

33 Rosenquist CJ, Lindfors KK. Screening mammography beginning at age 40 years. A reappraisal of cost-effectiveness. Cancer. 1998;88:2235–40

34 v. Ineveld BM, v. Oortmarssen GJ, de Konig HJ et al. How cost-effective is breast cancer screening in different EC countries? Eur J Cancer. 1993;29:1663

35 Elmore JG, Barton MB, Moceri VM et al. Ten-year risk of false positive screening mammograms and clinical breast examinations. N Engl J Med. 1998;16:1089–96

■ Suggested Reading

1 Fletcher SW, Black W, Harris R et al. Report of the International Workshop on screening for breast cancer. J Natl Cancer Inst. 1993;85:1644–56

2 Hendrick RE, Smith RA, Rutledge III JH et al. Benefit of Screening Mammography in Women Aged 40–49: A new meta-analysis of randomized controlled trials. Monogr Natl Cancer Inst. 1997;22:87–92

3 Kerlikowske K, Barclay J. Outcomes of modern screening mammography. Monogr Natl Cancer Inst. 1997:22:105–11

4 Nystrom L, Rutqvist LE, Wall S et al. Breast cancer screening with mammography: orverview of Swedish randomized trials. Lancet. 1993;341:973–78

5 Organising Committee and Collaborators: Breast-cancer screening with mammography in women aged 40–49 years. Int J Cancer. 1996;68:693–9

6 Peer PGM, v. Dijck JAAM, Hendriks JHCL et al. Age-dependent growth rate of primary breast cancer. Cancer. 1993;71:3547–51

7 Sickles EA, Kopans DB. Deficiencies in the analysis of breast cancer data. J Natl Cancer Inst. 1993;85:1621–4

8 Wilson JMG, Jungner G. Principles and practice of screening for disease. Geneva: World Health Organisation (WHO Public Health Paper 34), 1968.

22. Additional Diagnostic Evaluation of Screening Findings and Solving of Problems in Symptomatic Patients

Pathognomonic Findings

(Table 22.1)

■ Definition

The term pathognomonic refers to findings that, without further tests, are diagnostic of a certain histology and consequently do not require surgical confirmation.

■ Incidence

Pathognomonic findings are rare. Most fibroadenomas, for instance, fail to show the mammographically typical calcifications.

■ Typical Findings and Diagnostic Strategy

Pathognomonic findings have to be distinguished from typical findings, which are strongly suggestive of the underlying histology but cannot unequivocally prove it. For probably benign findings, comparison with previous examinations or follow-up mammography at half-year intervals is generally adequate. Malignant findings should be confirmed histologically by surgical or percutaneous biopsy before any therapy is initiated.

Table 22.1 Pathognomonic images

Histologic diagnosis	Characteristic mammographic findings
Lipoma	Focal, round, or oval lesion of fat density with delicate rim (capsule)
Hamartoma	Focal, smoothly outlined lesion containing areas of lipomatous and water density
Oil cyst	Focal radiolucency with surrounding rim (capsule) without/with eggshell-like calcifications
Lymph node	Focal, oval, smoothly outlined density, with — depending on the projection — central or marginal, round radiolucency
Galactocele	Focal, smoothly outlined lesion, composed of fatty components and water-equivalent structures (layering possible), history of pregnancy or lactation
Calcified fibroadenoma	Smoothly outlined, focal density with/without halo, oval, or polylobulated, if containing characteristic calcifications
Cyst containing milk of calcium	Smoothly outlined, focal, rund density with calcifications that project centrally in the craniocaudal view and layer inferiorly on the mediolateral view
Verruca	Smoothly outlined mass exhibiting a cauliflower-like structure (multilobulated) and frequently very sharp borders (soft-tissue–air)
	Characteristic sonographic findings
Cyst	Anechoic, smoothly outlined thin-walled lesion with good distal acoustic enhancement and good compressibility

Differential Diagnosis and Diagnostic Workup

Smoothly Outlined Density

(Fig. 22.**1**)

■ Diagnostic Question

A smooth outline of a density generally speaks for a benign lesion.

Smoothly outlined localized findings seen on screening mammography most frequently represent cysts or fibroadenomas, but 2–7% of all breast carcinomas can be expected to present as a nodule with a partially well-circumscribed margin and 2% with a well-defined outline.

Owing to displacement of surrounding fat by their growth, medullary, papillary, or mucinous carcinomas can give the impression of a capsule and even might have a halo sign (see Fig. 15.**2 e**). In some medullary carcinomas (Type I), the same phenomenon can result in a demarcating capsule-like zone of connective tissue. Furthermore, intracystic carcinomas, metastases, involved lymph nodes, lymphomas, or sarcomas can present as smoothly outlined focal lesions.

■ Diagnostic Strategy

1. The first step of the evaluation addresses the question: Is the lesion within or outside the parenchyma?
   - This can sometimes be answered by inspection, palpation, or routine imaging.
   - If this cannot be unequivocally answered, the tangential coned-down view should be obtained after marking the skin (Fig. 22.**2**).
     Concerning skin changes, see Chapter 17.
   - Overlying structures such as the incidentally visualized contralateral nipple (Fig. 22.**3**) or even the tip of the nose (Fig. 19.**1 f**) are typical artifacts seen as semicircular density in one view only.
2. The smoothly outlined intraparenchymal lesion is further evaluated as to radiodensity.
   - Fat-containing lesions are pathognomonic (lipoma, oil cyst, hamartoma, galactocele, lymph node) and do not require any further diagnostic evaluation.
   - Solitary, smoothly outlined lesions are pathognomonic as long as they exhibit

calcifications characteristic of fibroadenomas. But this is only applicable to a small number of patients. They are observed by follow-up mammography with the intervals determined by the overall observation period available. If no previous films exist, follow-up is usually recommended after 6, 12, 24, and 36 months.

3. The well-circumscribed or fairly well-circumscribed lesion of soft-tissue density needs further evaluation.
   - The simplest approach is the comparison with previous mammograms.[1-4]
   - If a lesion is stable for more than 3 years, no special diagnostic evaluation is necessary. For lesions with shorter observation periods, further follow-up is indicated.
     Since some smoothly outlined malignancies can grow slowly, it is advisable to check a newly discovered lesion at 6, 12, 24, and 36 months to establish stability for a period of 3 years. During this follow-up, it is advisable to always compare with the initial films as well, and not only with the most recent films.
   - A growing lesion or a new well-circumscribed lesion should be evaluated by sonography to determine if it is a simple cyst.
   - If sonography proves a cyst, no further evaluation is needed.
   - If the cystic nature is equivocal, aspiration is indicated.[5]
   - If a sonographically solid lesion is well-circumscribed on mammography and more than 75% of its contour clearly visible without superimposition, short-interval follow-up mammograms are adequate.[6]
   - For the other smoothly outlined solitary lesions found to be solid, further evaluation is needed. Most masses, especially those larger than 5 mm in diameter, should be subjected to percutaneous biopsy for histologic evaluation. If the histology is compatible with a benign entity, further mammographic observation or routine following is adequate.
   - Multiple smoothly outlined lesions indicate benignity, but this is not definitive

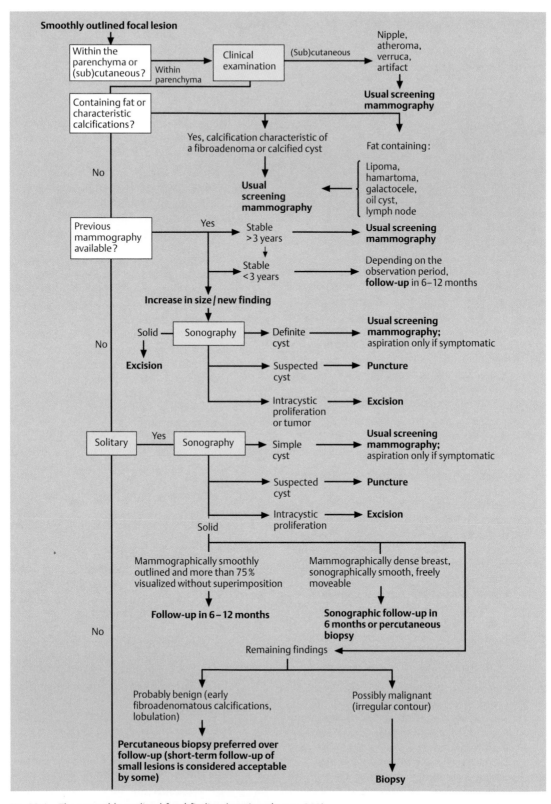

Fig. 22.**1** The smoothly outlined focal finding (continued on p. 399)

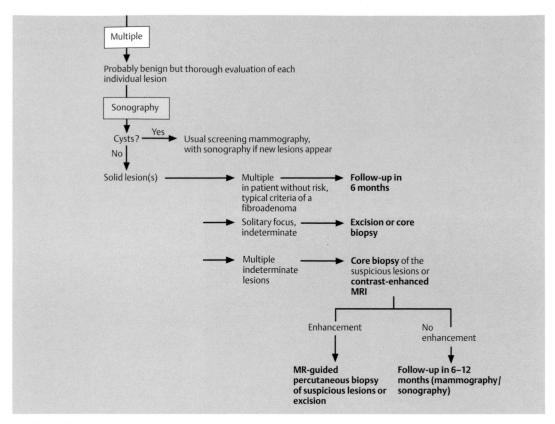

Fig. 22.**1**   (Cont.)

since nodular lesions can, albeit rarely, be the manifestation of multicentric or metastatic disease. Moreover, thorough mammographic–sonographic analysis should be conducted so that a carcinoma is not overlooked amidst multiple benign lesions (Fig. 22.**4**). In individual cases with multiple lesions of concern, MRI may be helpful in demonstrating absence of enhancement (in fibrous fibroadenomas) or in guiding biopsy to the most suspicious lesion (Fig. 22.**5a–d**).[7]

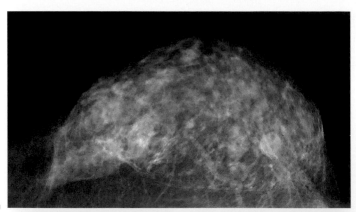

a

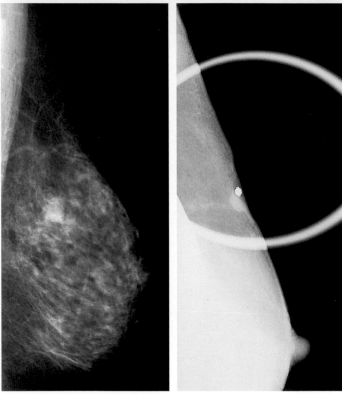

b   c

Fig. 22.**2 a–c**
a The craniocaudal view shows a
10 mm round lesion projecting on the
medial half of the breast, which can
be localized in the upper half of the
breast in the mediolateral view (**b**)
c A tangential compression spot view
after marking of the palpable
atheroma shows superimposition of
marker and lesion (underexposed view
to visualize the skin)

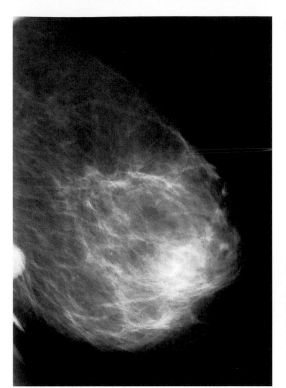

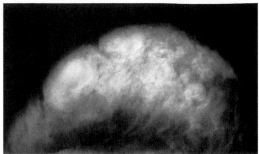

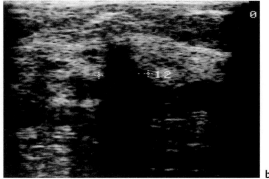

Fig. 22.**3** Incidental visualization of the contralateral nipple, seen as convex density close to the chest wall (mediolateral view)

Fig. 22.**4a** and **b**
a Patient with known fibrocystic changes. Mammography shows lumpy, dense breast tissue unchanged since films. The lumps could be confirmed as representing simple cysts by sonography
b In addition, an irregularly outlined hypoechoic lesion with distal shadowing, measuring 9 mm in diameter, is visualized sonographically within dense surrounding tissue. *Histology:* infiltrating lobular carcinoma

Fig. 22.**5 a–d** Multiple round lesions. This patient had supraclavicular nodal metastases and came for primary tumor search
a and **b** Mammographically (craniocaudal view), several indeterminate masses are seen in the outer quadrants

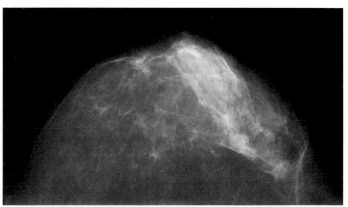

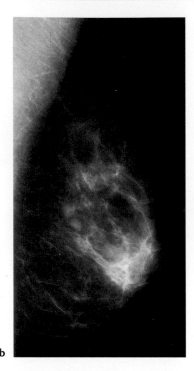

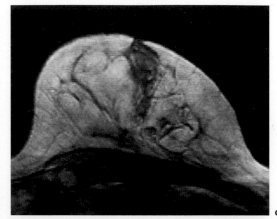

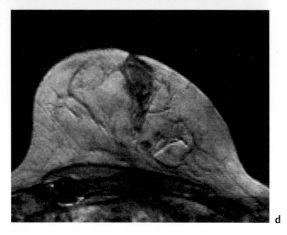

Fig. 22.**5 b–d** A representative MRI section shows two nodules before (**c**) and after (**d**) i.v. administration of Gd-DTPA. Neither nodule shows any appreciable enhancement. These findings are compatible with old fibroadenomas. An excisional biopsy was deferred. Follow-up mammography revealed the lesion to be stable. Further tumor search discovered a gastric carcinoma

Lesions Not Smoothly Outlined

(Fig. 22.**6**)

■ **Diagnostic Problems**

The spectrum of densities not smoothly demarcated includes parenchymal lobules, benign tumors (cyst, fibroadenoma, phyllodes tumor, papilloma, nodular adenosis), localized post-traumatic and post-therapeutic changes (hematoma, fat necrosis, scar), and carcinomas.

■ **Diagnostic Strategy**

1. First, it must be decided whether the finding represents a true lesion or is caused by superimposition or summation.
   - A true mass must be unambiguously as-

signed a spatial dimension in both projections.
   - If seen in one projection only, its focal nature can be confirmed or excluded by one or several spot compression views.
   - Further projections might be helpful, especially the rolled view.

2. If the presence of a real mass is confirmed, previous mammograms should be obtained for comparison of size and radiodensity.[1–3]
   - A finding stable over more than 3 years favors a benign process. For shorter observation periods, further follow-up at 6 to 12-month intervals is necessary.
   - Lesions that are clearly suspicious always need further workup (core or surgical biopsy), even if short-term follow-up shows no change.
   - Any increase in size mandates further evaluation.

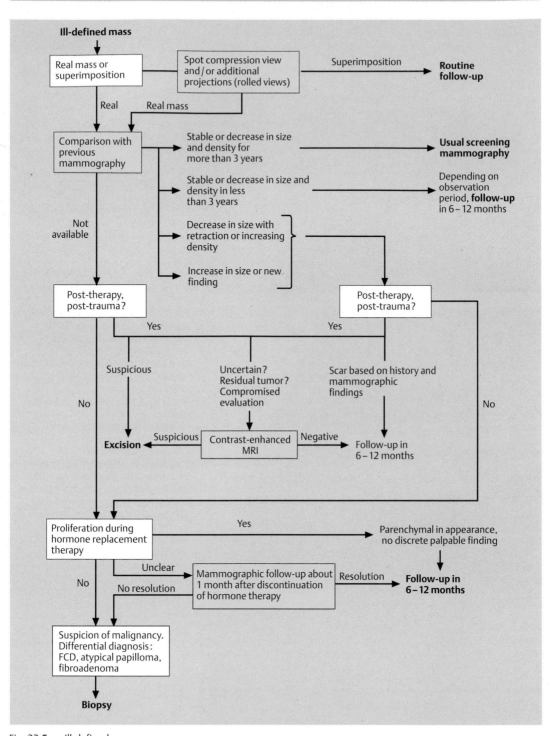

Fig. 22.**6 a**   Ill-defined mass

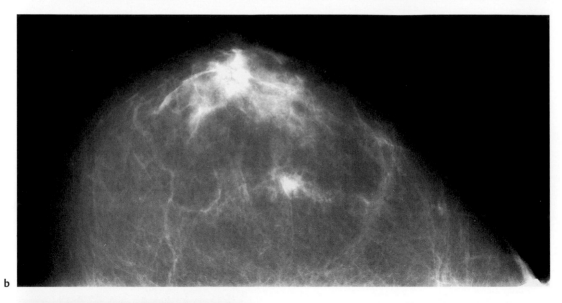

b

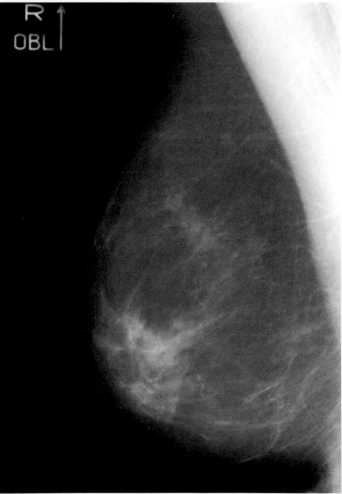

c

Fig. 22.**6 b, c** If an irregular density is noted, it must first be decided, whether this is a mass or superimposed structures.

b On the cc-view there is a somewhat striking density laterally, about 6 cm behind the nipple

c On the MLO-view it becomes clear that the density that was visible on the cc-view is composed of faint densities, which with cc-compression are by chance superimposed.

Based on just 2 views it could be decided that the abnormality turned out to be a composite density, not a mass. If densities resolve completely in further views, no further work-up is indicated. The finding is compatible with superimposition of benign breast tissue.

(*Diagnosis* proven by >3 year follow-up.)

3. Before unnecessary surgery is recommended, it should be determined if a lesion could be hormone-induced.
   - In postmenopausal patients, hormone replacement therapy can induce the growth of cysts or fibroadenomas otherwise not observed in this age group.[8, 9] After hormone therapy has been discontinued, the hormone-stimulated parenchyma very rapidly undergoes involution, usually accompanied by a mammographically visible decrease in size and density of the hormonally induced focal finding.
   - If the focal finding persists after discontinuation of the hormone therapy, biopsy is indicated to establish the diagnosis.

4. Clinical history and physical examination determine whether the findings are post-traumatic or post-therapeutic. In the presence of scarring, the following approach is recommended:
   - As long as clinical and mammographic findings concur, follow-up examinations are adequate.
   - If serial examinations reveal an increase in size, progressing radial configuration, or suspicious microcalcifications, biopsy is indicated.
   - In case of questionable findings or impaired mammographic evaluation or both, MRI can be very helpful since it is able to detect tumor, even within severe scarring, and since it can readily differentiate between tumor and fibrosis.[7, 10–13]

Architectural Distortion

(Fig. 22.**7**)

■ **Diagnostic Questions**

Architectural distortion may be the only sign or an early sign of a carcinoma. Tubular carcinomas characteristically present as a spiculated mass. Absence of a central density is not a reliable sign of benignity. Neoplastic changes must be distinguished from summation effects caused by crossing Cooper's ligaments and from radial structures secondary to post-traumatic/post-therapeutic scarring. Differentiation from radial scars (synonym: sclerosing radial lesion infiltrating epitheliosis), which represent a special manifes-

tation of fibrocystic and proliferative changes, requires excisional biopsy since these can coexist with DCIS, tubular carcinoma, or invasive carcinoma.[14–16]

■ **Diagnostic Strategy**

(Fig. 22.**8** and 22.**9**)

1. First, a scar should be excluded by clinical history and physical examination. Even small incisions for abscess drainage can induce intraparenchymal scars.
   - If clinical and mammographic findings do not completely agree with this diagnosis, previous examinations, including pre-operative mammograms, should, if possible, be obtained for comparison. Knowing the original location of an excised finding is helpful. Periareolar scars are usually not helpful in localizing the site of prior breast surgery.
   - If previous mammograms are not available, if the region of interest is not included, or if the radial structure does not unequivocally coincide with the scar, contrast-enhanced MRI may be helpful (Fig. 22.**9**).
   - An evolving or progressing spiculation is an indication for biopsy. In addition to a carcinoma, post-traumatic fat necrosis must be considered, which can also be manifested as an ill-defined mass or as architectural distortion with or without central density.

2. Architectural distortions that cannot be explained by scarring should be biopsied, even if previous mammograms reveal stability. The reason is that several malignancies, especially tubular carcinoma and carcinoma in situ, present as architectural distortion that can be stable for a long time or can grow very slowly.

3. If architectural distortion is seen in one projection only, superimposition of structures must be excluded by spot compression views or by rolled views. If it is reproducible and remains undetectable in a second or third projectional plane, it must be searched for by spot compression or magnification views in additional projections.
   - Sometimes, supplemental sonography is helpful.[17] Small spiculated carcinomas are often sonographically visualized as irregu-

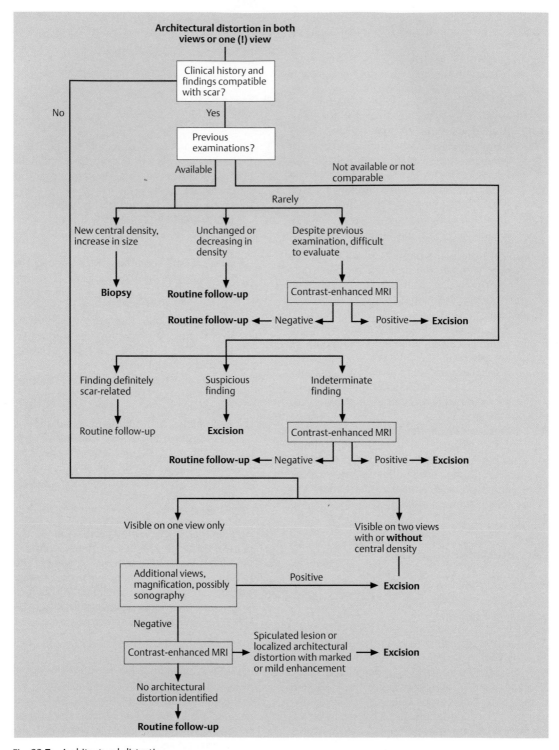

Fig. 22.**7**   Architectural distortion

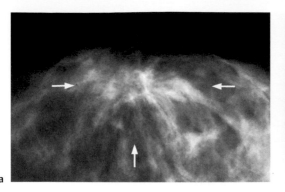

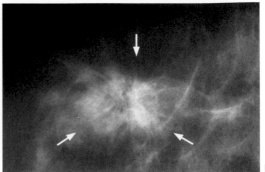

Fig. 22.**8 a–n** Differential diagnosis of architectural distortion

a Patient A: delicate architectural distortion in the retroareolar area, with interposed fat lobules centrally: periareolar scarring.

b Patient B: architectural distortion without central focal density. *Histology:* sclerosing adenosis

c Patient C: relatively thick extensions radiate from an irregularly outlined mass. *Histology:* regressively altered fibroadenoma

d Patient D. This spiculated mass without central density has the characteristic pattern of a radial scar. Biopsy confirmed this diagnosis

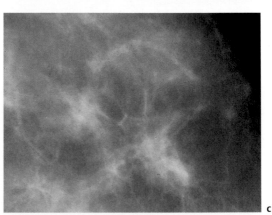

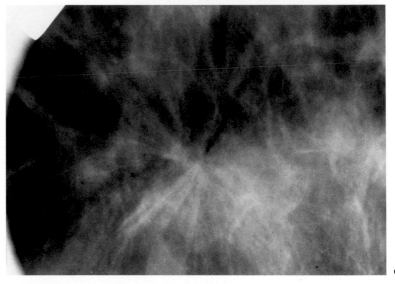

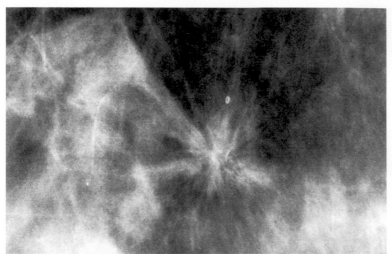

e

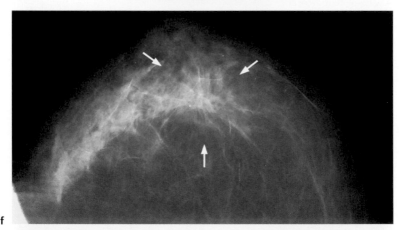

f

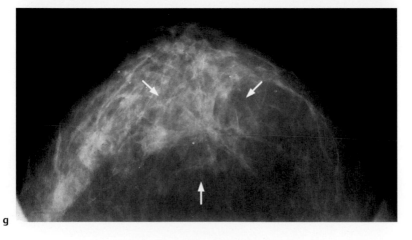

g

Fig. 22.**8 e–g**
e Patient E. This spiculated mass has a similar pattern. However, greater central density and thicker spicules suggest the true diagnosis of infiltrating ductal carcinoma. Definitive differentiation of malignancy from radial scar is not possible based on imaging findings. Biopsy needs to be done to make the final diagnosis.
f Patient F. Clinically, no palpable abnormality. Mammographically, marked architectural distortion
g The same patient, mammography 6 years later. The radial extensions are longer. *Histology:* radial scar

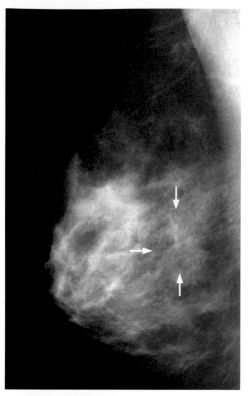

h

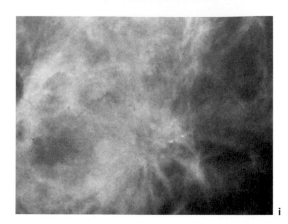

i

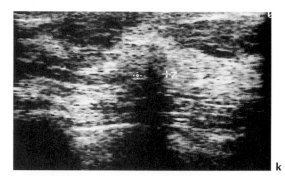

k

Fig. 22.**8 h–k**   Patient G
h Discrete architectural distortion in the upper half of the breast close to the chest wall with very few round calcifications
i Specimen radiography. The architectural distortion as well as the microcalcifications are clearly visible

k Sonographically, a hypoechoic irregularly outlined area, measuring 9 mm in diameter, with acoustic shadowing. *Histology:* atypical ductal epithelial hyperplasia with DCIS measuring 7 mm diameter, malignant lobular transformation

Fig. 22.**8 l**   Patient H: a small focus of distortion in the upper half of the breast. *Histology:* undifferentiated ductal carcinoma measuring 5 mm in diameter

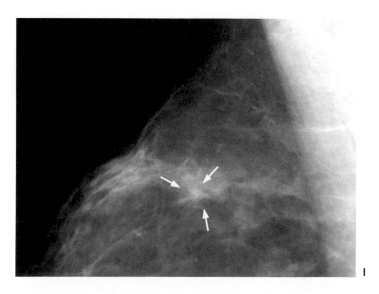

l

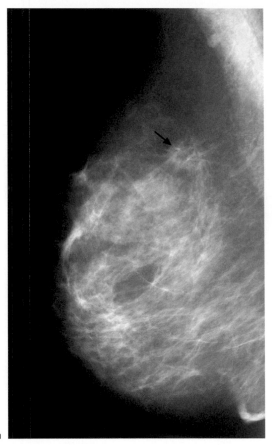

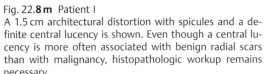

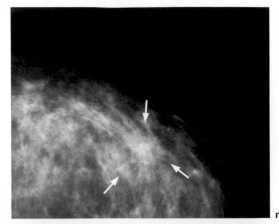

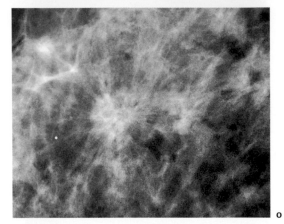

Fig. 22.**8 m** Patient I
A 1.5 cm architectural distortion with spicules and a definite central lucency is shown. Even though a central lucency is more often associated with benign radial scars than with malignancy, histopathologic workup remains necessary
Histology: Ductal carcinoma growing around a fat lobule

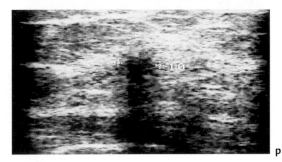

larly outlined, hypoechoic focal lesions with or without distal acoustic shadowing.

– If the exact location of an architectural distortion remains unclear, contrast-enhanced MRI may help by tomographic identification of the area of distortion or by displaying its enhancement behaviour. But it should be kept in mind that even faintly enhancing spiculated structures should be excised since radial scars can harbor carcinomas in situ that might not show strong enhancement.[1]

Fig. 22.**8 n–p** Patient K
n Architectural distortion in the medial half of the breast
o Specimen radiography
p Sonographically, a 10 mm hypoechoic irregularly outlined focus with acoustic shadowing corresponds to the mammographic finding. *Histology:* infiltrating lobular carcinoma measuring 13 mm in diameter

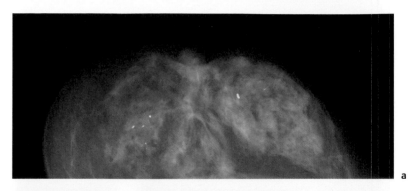

a

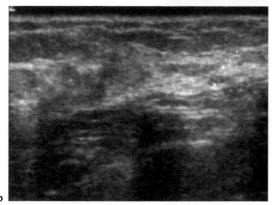

b

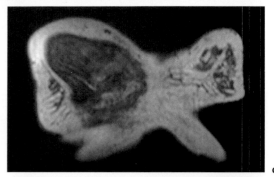

c

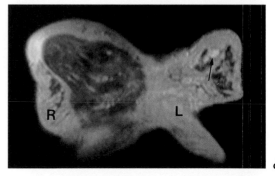

d

Fig. 22.**9 a–d**   Patient with extensive scarring
a–d Patient A
a In addition to extensive scarring, a suspicious nodular density is noted very close to the chest wall. Despite numerous attempts, this finding could not be reproduced in any other view because of compromised positioning due to scarring. This region was not included on previous mammograms. MRI was recommended for further localization of the finding after it could not be delineated sonographically because of scarring and resultant limited evaluation
b Sonographic visualization of scar tissue, no focal findings
c and **d** Prepectoral coronal slice of MRI before (**c**) and after (**d**) administration of contrast medium. While the pectoral muscle is predominantly seen on the right, a highly suspicious enhancement is seen on the left in the prepectoral parenchyma (arrow). The finding was successfully excised after MR-guided localization. *Histology:* ductal carcinoma, 1 cm

Asymmetry

(Fig. 22.**13**)

■ Diagnostic Questions

While asymmetry can be a subtle sign of malignancy, occasionally the only sign,[18] most asymmetry is due to normal breast parenchyma (Fig. 22.**10a–d**).

■ Diagnostic Strategy

If asymmetry is present, it should be closely scrutinized: previous mammograms, if available, can be helpful.

Correlation with the *findings of the physical examination*—which should be assessed with the mammographic findings in mind—is of utmost importance. Mammographic asymmetry due to diffuse growth of a carcinoma is often palpable. It should be remembered that diffusely growing

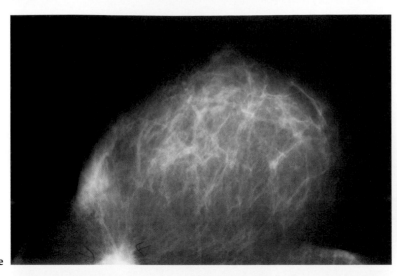

e

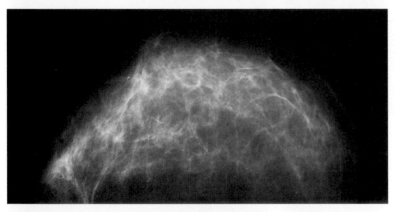

f

Fig. 22.**9 e–h**   Patient B: the role of contrast-enhanced MRI with a worrisome finding and with a preceding mammography, which for technical reasons is not helpful. This patient was referred 1 year after tumorectomy and radiotherapy because of a spiculated focal finding in two projections. (The primary carcinoma did not contain any microcalcifications)

e Current mammography delineates a spiculated density consistent with a scar, but recurrence could not be excluded

f The previous mammogram is of little value since the area is not included

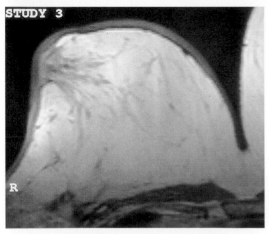

g

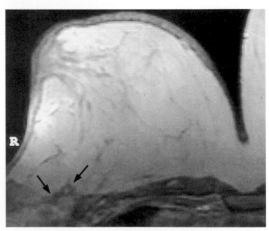

h

g Contrast-enhanced MRI, corresponding section before Gd-DTPA. A spiculated lesion is visualized with high signal in the center before administration of contrast medium. This high signal intensity can be attributed to resolving products of hemoglobinolysis

h The same section as in (**c**) after i.v. administration of Gd-DTPA. There is no appreciable increase in signal intensity, excluding a malignancy with a high degree of certainty. The finding corresponds to scarring with increased signal intensity due to centrally deposited products of hemoglobinolysis

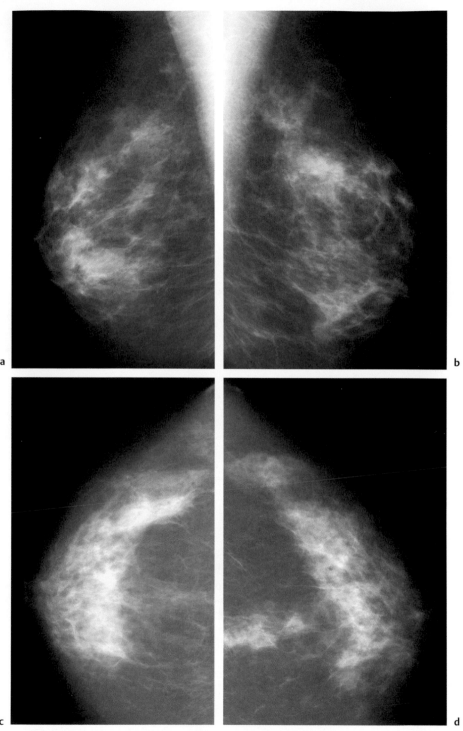

a

b

c

d

Fig. 22.**10 a–d**
a Mammography—oblique view, right
b Mammography—oblique view, left
c Mammography—craniocaudal view, right
d Mammography—craniocaudal view, left

Routine mammography reveals a definite asymmetry me-diocentrally on the left. The presence of regularly dis-tributed fat lobules and the absence of a sonographic and clinically palpable finding speaks against a malignancy with a high degree of certainty

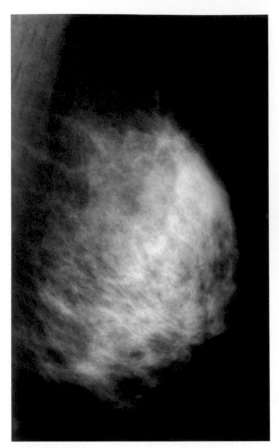
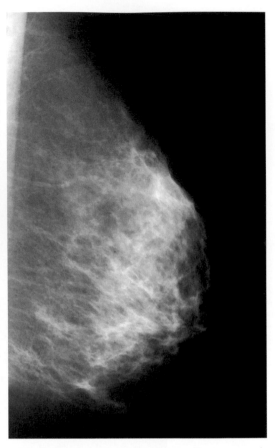

Fig. 22.**11 a** and **b** In this patient, asymmetry has increased during postmenopausal hormone therapy. Return to the initial findings, clinically as well as mammographically, 3 months after discontinuation of the hormone medication

a Mammography during postmenopausal hormone medication
b Mammography 3 months after discontinuation of the hormone medication

carcinomas, such as some lobular carcinomas, might not present as palpable focal lesions but as generalized rubbery, increased consistency or as a focal palpable ridge of tissue. Known asymmetry without a palpable abnormality speaks against an underlying malignancy. It can, however, be difficult to categorize a palpable finding in a diffusely nodular or dense breast.

Sonography[4-5] is a valuable supplemental examination by detecting

– (Or excluding) cysts as cause of the asymmetry
– Possible underlying focal findings in mammographically dense tissue

Postmenopausal hormone therapy[19-21] can produce a pronounced proliferation of the parenchyma, with formation of cysts, lumps, or renewed growth of fibroadenomas.[8, 9] This can accentuate known preexisting asymmetries or lead to the formation of new solid masses or cysts.[22] Since these changes regress after hormone withdrawal, diagnostic problems might be resolved by discontinuing any hormone administration (Figs. 22.**11 a–b**).

Some believe that any *asymmetry* judged *suspicious or indeterminate* should be subjected to *excisional biopsy*. Since diffusely growing carcinomas may be more difficult to successfully sample by percutaneous biopsy and since diffusely growing lobular carcinomas with faint or even lacking contrast enhancement have been reported, *excision should be considered* (Fig. 22.**12**).

The diagnostic approach to asymmetry is summarized in Fig. 22.**13**.

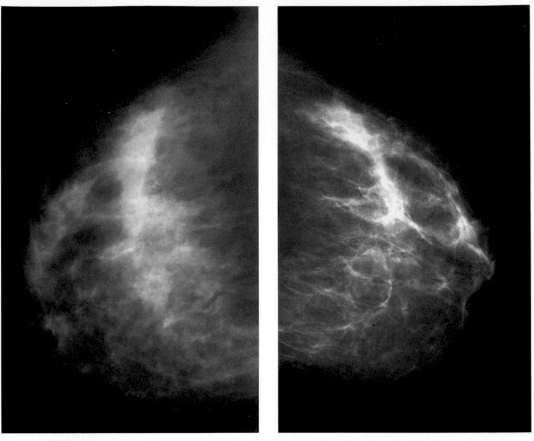

Fig. 22.**11 c** and **d**   The craniocaudal mammograms of a patient with a striking asymmetry are shown. The breast tissue on the right is denser and less distinct.
History: unilateral breast feeding for 2 years.

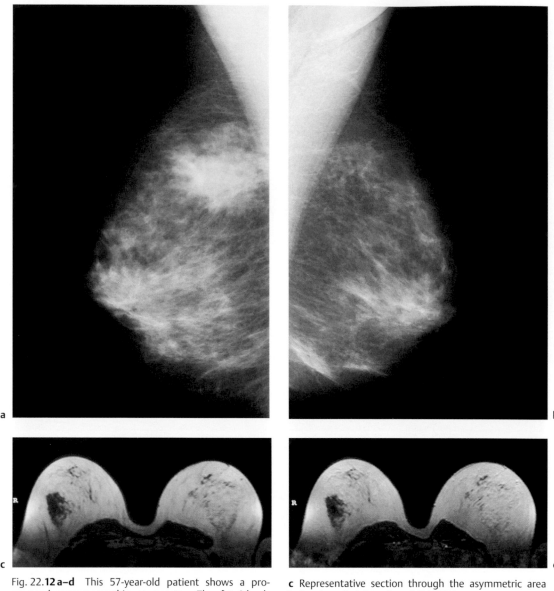

Fig. 22.**12 a–d** This 57-year-old patient shows a pronounced mammographic asymmetry. The fat islands
within the asymmetry as well as the palpable fibrocystic
finding speak for benignity
a and **b** Mammography shows a pronounced asymmetry
on the right in comparison to the left (**b**)

c Representative section through the asymmetric area
before i.v. administration of Gd-DTPA
d The same section as in (**b**) after i.v. injection of Gd-
DTPA shows no appreciable enhancement, supporting the
diagnosis of a benign asymmetry

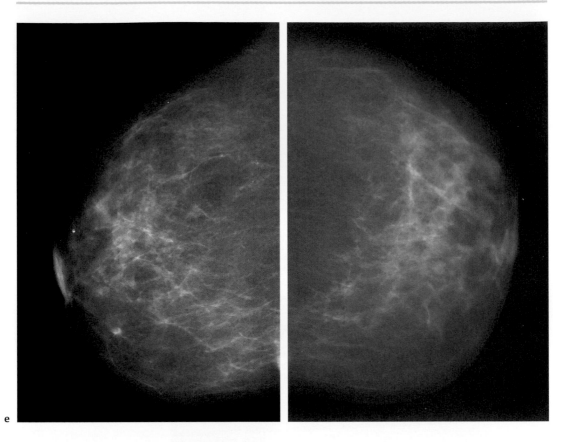

e

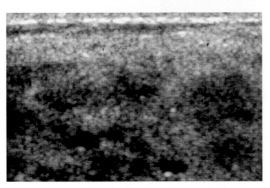

f

Fig. 22.**12 e–h**   This 68-year-old patient presented with a moderate palpable asymmetry and a striking mammographic asymmetry. No microcalcifications (**e**). Ultrasound showed dilated ducts, but was considered inconclusive (**f**).

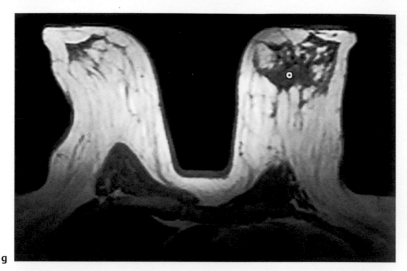

g

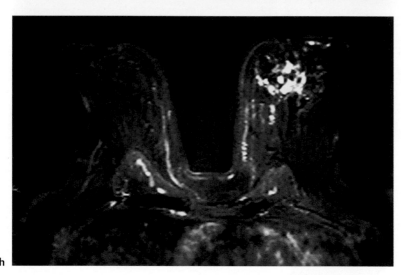

h

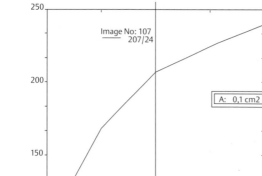

i

Fig. 22.**12 g–i** To determine the best area for percutaneous biopsy, an MRI was performed. A representative image before (**g**) intravenous application of Gd-DTPA is shown, as well as the subtraction image of the same slice (**h**) (= postcontrast minus precontrast)
Strong enhancement is seen which, however, exhibits a delayed enhancement curve (**i**). Even though enhancement is diffuse and delayed and therefore unspecific, malignancy may not be excluded, particularly in view of the striking asymmetry of enhancement. Histology revealed an invasive ductal carcinoma with an extended intraductal component. The latter may explain the unusually discrete clinical findings

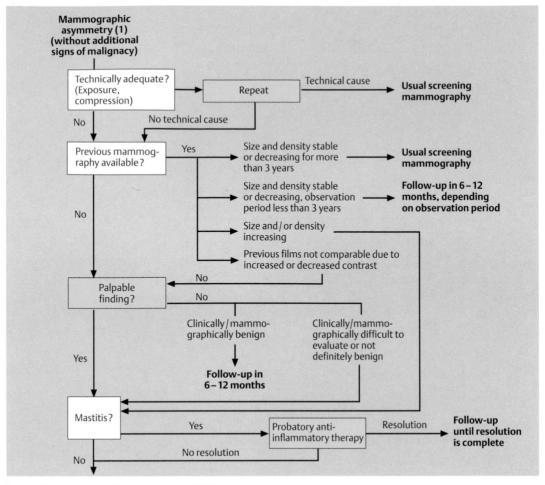

Fig. 22.**13** Asymmetry (continued on p. 420)

The Radiographically Dense Breast

Dense tissue is encountered in a high percentage of patients under the age of 40 years and with decreasing frequency in patients over the age of 50 years.

■ Diagnostic Questions

The problem of the mammographically dense breast is inherent in the inverse relationship between mammographic sensitivity of detecting carcinomas without microcalcifications and increasing radiographic density.[23–25]

■ Dense Breast in Asymptomatic Patients without Increased Risk

■ Diagnostic Strategy and Goals

The indication for imaging these patients is the same as for screening according to patient age and is summarized in Table 22.**2** (see also Chapter 21).

The routine application of sonography and contrast-enhanced MRI is not indicated in these patients.

Indications, possibilities, and limitations of the imaging methods for these patients will be reviewed.

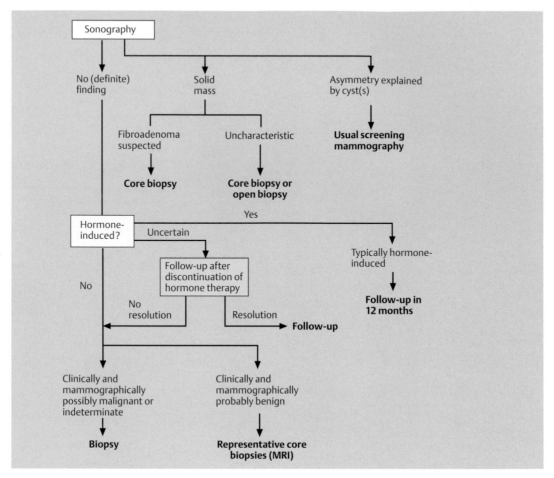

Fig. 22.**13** (continued)

Table 22.**2** Examination of the asymptomatic patient with dense breasts without increased risk, as recommended by the American Cancer Society and the American College of Radiology[117]

Examination for early detection	
Patient < 40 years →	No mammographic screening indicated
Patient ≥ 40 years →	Annual mammogram

■ Mammography

For asymptomatic *patients under the age of 40* without increased risk, screening with mammography is not recommended.

The reasons:

- Low incidence of breast carcinoma in this age group. The incidence of breast carcinoma is less than 1/10 000 for the 25-year-old woman, while it exceeds 10/10 000 for the woman over 50.[91]
- Limited sensitivity of mammography in this age group because of dense parenchyma.
- Increased radiosensitivity of the juvenile parenchyma (see also p. 454–5).

Screening of *women 40 to 50 years of age* is currently still under discussion. Since most of the initial randomized trials predominantly included women above age 50, fewer data existed. Furthermore—probably because the percentage of DCIS among the detected carcinomas is higher below than above age 50—the effect of screening on mortality reduction became apparent after a longer lag time (> 8 years) than for women below 50. In addition—due to the higher percentage of more aggressive faster growing breast tumors in

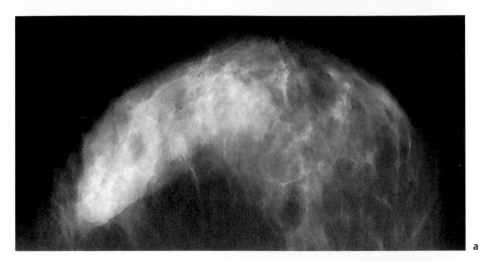

a

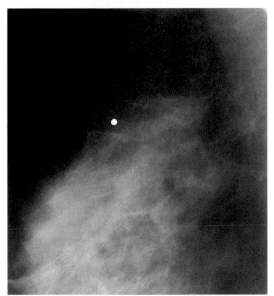

b

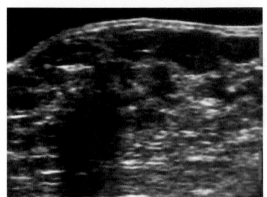

c

Fig. 22.**14 a–c**   Patient with suspicious palpable finding in the upper outer quadrant
a and **b** Mammography (**a** = craniocaudal, **b** = oblique view, coned magnification) shows dense tissue in the area (marked by lead BB) of a palpable mass. The tissue appears slightly less lucent than the contralateral side but without discernible focal finding or calcifications suggestive of malignancy
c Sonography of the palpable finding reveals a suscipious hypoechoic area measuring about 2 cm. *Histology:* ductal carcinoma, 2.1 cm in size

the 40–49-year-old patients—a screening interval of 12–18 months would probably be much more effective for mortality reduction than the screening interval of 2 years, which was used in most randomized trials.[27, 28] In spite of the described difficulties of interpretation, increasing data exist which do show significant mortality reduction for the 40–49-year-old women.[29–31]

From the medical standpoint, women should be included in a screening program beginning at the age of 40 years. Whether this is socioeconomically feasible is to be addressed separately.

Owing to the more rapid growth of premenopausal breast cancers, these women should be screened annually.[27, 28]

Asymptomatic *patients over the age of 50 years* should undergo mammographic screening at intervals of 1 to 2 years. In the United States, it is recommended that these women be screened annually.

Screening the mammographically dense breast is worthwhile. Even in the very dense breast, microcalcifications can be reliably detected as important evidence of a carcinoma. Noncalcified

Table 22.**3**   Further procedure depending on findings

Mammography and palpation unremarkable	→ No immediate further workup, age-dependent follow-up
Positive palpable finding	→ Figure 22.**19 a**
Positive mammographic finding: microcalcifications	→ Figure 22.**42**
smoothly outlined focal lesion	→ Figure 22.**1**
ill-definded mass	→ Figure 22.**6 a**
architectural distortion	→ Figure 22.**7**
asymmetry	→ Figure 22.**13**

carcinomas can become visible if they have induced retraction or parenchymal bulging, or if they are of increased density relative to the surrounding tissue, or located at the periphery of the cone of dense breast-tissue.

Because of the more difficult detection of small noncalcified carcinomas within mammographically dense tissue, physical examination of these patients plays a more important role.

■ **Supplemental Methods**

In mammographically dense tissue, using additional imaging methods is not indicated for asymptomatic patients. Because of the decreased sensitivity of mammography, it would be desirable to obtain additional information, but neither sonography nor contrast-enhanced MRI is suitable or approved to replace or routinely complement mammography.

Even though some interesting results have been presented by a few very experienced sonographers,[32, 33] there exists no validation yet that would justify the use of sonography for any type of screening. Sonography is operator-dependent. It is more time-consuming than mammography and the problem of quality assurance is not yet solved. There is no justification to use sonography instead of mammography, since—even with high resolution sonography—the sensitivity for small lesions and DCIS is too low.[34-38] Even if sonography were used in conjunction with mammography, numerous false positive calls might result per nonpalpable carcinoma detected in addition to mammography.[32, 33]

Contrast-enhanced MRI is not useful in this patient group. Apart from the high costs, an unacceptably large number of false positive findings can be expected in asymptomatic and younger patients. False negative findings can occur if the

threshold for diagnosing a carcinoma has been increased to avoid false positive findings.

■ **Further Approach Depending on the Findings**

If an asymptomatic patient turns out to be symptomatic because of a newly detected palpable or mammographic finding, further workup is indicated, as summarized in Table 22.**3**.

■ **Dense Breast in Asymptomatic Patients with High Risk**

■ **Diagnostic Strategy and Goals**

If the *risk of developing a breast carcinoma is definitely increased* because of the patient's clinical history (prior breast carcinoma or proliferative mastopathy with atypias) or family history (breast carcinoma in a mother, father, or sibling, especially if bilateral, several affected relatives, or premenopausal occurrence and especially if relatives were affected before age 30 (see pp. 3–7)), then an *individually tailored survey seems appropriate.* That is, yearly mammographic screening starting at a young age (depending on the individual risk) should be considered.

■ **Mammography and Clinical Findings**

Regular mammography is the most important prerequisite for an effective early cancer detection:

– Mammography—depending on the individual risk is beneficial even before the age of 40 years
– Beginning at the age of 40–50 years, annual mammography is recommended[29-31]
– Physical examination of the breast tissue plays an important role, in particular, if the parenchyma is very dense

Fig. 22.**15 a–d** Advantages of contrast-enhanced MRI for following the dense breast (increased risk). This patient is status after right-breast carcinoma and underwent bilateral mammography. Because of an indeterminate finding in the irradiated right breast, contrast-enhanced MRI was performed, incidentally visualizing a suspicious finding in the left breast

a Contrast-enhanced MRI before i.v. application of Gd-DTPA. This is the same slice as shown in (**b**). The section of the irradiated right breast is only partially imaged on this slice because of post-therapeutic volume loss and retraction towards the chest wall

b After i.v. injection of contrast medium, an early irregularly outlined and thus suspicious enhancement is seen at 12 o'clock in the left breast

c Craniocaudal mammography, left breast
Histology: 1 cm ductal carcinoma

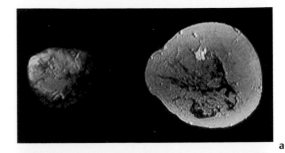

a

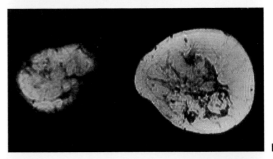

b

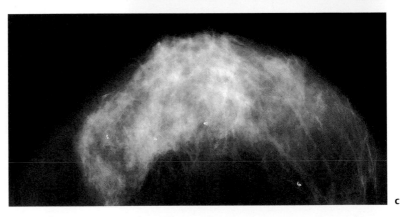

c

– The potential use of further imaging modalities, such as ultrasound and MRI is presently under investigation in several national studies.[40–44] It is recommended to refer patients at risk (definition, see p. 6) to such studies to allow evaluation of these methods (additional cancers detected, false negatives, false positives, additional workup initiated) and to thus offer the patient the most appropriate workup for the individual risk profile avoiding both under and overdiagnosis.

■ Sonography and Percutaneous Biopsy

To evaluate worrisome palpable findings, asymmetries, or densities, *sonography* and, when indicated, *percutaneous biopsy* should be generously employed in these patients.[32–39, 54–62]

■ Contrast-enhanced MRI

In mammographically dense tissue, combining mammography and contrast-enhanced MRI achieves the highest sensitivity *for detecting or excluding additional invasive foci* in the ipsilateral or contralateral breast (Figs. 22.**15 a–d**, 22.**16 a–d**, and 22.**18**; see also Figs. 15.**14 a** and **b**).[7, 50–53, 122–127] Since contrast-enhanced MRI has only a moderate specificity and consequently leads to numerous diagnostic biopsies, its usefulness in diagnosing the mammographically dense breast still needs further evaluation for the various risk groups:

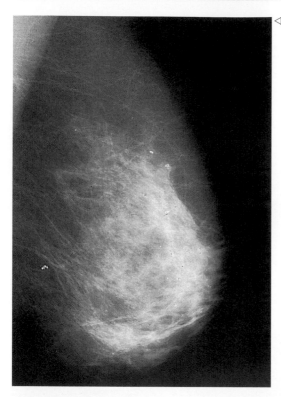

◁ Fig. 22.**15 d** Mediolateral view, left breast. Outside mammography, which was obtained without clinical suspicion, reveals no evidence of malignancy and would not have prompted any further investigation. Retrospectively reviewed, sonography reveals no focal finding. *Histology:* ductal carcinoma

Fig. 22.**16 a–d** Assessing extent of and detecting additional foci in the mammographically dense breast. *Histology:* multifocal papillary carcinoma. Patient with a suspicious palpable finding behind and medial to the nipple following excisional biopsy of a benign lesion 3 years ago. Though the area is sonographically hypoechoic and thus considered suspect, supplemental MRI was ordered because of impaired evaluation of the surgically altered retroareolar region
a and **b** Mammography, craniocaudal, and oblique views show very dense tissue with cicatricial retraction
c MRI section at the level of the palpable finding in the region of the scar before administration of Gd-DTPA
▽

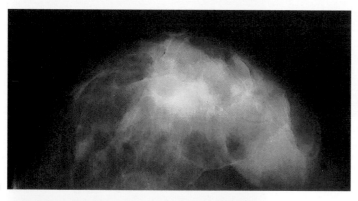

a

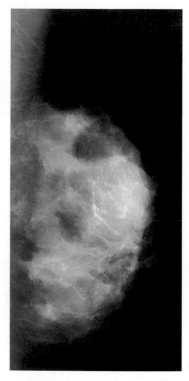

b

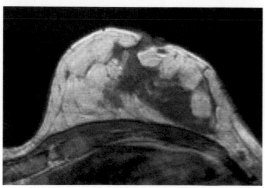

c

Fig. 22.**16 d** The same level after Gd-DTPA shows highly ▷
suspicious enhancement in the palpable finding. Also visualized are several additional foci of suspicious enhancement, neither suspected clinically nor by any other
method. *Histology:* multicentric lobular carcinoma

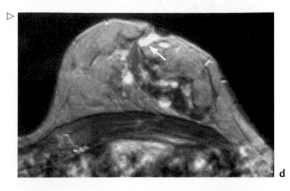

d

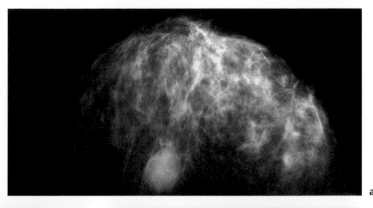

a

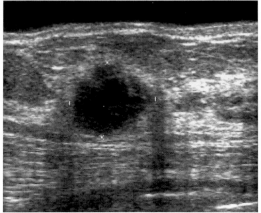

c

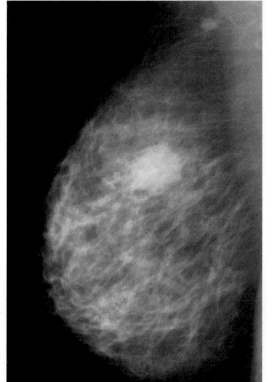

b

Fig. 22.**17** This 61-year-old patient presented with a palpable lump of approximately 3 cm. Based on the patient's
age, on its partly smooth borders, which were to some
degree superimposed by breast tissue, the lesion had to
be considered suspicious (BI-RADS 4)
b Craniocaudal and MLO outside mammogram
c Ultrasound was performed to guide percutaneous core
needle biopsy. No additional focus was noted
Fig. 22.**17 d–h** ▷

Fig. 22.**17 d–h**

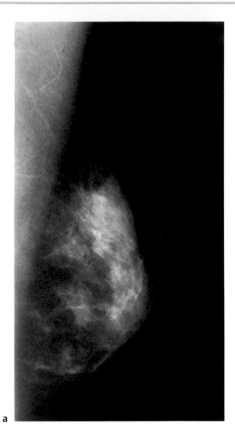

a

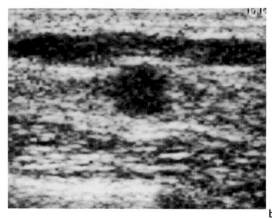

b

Fig. 22.**18 a** and **b** This is a 33-year-old patient with newly discovered palpable finding in the upper outer quadrant. *Histology:* phyllodes tumor
a The palpable finding is mammographically obscured within the very dense juvenile parenchyma, not excluding a tumor
b Sonographically round nodule, not completely well-demarcated within the hyperechoic parenchyma and indenting the subcutaneous space (not surrounded by reactive changes). Because of the round configuration with moderate moveability and an indistinct outline, an excisional biopsy was ordered

◁ Fig. 22.**17 d** Contrast-enhanced MRI was performed to check for multicentricitiy. (A coronal MR subtraction image is shown.) It demonstrates the fairly well-circumscribed main tumor at 12 o'clock and two small additional foci at 9 and 6 o'clock. (Further enhancing foci were noted in other areas as well)
e and **f** Small enhancing foci may be caused by malignancy or benign changes. Therefore, histologic proof is necessary before further therapeutic decisions are made
In this case, two representative foci were marked under MR guidance. First the breast is positioned in the biopsy coil using moderate compression and imaging is performed to find *lesion 1*(**e**) (arrow) and *lesion 2*(**f**). *Both lesions* are shown on transverse subtraction images (postcontrast minus precontrast)
g and **h** The needle is then positioned and another MR sequence is obtained showing the wire in place in *lesion 1*(**g**) and in *lesion 2* (**h**) Histology of the main tumor was invasive ductal carcinoma. The additional foci proved to be ductal carcinoma in situ. The patient decided against breast conservation and was treated by mastectomy and breast reconstruction.

- Initial trials evaluating the complementary role of contrast-enhanced MRI before surgery (exclusion of additional foci)[122–127] and in the follow-up care (status post radiation as well as concurrent evaluation of the contralateral breast)[7, 50, 127] suggest a diagnostic gain by detecting relevant additional cancers
- The potential role of contrast-enhanced MRI in genetic risk patients is presently under investigation.[40–44]

If contrast-enhanced MRI reveals suspicious enhancement in a nonpalpable finding, this has to be further evaluated by MR-guided core biopsy or by preoperative localization.[45–49] It would be inappropriate to recommend a biopsy without preceding localization or even a mastectomy on the basis of an MR-demonstrated enhancement, since enhancement can also be observed in benign changes.

■ Dense Breast with Palpable Finding

(Fig. 22.**19 a**)

■ The Role of the Palpable Finding and Diagnostic Problems in the Dense Breast

Palpable findings need to be worked up to determine their clinical relevance. Only about 20% of palpable masses that are excised turn out to be malignant. The imaging workup is undertaken to try to establish the diagnosis of the palpable mass and whether cancer is present elsewhere in the breast.

■ Diagnostic Strategy and Goals

Our customary approach for evaluating a palpable finding in a mammographically dense breast is summarized in Figure 22.**19 a**. As already mentioned, pragmatic deviations may be useful and can be applied depending on the experience and specific knowledge of the diagnostic team and the particular question posed by the individual case.

■ Mammography

Even in mammographically dense breasts, some palpable lesions can be characterized.
    Carcinomas can be detected in dense parenchyma if they

– contain microcalcifications (high sensitivity even of nonpalpable small carcinomas!), or
– cause increased density, parenchymal asymmetry, architectural distortion, or bulging of the parenchyma.

Opaque skin-markers should be placed over palpable lesions so they can be localized on the mammogram.
    If a palpable finding corresponds to a mammographic abnormality (rarely the case) that exhibits the pathognomonic features of a lipoma, calcified fibroadenoma, lymph node, galactocele, or oil cyst, mammography allows the positive exclusion of a malignancy even in the mammographically dense breast, and an excision can be avoided.
    The sensitivity of mammography for detecting a carcinoma without microcalcification decreases with increasing radiodensity of the tissue.[23–26]
    Therefore:
    A carcinoma cannot be excluded mammographically in radiodense tissue in the presence of a questionable or definite palpable abnormality (except for the rare benign findings that are pathognomonic). This applies to any area which is isodense to the parenchyma that is not fat equivalent.
    Mammography should not, however, be omitted in the woman with a dense breast with a palpable abnormality (exception: a very young patient with a recent mammogram). In the woman undergoing breast surgery, preoperative mammography is indicated to detect or exclude additional abnormal areas that should be sampled in the ipsilateral or contralateral breast.

■ Sonography

Since cysts are anechoic and most tumors hypoechoic and since dense glandular or fibrous tissue is hyperechoic, *sonography can provide relevant complementary information for the evaluation of palpable findings, especially in mammographically dense tissue.*
    Sonography is useful for all abnormal palpable findings in mammographic dense tissue since:

– Definitive demonstration of cysts can avoid unnecessary biopsy.[4, 5]
– Hypoechoic *lesions can be percutaneously biopsied under sonographic guidance.* By documenting the correct position of the needle to the lesion sonographically, accuracy can be considerably improved in comparison with conventional puncture of palpable lesions without image guidance. Otherwise, small and deep lying palpable lesions can be missed, as they may escape from the advancing needle.
– Very easily moveable, smoothly outlined lesions with a pseudocapsule, homogeneous echo texture, and good distal enhancement are very suggestive of a fibroadenoma.[5, 39] Primarily in very young patients, follow-up or—in case of any doubts—complementary percutaneous biopsy should be considered as appropriate care for these women.

But:

– For all other hypoechoic findings that are clinically not definitely benign as well as for findings without sonographic findings, sonography cannot exclude a malignancy. Therefore, percutaneous biopsy or excision should be considered for these cases (Figs. 22.**18a–b**, see also Figs. 15.**13c–d**).

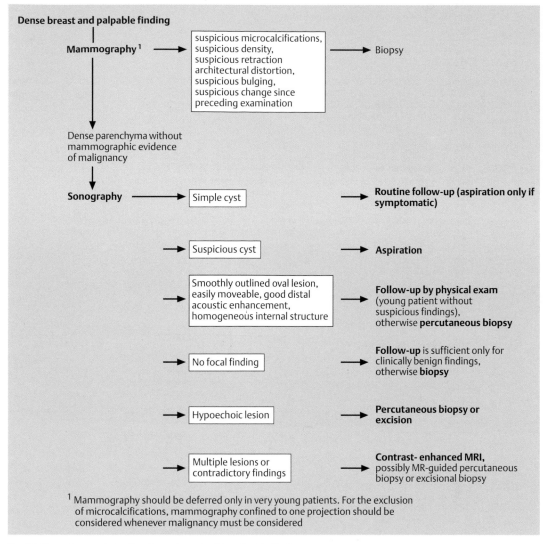

Fig. 22,**19 a** Approach to the dense breast with palpable finding

Since sonography cannot exclude a malignancy with sufficient certainty and, consequently, most noncystic lesions undergo percutaneous biopsy or excision anyhow, it may be tempting to omit sonography and proceed directly to percutaneous biopsy. This principle, however, forgoes the very simple noninvasive exclusion of a malignancy be demonstrating cysts or even a cluster of cysts.

■ Percutaneous Biopsy

Percutaneous biopsy is increasingly utilized for further evaluation of indeterminate findings palpated in mammographically dense breasts. In ex-

perienced hands, this can save costs by avoiding excisional biopsies of benign lesions.

The excellent accuracy described in recent literature (see Chapter 7) is essential for the diagnostic decision and can be achieved only when the following conditions are met:

- Adequate experience of the diagnostic team
- Optimal technique to ensure procurement of an adequate specimen (e.g., needle, diameter, length of the tissue cylinder, and insertion speed of the needle for biopsy see Chapter 7)
- Broad experience of the pathologist and—in particular, the cytologist—as well as of the

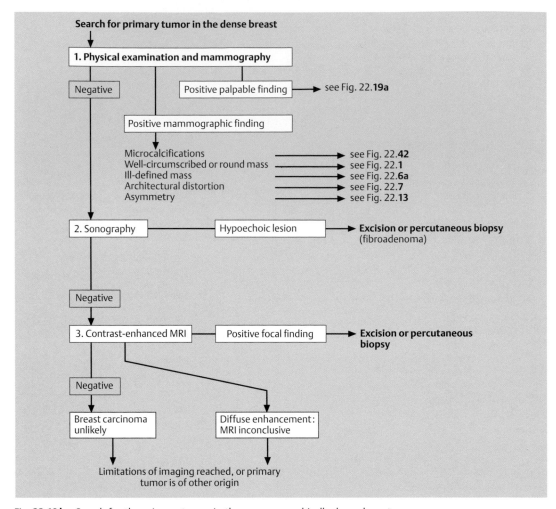

Fig. 22.**19 b** Search for the primary tumor in the mammographically dense breast

radiologist who performs the percutaneous puncture so that results comparable to those published in the literature can be obtained

● Quality assurance to maintain quality of care
● Adequate experience and direct communication between radiologist and pathologist/cytologist. This assessment considers:
– Whether an adequate specimen has been obtained
– Whether the obtained specimen corresponds to the finding in question, i.e., whether it is representative
– The known accuracy of the biopsy technique used
– Clinical and mammographic correlation

If these conditions are fulfilled, high accuracy approaching that of excisional biopsy can be expected.

It is important that *a suspicious finding should not be dismissed on the basis of a negative percutaneous biopsy.*

■ Contrast-enhanced MRI

Though the combination of mammography and contrast-enhanced MRI is highly sensitive and detects even small carcinomas, contrast-enhanced MRI should not be considered the primary method to supplement mammography in the evaluation of a palpable finding in the dense breast. The reasons are the considerably higher false positive rate of contrast-enhanced MRI in comparison with percutaneous biopsy and the relatively high proportion of patients (about 25%) with diffuse enhancement that precludes a definitive diagnosis, as well as the high cost of the examination.

The use of contrast-enhanced MRI is appropriate in patients with:

- Extensive scars and unclear palpable findings (status post surgery, implants, or radiation). A false positive diagnosis of cancer when the lesion represents old scar tissue (except for cases with fat necrosis) is rare with MRI. Small recurrences can be detected early.
- Multiple questionable findings, in particular when the results of other modalities are contradictory. The pattern of enhancement can serve to find or select suscipious areas for a targeted percutaneous biopsy.

■ Dense Breast and Special Considerations

■ Pain

Pain, especially when it varies with the menstrual cycle, is a frequent manifestation of fibrocystic alteration. It usually is bilateral and more severe in the upper outer quadrants. If a thorough mammographic and clinical evaluation is negative, the patient should be informed of the probable hormonal cause and be reassured. In general, this pain is not a manifestation of a malignancy.

If the patient complains of localized pain, experienced as "crawling ants" or a "creeping sensation" and it appears essentially unrelated to the menstrual cycle, it should be taken seriously and deserves further evaluation just like a palpable abnormality.

■ Search for Primary Tumor

In the woman with an axillary nodal metastasis and no palpable lesion in the breast to suggest a primary mammary carcinoma, clinical imaging in the usual order is indicated.

If mammography fails to identify the primary lesion in the breast, supplemental methods, such as sonography and, if sonography is negative, contrast-enhanced MRI can be helpful[50-53] (Figs. 22.**19**a and 22.**20**a–d).

If contrast-enhanced MRI is negative or inconclusive because of diffuse enhancement, breast imaging has reached its limitation, or the primary tumor is not in the breast. In the majority of these rare cases, the primary tumor is indeed found in other organs and, consequently, searching for a

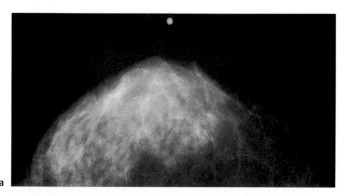

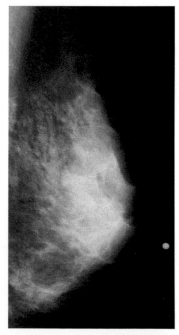

Fig. 22.**20**a–d   This patient with unremarkable mammographic, sonographic, and clinical findings was referred to MRI for search of a primary tumor because of metastatic axillary lymphadenopathy
a and **b** Slightly impaired evaluation because of mammographically moderately dense parenchyma (craniocaudal and mediolateral views). Sonography also failed to detect any underlying malignancy

Fig. 22.**20**c, d ▷

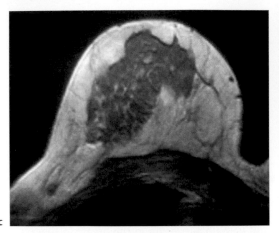

c

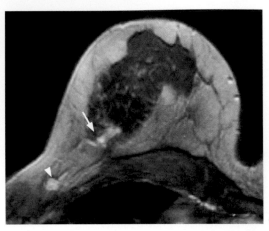

d

Fig. 22.**20 c** Representative section before administration of Gd-DTPA

d The same section as shown in (**c**) after administration of Gd-DTPA discloses within the nonenhancing parenchyma a highly suspicious, strongly enhancing lesion (arrow). An additional second strongly enhancing lesion with small extensions is noted in the prepectoral region. Both MRI-suspicious lesions were localized for the surgeon under MR-guidance. Histologically, a small ductal carcinoma (arrow) could be confirmed as well as an involved intramammary lymph node (arrowhead) (from Heywang-Köbrunner et al.[7])

primary tumor in other organs is appropriate in the presence of an axillary nodal metastasis. This also applies to adenocarcinomatous or even hormone-receptor positive metastases. (Depending on the method used for hormone-receptor analysis, carcinomas of other origin, rarely even lymphomas, can be hormone-receptor positive).

■ **Nipple Retraction**

Nipple retraction has to be evaluated carefully. Since a high percentage of new, unilateral nipple retraction is induced by an underlying carcinoma, supplemental mammographic views, sonography and, if needed, contrast-enhanced MRI, should be employed. (Figs. 22.**21** and 22.**22**, see also Figs. 15.**4 b**, 15.**5 a**).

■ **Discharge**

Discharge of the dense breast is guided by the same differential diagnostic considerations as discharge found in the breast of normal parenchymal density (see p. 453).

Fig. 22.**21 a–d**   This 61-year-old patient came for screening mammography. The patient had noticed the unilateral nipple retraction "for a long time." No evidence of a palpable finding or discharge
a Oblique view
b Craniocaudal view
A discrete architectural distortion was suspected in the retroareolar region on the craniocaudal view only. Because of this finding and the unilaterality of the nipple retraction, magnification views in two planes were performed

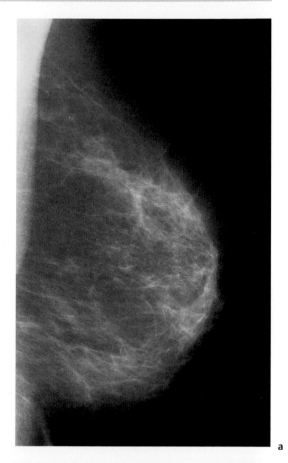

a

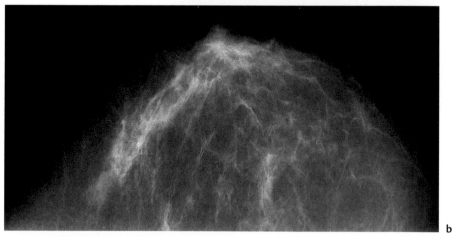

b

Fig. 22.**21 c** and **d** ▷

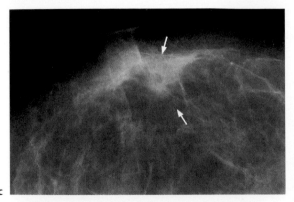

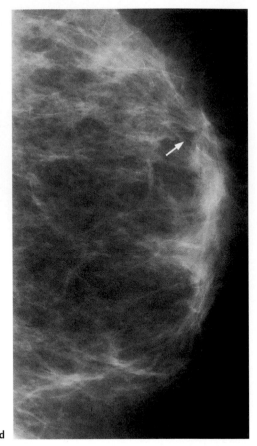

c

Fig. 22.**21 c** The spot compression clearly discloses the carcinoma as typical spiculated lesion

Fig. 22.**21 d** Only the magnification view in the oblique projection can positively localize the carcinoma (cranial) in the second plane. *Histology:* ductal carcinoma (mammography by Dr. D. Breuer, Halle, Germany)

d

Microcalcifications

(Fig. 22.**42**)

■ Possibilities and limitations of diagnostic methods

■ Mammography

Mammography is the only diagnostic method that can reliably detect calcifications suggestive for malignancy. Detecting calcifications is of great importance because about 30–40% of carcinomas harbor microcalcifications and since these carcinomas, because of the microcalcifications, are often discovered in a very early stage, frequently in a preinvasive stage (DCIS). The problem, however, is that a *considerable number of benign changes also contain microcalcifications.* The indiscriminate excision of all microcalcifications would yield a carcinoma in only every 10th to 20th specimen. Such a high number of diagnostic biopsies can be justified neither medically nor economically. Therefore, the presence of microcalcifications should not invariably lead to a recommendation to biopsy.

Technical Requirements for Mammographic Detection and Differential Diagnosis of Microcalcifications

Correct exposure is particularly important since underexposure can render microcalcifications undetectable within dense tissue (see p. 23).

Adequate compression is equally important since it improves sharpness and contrast (see pp. 39–40).

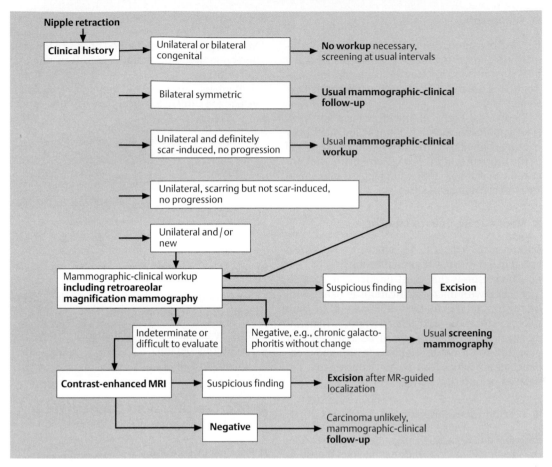

Fig. 22.**22** Nipple retraction of the mammographically dense breast

Magnification mammography. Its use yields a better morphologic evaluation and often the detection of additional fine calcifications. Thus, it improves the differentiation between calcifications judged to be benign or suspicious for malignancy, increases the identification of carcinomas, and helps to reduce the number of unnecessary biopsies. Moreover, *determining the exact extent* of the carcinoma may be decisively improved by magnification mammography.

Future Technical Improvements

The continued development of *digital imaging* may result in better visualization of masses and microcalcifications in the future. Digital imaging receptors can improve the image contrast within mammographically dense tissue through their linear characteristic curve and by largely elimi-

nating underexposures. Some digital receptors, which are approved for spot views, as well as some fulfield receptors, which are presently filing for approval, have excellent resolution. Whether a resolution that is far below 10 line pairs will prove satisfactory for routine clinical application, will require further testing. Whenever these most important questions ar solved it may be expected that the other advantages of digital systems can be fully used.

Computer-aided image analysis may help to increase the detection rate of microcalcifications and masses by eliminating misses caused by decreasing attention of the radiologist. For this purpose, computerized detection might be used for double reading. Such a software applied to digital images could highlight any areas of potential concern, attracting the radiologist's attention.

■ Sonography

Because of its poor detection of DCIS due to its inability to image microcalcifications, sonography does not provide any relevant diagnostic information to the differential diagnosis of microcalcifications.

Individual cases of microcalcifications with sonographic visualization of thickened ducts or of the larger microcalcifications have been reported in the literature, but this does not justify the conclusion that sonography can diagnose microinvasive or carcinomas in situ.

■ Magnetic Resonance Imaging

MRI does *not* appear to be suitable for the differential diagnosis of microcalcifications.

The reason is that most proliferative changes associated with microcalcifications enhance with a pattern similar to that of carcinomas in situ with microcalcification and are therefore indistinguishable. Furthermore, it can be assumed that only 80% to 85% of carcinomas in situ show enhancement (which can be uncharacteristic, i.e., delayed or diffuse).

■ Percutaneous Biopsy

Probably due to the discontiguous growth of DCIS, the accuracy of conventional needle biopsy is lower for the assessment of microcalcifications than for masses.[54–58]

Therefore, if conventional biopsy is used for assessment of microcalcifications, diligent correlation between imaging and histopathology is critical. A negative core biopsy or FNB cannot exclude malignancy or replace surgical biopsy. Vacuum biopsy has proven superior to conventional percutaneous biopsy;[59–62] but correlation with histopathology and follow-up (to check for complete or at least representative biopsy of a sufficiently large area) remain necessary.

Open biopsy after wire localization is recommended in indeterminate cases, if vacuum biopsy is not available or may not be appropriate (lesions close to the skin, extended areas of microcalcifications, very fine microcalcifications that possibly cannot be resolved by the digital image receptor).

The latest techniques using vacuum needles, which allow the removal of complete areas of suspicion, promise a further significant improvement of accuracy.

■ Summary

Mammography is the method of choice for the detection and differential diagnosis of microcalcifications.

Meticulous analysis of mammographically visualized microcalcifications is the prerequisite for

– Accurate detection of carcinomas
– Best possible assessment of the extent of carcinomas
– Avoiding high numbers of unnecessary biopsies of benign changes with microcalcifications

■ Analysis of Microcalcifications

The goal of analyzing calcifications is the categorization of calcifications as:

● Highly suspicious for malignancy
● Definitely benign
● Indeterminate

■ Microcalcifications Suggestive of Malignancy

■ Principal Classification

The systematic investigations of Lanyi and other authors[63–66] have shown that typically malignant microcalcifications arise almost exclusively in *invasive and noninvasive ductal carcinomas*, while lobular carcinomas calcify only very rarely and fail to develop a mammographically typical calcification pattern. These observations form the basis for considering calcifications that are ductal in distribution and configuration and are suggestive of malignancy.

Calcifications are analyzed as to

● Their location (malignant calcifications are implicitly intramammary)
● Their individual shapes
● Their distribution pattern

■ Typical Morphologies of Calcifications Suggestive of Malignancy

The following individual shapes are typical of carcinomas:

■ Linear and Branching Calcifications (Casting)

(Fig. 22.**23a–c**)

These calcifications, which can branch and assume *V-shapes or Y-shapes,* correspond to calcified casts of the small lactiferous ducts and are frequently a manifestation of a *comedo-type DCIS* or a comedo-type *invasive ductal carcinoma.* Their margins are irregular.

These calcifications are to be differentiated from the needle-like or branching calcifications of the so-called plasma cell mastitis that are generally larger and may have smooth parallel walls. Furthermore, sometimes secretory microcalcifications in benign fibrocystic changes may assume elongated shapes and exhibit some polymorphism (Figs. 22.**24–25**). Because the branching and casting microcalcifications are a frequent sign of carcinoma, the suspicion of malignancy should be raised whenever such calcifications are observed *within* a cluster of microcalcifications.

■ Pleomorphic and Larger Granular Calcifications

These microcalcifications are very variable in size, shape, and density and have been described as resembling crushed stone. The individual calcification within a group can be extremely *irregular,* sometimes even bizarre in shape (Figs. 22.**26** and 22.**27**) and ranges from fine to 2 mm in size. Usually each calcification is different from the others.

These calcifications have to be differentiated from the bizarre calcifications in fibroadenomas, which usually (but not always) are larger and coarser, frequently exhibit a different distribution pattern, and often are associated with a large, coarse dystrophic calcification. If such calcifications are contained in a completely well-circumscribed soft-tissue mass, this can be diagnostically helpful by indicating a fibroadenoma. However, any less characteristic soft-tissue density around microcalcifications is generally not helpful (see p. 452). In addition to fibroadenomas, the larger granular calcifications can be observed in certain proliferative fibrocystic changes and analyzing the distribution pattern may contribute to the differential diagnosis (see below).

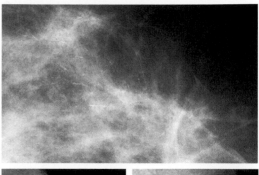

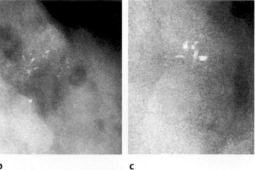

Fig. 22.**23 a–c**
a Multiple needle-like and fine microcalcifications in a ductal distribution (magnification view). *Histology:* DCIS, comedo-type
b Group of microcalcifications including several elongated or v-shaped calcifications: highly suspicious. *Histology:* DCIS, comedo type with microinvasion
c Group of elongated and very polymorphic, suspicious microcalcifications. *Histology:* DCIS, comedo-type

■ Fine-granular Calcifications

Fine-granular calcifications can occasionally be a manifestation of a carcinoma if they are extremely delicate and typically clustered in *small groups* or *segmentally distributed* (see below) (Fig. 22.**28a** and **b**). These distribution patterns suggest fine-granular calcifications in noncomedo DCIS. In the micropapillary and cribriform subtypes of the noncomedo DCIS and in the corresponding invasive carcinomas, these very fine-granular calcifications precipitate in the secretion-filled interspaces between the papillary or cribriform cellular proliferations.

Since fine-granular calcifications are frequently associated with benign changes, these calcifications have to be considered uncharacteristic of carcinoma. They should only raise a concern about malignancy if they exhibit a typical

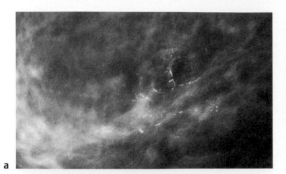

a

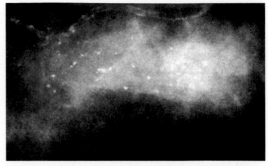

c

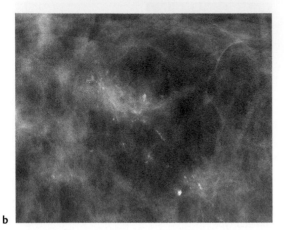

b

Fig. 22.**24 a–c** Though pleomorphic, linear calcifications must be considered strongly suggestive of malignancy, smooth, linear calcifications can be a manifestation of a benign condition
a Relatively coarse, elongated, partially v-shaped or y-shaped casting calcifications that grow along the ducts. In addition to these coarse calcifications, fine and tiny microcalcifications suggest the correct diagnosis: DCIS
b Calcifications with similar morphology and distribution as in (**a**). *Histology:* so-called plasma cell mastitis, no malignancy
c Diffusely distributed microcalcifications with slight polymorphism including individual elongated forms. *Histology:* fibrocystic disease including secretory type calcifications

malignant distribution pattern, as listed below, have increased in size, or are new. For small groups of fine-granular calcifications, the decision to perform a biopsy should be made reluctantly, as these are more likely due to benign proliferative changes.

■ **Typical Distribution Pattern of Malignant Calcifications**

■ **Ductal Arrangement of Calcifications Along the Lactiferous Ducts, Including Branching V-shaped and Y-shaped Figures**

(Figs. 22.**23a**, 22.**24a**, 22.**28a**)

This pattern is considered strongly suggestive of an intraductal origin of the calcifications and requires biopsy because of the high suspicion of malignancy. This pattern can be seen in malig-

nancy as well as in secretory disease where secretions are, however, much coarser and may exhibit parallel walls.

■ **Segmental Distribution of the Calcifications**

The suspicion of malignancy increases with the conspicuity of the segmental arrangement (Figs. 22.**23a** and 22.**29**). So-called club or butterfly forms of segmental arrangement have also been described by Lanyi.[63]

■ **Lack of Symmetry**

Malignant calcifications rarely appear in symmetrical location in the right and left breast[63]. Therefore, the suspicion of malignancy is strengthened if calcifications are found at one location in one breast only.

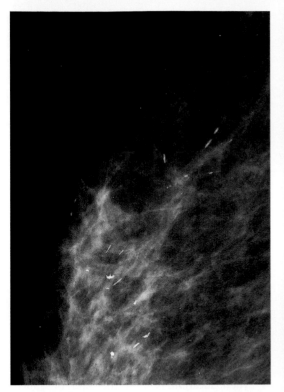

Fig. 22.**25**   Coarse needle-shaped calcifications, following the ducts and oriented toward the nipple: "Plasma cell mastitis"

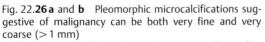

Fig. 22.**26 a** and **b**   Pleomorphic microcalcifications suggestive of malignancy can be both very fine and very coarse (>1 mm)
a The mediolateral view shows two groups of very fine pleomorphic microcalcifications, 4 cm apart, in the lateral aspect of the breast: multicentric DCIS
b Delineation of a small group of considerably coarser pleomorphic calcifications, so-called granular mircrocalcifications. Despite the accompanying soft-tissue density, these calcifications should not be mistaken for bizarre calcifications of a fibroadenoma. Furthermore, the somewhat irregular contour of the accompanying soft-tissue density should be noted. *Histology:* DCIS

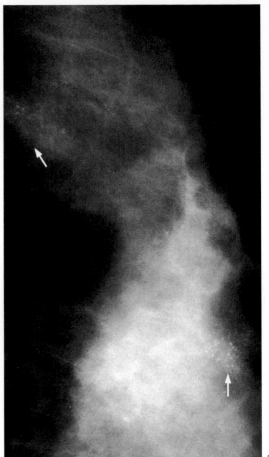

a

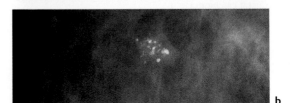

b

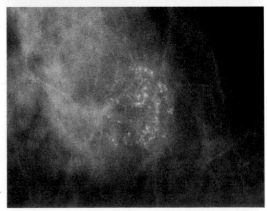

Fig. 22.**27**   Large group of polymorphic and casting mi- ▷
crocalcifications highly suspicious. *Histology:* DCIS

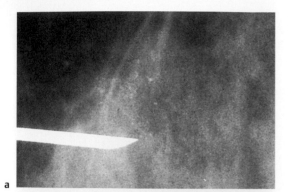

a

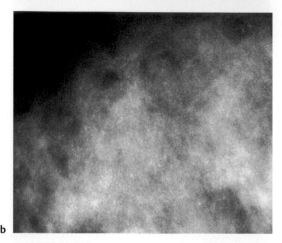

b

Fig. 22.**28 a** and **b**
a Fine-granular calcifications. The triangular arrangement is suggestive of malignancy. *Histology:* small invasive ductal carcinoma
b Very fine calcifications diffusely distributed throughout the entire breast, new since the previous examination and therefore suggestive evidence of a possible carcinoma. No palpable abnormality or difference compared to the contralateral side: *Histology:* ductal carcinoma diffusely spread throughout the breast

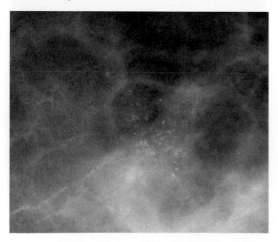

Fig. 22.**29** Typical triangular group, with its apex pointing toward the nipple (not imaged, right lower corner). *Histology:* DCIS, comedo-type

■ Summary

Malignant calcifications are always intramammary.
The following calcification patterns suggest— with a high degree of certainty—a malignancy:

● **Morphology:**
  – Linear irregular calcifications with branching
  – Pleomorphic granular and bizarre microcalcifications
  – (Multi)focal fine-granular calcifications if new or combined with a suspicious distribution pattern

● **Distribution pattern:**
  – Ductal arrangement
  – Segmental arrangement

■ Definitely Benign Calcifications

The benign nature of the calcifications can be deduced on the basis of

● Their location (within the skin or subcutaneous tissue)
● Their morphology
● Their distribution pattern

■ Extramammary Benign Calcifications and Artifacts

All calcifications located outside the breast parenchyma, i.e., intracutaneous and subcutaneous calcifications, as well as calcific densities and artifacts, are benign.

■ Extramammary Benign Calcifications

Dermal or subcutaneous calcifications are mostly in sebaceous glands of the skin. They are round, usually ring-like, sometimes dumb-bell–like, and correspond to the size of the skin pores (Fig. 22.**30**). They are often found in the dermis of the inner half of the breast.

In general, they can be easily diagnosed on the basis of their location and configuration. If they appear in groups, the diagnosis might be questioned, in particular when their round and ring-like contours are not clearly discernible. If a cutaneous origin (which could prove their benignity) is suspected, a *tangential view* should be obtained for clarification (Fig. 22.**31**) (p. 49).

■ Artifacts

Artifacts can occasionally mimic microcalcifications. Powder or ointment (Fig. 22.**32**) on the skin can produce characteristic, punctate, or streaky calcific densities arranged along dermal lines. Recognizing such structures is generally not problematic. The same applies to artifacts on the intensifying screen caused by fingerprints, dust, and defects of the screen (Fig. 22.**33**). Furthermore, dot-like or linear artifacts can be imprinted on the film by the rolls in the automatic processor.

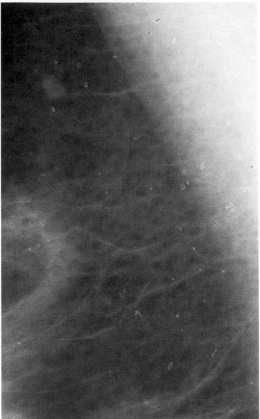

Fig. 22.**30** Punctate and ring-like calcifications projecting diffusely throughout the entire breast. Several of the calcifications can clearly be assigned to skin pores. Finding corresponds to calcifications in sebaceous glands

Fig. 22.**31 a–c**
a The craniocaudal view shows several round calcifications close together in the retroareolar region (arrow)
b These calcifications are projected over the subcutaneous region (arrow) in the tangential view
c Underexposed film copy of the tangential view with cutaneous calcifications of another patient. The relative underexposure (**b, c**) is necessary to illustrate the cutaneous location of the calcifications

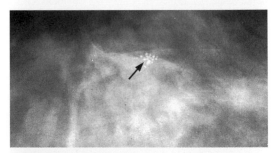

a

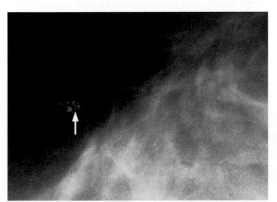

b

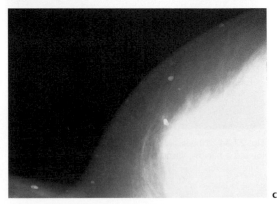

c

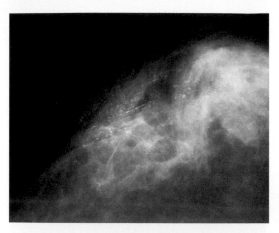

Fig. 22.**32** Artifacts caused by ointment applied to the skin

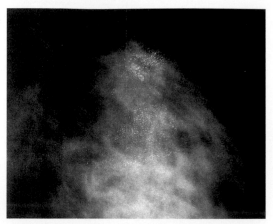

Fig. 22.**33** Artifact of the intensifying screen: fingerprint.

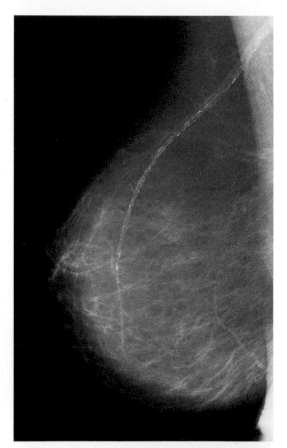

Fig. 22.**34** Linear and round calcifications directly following a narrow, vascular structure: arteriosclerosis

■ **Benign Intramammary Calcifications**

The analysis of the shape and distribution determines the correct diagnosis of benign intramammary calcifications.

■ **Typical Morphology of Benign Calcifications**

(Figs. 22.**34**–22.**40**)

Large (>1 mm), rounded calcifications with or without central radiolucency can develop in scars or fat necroses (subcutaneous without trauma, usually bilateral with calcifying liponecrosis), "plasma cell mastitis," and calcified fibroadenomas or papillomas (whereby the soft tissue density may or may not be visible).
They are invariably benign.

Semicircular or shell-like calcifications around radiolucent lesions can develop in oil cysts, scars, and fat necrosis, as part of a foreign-body reaction around droplets of silicone or wax injected for augmentation, in calcifying liponecrosis, and in "plasma cell mastitis."
They also are *always benign.*

These calcifications have to be distinguished from *shell-like calcifications along the periphery of lesions of soft-tissue density.*
They occur:

– *In fibroadenomas or papillomas.* Together with other evolving calcifications confined to an oval or round area or within a smoothly outlined soft-tissue density, the evolving peripheral calcification is relatively characteristic of

Fig. 22.**35 a–c**
a Multiple elongated, curved, crescentic, and ring-like calcifications following recurrent mastitis with abscess incision and drainage
b Almost symmetrically arranged "idiopathic" calcifying liponecrosis without known preceding trauma
c Large calcified fat necrosis following breast augmentation with transplanted autogenous adipose tissue (mediolateral view)

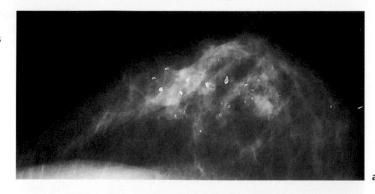

a

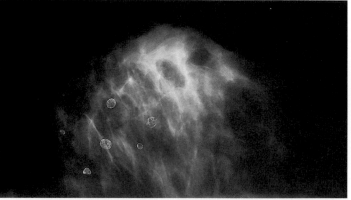

b

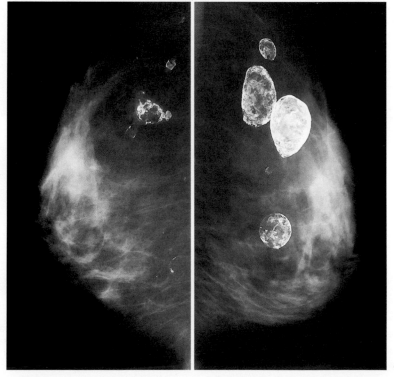

c

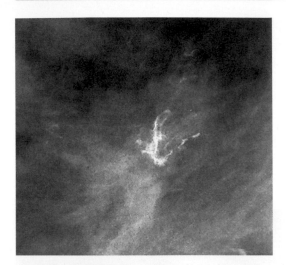

Fig. 22.**36** Elongated, in part linear, dystrophic calcifications within scar-induced architectural distortion

fibroadenomas or papillomas. Since small peripheral calcifications are not absolute proof, follow-up examinations at 6-, 12-, 24-, and 36-month intervals should be obtained for confirmation, showing progression to typical coarse calcifications.

In the case of additional suspicious findings (e.g., indistinctly outlined surrounding density), further evaluation of individual cases is indicated.

– *In cysts.* Calcifications in the wall can develop in oil cysts or milk of calcium cysts but can also indicate a complex cyst. If an oil cyst (radiographically visualized central radiolucency) or a simple milk of calcium cyst ("teacups" on mediolateral mammogram or, in the case of large cysts, sonographically moveable sedimentations) has been documented, further diagnostic steps are unneces-

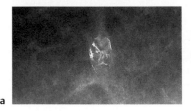

a

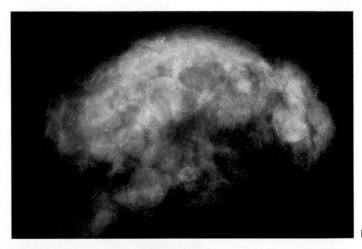

b

Fig. 22.**37 a** and **b**
a Fine eggshell-like calcifications projected over an oval radiolucency: calcifying oil cyst
b Subtle shell-like (in part, punctate) calcifications around drop-like deposits of wax, injected for augmentation

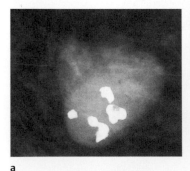

a

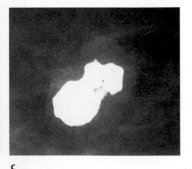

c

b

Fig. 22.**38 a–c**
a Several coarse, irregularly outlined calcifications within a lobulated lesion: typical fibroadenoma

b Barely discernible oval density with typical coarse bizarre fibroadenomatous calcifications
c Macrocalcifications of an almost completely calcified fibroadenoma

sary. Otherwise, further workup (aspiration or biopsy) is needed. The reason is that particularly hemorrhagic cysts, which can be a manifestation of a papilloma or carcinoma, have the tendency to form mural calcifications.

– As a foreign-body reaction around deposits of silicone or wax that have been injected for augmentation. These shell-like calcifications are *definitely benign*. The usually increased density due to fibrosis, silicone, and calcifications, however, compromises the overall evaluation of the breast tissue (Fig. 22.**37b**).

Coarse, popcorn-like, or bizarre calcifications larger than 2 mm can be found in fibroadenomas and papillomas. The larger these calcifications are, the more characteristic they are. Such *characteristic popcorn-like or bizarre calcifications support the diagnosis of a fibroadenoma or papilloma with a high degree of certainty.*

Only *if (very rare!) calcifications suggestive of malignancy are found next to these calcifications* or if coarse calcifications are surrounded *by an irregularly outlined density* must the differential diagnosis consider *necrotic calcifications in a carcinoma* or *a calcified fibroadenoma* surrounded by a carcinoma.

It is also important to keep in mind that *bizarre fibroadenomatous calcifications smaller than 2 mm can resemble pleomorphic granular calcifications found in carcinomas.*

Consequently, bizarre calcifications can only establish the diagnosis of a fibroadenoma if they are large enough and show an arrangement uncharacteristic of malignancy.

Coarse, needle-like calcifications can occur:

– *In so-called plasma cell mastitis.* Like ductal calcifications, they follow the ductal system. Histologically, they are intraductal and periductal. *Despite a ductal or segmental, V-shaped and Y-shaped arrangement, they can be clearly identified as benign as long as they are large, coarse, and smooth.* A central radiolucency within the needles or a combination with round, coarse calcifications with or without

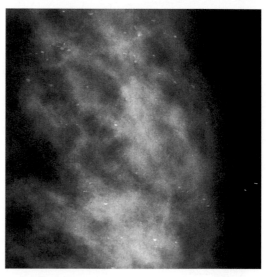

Fig. 22.**39** In part round, in part linear and multiple crescentic, teacup calcifications due to sedimentation of calcific particles within milk of calcium cysts, only seen in the mediolateral view

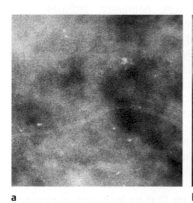
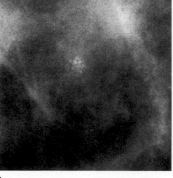
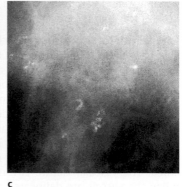

a   b   c

Fig. 22.**40 a–c**
a Punctate scattered calcifications in blunt duct adenosis

b Several punctate, clustered calcifications in a round group (morula-like): small cystic adenosis
c Typical image of multiple, morula-like calcifications with intralobular distribution in sclerosing adenosis

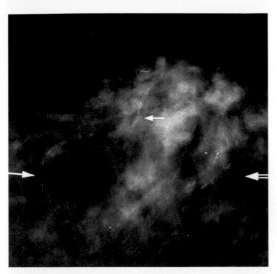

Fig. 22.**41**   Long arrow: calcifications as part of a plasma cell mastitis
Short arrow: vascular calcifications
Open arrow: segmentally arranged, pleomorphic calcifications of DCIS

radiolucency is considered definitive proof. Caution is advised when evaluating *needle-like, fine* calcifications since the differentiation between a primary ductal carcinoma and "plasma cell mastitis" can be difficult (Fig. 22.**24**).

– *In scars.* Mainly, *coarse needles* and *bizarre linear calcifications* are characteristically seen along the scars. Again, caution should be taken when evaluating *delicate* calcifications and possible ductal distribution since a new or residual carcinoma within or adjacent to the scar has to be excluded.

Parallel microcalcifications are characteristic of vascular calcifications. They do not follow (in two projections) the course of ductal structures. Even if these calcifications appear amorphous or fragmented, the correct diagnosis can usually be established as long as the outer border of the calcifications form two *parallel* lines that resemble railroad tracks. The outer contour of the lines is smooth, but the lines need not be completely calcified. The vascular nature is further supported when the vessels are delineated as tubular soft-tissue densities within the surrounding adipose tissue.

Small calcifications *that are round, punctate, or stippled and have a uniform shape* are *charac-*

teristically associated with various forms of fibrocystic changes. Most calcifications are diffusely distributed or are in a rosette-like arrangement (see below). Only with additional suspicion (existence of adjacent suspicious microcalcifications or masses) must malignancy coexisting with fibrocystic changes be excluded.

Calcifications that show a *teacup phenomenon* are characteristic of fibrocystic changes (Fig. 22.**39**).[63–66]

The teacup phenomenon is caused by sedimentation in microcysts (cysts containing milk of calcium) (see also p. 189). Since the teacup phenomenon may be detectable only on the 90° lateral view, *obtaining a 90° lateral view—if possible, with magnification—is mandatory for the assessment of indeterminate microcalcifications.*

In the craniocaudal view, these calcifications frequently appear amorphous, and accurate diagnosis cannot be made on this view. The teacup phenomenon is usually seen in some of the microcalcifications only. The diagnosis of a benign process can be made with a high degree of certainty if *neither calcifications suggestive of malignancy nor suscipious masses* (as evidence of a carcinoma that *coexists* with the described benign changes) are observed amidst these calcifications (Fig. 22.**41**).

■ Typical Distribution of Benign Calcifications

Solitary calcifications are characteristically benign. Several solitary calcifications can be observed in one or both breasts.

Diffuse (evenly distributed throughout the parenchyma, see also Fig. 22.**40**) **and symmetric distribution** favors benignity. Diffusely distributed, mostly symmetric calcifications are typically associated with certain types of fibrocystic changes, mainly sclerosing adenosis. The symmetric appearance of malignant microcalcifications is extremely rare.

The calcifications in benign changes are frequently punctate, stippled, or round.

If amorphous calcifications show a symmetric distribution, a predominantly monomorphic appearance and, in particular, the teacup phenomenon, the diagnosis of fibrocystic changes is supported.

It is important that *no branching or pleomorphic calcifications* are seen among *these calcifications* and that *segmental distribution* cannot be identified. Otherwise, a malignancy coexistent with benign changes must be considered.

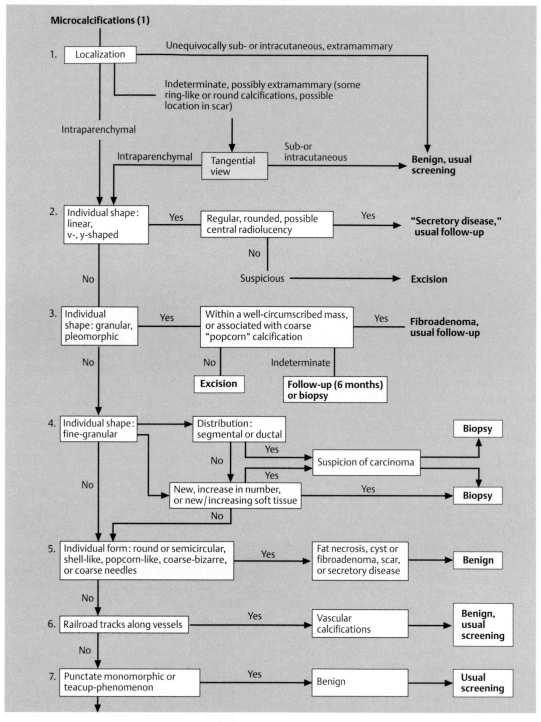

Fig. 22.**42**   Microcalcifications (continued on p. 448)

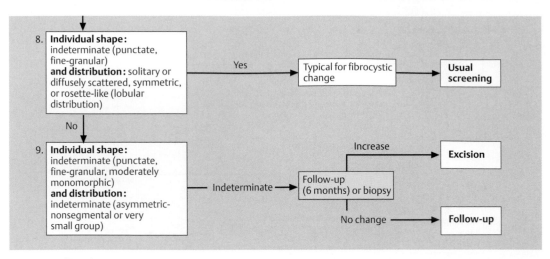

Fig. 22.**42** (Cont.)

Clustered calcifications should be carefully evaluated.

To determine whether microcalcifications are clustered, the cluster must be visualized *in two projections.* Only an evaluation in two projections can separate a true cluster from a coincidental superimposition of calcifications that are at different locations but seen next to each other in one view. Such *"pseudogroups"* are *not indicative of malignancy.*

Typical benign groups can be observed:
- In *calcifying liponecrosis* and subcutaneous calcifications. Benignity can be proved by documenting the subcutaneous location (tangential view) or by identifying a central radiolucency or round configuration.
- In a confined small area corresponding to a *fibroadenoma or papilloma* and exhibiting a typical morphology of the calcifications (see above) or, if the calcifications are within a smoothly outlined (see definition) soft-tissue density.
- *Along scars* as typical individual forms (coarse needles, ring-like, round calcifications) and lacking any malignant forms and distribution pattern.
- In *microcystic adenosis* (Figs. 22.**40b** and **c**). These calcifications characteristically are close to each other in a round, *rosette-like or morula-like* arrangement. They are in the lobule and, *because of their lobular location, are not indicative of malignancy.*

The diagnosis of benignity is further supported by the *multiplicity and symmetry* of such small groups and by relatively uniform morphology. Additional casting or pleomorphic calcifications in a ductal or segmental distribution have to be excluded. Otherwise, a carcinoma must be considered.

Track-like calcifications along vessels are definitely benign (see above).

■ **Summary**

(Fig. 22.**42**)

Extramammary calcifications, with their location proven by tangential views, are benign. Artifacts mimicking microcalcifications have to be excluded.
Intramammary calcifications are benign if they exhibit the following calcification pattern:

■ **Morphology**

- Coarse, with or without central radiolucency.
- Semicircular or shell-like calcifications around lesions with a central area of radiolucency. Examples: oil cysts, fat necrosis, calcifying liponecrosis.
- Relatively typical also are peripheral calcifications of fibroadenomas and papillomas.

- Coarse, popcorn-like, and large bizarre calcifications (in general >2 mm). Examples: fibroadenomas, papillomas, "plasma cell mastitis," scars.
- Railroad track vascular calcifications.
- Small and tiny calcifications that are round, punctate, or stippled monomorphic. Distribution: symmetric, diffuse, or in individual morula-like groups. Example: fibrocystic changes.
- Teacup calcifications. Examples: milk of calcium in microcystic benign changes.

■ Distribution Pattern

- Solitary calcifications.
- Diffuse and symmetrical distribution.
- Groups can be observed in the following conditions:
  - Calcifying liponecrosis (typical subcutaneous in location and ring-like or round in morphology).
  - In fibroadenomas and papillomas with typical shapes or with a typical surrounding well-circumscribed soft-tissue density.
  - In scars.
  - In blunt duct adenosis with typical lobular configuration: rosette-like and closely packed.
- Along the course of vessels.

■ Indeterminate Microcalcifications

■ Definition

Indeterminate microcalcifications are calcifications that are classified as not unequivocally benign or as suspicious because of

- Their location
- Their morphology
- Their distribution

These mainly include:

- Fine-granular and amorphous calcifications that do not follow a typical distribution pattern
- Calcifications with mild to moderate pleomorphism (Fig. 22.43)
- Calcifications that do not show a typical segmental or lobular arrangement, appear

asymmetric to the contralateral side, are found in one location only (Fig. 22.44) or appear to form groups
- Other calcifications that are neither typically benign nor typically malignant

In terms of numbers, indeterminate calcifications are unfortunately at least as frequent as characteristically benign or suspect calcifications.

■ Incidence

Indeterminate calcifications can be expected in the following conditions:

- Invasive *carcinoma* and *carcinoma* in situ: Some invasive carcinomas, most carcinomas in situ of the noncomedo type, and 20% of the carcinomas in situ of the comedo type show no characteristic microcalcifications or no microcalcifications at all.
- Since benign fibrocystic changes frequently represent an amalgamation of different proliferative changes of *ductal as well as lobular origin* and since the lobules themselves can be involved in sclerosing processes, the described typical benign forms and arrangements of microcalcifications are only found in a certain percentage. This means that pleomorphic or elongated shapes as well as worrisome distributions can be encountered in benign changes. Since these calcifications cannot be differentiated from malignant calcifications with sufficient certainty, a gray zone exists in which an unequivocal classification of the analyzed calcification cannot be achieved.
- With beginning *calcification of fibroadenomas*, small bizarre, linear, or punctate calcifications can appear. They cannot always reliably be differentiated from suspicious microcalcifications.
  Location of uncharacteristic calcifications *within a smoothly outlined soft-tissue mass* can be helpful in the differential diagnosis.
- Rare differential diagnostic problems arise when the calcifications in plasma cell mastitis are relatively delicate.
- Furthermore, calcifications in *fat necroses and scars* can occasionally be pleomorphic, containing elongated and more characteristically curved shapes. If the microcalcifications are still small or appear in groups, they cannot invariably be differentiated from suspicious ductal calcifications.

Fig. 22.**43** Punctate, linear, and pleomorphic microcalcifications in the upper outer quadrant (magnification mammography). *Histology:* Parenchyma containing matrix microcalcifications

Fig. 22.**44** Unilateral, relatively monomorphic, fine microcalcifications without typical distribution. *Histology:* simple fibrocystic changes without proliferations containing psammomatous calcifications

■ **General Aspects of the Differential Diagnosis of Indeterminate Microcalcifications**

In principle, it is not possible to detect *all* invasive carcinomas or carcinomas in situ, because only some of the invasive and even fewer of the carcinomas in situ contain microcalcifications. Some carcinomas only display indeterminate calcifications. Furthermore, typically benign calcifications can occasionally be associated with carcinomas

when the carcinoma arises in an area of benign disease. Such individual cases should not lead to the uncritical removal of all microcalcifications.

It is inappropriate to resect all indeterminate calcifications because only a small portion of the biopsies will be positive for malignancy. Diagnostic biopsies of benign calcifications will not only raise the costs to unacceptably high levels but also will compromise the outcome of future evaluations because of scarring secondary to multiple surgeries. Furthermore, too many diagnostic excisions of benign lesions will lead to a loss of confidence in diagnostic imaging and a loss of compliance.

■ **Considerations as to the Differential Diagnosis of Indeterminate Calcifications in the Individual Case**

The diagnostic decision, which should include a recommendation of how to continue with the workup, must *always* be *individualized.*

When deciding between *biopsy* and *follow-up examination,* it must be considered that calcifications in a carcinoma in situ can remain *stable* over several years. If situated within dense tissue, an associated mass might not be recognized. In general, follow-up examinations obtained at *6-month* intervals are considered totally adequate.

The decision process must incorporate:
● An assessment based on a meticulous analysis of the microcalcifications (location, individual form, distribution pattern)
● Supplemental information as to the surrounding soft tissue structures (asymmetries, retraction, prior surgeries, scars, etc.)
● Clinical history (family history, patient history as to previous breast cancer and other risk factors, prior surgery, scars, etc.)
● Clinical findings, e.g., discharge, retraction, scars, as well as palpable abnormalities, review of the mammographic findings
● Serial changes if previous mammograms are available

The radiologist should recognize that:

– New or increasing microcalcifications and a new or increasing contiguous soft-tissue density are an indication for biopsy
– Failure to observe any appreciable changes for less than 1–2 years raises the likelihood of a benign diagnosis only slightly

The decision to proceed with follow-up examinations, core, preferably vacuum biopsy, or ex-

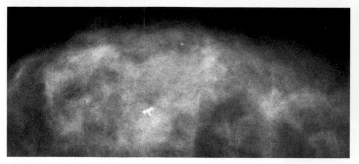 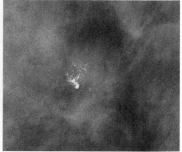

Fig. 22.**45 a** and **b**
a Very fine calcifications as well as a coarse calcification with a bizarre outline are seen within a barely discernible round density measuring 7 mm located within dense parenchyma

b Magnification mammography. Diagnosis: fibroadenoma, confirmed by increasing coarseness of the calcifications on follow-up

cisional biopsy has to incorporate all available data.

Considerations include:

● Follow-up examinations are advisable only when the compilation of all findings suggest a benign lesion with a high degree of certainty
● That the accuracy of percutaneous biopsies for the evaluation of microcalcifications depends on the ability to sample sufficient tissu including the calcifications at the time of biopsy

The presence of microcalcifications in cores should be documented with specimen radiography. Adequate material has to be obtained (see Chapter 7). The core biopsy can confirm a presumed benign or malignant finding. A negative core biopsy should not be used to dismiss a suspicion raised by imaging. The excisional biopsy is considered the most reliable method to evaluate continued suggestive or possibly malignant findings.

Comparable accuracy can be achieved if a sufficient number of cores ($\geq$ 20 cores, 11 G needles) are acquired by vacuum biopsy.

After any type of biopsy correlation of imaging before biopsy, of specimen radiographs, of imaging after biopsy (if available) and histology is indispensable.[68]

■ **Appendix: Differential Diagnostic Significance of a Soft Density Surrounding Microcalcifications**

(Figs. 22.**45**–22.**49**)

A surrounding or accompanying soft-tissue density is often not helpful. Presence or absence of a soft-tissue density can by no means substitute a meticulous analysis of the mircocalcifications.

A surrounding soft-tissue density is **contributory** if:

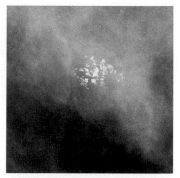

Fig. 22.**46 a** and **b**
a Pleomorphic bizarre calcifications in a subtle oval area. *Histology:* fibroadenoma
b Granular and irregular linear calcifications forming an oval group with a pointed extension. Note the calcifications outside the soft-tissue density. *Histology:* DCIS

– It is identifiable as a vessel (best if seen in two projections) with beginning mural calcifications
– It is round and entirely smooth in outline: this can also be considered as quite reliable evidence of a fibroadenoma

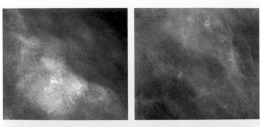

a

b

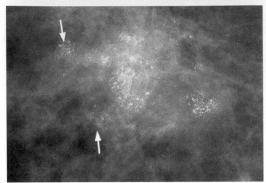

c

Fig. 22.**47 a–c**
a Specimen radiography. Round lesion measuring 8 mm, with multiple, somewhat pleomorphic calcifications that are closely aggregated: papilloma
b Specimen radiography. Multiple tiny round groups, almost forming a circle, of punctate calcifications: papillomatosis
c Specimen radiography. Multiple groups of microcalcifications are delineated within an indistinctly outlined soft-tissue density, with two groups unmistakably punctate. In addition, there are many granular, pleomorphic calcifications: papillary carcinoma

- It is ill-defined or spiculated and consequently unequivocally suspect
- It is of fat density and consequently has a pattern diagnostic of a benign entity, e.g., oil cyst

Less contributory is:

- Finding uncharacteristic densities around microcalcifications, since they may be caused by infiltration, reactive changes, uncharacteristic benign changes, or superimposition.
- Finding nodular densities around microcalcifications. They can—unless unequivocally smooth in outline—suggest an early calcifying fibroadenoma or papilloma. But this is not conclusive because invasive carcinomas or carcinomas in situ can be nodular and calcify.
- Finally, presence or absence of a soft-tissue density around microcalcifications permits no reliable differentiation between invasive carcinoma and carcinoma in situ. On one hand, a soft-tissue density accompanying an invasive carcinoma can be overlooked amidst surrounding dense parenchyma. On the other hand, a reactive fibrosis can produce a soft-tissue density around a pure carcinoma in situ.

Nipple Discharge

(Fig. 22.**50 a**)

■ Definition

A pathologic discharge refers to a spontaneous, usually unilateral, nonmilky secretion from one or a few lactiferous ducts.

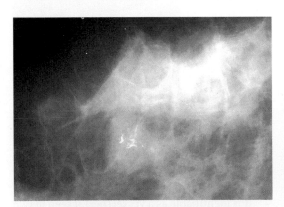

Fig. 22.**48** Oval, partially sharply outlined lesion measuring 11 mm, with relatively large, pleomorphic, bizarre calcifications centrally. Despite the relatively coarse structure, not a fibroadenoma but an intraductal carcinoma

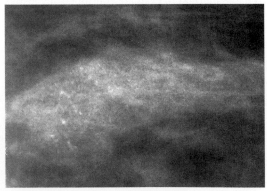

Fig. 22.**49** Multiple fine-granular microcalcifications. Biopsy recommended because of suggested segmental distribution (magnification × 3): DCIS
The density in the area of the microcalcifications is probably just caused by surrounding breast tissue, possibly also by some reactive fibrosis. It cannot be used as an indicator of invasion

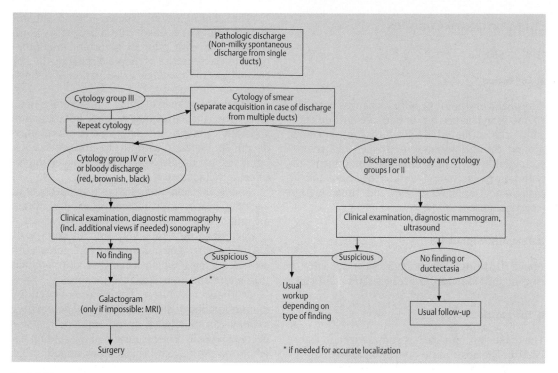

Fig. 22.**50 a**

■ **Diagnostic Problems**

An intraductal lesion presenting with nipple discharge can be localized and its extent determined by galactography. Neither galactography nor other imaging methods can ascertain the histopathology of the process. Therefore, any galactographically detected intraductal lesion must be surgically explored.

■ **Diagnostic Strategy**

1. Bilateral nonmilky discharge is generally a manifestation of a hormonal dysfunction and consequently not an indication for galactography. Only the case of a bilateral hemorrhagic or cytologically suspicious discharge warrants further evaluation. As a rule, any discharge calls for a cytologic smear. Only a positive cytologic smear is diagnostically useful. A negative cytologic smear can never exclude malignancy.

2. Unilateral discharge must be further evaluated whenever one or several lactiferous ducts secrete, whenever the color of the discharge may indicate malignancy (see below), or the cytologic smear is positive:

   – A discharge from several ducts usually has a hormonal cause, and checking the status of the endocrine system is recommended. If the cytology of the discharge is questionable or suggestive, one duct after the other has to be canalized for galactography.
   – If the discharge is brownish, greenish, or hemorrhagic, galactography is indicated.
   – Any discharge from one duct should be galactographically evaluated.
   – Any cytologically suggestive discharge is an indication for galactography.

3. Any filling defect with or without irregularities of the ductal wall or any truncated duct is a manifestation of an intraductal process that must be excised after prior localization. For galactographically documented ductectasia or a normal ductal system, follow-up mammography at the age-specific intervals is adequate.[69, 70]

4. If galactography is impossible, MRI may be able to demonstrate an enhancing lesion and guide biopsy.[7]

Inflammatory Changes

(Fig. 22.**50 b**)

■ **Definition**

If localized erythema or diffuse changes with erythema or hyperthermia, or both are noticed clinically, the differential diagnosis must center around the differentiation between malignancy (carcinoma with inflammatory component, inflammatory carcinoma, and, rarely, hematologic malignancy or metastases) and inflammation (mastitis, abscess).[71, 72]

■ **Diagnostic Problems**

Above all, the differentiation between subacute or chronic inflammatory processes can be difficult.

■ **Diagnostic Strategy**

The diagnostic approach is summarized in Figure 22.**50 b**. The possibilities and limitations of the individual methods can be briefly outlined as follows.

The *clinical history* speaks for an inflammatory origin in context with a pregnancy, with lactation, or with prior or recurrent inflammations. In the presence of nipple discharge, the microbiologic and cytologic examination of the discharge can be helpful.

Mammography is of special importance here. It is true that malignancy and inflammation generally cannot be distinguished in a focal mass or diffuse density without microcalcifications, but if suspicious *microcalcifications* can be indentified, a malignancy is very probable.

Sonographically demonstrated hypoechoic or anechoic spaces with fluctuation would indicate an inflammatory process. An abscess, which is characterized by a relatively smooth inner wall, has to be distinguished from a carcinoma with central necrosis, which usually exhibits nodular thickening and an irregular inner surface.

Without conclusive evidence provided by mammography or sonography, *anti-inflammatory therapy* can be tried if an inflammation is suspected clinically. The resolution of the finding has to be monitored until it becomes undetectable. The necessary short-term follow-up can be performed sonographically/clinically.

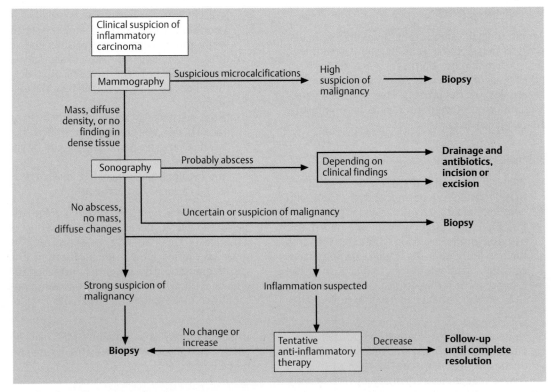

Fig. 22.**50 b** Inflammatory changes

Finally, it should be mentioned that some inflammatory processes fail to elicit any clinical inflammatory signs, as found in so-called cold abscesses (TB, fungus) and in some granulomatous conditions, as well as in chronic inflammations that may occur in association with fibrocystic changes. Their diagnosis is generally only established histologically after biopsy of a lesion that was discovered as a palpable finding or mammographic density.

The Young Patient

■ Special Considerations and Problems

Diagnosis of breast cancer can be more difficult in young patients (below 35–40 years) than in those who are older

There are several reasons for this:

- Very low incidence of breast cancer in this age group. Less than 7,5 % of all breast cancers occur before age 40.[73] In patients who are affected before age 30 hereditary breast cancer should be considered.[73–75]
- High incidence of benign breast disease (lumpiness, fibroadenomas)
- Decreased sensitivity of mammography in some of these patients
- Still small but, compared to older age groups, increased radiation risk at a young age. Whether the otherwise very low risk of radiation-induced breast cancer may be increased for certain hereditary types of breast cancer (due to specific gene changes), has lately been discussed.[76] Being the only method suitable for screening and the only method that can reliably detect DCIS, mammography remains indispensable in these patients.

These factors have led to an increased rate of delayed diagnoses of carcinoma among young patients compared to older patients. Furthermore, the positive biopsy rates (the number of carcinomas per recommended biopsies) are much lower in younger patients.[77–82]

Few women in this age group undergo mammographic screening. This is usually limited to women with first-degree relatives with premenopausal breast cancer, a history of treatment for Hodgkin disease, a prior breast biopsy revealing a high-risk lesion, or a previous history of breast cancer. In younger women, most cancers present as clinically evident masses, which need to be distinguished from the numerous benign masses and lumps detected in the young patient. These should be viewed with suspicion and the workup of these lesions individually tailored to each patient. The screening for the detection of lesions in these women is performed as in older women. A sensitivity to the real or perceived risk of radiation-induced cancer should be part of the treatment of these younger women. Even in pregnant women, however, suspicious lesions should be appropriately worked up.

■ Breast Changes in the Young Patient and Their Histology

The appearance of the normal breast beginning from childhood to adult age has been reviewed in Chapter 9. Based on age-related physiologic changes, the breast of the young patient on palpation is denser and lumpier than that of older patients (> 50 years). This higher consistency or lumpiness in itself does not imply disease. It does, however, impair clinical and—if performed—mammographic evaluation. Large individual variations exist; sometimes the breast of even very young patients (in their twenties) can contain ample amounts of fat.

The following benign entities are typically found in young patients.

Fibrocystic changes, hyperplastic and proliferative changes can occur. When proliferative changes with atypia are detected, this entity is associated with an increased risk of malignancy (see Chapter 10), as it is in older women.

Fibroadenomas. Even though fibroadenomas have a wide age distribution, the greatest incidence is in women between the ages of 25 and 35, and the fibroadenoma is the most frequent breast mass in children. Both pericanalicular and intracanalicular types are seen. In young patients, they largely consist of ample myxoid stroma with a high water content and are vascular. Some are cellular and adenomatous. Fibrosed fibroadenomas usually do not occur in young women. Multiple fibroadenomas are frequently encountered.

The juvenile fibroadenoma or *giant fibroadenoma* is a special type of fibroadenoma that occurs almost exclusively in young patients (maximum incidence around menarche). It is a well-circumscribed tumor, typically with rapid growth. Histologically, it consists of proliferating stroma and often epithelial hyperplasia. It is completely benign and not associated with an increased risk of malignancy.

The *phyllodes tumor* (see Chapter 17) is much rarer in the young patient than the juvenile fibroadenoma. It can, however, be encountered, albeit rarely, in the young patient as well as a rapidly growing, well-circumscribed mass.

Papillomas can occur in young patients.

Juvenile papillomatosis is an infrequent finding, which is typically diagnosed in adolescents and young women. Histologically, the lesion, which generally becomes apparent as a palpable mass or nipple discharge, is characterized by ductal papillomatosis, papillary apocrine hyperplasia, multiple (micro)cysts, often cellular atypia, and sometimes even necrosis. About 30–40% of the cases are associated with a family history of breast carcinoma. Local recurrence and bilaterality have been reported. Whether the individual risk of breast carcinoma is increased is debated. An association of juvenile papillomatosis and juvenile secretory carcinoma has been reported.[83–86]

Overall *malignancy* is less frequent in young patients than in the patient above 40 years of age. Various types of malignancy, including breast carcinomas, hematologic malignancy, and sarcomas, have been encountered.

During pregnancy the following benign and malignant entities can also be encountered:
Benign. The fibroadenoma is the most frequent benign mass occurring during pregnancy. It is followed by papillomas, fibrocystic disease, galactocele, abscess, puerperal mastitis, and (see Chapters 11 and 13, respectively), rarely, breast infarct or phyllodes tumor.

Many fibroadenomas increase in size during pregnancy, becoming apparent and necessitating further workup. Sometimes infarction may occur.

Breast infarct,[87, 88] which can affect any part of the breast tissue as well as sometimes a fibroadenoma,[89] is histologically characterized by a mass consisting of or containing coagulation necrosis. The exact etiology of breast infarcts during pregnancy is not known.

Malignant. About 1–2% of breast cancers are considered concurrent with pregnancy or lactation. These include cancers that are detected during or within 1 year of pregnancy. Unfortunately, diagnosis of these cancers is often too late, probably because of the difficult distinction between neoplastic growth versus physiologic changes during pregnancy and lactation.[90] Besides breast cancer, an association with pregnancy has been described for some rare lesions such as benign and malignant phyllodes tumor, Burkitt lymphoma, and angiosarcoma.

Risk of Breast Cancer

Breast cancer is an unusual disease in younger women. Even though malignancies have been described in the teenage group and women in their early twenties, a relevant increase of risk starts after about 25 years of age. At age 25, the incidence of breast cancer is about 1/10000. If a young woman (< age 30) has breast cancer, she has a significant risk of being a BRCA gene carrier. Genetic counseling may be indicated to offer optimum future monitoring to her and—if desired—her relatives.

After age 30 the risk of breast cancer in young women rises rapidly to about 1 : 1000 at age 40.[88, 91] Although malignant lesions are rare in these younger women, they do occur, and an attempt should be made to avoid unnecessary delay in diagnosis. In patients with genetic risk factors and in those with a family history of premenopausal breast cancer, the risk of breast cancer increases significantly even before 35–40 years of age.

The following paragraphs will summarize special issues in the diagnostic workup of young patients. Based on these considerations, recommendations of a diagnostic strategy will be suggested.

■ Clinical Findings

The great majority of young patients with breast problems present with a lump, lumpiness, localized pain, and occasionally with pathologic nipple discharge or other rare findings. Some young patients are referred because of an individual or strong family history of breast cancer or because of known genetic risk factors.

Benign causes of a palpable abnormality in the young patient include normal breast tissue, fibroadenoma, fibrocystic changes, papilloma, cyst, and, infrequently, juvenile papillomatosis. During pregnancy or lactation, benign causes include a galactocele, an abscess, puerperal mastitis, or a breast infarct.

Juvenile papillomatosis can present on palpation as an indeterminate mass or can be palpable like a fibroadenoma. Breast infarct becomes apparent as an indeterminate or suspicious mass of rubbery consistency.[88]

Unfortunately, in situ and invasive carcinoma, as well as other rare malignancies, have to be included in the differential diagnosis.

The differential diagnosis of very large masses should include the juvenile fibroadenoma, virginal hypertrophy, and rarely phyllodes tumor, lymphoma (e.g., Burkitt lymphoma during pregnancy), or sarcoma (periductal fibrosarcoma or angiosarcoma during pregnancy). The causes of pathologic discharge are similar to those in the older age-group and include papillomas, papillomatosis, duct ectasia, or fibrocystic changes, a lactating fibroadenoma (rarely), or, in about 10% of the cases, a carcinoma.

As in the older patients, sensitivity of the clinical examination for the detection of carcinoma varies with the lesion size and decreases strongly with smaller tumor size.[92, 93] As reported by Reintgen[33] on a large series of over 500 breast carcinomas, only about 50% of the carcinomas in the size range of 11–15 mm are palpable, and even experienced clinicians do not detect the majority of breast cancers until they are greater than 15 mm.

Overall, clinical evaluation of the young patient is more difficult because of the increased firmness and nodularity of the breast tissue. Because of even more pronounced nodularity and firmness of the breast tissue, evaluation frequently is significantly impaired during pregnancy and lactation.

Furthermore, the high prevalence of benign disease impairs assessment. During pregnancy and lactation, detection and diagnosis of malignancy and its differentiation from the physiological hypertrophic changes become even more difficult, as documented by the commonly encountered delays in diagnosis.[88, 90, 94–96]

■ Mammography

Mammographic evaluation in the young patient is often impaired by dense glandular tissue that can obscure both benign and malignant masses. Therefore, the value of mammography is limited. However, because of the variability of parenchymal patterns—about 30% of the patients have sufficient amounts of interposed fat to be well-assessed mammographically—and because of its unique capability to image microcalcifications (which may be the only sign of malignancy in about 30% of the carcinomas), mammography can

be useful (see Figs. 22.**54** and 22.**55**) below 35 years of age. It should therefore be utilized whenever indicated (see below).

When not obscured by dense tissue, **benign lesions** display large variations, as decribed in the respective chapters. Juvenile papillomatosis, an infrequent lesion seen predominantly in the young patient, usually cannot be distinguished from dense glandular tissue on mammography (Fig. 22.**51a**). This appearance together with the usual encountered palpable abnormality does not allow exclusion of malignancy. Breast infarct, a rare finding associated with pregnancy or lactation, can be obscured by dense tissue or present as an ill-defined mass or asymmetry mammographically. It usually cannot be distinguished from malignancy. For lesions with typical benign features (fat-containing lymph node, hamartoma, etc.), no further assessment is needed. For those with a high probability of benignity (>98%), follow-up is justified. In the other cases, which unfortunately constitute the large majority in the young patients, biopsy remains necessary.

As to detection and diagnosis of **malignancy**, many authors have reported a decreased sensitivity of mammography and a lower positive predictive value for patients under 35 years of age.[78, 97–107]

The increased number of reported false positive calls is explained by the high prevalence of benign lesions (nodular breast tissue or fibroadenomas), where malignancy cannot be excluded because of uncharacteristic appearance or overall high radiodensity (Fig. 22.**52a**).

Mammographic false negative interpretations have mainly been attributed to two facts:

– Owing to the higher amount of glandular or dense breast tissue, carcinomas without microcalcifications may be obscured (Fig. 22.**53a, b**)
– A relatively high percentage of carcinomas (15–20%) in young patients has been reported as having been misinterpreted as benign masses (like fibroadenomas) (Fig. 15.**13c, d**).[97, 99, 104–106]

In spite of these problems, mammography is able to detect nonpalpable carcinomas even in young patients[105, 107] (Fig. 22.**54a–d**):

– In those younger patients (circa 30%) who have fatty or mixed dense/fatty breast patterns, accuracy is comparable to that achieved in older patients

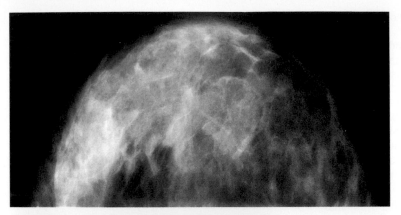

Fig. 22.**51 a** Fifteen-year-old patient with a family history of breast cancer. She presented with a palpable mass in the upper outer quadrant Mammogram cc-view. Dense breast tissue. No mass visible

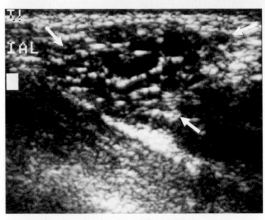

Fig. 22.**51 b** Sonogram displays a hypoechoic mass including small cystic spaces. *Histology:* juvenile papillomatosis

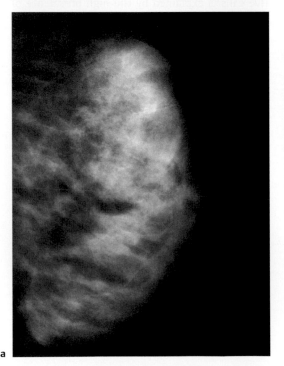

Fig. 22.**52** Eighteen-year-old patient with a palpable mass at 12 o'clock
a Mammographically the mass is obscured by dense tissue
b Sonographically a hypoechoic round mass with posterior enhancement is seen, fairly mobile. Core biopsy revealed a fibroadenoma.

- Detection of carcinomas presenting with suggestive microcalcifications is excellent in any breast type

During pregnancy and lactation, mammographic evaluation, which is only indicated in symptomatic patients, is even more difficult than in the nonpregnant young patient. This is caused by further increase in density due to glandular proliferation, increased water content, and hyperemia. Even though numerous lesions can be obscured mammographically and benign lesions can only rarely be unequivocally diagnosed by mammography, mammography should be applied in all indeterminate or suspicious lesions; mostly because of mammography's capability to image microcalcifications, a definite diagnosis of malignancy will be possible in at least some cases (Fig. 22.**55**). In these cases, mammography can accelerate the diagnosis of carcinoma. It is common for patients to be biopsied only after completion of pregnancy. Additionally, in the case of suspected malignancy, further foci may be detected, which can be important for adequate treatment planning.

When mammography is applied in the young patient, it must be remembered that the potential risk of radiation is higher for young patients than for older patients. Consideration of this potential increased risk of breast cancer is important when mammography is applied in asymptomatic patients. It is not important in those symptomatic patients whose symptoms cannot be explained by clinical or sonographic findings. Because of the low energy of the mammographically used X-rays, virtually no radiation will reach the fetus, particularly when the abdomen is shielded. Therefore, pregnancy is not a contraindication to mammography. To decrease mammographic density and thus improve mammographic evaluation during lactation, mammograms should be taken directly after breast feeding.

Based on the above considerations and the experiences reported in the literature, the following recommendations are given for the **use of mammography:**

- *Routine mammographic screening* is not advocated in the *asymptomatic normal risk patient younger than 40*.[100, 105, 108]
- In women with a first-degree relative with premenopausal breast cancer and in women with positive genetic testing, with a history of Hodgkin disease with a prior breast cancer, and mediastinal irradiation[109], or with a high-risk lesion of breast biopsy, routine screening before age 40 is indicated. In women with a first-degree relative with breast cancer, screening should begin at an age 10 years earlier than the cancer was diagnosed in that relative but not earlier than 25 years of age.[108, 110] In women treated for Hodgkin disease, screening should commence no later than 8 years after the completion of treatment.[109, 111]
- Considering the high prevalence of benign problems (e.g., cysts) that can at least partly be solved by ultrasound, *in symptomatic patients mammography should be used after sonography.*
- *In all symptomatic patients* without a definitely benign diagnosis established sonographically (cyst, galactocele, freely moveable typical benign solid mass as defined on pp. 100–101), *mammography is strongly recommended* since it may be able to detect suggestive microcalcifications or masses.
- This also applies to symptomatic patients during pregnancy. Pregnancy is no contraindication to mammography.
- In the case of *absent mammographic findings in dense tissue or potentially benign mammographic findings,* a negative mammogram should not dissuade from *further workup* of suspicious or indeterminate clinical findings.

■ Sonography

In view of the difficulties surrounding mammographic detection and diagnosis of breast cancer in the young patient, sonography has been proposed as the method of choice in young patients. Indeed, the use of sonography is recommended as the first method for the workup of symptomatic patients below the age of 35 years.[112] The reasons are as follows:

- Since sonography is not associated with any radiation, it is completely harmless for the patient.
- In the case of a simple cyst, a definitive diagnosis is possible by sonography, and no further workup is necessary.
- In patients with mammographically dense tissue, a hypoechoic suggestive mass detected in an area of an indeterminate palpable finding supports the diagnosis of malignancy and immediate further workup (Fig. 22.**53c**) and (Fig. 22.**54e**).

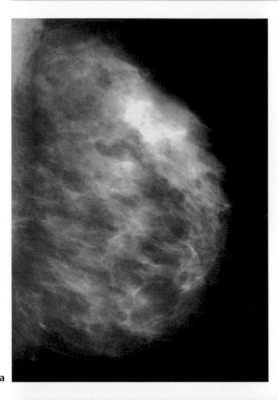

a

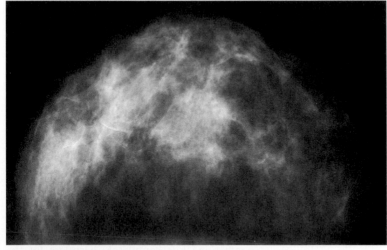

b

Fig. 22.**53**   Two months after a normal screening mammogram and normal clinical examination, this 38-year-old patient with a family history of breast cancer noticed a palpable mass in the upper outer quadrant of her left breast

a, b Oblique and cc mammogram 2 months before showed dense breast tissue, no mass

– In the pregnant or lactating patient, a galactocele can be suspected if a hypoechoic lesion shows fluctuation of the echoes with palpation or if septations are seen (Fig. 11.4). The diagnosis can easily be established by aspiration of milk.

As with mammography, many of the benign and malignant lesions unfortunately exhibit a wide range of sonographic findings and considerably overlap in their sonographic appearance (Fig. 15.13d, Fig. 22.51b, Fig. 22.52b).

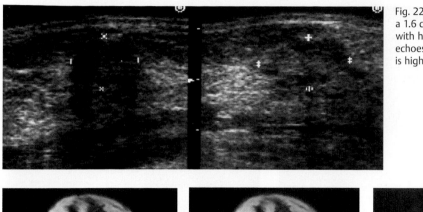

Fig. 22.**53c** Sonographically a 1.6 cm hypoechoic mass with heterogeneous internal echoes and distal shadowing is highly suspicious

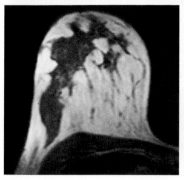 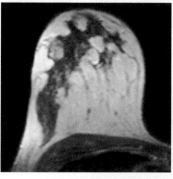 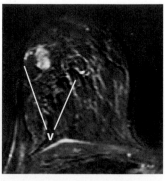

d   e   f

Fig. 22.**53d–f** Contrast-enhanced MRI, which was performed to exclude additional foci, confirmed the presence of an oval mass of about 1.8 cm with some irregularities. In spite of its delayed enhancement and fairly oval shape, the mass is suspicious. No further foci. (v = vessel)
d Precontrast image **e** Postcontrast image (3rd minute) **f** Subtraction of image (**e**) minus (**d**)
Histology: invasive ductal carcinoma NOS

Juvenile papillomatosis can present as a hypoechoic mass, which can be more or less well-circumscribed or can resemble a fibroadenoma. With high-resolution sonography, numerous, mostly small cysts and dilated ducts may be visible within the lesion (so-called typical Swiss-cheese appearance) that can be a hint to this diagnosis (Fig. 22.51b).[113] Since cystic spaces can also be encountered with fibrocystic changes and in phyllodes tumors, this appearance cannot be considered pathognomonic, and further workup remains necessary. Breast infarct presumably will present as an indeterminate hypoechoic mass or complex mass of mixed echogenicity and attenuation and can therefore not be distinguished from malignancy.

Overall, the sonographic appearance cannot be considered sufficiently characteristic for the majority of solid lesions to warrant a final diagnosis. Workup must be continued:

- If the abovementioned criteria of a simple cyst or typical fibroadenoma are not fulfilled.
- If there are no sonographic findings.
- As with older women, the general limitations of sonography concerning the detection of small and preinvasive carcinomas also apply to the young patients.[34–38, 101] In young and older patients, most investigators report only moderate sensitivity (about 70%) for the detection of early malignancy by sonography.[34–38, 98, 114]
- Sonographic differentiation between benign and malignant masses is usually not reliable (Fig. 15.**13d**).[37, 114–116]

■ Percutaneous Biopsy

Percutaneous biopsy appears a most valuable adjunct, particularly in young patients with indeterminate changes.[98, 104] Its increased use may help

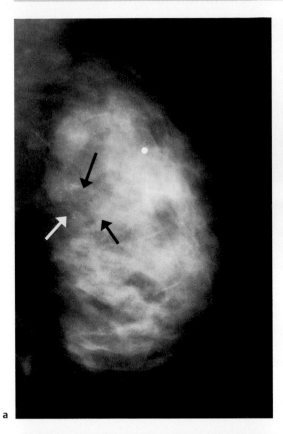

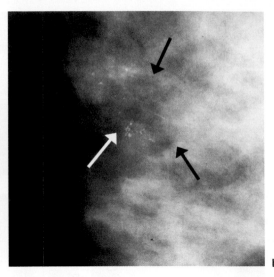

Fig. 22.**54** Breast cancer in young patients
a, b. Twenty-two-year-old patient who presented with bone metastases. Search for primary tumor revealed mammographically suggestive microcalcifications, which are excellently seen in spite of the dense tissue
a Oblique view
b Magnification of the area of microcalcifications

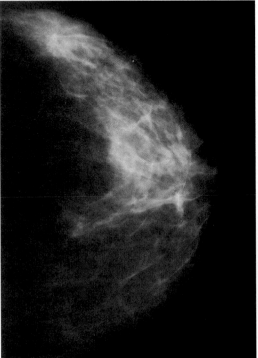

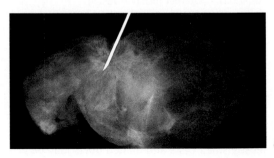

Fig. 22.**54 c–f** Thirty-two-year-old patient with carcinophobia
c Suggestive architectural distortion in the upper outer quadrant
d Specimen radiograph reveals a radiolucent center, which, however, does not prove benignity

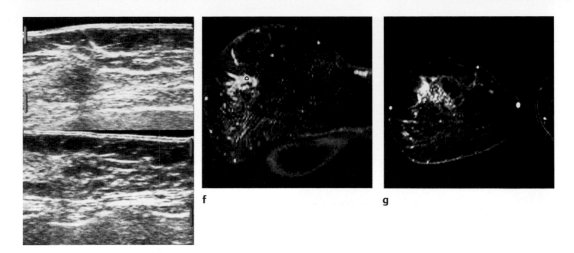

e

e Sonogram in two planes shows architectural distortion
f MR subtraction (post-CM minus pre-CM): a star-like enhancement is shown in the area of suspicion
g MR subtraction of another slice, 1 cm from slice (**e**).
Further areas of enhancement are seen in other slices as
well.

Histology: sclerosing adenosis, associated with non-
comedo DCIS. The enhancement on the adjacent slices
only corresponded to areas of adenosis

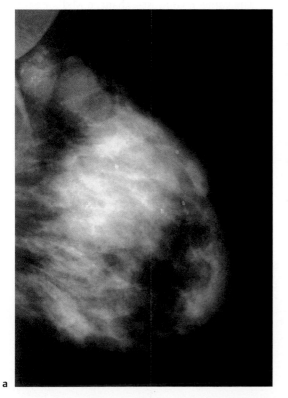

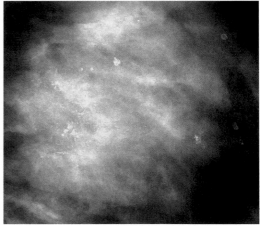

Fig. 22.55 Forty-two-year-old lactating patient with left
breast lump
a–c A large area with suspicious microcalcifications (arrows) is shown. Note microcalcifications within two suspicious lymph nodes in the axillary tail.
Histology: invasive ductal carcinoma

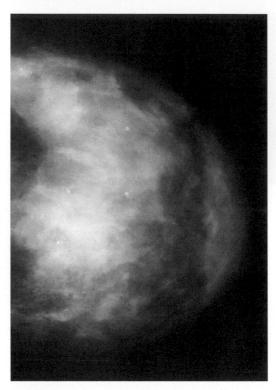

Fig. 22.**55 c**

to both avoid a large number of diagnostic excisional biopsies and decrease the cases with a delayed diagnosis.

Owing to the widely varying sensitivity of fine-needle aspiration,[117-121] core biopsy or vacuum biopsy[54-62] may be the more appropriate procedure at most facilities. Sufficient material must be obtained, and the results of percutaneous biopsy must be counterchecked with the clinical and imaging findings.

In case of indeterminate results, insufficient material, or results that are not concordant with imaging findings, repeat biopsy must be undertaken.

During pregnancy or lactation, an increased tendency to bleed exists due to the physiological hyperemia. This can usually be taken care of by firm compression, even during the procedure. An increased risk of infection or milk fistulas, as reported for surgical biopsy, has not been encountered.[117] However, it may be best taken care of by cessation of breast feeding before biopsy.[88] The radiologist should be aware of the possibility of fistula formation if biopsy of a galactocele is attempted.

Magnetic Resonance Imaging

Contrast-enhanced MRI is not indicated as a screening method for young patients with dense or lumpy breast tissue.

The reasons are:

- MRI has a high sensitivity for detection of occult benign changes (e.g., fibroadenomas, areas of adenosis) in at least 20% of patients (Fig. 22.**54f, g**)
- Areas of transient enhancement due to hormonal influences, which may be another cause of false positive calls, appear to the more frequent in this age group.[7]
- At the same time, the prevalance of malignancy is lower than that of benign disease by a factor of about 1000

Therefore, contrast-enhanced MRI might necessitate an unacceptably high number of workups for benign changes, while detecting very few, if any, malignancies.

Finally, MRI is generally not necessary for evaluation of palpable, mammographically or sonographically visible masses, since percutaneous biopsy—due to its lower false positive rate—is much more cost-effective.

The value of contrast-enhanced MRI for early detection of malignancy in very high-risk young patients with dense tissue is presently being evaluated (Figs. 22.**53d–f**). First results indicate that MRI may be able to play an important role in this field.[40-44]

Diagnostic Strategy

Based on the different situations concerning prevalence of breast cancer and the capabilities of each method and based on different estimations of potential radiation hazards in this age group, the following diagnostic strategy should be adapted:

- Screening is not recommended for asymptomatic patients without significantly increased risk.
- In high-risk patients, screening mammography before age 40 may be useful. Whether additional sonography or MRI may be able to increase the detection rate of malignancy at acceptable false positive rates in such high-risk patients is under investigation.
- For the evaluation of palpable masses in patients under 35 years of age, sonography

should be used first. If a benign diagnosis can be made with a high degree of accuracy, no further workup is necessary, and follow-up is sufficient.

– In all other cases, a mammogram should follow. A single-view mammogram for detection of microcalcifications may be sufficient. Additional views should be obtained as needed.

– Pregnancy or lactation is no contraindication to mammography. During lactation, mammography should be performed immediately after breast feeding because the breast density is lower than before breast feeding. Based on its capability to visualize suspicious microcalcifications, mammography, even in very dense breasts, can help to avoid a delay in diagnosis or may be able to detect additional foci. It should therefore be used whenever indicated.

– In all cases with negative or benign-appearing findings with imaging, the diagnosis must be critically correlated with the clinical findings. In view of the limited sensitivity of all modalities in young patients, percutaneous biopsy should be generously used in case of any doubt.

– As usual, percutaneous biopsy has to be performed diligently and its results critically checked to determine whether the diagnosis is appropriate for the imaging and clinical findings.

■ References

1 Tabar L; Gad A, Holmberg L et al. Significant reduction in advanced breast cancer: results of the first seven years of mammography screening in Kopparberg, Sweden. Diagn Imag Clin Med. 1985;54:158–64
2 Sickles EA, Ominsky SH, Sollitto RA et al. Medical audit of a rapid-throughput mammography screening practice: methodology and results of 27,114 examinations. Radiology. 1990;175:323–7
3 Frankel SD, Sickles EA, Curpen BN et al. Initial versus subsequent screening mammography: comparison of findings and their prognostic significance. AJR. 1995;164:1107–9
4 Bird RE, Wallace TW, Yankaskas BC. Analysis of cancers missed at screening mammography. Radiology. 1992;34:1949–52
5 Stavros AT, Thickman D, Rapp CL et al. Solid breast nodules: use of sonography to distinguish between benign and malignant lesions. Radiology. 1995;196:123
6 Sickles EA. Nonpalpable, circumscribed, non-calcified solid breast masses: likelihood of malignancy based on lesion size and age of patient. Radiology. 1994;192:439
7 Heywang-Köbrunner SH, Beck R. Contrast-enhanced MRI of the Breast. 2nd ed. Heidelberg, New York: Springer; 1995
8 Kavaknagh AM, Mitchell H, Gilles GG et al. Hormone re-

placement therapy and accuracy of mammographic screening. Lancet. 2000;355:270–4
9 Harvey JA. Use and cost of breast imaging for postmenopausal women undergoing hormone replacement therapy. AJR. 1999;172:1615–9
10 Krämer S, Schulz-Wendtland R, Hagedorn K et al. Magnetic resonance imaging in the diagnosis of local recurrences in breast cancer. Anticancer Res. 1998;18:2159–61
11 Viehweg P, Heinig A, Lampe D et al. Retrospective analysis for evaluation of the value of contrast-enhanced MRI in patients with breast conservative therapy. MAGMA (Magnetic Resonance Materials in Physics, Biology and Medicine). 1998;7:141–52
12 Fischer U, Kopka L, Grabbe E. Magnetic resonance guided localization and biopsy of suspicious breast lesions. Topics in Magnetic Resonance Imaging. 1998;9:44–59
13 Heinig A, Heywang-Köbrunner SH, Viehweg P et al. Wertigkeit der Kontrastmittel-Magnetresonanztomographie der Mamma bei Wiederaufbau mittels Implantat. Der Radiologe. 1997;37:710–7
14 Dessole S, Meloni GB, Capobianco G et al. Radial scar of the breast: mammographic enigma in pre-and postmenopausal women. Maturitas. 2000;34:227–31
15 Orel SG, Evers K, Yeh IT et al. Radial scar with microcalcifications: radiologic–pathologic correlation. Radiology. 1992;183:479
16 Alleva DQ, Smetherman DH, Farr GH et al. Radial scar of the breast: radiologic–pathologic correlation in 22 cases. Radigraphics. 1999;19:27–35
17 Cohen MA, Serlazza SJ. Role of sonography in evaluation of radial scars of the breast. AJR. 2000;174:1075–8
18 Harvey JA, Fajardo LL, Innis CA. Previous mammograms in patients with impalpable breast carcinoma: retrospective vs. blinded interpretation. AJR. 1993;161:1167
19 Greendale GA, Reboussin BA, Sie A et al. Effects of estrogen and estrogen-progestin on mammographic parenchymal density. Postmenopausal Estrogen/Progestin Interventions (PEPI) Investigators. Ann Intern Med. 1999:130: 262–9
20 Laya MB, Larson EB, Taplin SH et al. Effect of estrogen replacement therapy on the specificity and sensitivity of screening mammography. J Natl Cancer Inst. 1996;88:643–9
21 Litherland JC, Stallard S, Hole D et al. The effect of hormone replacement therapy on the sensitivity of screening mammograms. Clin Radiol. 1999;54:285–8
22 Doyle GJ, McClean L. Unilateral increase in mammographic density with hormone replacment therapy. Clin Radiol. 1994;49:50
23 Mandelson MT, Oestreicher N, Porter PL et al. Breast Density as a Predictor of Mammographic Detection: Comparison of Interval- and Screen-Detected Cancers. J Natl Cancer Inst. 2000;92:1081–7
24 van Gils CH, Otten JD, Hendricks JH et al. High mammographic breast density and its implications for the early detection of breast cancer. J Med Screen. 1999;6:200–4
25 Jackson VP, Hendrick RE, Feig SA, Kopans DB. Imaging of the radiographically dense breast. Radiology. 1993;1993:297
26 Morrone D, Ambrogetti D, Bravetti P et al. Diagnostic errors in mammography. I. False negative results. Radiol Med Torino. 1991;82:212
27 Tabar L, Vitak B, Chen HH et al. Update of the Swedish Two-County Trial of breast cancer screening: histologic grade-specific and age-specific results. Swiss Surg. 1999;5:199–204
28 Michaelson JS, Hapern E, Kopans DB. Breast cancer: computer simulation method for estimating optimal intervals for screening. Radiology. 1999;212:551–60

29 Hendrick RE, Smith RA, Rutledge JH III et al. Benefit of screening mammography in women aged 40–49: a new meta-analysis of randomized controlled trials. In: Journal of the National Cancer Institute Monographs. No. 22. Washington, D.C.: Government Printing Office, 1997:87–92

30 Andersson I, Janzon L. Reduced breast cancer mortality in women under age 50: updated results from the Malmo Mammographic Screening Program. In: Journal of the National Cancer Institute Monographs. No. 22 Washington, D.C.: Government Printing Office, 1997:63–7

31 Bjurstam N, Bjorneld L, Duffy SW et al. The Gothenburg Breast Cancer Screening Trial: preliminary results on breast cancer mortality for women aged 39–49. In: Journal of the National Cancer Institute Monographs. No. 22 Washington, D. C.: Government Printing Office, 1997:53–5

32 Kolb TM, Lichy J, Newhouse JH. Occult cancer in women with dense breasts: Detection with screening US—diagnostic yield and tumor characteristics. Radiology. 1998;207:191–9

33 Buchberger W, De Koekkoek-Doll P, Springer P et al. Incidental findings on sonography of the breast: clinical significance and diagnostic workup. AJR. 1999;173:921–7

34 Cantarzi S, Guiseppetti GM, Rizzato G et al. A multicenter study for the evaluation of the diagnostic efficiency of mammography and echography in nonpalpable breast neoplasms. Radio Med Torino. 1993;84:193

35 Balu-Maestro C, Bruneton JN, Melia P et al. High frequency ultrasound detection of breast calcifications. Eur J Ultrasound. 1994;3:247

36 Ciatto S, Roselli-del-Turco M, Catarzis M et al. The diagnostic role of breast echography. Radiol med. 1994;88:221

37 Pamilo M, Soiva M, Anttinen et al. Ultrasonography of breast lesions detected in mammography screening. Acta Radiol. 1991;32:220

38 Potterton AJ, Peakman DJ, Young IR. Ultrasound demonstration of small breast cancers detected by mammographic screening. Clin Radiol. 1994;49:808

39 Tohno E, Cosgrove DO, Sloane UP. Ultrasound diagnosis of breast diseases. Edinburgh: Churchill Livingstone; 1994

40 Leach M. Assessing contrast enhanced MRI as a method of screening women at genetic risk of breast cancer: study design, methodology and analysis. Proc ISMRM. 1998:226

41 Bick, U. Integriertes Früherkennungskonzept bei Frauen mit genetischer Präposition für Brustkrebs. Radiologe. 1997;37:591–3

42 Breast MRI Protocol, Study 6883 of the National Cancer Institute, Washington D.C., August 27, 1996

43 Stoutjesdijk MJ, Boetes C, Van Die LE et al. Magnetic resonance mammography for breast cancer screening of patients from high risk populations: results of a prospective pilot study. Radiology. 1999;213(P):454

44 Kuhl CK, Schmutzler R, Leutner CC et al. Breast MR screening in 192 women proved or suspected to be carriers of a breast cancer susceptibility gene: preliminary results. Radiology. 2000;215:267–79

45 Heywang-Köbrunner SH, Hyynh AT, Viehweg P et al. Prototype breast coil for MR-guided needle localization. J Comput Assist Tomogr. 1994;18:876–881

46 Orel SG, Schnall MD, Newman RW et al. MR imaging-guided localization and biopsy of breast lesions: initial experience. Radiology. 1994;193:97–102

47 Kuhl, C, Elevelt A, Leutner C et al. Interventional breast MR imaging: clinical use of a stereotactic localization and biopsy device. Radiology. 1997;204:667–75

48 Heywang-Köbrunner SH, Heinig A, Schaumlöffel U et al. MR-guided percutaneous excisional and incisional biopsy of breast lesions. Eur Radiol. 1999;9:1656–65

49 Heywang-Köbrunner SH, Heinig A, Pickuth D et al. Interventional MRI of the breast: lesion localization and biopsy. Eur Radiol. 2000;10:36–45

50 Heywang-Köbrunner SH, Viehweg P, Heinig A, Küchler C. Contrast-enhanced MRI of the breast—accuracy, value, controversies, solutions. Europ J Radiol. 1997;24:94–108

51 Morris EA, Schwartz LH, Dershaw DD et al. MR imaging of the breast in patients with occult primary breast carcinoma. Radiology. 1997;205:437–40

52 Schorn C, Fischer U, Luftner-Nagel S et al. MRI of the breast in patients with metastatic disease of unknown primary. Eur Radiol. 1999;9:470–3

53 Orel SG, Weinstein SP, Schnall MD. Breast MR imaging in patients with axillary node metastases and unknown primary malignancy. Radiology. 1999;212:543–9

54 Brenner RJ, Fajardo L, Fisher PR et al. Percutaneous core biopsy of the breast: effect of operator experience and number of samples on diagnostic accuracy. AJR. 1996;166:341–6.

55 Liberman L, Dershaw DD, Glassman JR et al. Analysis of cancers not diagnosed at stereotactic core breast biopsy. Radiology. 1997;203:151–7

56 Meyer JE, Smith DN, Lester SC et al. Large core needle biopsy: nonmalignant breast abnormalities evaluated with surgical excision or repeat core biopsy. Radiology. 1998;206:717–9

57 Jackman RJ, Nowels KW, Rodriguez-Soto J et al. Stereotactic, automated, large-core needle biopsy of nonpalpable breast lesions: false-negative and histologic underestimation rates after long-term follow-up. Radiology. 1999;210:799–805

58 Maniero MB, Philpotts LE, Lee CH et al. Stereotaxic core needle biopsy of breast microcalcifications correlation of target accuracy and diagnostic with lesion size. Radiology. 1996;198:665–9

59 Jackman RJ, Marzoni FA, Nowels KW. Percutaneous removal of benign mammographic lesions: comparison of automated large-core and directional vacuum-assisted biopsy techniques. AJR. 1998;171:1325–30

60 Heywang-Köbrunner SH, Schaumlöffel U, Viehweg P et al. Minimally invasive stereotactic vacuum core breast biopsy. Eur Radiol. 1998;8;377–85

61 Zannis VJ, Aliano KM. The evolving practice pattern of the breast surgeon with disappearance of open biopy for nonpalpable lesions. Am J Surg. 1998;176:525–8

62 Götz L, Amaya B, Häntschel G et al. Mammographically guided vacuum biopsy: experiences with 700 cases. Eur Radiol. 2000;10(2 Suppl):329

63 Lanyi M. Formanalyse von 5641 Mikroverkalkungen bei 101 Milchgangskarzinomen: die Polymorphie. Fortschr Röntgenstr. 1983;139:240

64 LeGal M, Chavanne D, Pellier D. Valeur diagnostique des microcalcifications groupées découvertes par mammographies. A propos de 227 cas avec vérification histologique et sans tumeur du sein palpable. Bull Cancer (Paris). 1984;71:57–64

65 a) Sickles EA. Breast calcifications: mammographic evaluation. Radiology. 1986;160:289
   b) Lafontan DB, Daures JP, Salicru B et al. Isolated clustered microcalcifications: diagnostic value of mammography—series of 400 cases with surgical verification. Radiology. 1994;190:479

66 Bassett LW. Mammographic analysis of calcifications. Radiol Clin North Am. 1992;30:93–105

67 Breast Imaging Reporting and Data System (BIRADS ™) 3rd ed. Reston, Va. American College of Radiology.

68 Heywang-Köbrunner SH, Schreer I, Müller-Schimpfle M et al. Recommendations of the German Roentgen Ray Society for Breast Imaging and Intervention. Stuttgart–New York: Thieme 2000, in preparation

69 Tabar L, Dean PB, Pentek Z. Galactography: The diagnostic procedure of choice for nipple discharge. AJR. 1983;149:31–8

70 Kindermann G. Diagnostic value of galactography in the detection of breast cancer. In: Zander J, Baltzer J, eds. Early Breast Cancer. Berlin: Springer; 1985:136–9

71 Tardivon AA, Viala J, Corvellec Rudelli A et al. Mammographic patterns of inflammatory breast carcinoma: a retrospective study on 92 cases. Eur J Radiol. 1997;24:124–30

72 Kushwaha AC, Whitman GJ, Stelling CB et al. Primary inflammatory carcinoma of the breast: retrospective review of mammographic findings. AJR. 2000;174:535–8

73 Winchester DP. Breast cancer in young women. Surg Clin North Am. 1996;76:279–87

74 Kutner SE. Breast Cancer Genetics and Managed Care. Cancer suppl. 999;86:2570–4

75 Boice JD Jr, Preston D, Davis FG, Monson RR. Frequent chest X-ray fluoroscopy and breast cancer incidence among tuberculosis patients in Massachusetts. Radiat Res. 1991;125:214–22

76 a) Sharan SK, Morimatsu M, Abrecht U et al. Embryonic lethality and radiation hypersensitivity mediated by Rad51 in mice lacking BRCA 2. Nature. 1997;386:804–10
b) Bebb G, Glickman B, Gelmon K et al. „At risk" for breast cancer. Lancet. 1997;349:1784–5
c) Den Otter W, Merchant TE, Beijerinck D et al. Breast cancer induction due to mammography screening in hereditarily affected women. Anticancer Res. 1996;16:3173–5

77 Bassett L, Ysrael M, Gold R, Ysrael C. Usefulness of mammography and sonography in women less than 35 years of age. Radiology. 1991;180:831

78 Bennett JC, Freitas R Jr, Fentiman IS. Diagnosis of breast cancer in young women. Aust N Z J Surg. 1991;61:284

79 Kerlikowske K, Grady D, Barclay I et al. Positive predictive value of screening mammography by age and family history of breast cancer. JAMA. 1993;270:2444

80 Lamin DR, Harris RP, Swanson FH et al. Difficulties in diagnosis of carcinoma of the breast in patients less than 50 years of age. Surg Gynecol Obstet. 1993;177:457

81 Gajdos C, Tartter PI, Bleiweiss IJ et al. Stage O to stage III breast cancer in young women. J Am Coll Surg. 2000;190:523–9

82 Gillett D, Kennedy C, Carmalt H. Breast cancer in young women. Aust N Z J Surg. 1997;67:761–4

83 Rosen PP, Holmes G, Lesser ML et al. Juvenile papillomatosis and breast carcinoma. Cancer 1985;55:1345

84 Bazzocchi F, Santini D, Martinelli G et al. Juvenile papillomatosis (epitheliosis) of the breast: a clinical and pathological study of 13 cases. Am J Clin Pathol. 1986;86:745

85 Tokunaga M, Wakimoto J, Muramoto Y et al. Juvenile secretory carcinoma and juvenile papillomatosis. Japan J Clin Oncol. 1985;15:457

86 Ferguson TM, McCarty KS, Filston HC. Juvenile secretory carcinoma and juvenile papillomatosis: diagnosis and treatment. J Pediatr Surg. 1987;22:637

87 Hasson J, Pope CH. Mammary infarcts associated with pregnancy presenting as breast tumors. Surgery. 1961;49:313

88 Harris JR, Hellman S, Henderson C, Kinne DW. Breast Diseases. 2nd ed. Philadelphia: JB Lippincott; 1991

89 Wilkinson S, Green WO Jr. Infarction of breast lesions during pregnancy and lactation. Cancer. 1964;17:1567

90 Gorins A, Lenhardt F, Espie M. Breast cancer during pregnancy. Epidemiology—diagnosis—prognosis. Contracep Fertil Sex. 1996;24:153–6

91 Maass, H. Mammakarzinom: Epidemiologie. Gynäkologe. 1994;27:3

92 Ciatto S, Roselli-del-Turco M, Cantarzi S et al. Causes of breast cancer misdiagnosis at physical examination. Neoplasma. 1991;38(5):523

93 Reintgen D, Berman C, Cox C et al. The anatomy of missed breast cancers. Surg Oncol. 1993;2(1):65

94 Applewhite RR, Smith LR, De Vincenti F. Carcinoma of the breast associated with pregnancy and lactation. Am Surg. 1973;39:101

95 Fleming U, Sheridan B, Atkinson L et al. The effects of childbearing on carcinoma of the breast. Med J Aust. 1970;1:1252

96 Treves N, Holleb AI. A rport of 549 cases of breast cancer in women 35 years of age or younger. Surg Gynecol Obstet. 1958;107:271

97 Meyer J, Kopans D, Oot R. Breast cancer visualized by mammography in patients under 35. Radiology. 1983;147:93

98 Ashley S, Royle G, Corder A et al. Clinical, radiological and cytological diagnosis of breast cancer in young women. Br J Surg. 1989;76:835

99 Harris V, Jackson V. Indications for breast imaging in women under age 35 years. Radiology. 1989;172:445

100 Jeffries D, Adler D. Mammographic detection of breast cancer in women under the age of 35. Invest Radiol. 1990;25:67

101 Bassett LW, Kimme-Smith C. Breast sonography. AJR. 1991;156:449

102 Joensuu H, Asola R, Holli K et al. Delayed diagnosis and large size of breast cancer after a false negative mammogram. Eur J Cancer. 1994;30A(9):1299

103 Yelland A, Graham MD, Trott PA et al. Diagnosing breast carcinoma in young women. BMJ. 1991, Mar 16;302(6777):618

104 Dawson AE, Mulford DK, Taylor AS et al. Breast carcinoma detection in women aged 35 years and younger: mammography and diagnosis by fine-needle aspiration cytology. Cancer. 1998;84:163–8

105 de Paredes ES, Marsteller L, Eden B. Breast cancers in women 35 years of age and younger: mammographic findings. Radiology. 1990;177:117

106 Gilles R, Gallay X, Tardivon A et al. Breast cancer in women 35 years old or younger: clinical and mammographic features. Eur Radiol. 1995;5:630

107 Olivetti L, Bergenzini R, Vanoli C et al. Is mammography useful in the detection of breast cancer in women 35 years of age or younger? Radiol Med (Torino). 1998;95:161–4

108 Liberman L, Dershaw DD, Deutch BM et al. Screening mammography: value in women 35–39 years old. AJR. 1993;161(1):53

109 Cutuli B, Dhermain F, Borel C et al. Breast cancer in patients treated for Hogkin's disease: clinical and pathological analysis of 76 cases in 63 patients. Eur J Cancer. 1997;33:2315–20

110 Moskowitz M. Breast cancer screening: all's well that ends well, or much ado about nothing? AJR. 1988;151:659

111 Dershaw DD, Yahalom I, Petzek JA. Mammography of breast carcinoma developing in women treated for Hodgkin's disease. Radiology. 1992;184:421–3

112 Kossoff MB. Ultrasound of the breast. World J Surg. 2000;24:143–57

113 Kersschot EAJ, Hermans M, Pauwels C et al. Juvenile papillomatosis (Swiss cheese disease) of the breast: sonographic appearance. Radiology. 1988;169:631

114 Jackson V. The role of US in breast imaging. RAdiology. 1990;177:305

115 Adler DD, Heyde DL, Ikeda DM. Quantitative sonographic parametersa as means of distinguishing breast cancers from benign solid masses. J Ultrasound Med. 1991;10:505

116 Fornage BD, Lorrigan JG, Andry E. Fibroadenoma of the breast: sonographic appearance. Radiology. 1989;172:671

117 Michaelson JS, Kopans DB, Cady B. The breast carcinoma screening interval is important. Cancer 2000;88:1282–4

118 Harris, J, Lippmann M, Veronesi U, Willett W. Breast cancer. N Engl J Med. 1992;327:319

119 Dent DM, Kirkpatrick AE, McGoogan E, Chetty U, Anderson TJ. Stereotaxic localization and aspiration cytology of impalpable breast lesions. Clin Radiol. 1989;40:380

120 Dowlatshahi K, Yaremko ML, Kluskens LF, Jokich PM. Nonpalpable breast lesions: findings of stereotaxic needle-core biopsy and fine-needle aspiration cytology. Radiology. 1991;185;639

121 Dempsey P, Rubin E. The roles of needle biopsy and periodic follow-up in the evaluation and diagnosis of breast lesions. Semin Roentgenol. 1993;28:252

122 Krämer S, Schulz-Wendtland R, Hagedorn K et al. Magnetic resonance imaging and its role in the diagnosis of multicentric breast cancer. Anticancer Res. 1998;18:2163–4

123 Boetes C, Mus RD, Holland R et al. Breast tumors: Comparative accuracy of MR imaging relative to mammography and ultrasound for demonstrating extent. Radiology. 1995;197:743–7

124 Oellinger H, Heins S, Sander B et al. Gd-DTPA-enhanced MR breast imaging: the most sensitive method for multicentric carcinomas of the female breast. Eur Radiol. 1993;3:223–8

125 Harms SE, Flaming DP, Hesley KL et al. MR imaging of the breast with rotating delivery of excitation off resonance: Clinical experience with pathologic correlation. Radiology. 1993;187:493

126 Mumtaz H, Hall-Craigs MA, Davidson T et al. Staging of symptomatic primary breast cancer with MR imaging. AJR. 1997;169:417–24

127 Fischer U, Kopka L, Grabbe E. Breast carcinoma: effect of preoperative contrast-enhanced MR imaging on the therapeutic approach. Radiology. 1999;213:881–8

Appendix 1

■ TNM Classification of Breast Carcinomas (1)

Breast cancers are classified based on histopathology of the primary tumor (T stage), regional nodal status as confirmed by histopathology (N stage), and distant metastases (M stage).

In case multiple simultaneous carcinomas exist in one breast, T stage is determined by the carcinoma with the highest T stage. If carcinomas exist in both breasts, each breast is staged separately. The size of invasive carcinomas is determined based on the size of the invasive component only.

TX	Primary tumor cannot be assessed (for example: no histology available)
TO	No primary tumor detected (p is added if tissue was histopathologically assessed)
pTis	ductal carcinoma in situ (DCIS) or lobular carcinoma in situ (LCIS) or Paget's disease of the nipple without DCIS, LCIS, or invasive tumor in the breast. (If invasive tumor, DCIS, or LCIS is detected in the breast, the disease is staged based on these entities)
pT1	tumor ≤20 mm
T1mic	microinvasion: The basal membrane has been exceeded in one or more foci. No focus exceeds 1 mm in size
pT1a	≤5 mm
pT1b	5 mm < tumor ≤10 mm
pT1c	10 mm < tumor ≤20 mm
pT2	20 mm < tumor ≤50 mm
pT3	tumor >50 mm
pT4	tumor of any size that invades skin or chest wall*
pT4a	invasion of chest wall*
pT4b	skin edema, ulceration, or cutaneous satellite nodule**
pT4c	T4a + b
pT4d	inflammatory carcinoma (inflammatory carcinoma without proof of in-breast tumor and with negative skin biopsy is classified as pTX)
N	concerns histopathologic staging of the regional lymph nodes (lymph-node groups, see Appendix 2). So far this included at least sampling of ≥ six lymph nodes of level I.
NX	regional lymph nodes cannot be assessed (for example: had been removed before or were not sampled)
pN0	no regional lymph-node metastases
pN1	mobile metastatic lymph node(s) of the ipsilateral axilla
pN1a	only micrometastases (≤2 mm)
pN1b	at least one metastasis >2 mm
i	one or more metastases in 1–3 lymph nodes all < 20 mm
ii	≥ 4 lymph nodes with all foci < 20 mm
iii	metastatic involvement exceeds lymph-node capsule, but all foci < 20 mm
iv	metastatic focus or foci ≥ 20 mm
pN2	metastatic lymph nodes located in the ipsilateral axilla and fixed to one another or to surrounding structures
pN3	metastatic involvement of internal mammary lymph nodes
M1	–involvement of supraclavicular, cervical, or contralateral lymph nodes –distant metastases

■ References

Hermanek P. TNM atlas. Berlin, Heidelberg, New York: Springer; 1998

---

* The chest wall includes ribs and intercostal muscles, but not the pectoral muscles.
** Skin retraction alone does not lead to a T4 classification

Appendix II

■ Definitions of Anatomic Locations (1)

■ Breast

The breast is subdivided into 7 different regions, as shown below:

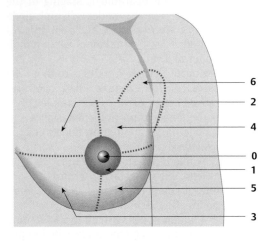

0. Nipple (ICD Code: C 50.0)
1. Central part (ICD-Code: C 50.1)
2. Upper inner quadrant (ICD Code: C 50.2)
3. Lower inner quadrant (ICD Code: C 50.3)
4. Upper outer quadrant (ICD Code: C 50.4)
5. Lower outer quadrant (ICD Code: C 50.5)
6. Axillary tail (ICD Code: C 50.6)

■ Lymph Nodes

The regional lymph nodes include axillary lymph nodes of level I–III and the ipsilateral internal mammary lymph nodes.

The *axillary* lymph nodes accompany the axillary vein and its branches and are subdivided, as follows:

Level I (lower axilla): lymph nodes lateral to the lateral margin of the pectoral minor muscle

Level II (mid axilla): lymph nodes deep to the pectoral minor muscle

Level III (upper axilla): lymph nodes medial to the medial margin of the pectoral minor muscle (including the subclavicular, infraclavicular, and the apical lymph-node groups

Apart from axillary lymph nodes only the *ipsilateral internal mammary lymph nodes* belong to the regional lymph nodes.

If lymph nodes other than the above-mentioned ones are involved, these are considered distant metastases.

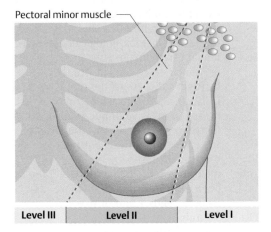

Pectoral minor muscle

| Level III | Level II | Level I |

■ References

Hermanek P. TNM atlas. Berlin, Heidelberg, New York: Springer; 1998

Index

Page references in **bold type** refer to illustrations.

A

abnormalities, 171–175
  summary, 175
abscesses, 242–243, **244**, 245
  clinical findings, 242
  histology, 242
  mammography, 243, **244**
  MRI, 243, **244**
  percutaneous biopsy, 245
  sonography, 243, **244**
  summary, 245
accessory breast tissue, **172**, 173
accordion effect, 139
accuracy
  mammography, 14–15
    ductal carcinoma in situ, 262
    fibroadenoma, 217
  MRI, 103–104
    ductal carcinoma in situ, 263
    fibroadenoma, 222–223
  percutaneous biopsy, 133–134, 307, 308–309
  sonography, 301–302
    cysts, 201
    ductal carcinoma in situ, 262
    fibroadenoma, 220–222
acoustic shadows, in benign breast disorders, **190**, 191
ACR, see American College of Radiology
adenofibrolipoma, 209–210
adenofibroma, 210–224
adenoma, 211
  papillary, of nipple, 224
adenopathy
  axillary, 283, **317**
  metastatic, 315–317, **316**, **317**, **318**
  other causes, 319, **319**
adenosis, 182
  nodular, **186**
ADH, see atypical ductal hyperplasia
adolescent breast, 163, **164**
  see also young patients
age, and radiation risk, 37
air-gap technique, 21
American College of Radiology (ACR)
  film labeling requirements, 46–47

imaging recommendations, 69
mammography equipment requirements, 60–62
anatomy
  definitions of locations, 468
  lactiferous duct, **162**, 163
  locations, 468
  lymph nodes, 313
  normal breast, **162**, 162–163
angioma, 231–232
angiosarcoma, 328
  postmastectomy, 329
anisomastia, 171
appearance, 161–386
  benign breast disorders, 181–196
  benign tumors, 209–235
  carcinoma in situ, 252–265
  cysts, 197–208
  inflammatory conditions, 236–251
  invasive carcinoma, 266–312
  lymph nodes, 313–324
  male breast, 382–386
  malignant tumors, 325–338
  normal breast, 162–180
  post-surgical changes, 339–349
  post-therapeutic changes, 349–373
  post-traumatic changes, 339–349
  semi-malignant tumors, 325–338
  skin changes, 375–381
application of diagnosis, 387–468
architectural distortion, **444**
  diagnostic workup, 405, **406**, **407**–**410**, **411**–**412**
  differential diagnosis, 294–295
  sonography, 299
arteriosclerosis, and calcification, 442, **442**
arteritis, giant cell, 245
artifacts
  and calcification, 441, **442**
  evaluation, 64
  in MRI, 106, 107
aspiration of cysts, 201–202
asymmetry, 171, **172**
  calcifications, 438
  differential diagnosis, 411, **413**, 414, **414**–**415**, **416**–**418**, **419**–**420**

attenuation, invasive carcinoma, 296, 299
atypia, 182
atypical ductal hyperplasia (ADH), 139, 149, 182, **409**
augmentation surgery, 368–371
  summary, 371–372
autoimmune disease, and granuloma, 250
automatic exposure, mammography, 24–25, **25**, 30, 32–34
  control system, 61–62
  performance assessment, 64
axillary lymph nodes, and invasive carcinoma, 270
axillary view, **50**

B

bar pattern, 61
BCDDP, see Breast Cancer Detection Demonstration Project
B-cell lymphoma, 332
benign disorders/lesions, 181–196, 209–235
  calcifications, typical, 188–189
  definition, 181
  histopathology, 181–183
  incidence, 181
  mammography, 184, **185**–**188**, 188–189, 191
  MRI, 111, **192**, 192–195, **193**
  pathogenesis, 181
  percutaneous biopsy, 195
  sonographic patterns, 100–101, **101**
  sonography, **190**, 191–192
  summary, 195–196
biopsy
  and asymmetry, 414
  imaging guidance, 132
  localizing clip, 139, **140**
  mastitis, 241
  open, 184
  percutaneous, see percutaneous biopsy
  skin thickening, 380

biopsy
  stereotactic, 141–142, **144**, 144–146, 145
  ultrasound-guided, 140–141, **141**
biopsy coil, **147**
biopsy guns, **138**
BI-RADS, *see* Breast Imaging Reporting and Data System
blunt duct adenosis, 182
blurring, 26–27
breast
  anatomic locations, definitions, 468
  compression, 21, 31–32, 39–40, **41**
  contour, 9
  density, *see* breast density
  examination technique, 9–13
  female
    adolescent, 163, **164**
    mature, 163, 165
  implants, *see* implants
  male, 382–386
  normal, 162–180
    anatomy, **162**, 162–163
  size, 9
  symmetry, 9
    see also asymmetry
breast cancer
  genetic screening, 6
  in men, 384–386, **385**, **386**
  risk factors, 3, 6–7
    see also carcinoma; tumors;
      specific lesions
Breast Cancer Detection Demonstration Project (BCDDP), 390–391
breast coil, MRI, 106
breast-conserving therapy, definition, 349
breast density
  and automatic exposure, 33
  changes, 188
  and contrast, 29
  diagnostic workup
    not smoothly outlined, 402, **403**, **404**, 405
    smoothly outlined, 397, **398–399**, 399, **400**, **401–402**
  and hormone replacement therapy, **179**
  invasive carcinoma, 274
  and radiation dose, 38–39
  and scatter reduction, 21
    see also dense breast
Breast Imaging Reporting and Data System (BI-RADS), 68
  and benign breast disorders, 195
  and biopsy interpretation, 149
  classification, 68
breast implant, *see* implants
bucky, positioning, in mediolateral oblique view, **43**
Burkitt lymphoma, 332

C

CAD, *see* computer-assisted detection
calcifications
  adenopathy, metastatic, **318**
  asymmetry, 438
  benign, **185**, 188–189, 440–441, **441**
    distribution, 446, 448
    morphology, 442, **442**, **443**, 444–445, **444–445**, 446
  branching, 437, **437**
  after breast-conserving therapy, 355
  casting, 437, **437**, **439**
  in cysts, 444
  dystrophic, 340, 342
  eggshell-like, **444**
  in fibroadenoma, 216–217
  fine-granular, 437–438, **440**
  granular, **188**, 437
  linear, 437, **437**, **438**
  malignant, 438
    summary, 440
  morphology, **69**
  needle-like, 445
  nodal, 319–320, **320**
  pleomorphic, 437, **439**
  post-surgical, 342, **344–345**, **345**
  after reduction surgery, **373**
  reporting and documentation, 68–69
  segmental distribution, 438
  summary, 448
    see also microcalcifications
calcium, *see* milk of calcium
cancer
  detection, 40, **41**
  risk of mammography, 37
    see also carcinoma; *specific lesions*
cannulation, nipple, 75–76
capsular fibrosis, MRI, 124
carbon solution, for preoperative marking, 158
carcinoma
  comedo, 255
  cribriform, 254, 255, **259**, 272
  diffusely growing
    mammography, **288**
    signs, 287–288
    sonographic appearance, **300**
  Doppler imaging, 94–95, **95**, **96**
  ductal, **279**, **280**, **281**, **282**, **285**, **408**, **410**
    diffusely growing, **288**
    histology, 292
    invasive, 271, **462**
    mimicking lobular, **278**
    MRI, **305**
    multifocal, **290**
    scirrhous, **277**
    in situ, *see* ductal carcinoma in situ
    sonographic appearance, **298**, **299**

inflammatory, 272–273, **289**, 292, 301
  diagnostic workup, **453**, 454
  signs, 288
intraductal, **283**, **290**
  MRI, **304**
invasive, *see* invasive carcinoma
lobular, **279**, **289**, **300**, 301, **401**, **410**
  histology, 292
  invasive, 271
  scirrhous, **306**
  in situ, *see* lobular carcinoma in situ
medullary, 272, 292, **293**, 301
and microcalcifications, classification, 436–438, 440
micropapillary, 254–255, 255, **259**
and MRI enhancement, 111, 124
mucinous, 272, **282**, 292, 301
  sonographic appearance, **299**
noncalcifying, 287
non-comedo, 254–255, **285**
Paget, 272
papillary, 255, **259**, **260**, **261**, 272, 292, **293**, 301
  and microcalcifications, **452**
screening detection rate, 390
and silicone implant, **369**
in situ, 252–265
  definition, 252
  ductal, *see* ductal carcinoma in situ
  lobular, *see* lobular carcinoma in situ
  papillary, 255
  summary, 264
solid, 254, 255
sonography
  diagnosis, 87–88
  patterns, **99–100**
TNM classification, 467
tubular, 272, **291**, 292
types, 271–273
  see also focal lesions; lesions;
    malignancy; masses; metastases;
    recurrences; tumors; *specific lesions*
CCD, *see* charge-coupled devices
changes
  post-surgical, 339–349
  post-therapeutic, 349–373
  post-traumatic, 339–349
    see also skin changes
characteristic curve, film contrast, 23, **24**, 25
charge-coupled devices (CCDs), 71
chemotherapy, neoadjuvant, 105
chondroma, 231
chondrosarcoma, 329
classifications
  Breast Imaging Reporting and Data System (BI-RADS), 68
  ductal carcinoma in situ, 255
  Holland, 255

microcalcifications, 436–438, 440
TNM, 467
Van Nuys, 255
cleavage view, 50, **50**
clinical examination
    asymmetry, 171
    cysts, 197–198
    invasive carcinoma, 267
    inverted nipple, 174
    involution, 170
    macromastia, 173
    mature breast, 163, 165
    polymastia, 173
    in pregnancy, 175
clinical findings, 9–13
    abscess, 242
    benign breast disorders, 183
    breast cancer in men, 385
    after breast-conserving therapy
        with irradiation, 350
        without irradiation, 349–350
    cysts, 197
    ductal carcinoma in situ, 255
    fibroadenoma, 211
    fistula, 242
    granuloma, 246
    gynecomastia, 382
    hamartoma, 209
    hematologic malignancies, 332
    invasive carcinoma, 273–274
    lipoma, 230
    lobular carcinoma in situ, 253
    male breast, 382
    mastitis, 237
    metastases, 335
    nodular skin changes, 375
    papilloma, 225
    phyllodes tumor, 325
    post-surgical changes, 339
    post-traumatic changes, 339
    reporting and documentation, 65,
        66
    sarcomas, 329
    skin thickening, 378–379
    work sheet, **11**
    young patients, 456
clock face documentation, 66
clusters, microcalcifications, 189
coffee-bean shape, lymph nodes, 314,
    314, **315**
collimation assessment, 64
comedo ductal carcinoma in situ,
    254, 255, 256–258, **257**, **258**, **284**
complications, percutaneous biopsy,
    135–136
compression
    and breast implants, 58, **59**
    quality control, 65
    sonography, **93**
    see also spot compression
compression paddle
    positioning
        in craniocaudal view, 42
        in mediolateral oblique view, 42
    X-ray attenuation, 61

compression plate, 153, **154**
computed tomography (CT), internal
    mammary nodes, 322
computer-aided image analysis, 435–
    436
computer-assisted detection (CAD),
    71, 72–73
contour of breast, 9
contraindications
    galactography, 74
    percutaneous biopsy, 135
    pneumocystography, 81
contrast
    and automatic exposure, 32–34
    and breast compression, 31–32, 40
    digital sensors, 73
    and exposure, 32
    film processing, 35–36
    film selection, 35
    and grid technique, 32
    in mammography, 23, 27–36, **31**,
        34
        definition, 27
        factors determining, 29
        optimizing, 30
    and manual exposure, 34–35
    MRI media, 107
    and peak kilovoltage, 30–31
    and photocell position, 34
    and radiation quality, 29
    radiation spectrum, 18
    and scattered radiation, 31, 32
    in sonography, 90–91, **91**
    and target/filter combination, 30–
        31
Cooper ligaments
    and invasive carcinoma, 283, **285**
    and involution, **170**
    and mobility, 300
    sonography, 166, **168**
    thickening, 274, 287, 288
core needle biopsy, 132, 134–135
    accuracy, 133
    microcalcifications, 436
    technique, 137, **138**
    ultrasound-guided, 140–141, **141**,
        142, **143**
cost-effectiveness of screening, 393–
    394
craniocaudal view, **42**, **44**, 44–45
    tumor localization, **67**
CT, see computed tomography
cysticercosis, 245
cystosarcoma phyllodes, see phyl-
    lodes tumor
cysts, 182, 197–208
    aspiration, 201–202
    in benign breast disorders, 191
    and calcification, 444
    clinical examination, 197–198
    clinical findings, 197
    compressibility, 94
    diagnosis, 198
    histology, 197
    mammography, 202, **203**

pathognomonic findings, 396
pneumocystography, 81–83, **82**, **83**
simple vs. complex, **97**
sonography, 87, 198, **199–201**
    findings, **97**, 97–98, **98**
    summary, 204–205
    typical appearance, 198, **199–201**,
        201, 202, 203–204
    see also milk of calcium cyst; oil
        cysts; pneumocystography
cytology
    invasive carcinoma, 273
    nipple discharge, 225

D

darkroom
    cleanliness, 63, 64
    fog, 65
data storage, 73
DCIS, see ductal carcinoma in situ
definitions
    anatomic locations, 468
    augmentation, 368–369
    benign breast disorders, 181
    breast cancer in men, 384
    breast-conserving therapy
        with irradiation, 350
        without irradiation, 349
    carcinoma in situ, 252
    contrast in mammography, 27
    cysts, 197
    ductal carcinoma in situ, 254
    galactocele, 205
    galactography, 74
    gynecomastia, 382
    indeterminate microcalcifications,
        449
    intramammary lymph nodes, 234
    invasive carcinoma, 266
    oil cyst, 205
    pathognomonic findings, 396
    percutaneous biopsy, 132
    pneumocystography, 81
    preoperative localization, 152
    reconstruction, 364
    reduction, 371
    screening, 388
demarcation, sonographic, 296
dense breast, diagnostic workup
    high risk, 422, **423–424**
    without high risk, 415, 419–422
    and nipple retraction, 431
    with palpable finding, 423, **425**,
        426, **426–428**, 429–430, **430**
    and search for primary tumor, 431,
        431
    see also breast density
density, see breast density; film
depth localization, percutaneous bi-
    opsy, 141, **144**
desmoid, extra-abdominal, 338
detection quantum efficiency (DQE),
    72

diabetic mastopathy, 232–233
  mammography, 232–233, **233**
  summary, 233
diagnosis
  application, 387–468
  after augmentation, 369–370
  benign breast disorders, 183–184
  after breast-conserving therapy,
    350, 351
  cysts, 198
  differential, *see* differential diagno-
    sis
  ductal carcinoma in situ, 256
  fibroadenoma, 223
  fistula, 242–243
  granulomas, 246
  gynecomastia, 382–383
  hematologic malignancies, 332
  invasive carcinoma, 266–270, 270
  lipoma, 230
  mammography, categories, 69–70
  mastitis, 237
  metastases, 335
  nodular skin changes, 375
  papilloma, 225
  phyllodes tumor, 325–326
  post-surgical changes, 339–340
  post-traumatic changes, 339–340
  after reconstruction, 365
  after reduction surgery, 371
  sarcomas, 329
  skin thickening, 378
  sonographic, 87–88
  in young patients, 464
  see also diagnostic algorithms; di-
    agnostic workup
diagnostic algorithms
  architectural distortion, **406**
  asymmetry, **419–420**
  dense breast
    with palpable finding, **430**
    search for primary tumor, **431**
  focal lesion
    not smoothly outlined, **403**
    smoothly outlined, **398–399**
  microcalcifications, **447–448**
  nipple retraction, **435**
diagnostic workup
  architectural distortion, 405, **406**,
    407–410, 411–412
  asymmetry, 411, **413**, 414, **414–415**,
    416–418, **419–420**
  dense breast
    with high risk, 422, **423–424**
    without increased risk, 415, 419–
      422
    with palpable finding, 423, **425**,
      426, **426–428**, 429–430, **430**
  inflammatory changes, **453**, 454
  lesions not smoothly outlined, 402,
    403, **404**, 405
  microcalcifications, 434–452
  nipple discharge, 452–454
  nipple retraction, 431, **433–434**,
    435

smoothly outlined density, 397,
  398–399, 399, **400**, **401–402**
dielectric properties, 130
differential diagnosis
  architectural distortion, 405, **406**,
    407–410
  asymmetry, 411, **413**, 414, **414–415**,
    416–418, **419–420**
  benign breast disorders, MRI, 194–
    195
  dense breast
    with high risk, 422, **423–424**
    without increased risk, 415, 419–
      422
    with palpable finding, 423, **425**,
      426, **426–428**, 429–430, **430**
  diffuse changes, 294
  inflammatory changes, **453**, 454
  invasive carcinoma, 294–295
  lesions not smoothly outlined, 402,
    403, **404**, 405
  microcalcifications, 434–452
    indeterminate, 450–451
  nipple discharge, 452–454 ,
  nipple retraction, 431, **433–434**, **435**
  skin thickening, 378
  smoothly outlined density, 397,
    398–399, 399, **400**, **401–402**
  sonographic, invasive carcinoma,
    301–303
diffuse enhancement, MRI, 112
digital imaging
  mammography, 71–74
  summary, 73–74
directional vacuum assisted biopsy
  (DVA), **138**
discharge
  in benign breast disorders, 183
  and dense breast, 434
  and invasive carcinoma, 273
  spontaneous, 7
documentation
  invasive carcinoma, 268
  mammography, 66–70
Doppler imaging, 94–95, **95**, **96**
DQE, *see* detection quantum efficiency
duct
  dilated, 281
  ectasia, 76, **77**, 191
  hyperplasia, 182, **409**
ductal carcinoma in situ (DCIS), 254–
  264, **409**
  clinical findings, 255
  comedo, *see* comedo ductal carci-
    noma in situ
  definition, 254
  diagnosis, 256
  follow-up mammography, **291**
  histology, 254
  incidence, 254
  mammography, 256–259, **257**, **258**,
    259, **260**, **261**, 262
  and microcalcification, 256, 258,
    258, **259**

MRI, 262–263
  sensitivity, 104
  nipple discharge, **261**
  non-comedo, **113**
  papillary, 255, **259**, **260**, **261**
  percutaneous biopsy, 263–264
  sonography, 262, **263**
  summary, 264
DVA, *see* directional vacuum assisted
  biopsy
dye marking, 158

E

echo
  reverberation, **91**, **199**
  scatter, 93
  specular, 92–93
echogenicity, invasive carcinoma,
  296, **297**
elasticity, sonographic, invasive carcinoma, 300
elastography, 129
electrical impedance, 130
enhancement, MRI, 111, 124
epithelial hyperplasia, **409**
  forms, 182–183
equipment
  mammography, 60–62
  MR-guided biopsy, **147**
  MRI, 106
  sonography, 88–92
exaggerated lateral craniocaudal
  view, 45, 47, **48**
exaggerated medial craniocaudal
  view, 45, 47
examination technique
  clinical, 9–13
  cysts, MRI, 202–203
  MRI, 108–110
  sonography, 92–96
exposure
  automatic, 24–25, **25**, 30, 32–34
  and contrast, 32
  mammography, 23–25, **24**, 61–62
  manual, 34–36
  optimizing, dose-related, 38

F

fat necrosis, 339, 342, 346, 360
fat signal, in MRI, 107
fatty hilum, 317
  lymph nodes, 314, **314**, **315**
FDG-PET, *see* positron emission tomography
fibroadenoma, 210–224, **331**, **407**
  and calcification, **444**
  calcified, pathognomonic images,
    396
  clinical findings, 211
  diagnosis, 223
  histology, 211
  juvenile, 211, 215, **216**

mammography, 211, **212–215**
and mobility, 94, **94**
MRI, 111, 222–223
old, **220**
percutaneous biopsy, 222
vs. phyllodes tumor, 150
sonography, 217, **218–219**, 220, 220–221, **221**
pattern, **101**
summary, 224
in young patients, 455
fibroepithelial mixed tumors, 210–224
fibromatosis, 337
fibrosarcoma, 328
fibrosis, 352
benign, 232–234
focal, 182
fibrosis mammae, 233–234
filling defects, galactography, 76, **77**
film
cassette positioning, 42
characteristic curve, 23, **24**, 25
density
ACR standards, 62
and radiation dose, 39
range, 23
fixture retention, 65
labeling, 46–47
processing, 25–26
and contrast, **35**, 35–36
and image quality, 62–63
and radiation dose, 39
processor, quality control, 64–65
selection, and contrast, 35
storage, 71, 72
X-ray attenuation, 61
film-screen system, *see* screen-film systems
filtering, radiation spectrum, 19
fine focus technique, 56, 71
fine needle aspiration biopsy, 132, 134
accuracy, 133
technique, 136, **137**
ultrasound-guided, 141
fistula
clinical findings, 242
diagnosis, 242–243
histology, 242
mammography, 243
MRI, 243
sonography, 243
summary, 245
Fixmarker, 159
FLASH 3D sequences, 106
normal breast, **169**
focal fibrosis, 182, 233–234
focal lesions
in benign breast disorders, 191
diagnostic workup
not smoothly outlined, 402, **403**, **404**, 405
smoothly outlined, 397, **398–399**, 399, **400**, **401–402**

MRI, 111
reporting and documentation, **66**
focal spot
performance evaluation, 64
size, 17
focus, in sonography, 90, **90**, 93
fog
darkroom, 65
and film processing, 35
follow-up studies, 288–289, **290–291**, 292
intervals, 292
foreign body granuloma, 246
fullfield mammography, 71, 73
fungal infection, 245, 250

G

gadolinium oxysulfide, 23
see also Gd-DTPA
galactocele, 205–206, **206**
pathognomonic images, 396
galactography, 74–80
contraindications, 74
and ductal carcinoma, **261**, **294**
findings, 76
indications, 74
invasive carcinoma, 268, 273
normal, **76**
papilloma, 227
preoperative localization, 158
preoperative marking, 76
procedure, 75
side effects, 74
vs. sonography, lactiferous ducts, 78, **78–80**
summary, 78
Gd-DTPA, 3, 107
generator power, 60–61
genetic screening, breast cancer, 6
geometric blurring, 26, 27
giant cell arteritis, 245
giant fibroadenoma, 215, **216**, 455
glandular tissue, sonography, 166
granular cell tumor, 232, **232**
granuloma, 245–250
clinical findings, 246
diagnosis, 246
histology, 245
lipophagic, 342, 355, **358**, 360
mammography, 246–247, **247**, **248**
MRI, **248**, 249–250
percutaneous biopsy, 250
and scarring, 246, **247**, 249
silicone, 245, 246, 247, **248**, 249
sonography, 247, **247**, **248**, 249
summary, 250
grid technique
and radiation dose, 39
scatter reduction, 20–21, 31, 32, **33**
X-ray attenuation, 61
gynecomastia, 382–384, **383**, **384**
definition, 382
summary, 386

H

half-value layer measurement, 63, 64
halo sign, 397
hamartoma, 209–210, **210**
clinical findings, 209
pathognomonic images, 396
hardware, and image quality, 60–62
Health Insurance Plan (HIP) of Greater New York study, 389
vs. BCDDP study, 390
heel effect, X-ray tube, 19, **21**
hemangioendothelioma, 338
hemangiopericytoma, 338
hematologic malignancies, 332–334, **333**, **334**
summary, 334
hematoma, 339, 340, **340**, 342, 344, **347**
MRI, 349
old, 339
histiocytoma, malignant fibrous, 328, **330**
histology
abscess, 242
benign breast disorders, 181–183
breast cancer in men, 384
cysts, 197
diabetic mastopathy, 232
ductal carcinoma in situ, 254
fibroadenoma, 211
fistula, 242
granuloma, 245
gynecomastia, 382
interpreting, 149–150
invasive carcinoma, 270–273, 309
involution, 170
lobular carcinoma in situ, 252
and mammographic presentation, 292–293
mature breast, 163
metastases, 335
papilloma, 224
phyllodes tumor, 325
post-surgical changes, 339
post-traumatic changes, 339
in pregnancy, 175
sarcomas, 328–329
vs. sonography, invasive carcinoma, 301, **302**
young patient, beast changes, 455
histoplasmosis, 245
history
family, and risk of breast cancer, 3, 6
medical, and image interpretation, 7
personal, and risk of breast cancer, 3
Holland classification, 255
Homer wire, 159
hormone replacement therapy, 7, 177, **178–179**, 180
and asymmetry, 414, **414**
hyperemia, 352

I

ill-defined mass, diagnostic workup, 402, **403**, **404**, 405
image noise, 26
image quality
  evaluation, 64
  and film processing, 62–63
  and screen-film system, 62
  sonography, 89–91
    near field, 90–91
image receptor system, 21, 23, 27
image sharpness, mammography, 26–27
imaging guidance, biopsy, 132
imaging studies
  comparison with previous, 7, 67, 288–289, **290–291**, 292
  follow-up, 288–289, **290–291**, 292
  lymph nodes, 313
  techniques, new, 128–131
impedance imaging, 130
implants, 364–365, **365**–366
  and breast positioning, 56, 58–59, **59**
  failure, unenhanced MRI, 104
  leaks, MRI, 107
  normal findings on MRI, 124
  and positioning, 56, 58–59, **59**
  rupture, 124–125, **365**, **366**, 367
  silicone, 364–365
    and carcinoma detection, **369**
    and granuloma, 245, 246, 247, **248**, 249
    MRI assessment, 105
incidence
  ductal carcinoma in situ, 254
  indeterminate microcalcifications, 449
  lobular carcinoma in situ, 252
  skin thickening, 376, 378
indications
  galactography, 74
  mammography, 14
  MRI, 307
    contrast-enhanced, 104–106
    unenhanced, 106
  percutaneous biopsy, 134
    invasive carcinoma, 309
  pneumocystography, 81, 202
  preoperative localization, 152–153
  scintimammography, 128
  sonography, in invasive carcinoma, 295–296
inflammatory conditions, 236–251
  carcinoma, *see* carcinoma, inflammatory
  diagnostic workup, **453**, 454
inspection, visual, 9–10
  equipment, 65
  reporting and documentation, 65
intensifying screens, 21, **22**, 23
intraductal carcinoma, *see* ductal carcinoma in situ
intraductal mass, 75
  sonographic imaging, 78, **78–80**

intramammary lymph nodes, 234, 315
invasive carcinoma, 266–312
  additional foci, 270
  clinical examination, 267
  clinical findings, 273–274
  definition, 266
  diagnosis, 266–270, 295
  differential diagnosis, 294–295
  extent, 269
  focal
    direct signs, 276, 278, 281, 283
    indirect signs, 283, **285**, **286**, 287
  galactography, 268
  histology, 270–273
  imaging methods, 267–268
  and lymph nodes, 270
  mammography, 267, 268, 274–295
    signs, 274
  MRI, 268, **303**, 303–304, **304–306**, 306–307
    indications, 307
  percutaneous biopsy, 268, 307–309
  screening, 266, 267
  sonography, 268, 295–296, **297**, **298**, **299**, 299–303, **300**, **302**
    signs, 296, **297**
  summary, 309–310
  therapy, 269
inverted nipple, 174, **175**
involution, 170–171
iron oxide contrast, in lymph node imaging, 321–322
irradiation
  after breast-conserving therapy, 350
  changes after, 350–364
  see also radiation

J

Jackson sign, 10, 65
juvenile fibroadenoma, 455
juvenile papillomatosis, 455

K

keyhole sign, 124

L

labeling
  mammography film, 46–47
  sonography images, 95
lactation, **175–176**, 175–177
lactiferous ducts
  anatomy, **162**, 163
  kinked, 76
  sonographic imaging, 78, **78–80**
lateral view, 90°, 45–46, **46**, 47
LCIS, *see* lobular carcinoma in situ
legal aspects, invasive carcinoma, 268
leiomyoma, 231, **231**

leiomyosarcoma, 329, **331**
lesions
  mobility, 94, **94**
  multicentric, MRI assessment, 105
  reporting and documentation, 68
  solid, differentiating, 87
  see also carcinoma; focal lesions; masses
leukemia, chronic lymphocytic, 317
light transmission, 129
lipoma, 230, **230**
  pathognomonic images, 396
liponecrosis, calcifying, 442, **443**
liposarcoma, 328
litigation, and invasive carcinoma, 268
lobular carcinoma in situ (LCIS), 149, 252–254
  clinical findings, 253
  histology, 252
  incidence, 252
  mammography, 253, **253**
  MRI, 253
  percutaneous biopsy, 253
  summary, 264
  treatment, 253–254
lobular hyperplasia, 182
lobulated mass, 274, **275**
  differential diagnosis, 294
localization
  manual, **154**, 155
  preoperative, *see* preoperative localization
  stereotaxic, 153–154
localizing clip, at biopsy, 139, **140**
lymphedema, after radiation therapy, **360**
lymph nodes, 313–324
  anatomy, 313
  calcifications, 319–320, **320**
  definitions of anatomic locations, 468
  imaging, 313
  internal mammary, 322
  intramammary, 234, 315
  and invasive carcinoma, 270
  normal, 313–315, **314**, **315**
  pathognomonic images, 396
  percutaneous biopsy, 321
  sentinel node imaging, 320–321, **321**
  summary, 323
lymphoma, 332

M

macromastia, 173
magnetic resonance imaging (MRI), 3, 103–127, 174
  abscess, 243, **244**
  accuracy, 103–104
    ductal carcinoma in situ, 263
  benign lesions/disorders, **192**, 192–195, **193**

differential diagnosis, 194–195
typical signs, **122–123**
biopsy guidance, 146–147, **147**,
148, 149
after breast-conserving therapy,
361, **362**, 363, **363**
contrast-enhanced, 103–104
accuracy, 103–104
examination procedure, 108, 109
guidelines, 112
indications, 104–106
interpretation, 109–112, 124
technical requirements, 106–107
cysts, 202–203
dense breast, 422, **423**
with palpable finding, 429–430
ductal carcinoma in situ, 262–263
fibroadenoma, 222–223
fistula, 243
granuloma, **248**, 249–250
hematologic malignancies, 334
hematoma, 349
implant failure, 104
indications, 104–106
interpretation, 109–112, 124–125
invasive carcinoma, 268, **303**, 303–
304, **304–306**, 306–307
involution, 170–171
lobular carcinoma in situ, 253
lymph nodes, 321–322, **322**
malignancy
highly suspicious signs, **113–114**
suspicious signs, **115–117**
untypical signs, **118–121**
mastitis, **239**, 241
mastopathy, **286**
and menstrual cycle, 169
metastases, 336
normal findings, 124, 168–169, **169**
papilloma, 227, **229**
phyllodes tumor, 327, **327**
pitfalls, 307
polymastia, 173
post-surgical changes, 347, 349
preoperative localization, 157–158
after reconstruction, 368, **369**
sarcomas, 330
skin thickening, 380
slice thickness, 106, 107
technical requirements, 106–107
and tumor extent, 269, 270
unenhanced
accuracy, 104
examination procedure, 108–109
indications, 106
interpretation, 110, 124
technical requirements, 107
in young patients, 463–464
magnetic resonance spectroscopy,
129
magnification mammography, 27, 32,
45
and biopsy, 145
ductal carcinoma in situ, **259**, **260**
hematoma, **347**

microcalcifications, **187**, 435
post-surgical changes, **345**
technique, 51–56, **57**, **58**, 61
male breast, 382–386
summary, 386
malignancy, 325–338
and MRI enhancement, 110–111
sonographic patterns, **99–100**, 100
in young patients, 455
see also carcinoma
mammary gland, *see* breast
mammography, 14–86
abscess, 243, **244**
accuracy, 14–15
ductal carcinoma in situ, 262
adolescent breast, **164**
asymmetry, 171, **172**
after augmentation, 370
benign breast disorders, 184, **185–**
188, 188–189, 191
breast cancer in men, 385
after breast-conserving therapy,
351–353, **353**, **354**, 355–357,
355–360
comparing with previous studies,
7, 67, 288–289, **290–291**, 292
components, 17–26
contrast, 27–36, **34**
cysts, 202, **203**
dense breast, 419–420, 422, **423–**
424
with palpable finding, 423, 426
diabetic mastopathy, 232–233, **233**
diagnostic categories, 69–70
diffusely growing carcinoma, **288**
digital, 71–74
ductal carcinoma in situ, 256–259,
257, **258**, **259**, **260**, **261**, 262
equipment, 60–62
quality control, 64–65
fibroadenoma, 211, **212–215**, 224
fibromatosis, 338
fistula, 243
follow-up studies, 288–289, **290**,
290–291, 292
form for patient, **4**
fullfield, 71, 73
granuloma, 246–247, **247**, **248**
gynecomastia, 383, **383**, **384**
hematologic malignancies, 332–
333, **333**, **334**
and histology, 292–293
and hormone replacement therapy,
177, **178–179**, 180
image sharpness, 26–27
indications, 14
invasive carcinoma, 267, 268, 274–
295
signs, 274, **275**
involution, 170, **171**
lipoma, 230
lobular carcinoma in situ, 253,
253
lymph nodes, normal, **314**
macromastia, 173

magnification, *see* magnification
mammography
male breast, 382, **383**
mastitis, 237, **238**, 239–241
metastases, 335–336, **336**, **337**
microcalcifications, 434
motion blurring, 26–27
nipple, inverted, 174, **174**
nodular skin changes, 375
normal glandular tissue, 165, **165**
papilloma, 225, **226**, 226–227
phyllodes tumor, 326, **326**, **328**
polymastia, 173
positioning, 40–46
in pregnancy, 175, **175–176**
preoperative, 153–155, 262
problem solving, 15–16
quality assurance, 63–65
quality factors, 60–65
questionnaire for patient, **4**
radiation dose, 36–39
after reconstruction, **365–366**,
365–367, **367**, **368**
recurrences, **359–360**
reporting and documentation, 66–
70
sarcomas, 329, **330**
screening, 15
sensitivity and specificity, 293–294
serial, 289
skin thickening, 379
slit, 32
technique
components, **17**
requirements, 16–17
viewing image, 26
views, 40–46
in young patients, 456–460, **457**,
458, **459–460**
see also specimen radiography
Mammography Quality Assurance
Act, 63
manual exposure, 34–36
manual localization, **154**, 155, **155**
mapping, sentinel nodes, 321
margins, sonographic, invasive carcinoma, 296
marking
dye, 158
galactographic findings, 76
microcalcifications, 269
scar-related change, 341
see also preoperative localization
masses
ill-defined, diagnostic workup,
402, **403**, **404**, 405
reporting and documentation, 68
solid, sonographic findings, 98–101
benign *vs.* malignant, **101**
see also carcinoma; lesions
mastitis, 236–241
acute, 236, **238**
biopsy, 241
chronic, 236, **239**, **240**
mammography, 237, **238**, 239–241

mastitis
  MRI, **239**, 241
  plasma cell, 437, **438**, **439**, 442, 445, **446**
  plasma-cell, 236, **240**
  puerperal, 236
  sonography, **238**, **239**, 241
  subacute, 236
  tuberculous, 246
mastodynia, 183
mastopathy, **286**
  diabetic, 232–233
medical physicist, responsibilities, 63–64
mediolateral oblique (MLO) view, 40, 42, **43**
  tumor localization, **67**
menstrual cycle
  and mammography scheduling, 2
  and MRI, 169
    benign breast disorders, 194
metastases, 334–337, **336**, **337**
  breast cancer, 315–317, **316**, **317**, **318**
  summary, 337
methods of diagnostic imaging, 1–160
microbiology, granuloma, 245
microcalcifications, **186**, **187**, 262, 270
  and additional foci, 270
  analysis, 436
  in benign breast disorders, 188–189
  diagnostic algorithm, **447–448**
  differential diagnosis, 294
  and diffusely growing carcinoma, 287
  distribution, **276**
  and ductal carcinoma in situ, 256, 258, **258**, **259**
  indeterminate, 449–452
  and malignancy, 281, 283, **284**, **285**
  malignant, 274, **275**
  monomorphic, **450**
  parallel, 446
  pleomorphic, **450**
  post-surgical, **345**
  and recurrence, 357, **359**
  reporting and documentation, **66**
  suggesting malignancy, classification, 436–438, 440
  summary, 436
  in young patient, **462–463**
microcysts, 182
microfocus technique, 56
microglandular adenosis, 182
micropapillary carcinoma, 254–255, 255
milk of calcium cyst, 188–189, 444
  pathognomonic images, 396
MLO, *see* mediolateral oblique view
mobility of lesions, 94, **94**
  invasive carcinoma, 300–301
modulation transfer function (MTF), 27, **29**

molybdenum, target/filter combinations, 19, **31**
Mondor disease, 10, 376
monitor resolution, 73
motion blurring, mammography, 26–27
MRI, *see* magnetic resonance imaging
MTF, *see* modulation transfer function
multicentric lesions, MRI assessment, 105
myoblastoma, 232, **232**
myocutaneous flap, 367, **368**

N

necrosis, 339
  calcifying, **443**
neurilemmoma, 231
neurofibroma, 231
nipple
  cannulation, 75–76
  changes, 7
  discharge, *see* nipple discharge
  and invasive carcinoma, 273
  inversion, 10, 174, **175**
  palpation, 65
  papillary adenoma, 224
  positioning, in craniocaudal view, 44
  retraction, **286**, 287, 431, **433**
    diagnostic workup, 431, **433–434**, **435**
    and invasive carcinoma, 283
    malignant, 289
nipple discharge
  and carcinoma, 293
  cytology, 225
  differential diagnosis, 452–454
  and ductal carcinoma in situ, **261**
  galactography, **294**
nodal calcifications, 319–320, **320**
nodular changes/lesions, **185**, **186**, **187**, 275
  skin, 375
  sonographic appearance, **297**
noise
  in mammography, **28**
  minimizing, 36
non-comedo carcinoma, 254–255, 258
non-Hodgkin lymphoma, 332, **333**
normal breast, 162–180
  galactography, **76**
  mammography, 165, **165**
  MRI, 168–169, **169**
  sonography, **94**, 96, 166, **166–168**
  summary, 171
nucleoside triphosphates, 129

O

oblique view, 45
  with customized settings, **50**
oil cysts, 205–206, **207**, 355, 360
  pathognomonic images, 396

optical density range, 23
  ACR standards, 62
osteochondrosarcoma, 329
osteoma, 231

P

PACS, *see* picture archiving and communications systems
Paget disease, 272, 292
pain
  in benign breast disorders, 183
  dense breast, 430
palpation
  findings, 10, 12
  invasive carcinoma, 273
  problems, 12
  reporting and documentation, 65
  technique, 10
papilloma, 224–230
  clinical findings, 225
  diagnosis, 225
  galactography, 227
  mammography, 225, **226**, 226–227
  and microcalcifications, **452**
  MRI, 227, **229**
  percutaneous biopsy, 229
  sonography, 227, **228**
  summary, 229–230
papillomatosis, **79**
  juvenile, 224, 455
  and microcalcifications, **452**
parasitosis, 245, 250
parenchyma
  diffuse changes after therapy, 352, **353**, **354**
  localized changes after therapy, 352–353
  pattern, 68
pathognomonic findings, 396
patient history, 2–8
patient information
  interventions, 3
  mammography, 2
  MRI with contrast, 3
  percutaneous biopsy, 136
  sonography, 2–3
patients, high-risk, MRI assessment, 105
peak kilovoltage (kVp), 19
  accuracy, 64
  and contrast, 30–31, **31**
penetration, radiation spectrum, 18
percutaneous biopsy, 132–150
  abscess, 245
  accuracy, 133–134, 307, 308–309
  after augmentation, 370–371
  in benign breast disorders, 184, 194–195
  complications, 135–136
  contraindications, 135
  dense breast, with palpable finding
  depth localization, 141, **144**
  ductal carcinoma in situ, 263–264

fibroadenoma, 222
granuloma, 250
hematologic malignancies, 334
and hormone replacement therapy, 180
indications, 134
    invasive carcinoma, 309
interpreting, 149–150
intramammary lymph nodes, 234
invasive carcinoma, 268, 307–309
lobular carcinoma in situ, 253
lymph nodes, 321
metastases, 337
MR-guided, 146–147, **147**, **148**, 149
papilloma, 229
and post-therapeutic changes, 364
and sarcoma, 330
scar tissue, 349
specimen handling, 147, 149
stereotactic, 141–142, **144**, 144–146, **145**
young patients, 463
phantom images, 33, 63, 65
phosphomonoesters, 129
phosphor spectroscopy, 129
phosphor storage screens, 72
photocell, 24–25, **25**
    positioning, 34
    in craniocaudal view, 45
phyllodes tumor, 323–328, **326**–**328**
    vs. fibroadenoma, 150
    mammography, 326, **326**, **328**
    MRI, 327, **327**
    sonography, 326, **327**, **328**
    summary, 327–328
    in young patients, 455
physician's work sheet, **11**
physicist, medical, 63–64
picture archiving and communications systems (PACS), 72
pitfalls, MRI and invasive carcinoma, 307
plasma cell mastitis, 437, **438**, **439**, 442, 445, **446**
pneumocystography, 81–83, **82**, **83**, 202, **204**
    contraindications, 81
    definition, 81
    indications, 81
    procedure, 81–82
    side effects, 81
    summary, 83
polyarteritis nodosa, 245
polymastia, **172**, 173
positioning
    breasts with implants, 56, 58–59, **59**
    mammography, 40–46
    sonography, **93**
positron emission tomography (PET), 129, 321–322, **322**
postprocessing, 72
pregnancy, 175–177, **176**
    and lesions in young patients, 455
preoperative localization, 152–160

definition, 152
galactographic guidance, 158
indication, 152–153
mammographic guidance, 153–155
materials, 158–159
MR guidance, 157–158
problems, 159–160
side effects, 152–153
summary, 160
technique, 153–160
ultrasound guidance, 155–157
previous imaging studies, 7, 67, 288–289, **290**–**291**, 292
problem solving, mammography, 15–16
prone table, 142, 144, **145**
prostheses, 364–366
punch biopsy, skin thickening, 380

Q

quality assurance, in mammography, 63–65
quality control, sonography equipment, 91
quality criteria
    craniocaudal view, 45
    mediolateral oblique view, 42
quality factors, in mammography, 60–65

R

radial scar, 149, 182, **186**, **407**, **408**
radiation
    carcinogenicity, 37
    protection, ACR recommendations, 61
    quality, 29, 38
        ACR recommendations, 61
    scattered, 20, 31
    spectrum, 18–19
        target/filter combinations, **20**
radiation dose
    and breast thickness, 38–39
    and exposure optimization, 38
    and grid, 39
    mammography, 36–39
    minimizing, 38
radiation therapy
    and image interpretation, 7
    and sarcoma, 329
    see also irradiation
radiography, see mammography; specimen radiography
radiology technologist, responsibilities, 63, 64–65
radiotherapy, see radiation therapy
reconstruction surgery
    changes after, 364–368
    summary, 371–372
recurrences, 351, 355–357
    focally growing, 356–357, **359**–**360**
    mammography, **359**–**360**

microcalcifications, 357, **359**
    after reconstruction, 367, **367**
reduction surgery, 371, **371**–**373**
    summary, 371–372
reporting and documentation
    Breast Imaging Reporting and Data System (BI-RADS), 68
    example reports, 70
    mammography, 66–70
    storage, 71, 72
resolution, 26
    ACR requirements, 60–61, 61
    MRI, 106
    sonography, 89–91
retraction, see nipple
reverberation echo, **91**
    cysts, **199**
reverse C sign, 124, **125**
rhabdomyosarcoma, 329
rhodium, target/filter combinations, 19
risk
    breast cancer in young patients, 455–456
    radiation dose in mammography, 37
    of screening, 392
risk factors, 3, 6–7
rolled views, 50, **51**
round changes, differential diagnosis, 294
round lesions, multiple, **401**
rupture, implant, 124–125

S

salad oil sign, **115**, 125
sarcoidosis, 245, 250
sarcomas, 328–330, **330**–**331**
    clinical findings, 329
    histology, 328–329
    mammography, 329, **330**
    MRI, 330
    sonography, 329, **330**
    summary, 330
scar formation, 347, 352, 360
    within breast, 340, **343**
    diagnosis, 340
    and granuloma, 246, **247**, 249
    MRI assessment, 105
    percutaneous biopsy, 349
    radial, see radial scar
    after reduction mammoplasty, **371**
    skin, 340, **341**
    sonography, **348**
scatter echoes, 93
scattered radiation, 20, 31
scatter reduction
    air-gap technique, 21, 31
    compression, 21, 31
    grids, 20–21, 31, 32, **33**
    other techniques, 32
scheduling, mammography, 2
scintimammography, 128

sclerosing adenosis, 182
screen, intensifying, 21, **22**, 23
screen cleanliness, 65
screen-film blurring, 26
screen-film contact, quality control, 65
screen-film systems, 21, **22**, 23
    and contrast, **34**, 35, **35**
    and image quality, 62
    and radiation dose, 39
    resolution, 27
screening, 388–395
    benefit-costs, 393–394
    benefit-risk, 392–393
    controversies, 391
    cost-effectiveness, 393–394
    and ductal carcinoma in situ, 255
    evaluation of findings, 396–466
    and invasive carcinoma, 266, 267
    mammography, 15
    MRI, 104
    and radiation risk, 37
    recommendations, 394
    reporting and documentation, 70
    sonography, 88
    studies
        case-control, 389–390
        randomized, 388–389
    summary of study results, 392
    in young patients, 458
screen speed, 64
semi-malignant tumors, 325–338
sensitivity, mammography, 14–15
sentinel node imaging, 320–321, **321**
seroma, 339, 340, **340**, 344
Sestamibi, 128
shadows, acoustic, **190**, 191
sharpness, mammography, 17–18
SID, *see* source to image-receptor distance
side effects
    galactography, 74
    pneumocystography, 81
    preoperative localization, 152–153
silicone implants, *see* implants
single photon emission computed tomography (SPECT), 128
size of breast, 9
skin changes, 7, 9–10, 375–381
    and invasive carcinoma, 273
    localized, after therapy, 352–353
    nodular, 375
    scars, 340, **341**
skin infiltration, 301
skin thickening, 283, 301, 375–376, **376–377**, 378–379, **378–380**
    causes, 376–377
    definition, 375–376
    diagnosis, 378
    differential diagnosis, 295
    incidence, 376, 378
    resolution, 359
    summary, 381
slice thickness
    MRI, 106, 107

sonography, 91
slit mammography, 32
sonography, 87–102
    abscess, 243, **244**
    accuracy, 301–302
    adolescent breast, **164**
    after augmentation, 370
    benign breast disorders, **190**, 191–192
    breast cancer in men, 385–386
    after breast-conserving therapy, 359–361, **360–361**
    cysts, 198, **199–201**
    dense breast, with palpable finding, 426, **426**, **427**, 429
    differential diagnosis, 301–303
    and ductal carcinoma in situ, 262, **263**
    equipment, 88–92
    examination technique, 92–96
    fibroadenoma, 217, **218–219**, 220, 220–221, **221**, 224
    fibromatosis, 338
    fistula, 243
    and granuloma, 247, **247**, **248**, 249
    hematologic malignancies, **333**, 333–334
    vs. histology, invasive carcinoma, 301, **302**
    and hormone replacement therapy, 180
    image quality, 89–91
    interpretation, 96–101
    invasive carcinoma, 268, 295–296, **297**, **298**, **299**, 299–303, **300**, **302**
    involution, 170
    lactiferous ducts, 78, **78–80**
    lymph nodes, normal, **315**
    macromastia, 173
    mastitis, **238**, **239**, 241
    metastases, 336, **336**
    microcalcifications, 436
    nipple, inverted, 174, **174**
    normal breast, 166, **166–168**
    papilloma, 227, **228**
    patterns
        benign lesions, 100–101, **101**
        malignancy, **99–100**, 100
    phyllodes tumor, 326, **327**, **328**
    polymastia, 173
    positioning, **93**
    post-surgical changes, 342, 344, 345, 347
    post-traumatic changes, 342, 344, 345, 347, **347**
    in pregnancy, **176**, 177
    after reconstruction, 368
    resolution, 89–91
    sarcomas, 329, **330**
    scar formation, **348**
    skin thickening, 380
    sound beam, **89**
    summary, 88
    in young patients, 460, **462**, 463

sound beam, sonography, **89**
source to image-receptor distance (SID), 17–18, **18**
specificity, mammography, 14–15
specimen handling, percutaneous biopsy, 147, 149
specimen radiography, 59–60, **60**, **187**, 262, **409**
    ductal carcinoma in situ, **260**
SPECT, *see* single photon emission computed tomography
spectroscopy, 129
specular echoes, 92–93
spiculated masses, 274, **275**, **277**, **407**
    differential diagnosis, 294
spindle cell tumor, benign, 231
spot compression technique, 45, 50–51, **53–54**, **55–56**
staging, invasive carcinoma, 269
    see also TNM
stand-off pad, **90**, **91**
stereotactic biopsy, 136, 141–142, **144**, 144–146, **145**
stereotactic localization, 153–155
structural changes, 188
summaries
    abnormalities, 175
    abscess, 245
    augmentation surgery, changes after, 371–372
    benign breast disorders, 195–196
    calcifications, 448
        malignant, 440
    carcinoma in situ, 264
    clinical findings, 12
    diabetic mastopathy, 233
    digital imaging, 73–74
    ductal carcinoma in situ (DCIS), 264
    fibroadenoma, 224
    fistula, 245
    galactography, 78
    granuloma, 250
    gynecomastia, 386
    hematologic malignancies, 334
    intramammary lymph nodes, 234
    invasive carcinoma, 309–310
    lobular carcinoma in situ (LCIS), 264
    lymph nodes, 323
    male breast, 386
    mammography, requirements, 16
    metastases, 337
    microcalcifications, 436
    normal breast, 171
    papilloma, 229–230
    phyllodes tumor, 327–328
    pneumocystography, 83
    post-therapeutic changes, 364
    preoperative localization, 160
    reconstruction surgery, changes after, 371–372
    reduction surgery, changes after, 371–372
    sarcomas, 330